# Complementary and Integrative Medicine in Cancer Care and Prevention

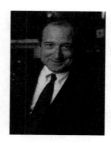

**Marc S. Micozzi, MD, PhD,** is a physician-anthropologist who has worked to create science-based tools for the health professions to be better informed and productively engaged in the new fields of complementary and alternative (CAM) and integrative medicine. He was the founding editor-in-chief of the first U.S. journal on CAM (1994) and of the first review journal (2002). He organized and edited the first U.S. textbook, *Fundamentals of Complementary & Integrative Medicine* (1996), now in a third edition (2006). It has been translated into Spanish and Japanese. He serves as series editor for Medical Guides to Complementary and Alternative Medicine with eighteen titles in print on a broad range of therapies and therapeutic systems within the scope of CAM. He organized and chaired continuing education conferences on the theory, science, and practice of CAM in 1991, 1993, 1995, 1996, 1998, and 2001.

Dr. Micozzi has conducted and published original research on diet, nutrition, and cancer. He worked as a Senior Investigator in the Cancer Prevention Studies Branch of the National Cancer Institute from 1984–86. He continued this line of research in collaboration with NIH colleagues when he was appointed Associate Director of the Armed Forces Institute of Pathology in 1986.

His early work on carotenoids (including lycopene), iron and cancer (with Nobel laureate Baruch Blumberg), anthropometric methods for age-related assessment of nutritional status, and other research made important contributions to this field. He received the young investigator award at Walter Reed Army Medical Center in 1992, at which time he was jointly appointed as a Distinguished Scientist in the American Registry of Pathology. During this time he coedited two comprehensive technical volumes on application of clinical trials methods to new investigations of the role of micronutrients and macronutrients in cancer. He has published 275 articles in the medical, scientific, and technical literature.

In 1995, he returned to Philadelphia (where he had completed his medical and graduate training at the University of Pennsylvania from 1974–83) to serve as Executive Director of the College of Physicians of Philadelphia, including creation of the C. Everett Koop Community Health Information Center. The White House Commission recognized this work in 2001. He has been a frequent speaker, as well as an effective spokesperson with the print and broadcast media.

In 2002, he became Founding Director of the Policy Institute for Integrative Medicine in Washington, DC. From 2003–2005, he accepted an interim appointment as Director of the Center for Integrative Medicine at Thomas Jefferson University Hospital in Philadelphia. He is presently a Senior Fellow of the Health Studies Collegium and maintains a part-time consulting practice in forensic medicine. He lectures at major universities in Philadelphia, San Diego, and Washington, DC. He can be contacted at marcmicozzi@aol.com.

# Complementary and Integrative Medicine in Cancer Care and Prevention

## Foundations and Evidence–Based Interventions

Editor

## Marc S. Micozzi, MD, PhD

Former Senior Investigator, National Cancer Institute, and Director, Center for Integrative Medicine, Thomas Jefferson University

SPRINGER PUBLISHING COMPANY

New York

Springer Publishing Company, LLC
11 West 42nd Street, 15th Floor
New York, NY 10036-8002

Acquisitions Editor: Sheri W. Sussman
Production Editor: Peggy M. Rote
Cover Designer: Joanne E. Honigman
Composition: Techbooks

07 08 09 10/5 4 3 2 1

---

**Library of Congress Cataloging-in-Publication Data**

Micozzi, Marc S., 1953–
Complementary and integrative medicine in cancer care and prevention : foundations and evidence-based interventions/edited by Marc S. Micozzi.—1st ed.
    p. ; cm.
  Includes bibliographical references and index.
  ISBN 0-8261-0305-7 (hardback)
1. Cancer—Alternative treatment. I. Title.
  [DNLM: 1. Neoplasms—therapy. 2. Complementary Therapies—methods.
  QZ 266 M626c 2007]
RC271.A62M53 2007
616.99′406—dc22                                        2006029898

---

Printed in the United States of America by Edwards Brothers.

*In Memory of David Larson*

# Contents

List of Figures & Illustrations   xv
List of Tables   xvii
Contributors   xix
Preface   xxi

## Part 1: Biology and Ecology of Cancer

**1   Cancer as a Cellular Phenomenon   3**
*Marc S. Micozzi*

Etiology and Epidemiology   4
Cellular Affinity   5
Cellular Differentiation   5
Carcinogenesis   6
Drugs in the Treatment of Malignant Diseases   7
Cancer Chemotherapy   9
Summary   10

**2   Cancer as a Biologic Phenomenon   13**
*Marc S. Micozzi*

Cancer and Human Biology   13
Models of Carcinogenesis   14
Cancer as Adaptation   15
Host Factors   17
Chemotherapy and Chemosensitivity   18
Conclusion   19

**3   Antiquity and Ecology of Cancer   21**
*Marc S. Micozzi*

Why Study Cancer in Antiquity?   22
How to Study the Antiquity of Cancer   23
Preservation of Human and Animal Remains   24

Paleopathologic Evidence From Human and Animal Remains   25
Documentary Evidence for Cancer in Antiquity   29
Cancer in Contemporary Societies   30

# Part 2: Mind/Body Approaches

4     **Mind/Body Modalities**   37
      *Carolyn Fang*

      Introduction   37
      Hypnosis   38
      Meditation   48
      Biofeedback   51
      Conclusion   57

5     **Guided Imagery**   65
      *Martin L. Rossman*

      Can Guided Imagery Treat Cancer Successfully?   65
      Evidence for Treating the Patient   67
      What Is Imagery and Why Is It Important?   67
      Treatment and Self-Care Options With Imagery   68
      Advantages of Interactive Guided Imagery   69
      Specific Uses of Interactive Guided Imagery in Cancer
         Care   70
      Precautions and Contraindications for Using Imagery With
         Cancer Patients   74
      Training, Certification, and Issues of Quality Assurance   75
      Reimbursement Status   76
      Relations With Conventional Medicine   76
      Summary   76

6     **Expressive Therapies**   81
      *Ilene Serlin*

      Introduction   81
      What Is Expressive Therapy?   82
      Origins of Expressive Therapies   83
      Storytelling as Healing Art   84
      Applications of Expressive Therapy   84
      How Does Expression Affect Health?   85
      Patients as Partners in Their Treatment Process   86
      Releasing Creative and Sexual Energy   87
      Cancer as a Metaphor   88
      Healing the Family   89
      Ecologic Body   89
      Healing Rituals in the Community   90

Movement Choirs    90
Conflict Resolution    91
Tamalpa Institute    91
UCSF Cancer Support Group    91
Art for Recovery    92
Art With Children    92
Summary    92

7    **Religion and Spirituality    95**
     *Kent C. Shih and David Larson*

     Introduction    95
     Cancer in America    96
     Spirituality and Religion in America    97
     Cancer Among Religious Groups    97
     Religious Commitment and Cancer    100
     Religion and Coping    102
     Biologic Mediating Factors    106
     Religion and Negative Health Outcomes    111
     Clinical Implications    112
     Summary    115

# Part 3: Diet, Nutrition, and Natural Products

8    **History of Diet and Cancer in Human Evolution    123**
     *Marc S. Micozzi*

     Introduction    123
     An Evolutionary Perspective on Diet and Cancer    124
     Cancer and Biologic Adaptation    125
     Energy Imbalance    127
     Specific Deficiencies    129
     Diet and Cancer in Modern Perspective    130
     Two-Stage Model of Cancer    131
     Specific Cancer Factors    132
     Modifying Factors    135
     Summary    137

9    **Diet, Biology, and Breast Cancer    141**
     *Marc S. Micozzi*

     The Problem of Breast Cancer    142
     Risk Factors for Breast Cancer: Early Nutrition
        and Breast-feeding    146
     Dietary Fat Intake    149
     Dietary Protein Intake    150

Energy Intake    150
Lactose Intolerance    151
Overview of Overnutrition    152
Reproductive Biology and Breast-feeding    152
Endogenous and Exogenous Hormones    154
Body Fat and Hormones    155
Breast Biology and Apocrine Gland Function    156
Breast Fluid Composition    157
Breast Tissue Microenvironment    158
Summary    159

10    Prevention of Cancer With Nutrients and Whole Foods    167
      *Marc S. Micozzi*

Introduction    167
Cancer as a Preventable Disease    168
Prevention of Cancer by Nutrients    168
Nutritional Inhibition of Cancer by Selected
      Nutrients    170
Process of Carcinogenesis    170
Vitamin A and Retinoids    171
Beta-Carotene and Carotenoids    177
Vitamin C (Ascorbic Acid)    178
Vitamin D and Calcium    187
Vitamin E (Alpha-Tocopherol)    188
B Vitamins and Choline    193
Copper and Zinc    194
Selenium    194
Dietary Fiber    198
Other Dietary Constituents    203
Whole Foods    204
Epidemiological Studies    205
Summary    209

11    Treatment of Cancer With Nutrients    213
      *Marc S. Micozzi*

Introduction    213
Vitamins A, C, and E Supplements    213
Vitamin A (Including Beta-Carotene and Retinoids)    214
Vitamin C    216
Vitamin E    219
Summary: Use and Combination of Vitamins    220

12    History of Alternative Cancer Diets    225
      *Marc S. Micozzi*

Macrobiotic Diet    225
Gerson Diet    230
Other Perspectives    233

Adjunctive Treatment    234
Contemporary Concerns    235
Livingston–Wheeler Diet    235
Issel's Whole Body Therapy    238
Kelley–Gonzalez Diet    238
Other Enzymatic Diets    241
Other Alternative Nutritional Treatments    241

13    Natural Products in Cancer Care and Treatment    243
*Marc S. Micozzi*

Introduction    243
Iscador (Mistletoe)    243
Green Tea    248
Red Tea    250
Pacific Yew and Hazelnut    250
Garlic    252
Camphor    255
Essiac    258
Hoxsey Method    262
Red Clover    262
Chinese Herbal Mixtures    264
Safety and Herb/Drug Interactions    265
Mushrooms and Mushroom Extracts    269
Essential Oils Therapy    270

# Part 4: Alternative Systems of Medicine

14    Naturopathy    281
*Marc S. Micozzi*

Introduction    281
History of Natural Medicine    283
Medical Eclecticism    284
Naturopathy and Cancer    292
Naturopathic Principles in Practice    294
Clinical Approach    300
Management of Preneoplastic Conditions    300
Summary    301

15    Chinese Medicine and Cancer Care    303
*Harriet Beinfield, Efrem Korngold, and Marc S. Micozzi*

Historical Origins    305
Why History Matters    305
Western References    306
Current Utilization    307

Chinese Traditional Medicine on Its Own Terms    308
Chinese Medicine and Cancer: Ancient and Modern Concepts    311
Cancer Types: Diagnostic Patterns    314
Chemotherapy and Radiation: A Yin-Yang Perspective    315
Acupuncture    316
Modern Chinese Herbal Research    319
Individual Herbs    320
Research Investigations    329
Enhancing Conventional Protocols    330
Safety and Herb/Drug Interactions    334
Anecdotal Reports    336
Summary    338
Acknowledgments    338

**16    Ayurvedic Medicine    345**
*Marc S. Micozzi*

Free Radicals, Cancer, and Transcendental Meditation    345
Clinical Results    347
Diet and Digestion    349
Behavioral Rasayanas    351
Bedside Manner    352
Active Ingredients, Free Radicals, and Herbal Medicines    352
Herbal Formulations as Anticancer Agents    353
Free-Radical Defenses    355
Finding Balance    356
Herbal Rasayanas    357
Synergism    359
Free-Radical Scavenging Effects    360
Enhancing Immunity    362
Controlling Free-Radical Effects on the Immune System    362
Cancer Prevention and Regression    363
Reduced Chemotherapeutic Toxicity    365
Aging    367
Redifferentiation and Rejuvenation in Cancer    368
Complications of Cancer    368
Other Herbs    370
Ayurvedic Clinical Approach    372
Summary    374

**17    Homeopathy    377**
*Joyce Frye*

Introduction    377
Background    377
The Medicines    378
Remedy Selection    379
The Cancer Prescription    380

Adjunctive Therapy    382
Palliation    382
Prevention    383
Summary    383

# Part 5: Alternative Therapies and Practices

18    **Controversial Therapies    387**
       *Marc S. Micozzi*

       Antineoplastons for Cancer Treatment    387
       Hydrazine Sulfate    391
       Additional Alternative Treatments    394

19    **Legal and Regulatory Access to Alternative Cancer Treatments    399**
       *Alan Dumoff*

       Introduction    399
       Some Historical Notes    401
       Barriers to Access    407
       Bias in Research Design, Interpretation, and Funding    411
       Judicial Reluctance to Recognize Health Care Freedom    415
       Direct Barriers to Practice    423
       Personal Import    429
       Federal, State, and Private Regulation of Payment    433
       State Regulation of Medical Practitioners    437
       Summary    440

20    **A Patient's Experience and Perspective    445**
       *Anonymous*

       Choosing Between Conventional and Alternative Cancer
          Treatments    447
       Getting Started    448
       Leaving the United States for Treatment    449
       Off to the Bahamas    452
       Complete Remission and Cure    454

Index    457

# List of Figures & Illustrations

Figure 1.1    The Periwinkle Plant (*Vinca major*). Source of the vinca alkyloids, early chemotherapeutic agents, vinblastin, and vincristine.   8

Figure 4.1    Mesmerism and hypnotism were the object of criticism during the 19th century.   39

Figure 4.2    Overlap of objective and subjective therapeutic benefits.   48

Figure 4.3    Brain-immune pathways of complementary and alternative medicine.   56

Figure 13.1   Horse Chestnut (*Aesculus hippocastannum*).   244

Figure 13.2   Garlic (*Allium sp.*).   253

Figure 13.3   Ginseng (*Panax sp.*).   264

Figure 13.4   Ginger (*Zingiber officinale*).   267

Figure 14.1   Dr. John Harvey Kellogg, brother of the Kellogg of the breakfast cereal company.   286

Figure 14.2   Samuel Thomson (1769–1843).   289

Figure 15.1   The pathogenesis of cancer.   313

Figure 15.2   The treatment of cancer.   314

Figure 16.1   The limbic system.   348

Figure 17.1   Commonly sold homeopathic dilutions relative to Avogadro's number.   378

Original line drawings for Chapters 1 and 13 by Alicia M. Micozzi.

# List of Tables

Table 8.1    High Risk or "Toxic" Diets    127

Table 8.2    Framework for an Original Human Diet    137

Table 9.1    Demographic Transition, Fertility, and Breast Cancer Rates    142

Table 9.2    Major and Minor Risk Factors for Breast Cancer    144

Table 9.3    Rates of Breast Cancer in Japanese-American Women Over Time    145

Table 13.1    Research Questions on Garlic    252

Table 13.2    PC-SPES Formula Composed of Eight Herbs    265

Table 13.3    Chemical Components of Essential Oils and Their Therapeutic Actions    273

Table 13.4    Utilization of Aromatherapy for Medical Purposes    273

Table 14.1    Phases of Naturopathy    282

Table 15.1    Debu Tripathy Herbal Examples Diagram    322

# Contributors

Harriet Beinfield, LAc
Codirector, Acupuncturist
Chinese Medicine Works
San Francisco, CA

Alan Dumoff, JD
Private Practice
Rockville, MD

Carolyn Fang, PhD
Associate Member
Population Science Division
Fox Chase Cancer Center
Cheltenham, PA

Joyce Frye, DO
Postdoctoral Fellow
Center for Clinical Epidemiology
and Biostatistics
University of Pennsylvania
Philadelphia, PA

Efrem Korngold, LAc, OMD
Codirector, Acupuncturist
Chinese Medicine Works
San Francisco, CA

David Larson, PhD (deceased)
President
National Institute for Healthcare Research
Rockville, MD

Martin L. Rossman, MD
Director and Founder
Collaborative Medicine Center
Mill Valley, CA

Ilene Serlin, PhD, ADTR
Licensed Psychologist, Registered
Dance/Movement Therapist
Mill Valley, CA

Kent C. Shih, MD
Oncologist
Louisiana Hematology Oncology
Associates
Baton Rouge, LA

This volume on complementary and integrative therapies (CIM) and cancer addresses a difficult but important subject. The largest, most comprehensive survey on utilization of CIM in the United States has shown that 80% of patients with cancer use complementary, alternative, and integrative treatments (Barnes, Powell-Griner, McFann, & Nahin, 2004). Virtually all these patients are also under treatment by oncologists, radiation therapists, and many other medical specialists. These patients come to their regular physicians seeking answers and guidance about what CIM may have to offer them. They prefer not to be told there is nothing they can do. However, what advice can be responsibly provided? Evidence indicates that a blanket rejection of CIM is no longer appropriate.

On the one hand, it is widely acknowledged in medicine that it is very important to develop new ideas and approaches to the prevention, treatment, and control of cancer. On the other hand, complementary and integrative medicine in cancer is fraught with unproven remedies, marketing claims, and unusual and idiosyncratic approaches that have generally shed more heat than light on the subject. The basic approach to cancer therapy in the 20th century had been to kill cancer cells in a manner that would be less toxic to noncancerous cells in the human body. At the end of the 19th century, the understanding and acceptance of the germ theory of disease led to the control of bacterial agents through the development of "magic bullets" to kill bacteria (bactericidal compounds) or to interfere with their reproduction (bacteriostatic drugs). Antibiotics have proven to be extremely successful in helping to cure bacterial infections, usually without unduly harming the human host. Until the development of antibiotic drug resistance, which turned "magic bullets" into "friendly fire," such approaches were seen as an unalloyed achievement in medicine and public health.

In cancer treatment, we have likewise harbored the hope that magic bullets can be developed but in the meantime rely on surgery, radiation therapy, and chemotherapy. In this manner, the medical historian may be reminded of the preantibiotic approach to infectious diseases—when bleeding, blistering, puking, and purging were the four modalities of choice to rebalance the bodily humours. Can complementary and integrative medical modalities, with their promise of gentler, less invasive, "more natural" approaches, hold promise for cancer treatment, prevention, or control?

Cancer is clearly a challenging area of medicine for the application of CIM. The amount of misinformation often seems to exceed the amount of real clinical scientific information available. Irresponsible marketing claims and appeals to desperate patients with "incurable" disease create a climate of reluctance for physicians to engage themselves or their patients in this troubling arena (Part 5).

As a medical examiner in 1983, I had the opportunity to investigate a cancer death in a woman with breast cancer under treatment with alternative (but not conventional) therapies. I investigated this category of remedy (that was employed subsequently in research at the National Institutes of Health) and have done "field investigations" in the office of the alternative practitioner in question. Keeping an open mind, I cannot determine whether the death was consistent with essentially untreated breast cancer or whether the alternative treatment ultimately had a negative or positive effect on the course of the disease. Scientific investigation is the only answer to questions such as these. Unfortunately, the lack of access of alternative practitioners to the mainstream medical system, especially for treatment of cancer, the devotion of practitioners and their patients to these alternative therapeutic modalities, the desire for "freedom" in "health choices," and the resulting lack of scientific attention, funding, and studies all contribute to a potentially confusing picture for the medical practitioner.

In addition to these practical concerns, there is a theoretical concern. One of the basic tenets of much of complementary and integrative medicine is that human societies over time are able to develop useful therapies and application of *materia medica* to the alleviation of human suffering and treatment of illness. Much of what we have called "complementary/alternative" medicine today actually represents the "traditional" medicine of other human societies (what anthropologists call ethnomedicine). Certainly the use of many medicinal plants by traditional cultures has been repeatedly validated by scientific study. Diseases that have been part of human heritage since earliest documented times, as proven by paleopathologic studies, yield opportunity and motivation for cultures to develop remedies as has clearly been the case in Ancient Egypt, China, India, Greece, and Rome, as well as indigenous societies in Asia, Africa, and the Americas (Part 4). Although many common diseases have been documented in ancient and prehistoric populations, there is very sparse evidence for cancer, which may be considered to be a "disease of modernization" or a "disease of modern civilization" (Chapter 3). If cancer was not there to be treated, on what basis could effective alternative treatments have been developed in the context of traditional cultures?

However, there is developing clear evidence that many CIM therapies may be effectively used in an adjunctive and supportive role in the cancer patient for the management of both complications of the disease and complications of medical treatment. There is evidence that CIM modalities may help improve quality of life and even help prolong survival in cancer patients (Part 2). Evidence that CIM may prevent or "cure" cancer has been more problematic, although some traditional (ethnomedical) herbal remedies from China (Chapter 15) and India (Chapter 16) appear to have the ability, in laboratory studies, to transform cancer cells through redifferentiation (as has been postulated for the role of vitamin A and its derivatives; for example, see Part 3). These properties are in contrast to the approach of seeking cures for cancer in nature by assessing only cytotoxicity against cancer cells (as with chemotherapy).

Aside from these considerations, CIM clearly may help patients reduce proven risk factors for cancer and other chronic diseases related to diet, smoking, and other behaviors, as has been the subject of serious epidemiologic study for over 25 years (Part 3).

Finally, the dictum that cancer is "not one disease, but many diseases" has proven useful for research and public health efforts. However, this book addresses various cancer sites taken together (with the exception of Chapter 9), partially in light of the limitations of evidence for most site-specific cancers and partially because the probable biological basis of carcinogenesis often does not hold significance when distinguished by site with regard to the possible applications of supportive CAM modalities.

The active participation of the medical and scientific community is essential to appropriately analyze and apply the possible benefits of CIM modalities for cancer prevention, treatment, and control. This volume is intended to provide a useful tool toward that goal.

## REFERENCE

Barnes, P. M., Powell-Griner, E., McFann, K., & Nahin, R. L. (2004). Complementary and alternative medicine use among adults: United States, 2002. *Seminars in Integrative Medicine, 2:* 54–71.

Marc S. Micozzi, MD, PhD
*Bethesda, Maryland*

# 1

# Biology and Ecology of Cancer

he term *cancer* (Latin for "crab") represents not a single disease entity but a mixed group of perhaps 600 or more types of diseases that involve abnormal cellular proliferation—*neoplasm*. A neoplasm, or tumor, is an abnormal new growth of cells. These diseases have the propensity to invade adjacent normal tissues and to spread to sites distant from the original location of disease. These two properties, (1) invasion and destruction of normal tissues at the site of origin and (2) growth at distant sites of spread (metastasis), distinguish the malignant cells of a cancer from the cells that comprise benign (or nonmalignant) growths (Abeloff et al., 2000).

For the sake of completeness, it should be noted that the functional distinction between malignant and benign neoplasms may be unclear as in the case of a fibroma (a benign fibrous tissue proliferation), for example, which grows larger and larger and may eventually kill the individual (if untreated) without ever metastasizing. Similarly, gliomas (a type of malignant brain tumor) are locally invasive and destructive tumors that rarely metastasize outside the central nervous system but rapidly kill the patient by local invasion and increased intracranial pressure.

Beyond the defining characteristics of invasion and metastasis, the different forms of cancer may vary in site of origin, histologic and pathologic features, etiology and epidemiology, natural history, and effectiveness of therapy. For example, the chances of long-term survival of a small basal cell carcinoma of the skin, or Stage 1 of Hodgkin's lymphoma, approach 100%, whereas the chances of long-term survival of advanced lung cancer are extremely low (American Cancer Society, 2004; Greenlee et al., 2000). Therapies for various malignancies vary widely, from combined or single-modality chemotherapy to radiation therapy and/or surgery.

# Etiology and Epidemiology

In Chapter 1, various theories on the origin of cancer are discussed. In Chapter 2 the basic principles of cancer epidemiology and the epidemiology of certain common forms of cancer are introduced.

Poorly understood events that take place within normally functioning cells may cause them to become aberrant. Abnormality in the genetic material transforms uniform, "law-abiding" cells into disorganized, "wild-growing" cells. These genetically transformed cells become immortal—they lose the ability to die naturally (Johnson, 2000). A neoplasm (new growth) is the result of such unrestrained cell growth. This new growth, or tumor, interferes with normal tissue function and is characterized by the capacity to invade normal tissue, blood vessels, and other organs (DeClerck, 2000). The cancerous growth draws in nutrients, leaving normal cells starving. The degree of damage may vary according to the speed of neoplastic development and spread. The potential for saving the life of the cancer patient often depends on the invasiveness and rate of cellular proliferation of the tumor.

The normal cell operates in a rather narrowly defined range of function, dependent on genetic regulation and tissue differentiation (Deng & Brodie, 2000). Such a normal cell is part of an organized entity in the form of a tissue or organ. These cells normally interact with each other in an orderly fashion. The sum total of cells and their activity adds up to form a functional organism. Cells are able to adapt to environmental factors and may change somewhat without losing their identity or functional ability. Comparison between normal cells and cancer cells is useful in gaining an understanding of cancer chemotherapy, which is based on differential destruction of cancer cells with intended survival of normal cells. However, cancer can be very difficult to treat because of the occurrence of metastases. It is thought that even a single cancer cell anywhere in the body may produce new cancerous growth.

The neoplasm or new growth of an abnormal mass of tissue that characterizes cancer is uncoordinated and persistent. There is no teleologic purpose to this growth. Neoplasms are autonomous and are not regulated by the host for food, oxygen, or removal of waste. Thus, the neoplastic cells compete with normal body cells for oxygen and food.

---

*The Terminology of Cancer*

**Tumors** are synonymous with neoplasm to a **certain** point. The term originally referred to the Latin "swelling."

**Oncos** means "tumor" in Greek.

**Oncology** is the science that deals with the study of tumors or cancer.

**Cancer** is the term that refers to malignant tumors.

---

Characteristics of normal cells and cancer cells are compared in the following.

# Cellular Affinity

Normal cells of any given type show affinity for other cells of the same type and little or no affinity for other types of cells. For example, liver cells will stick to other liver cells, but not to kidney cells, when these cells are placed together. On the contrary, cancer cells will exhibit affinity for any other cells, no matter what the origin of these cells may be. When placed in a solution, cancer cells will adhere to the normal cells available regardless of their origin.

The cell membrane plays an important role in the maintenance of cellular integrity. Contact between cells exists only in specialized areas of cell membranes. These contact specializations differ in size and shape, but one of their important functions is to contain cellular growth. Thus, cell growth *in vitro* is usually seen as one single layer, whereas growth and cell division *in vivo* stops when the organ attains its specific size and shape. These cellular projections are responsible for keeping cells in one area and restraining them in their size and growth patterns, thus maintaining the integrity of tissues and organs.

Cancer cells do not possess the contact specializations of normal cell membranes. They grow *in vitro* by division into mounds with cells piling on top of each other. Cancer cells stick to other cells but not to solid surfaces. The changes that occur in cancer cell surfaces may account for the lack of restraint in growth responsible for unchecked cellular proliferation. The lack of contact specializations between cancer cells is possibly responsible for the ability of these cells to break loose from the site of origin and travel via the bloodstream or lymphatic channels to distant sites, where they attach to other cells, initiating distant growth or metastases. Many scientific studies deal with the surface changes of cancer cells, presenting one possibility for understanding an important mechanism of carcinogenesis (Bode & Dong, 2004; DeClerck, 2000; Deng & Brodie, 2000).

# Cellular Differentiation

Cells in normal tissues differentiate from embryonic primitive stem cells. There is a wide range of changes that occur from the beginning of development to the final form, location, and function of cells. After cell transformation, the differentiated cell is recognized as a liver or kidney cell, a red blood cell, a lymphocyte, and so on. The term *dedifferentiation* was first used by histologists to relate a backwards change of a cell from differentiated to undifferentiated, or embryonic, type.

Cell dedifferentiation is also one of the criteria used by pathologists in relation to neoplasia. Most cancer cells show a degree of reverse differentiation. *Pleomorphism*, or variations in cellular size, is also characteristic of tumor cells. Some are small and others large, with variable amounts of DNA observed in the nuclei, which also vary in size and shape. The degree of differentiation of tumor cells has been related to the prognosis of the disease. The more differentiated the cellular component, the better the prognosis. However, this concept is not universal. Gastrointestinal tumors, for example, may show marked differentiation of cellular components but may still have high rates of cell proliferation.

The normal cytoplasmic to nuclear ratio is 1:4 or 1:6. The cancer cell shows a proportion of 1:1 with nuclei of highly variable form (nuclear disproportion). In general, the larger the nuclear size the more malignant the cell. Mitosis is usually atypical. Cancer cells are not organized into layers but show a disorganized anatomical structure with necrotic areas because of outgrowth of blood supply. Although cancer cells produce chemical factors that stimulate ingrowth of blood vessels into tumor tissue, this blood supply may be outstripped by uncontrolled growth, or the ingrowth of blood vessels may be inhibited by anticancer factors (Pazgal et al., 2003; Talks & Harris, 2000). Radiation treatment is effective in well-oxygenated tissues because of the reliance on oxygen for free-radical formation, one pathway that can trigger cell death (Taper et al., 1996). Conversely, radiation may also cause cancer by conversion of free-radical ions in the presence of oxygen (oxidation) with subsequent damage to normal cells. Chemotherapy, as with radiation therapy, may also be carcinogenic for similar reasons.

Invasiveness is also typical of cancer growth. Cancerous growths do not possess an outer capsule; encapsulation is present only in benign tumors. Enzyme synthesis often decreases in cancer cells, but it also can be the same as that in normal cells, and increased levels of abnormal enzymes may be produced. The rate of growth of cancer cells differs or varies from one cancer to another, from slow- to fast-growing forms.

# Carcinogenesis

Some information is available concerning the etiology of cancer in human populations. The study of world distribution of cancer and comparative evaluation of human populations, diets, living conditions, and environment has shed some light on possible causes of cancer (see Chapters 3, 13, and 14).

According to some epidemiological studies, cancers may be caused by factors present in the environment. Some forms of cancers are prevalent in certain parts of the world. In Japan the incidence of cancer of the stomach is much higher than that in Japanese immigrants to the United States, and it is even lower in their offspring. Among individuals of Jewish extraction, those born in Israel have a lower incidence of cancer than those born in the United States (the latter incidence is similar to that of the population of the United States in general).

Certain cancers have been associated with occupational hazards. The classic example is cancer of the scrotum, formerly prevalent in chimney sweeps. Chimney soot is implicated as a carcinogen in individuals exposed to it in their childhood or adolescence. Certain occupational cancers have been found to be related to chemicals and radioactive dyes in industry. Watch dial painters using radioactive radium dye were found to suffer from cancer of the lip, because of frequent moistening of the tip of the brush to obtain a fine point used in painting of the dial.

Carcinogens are substances that have been shown experimentally, or through observation, to produce cancer in animals and humans. Many cancer-causing agents are present in the environment to which we are exposed on a daily basis. Synthetic dyes, pesticides, weed killers, solvents, and other everyday chemicals have been tested and proven to be carcinogenic. Factory workers may be especially vulnerable to exposure to high levels of carcinogens.

A carcinogen may produce cancer many years after exposure and, in special cases, may even cause neoplasia in the offspring of mothers exposed, as in the case of diethylstilbestrol. The offspring of these daughters may also manifest abnormalities. The difficulty and possible uncertainty about a compound being carcinogenic may come from lack of evidence, from poor evidence, or from the limitations of human-based data. Research on cancer-producing compounds is mainly based on animal work, and, therefore, it may not be possible to prove an effect on human beings. The Toxic Substances Control Act, passed in 1976, requires testing of chemicals as possible health-endangering compounds for protection of workers and the population in general.

Certain viruses have been implicated as causative factors in cancers in animals such as mice, frogs, and especially chickens. Moreover, tissues containing these viruses cause cancer when injected into healthy animals. It has been postulated that viruses may infect embryonic cells. After a long period of time, the presence of the virus becomes evident, producing a "turn-on" effect and starting abnormal cellular transformation and proliferation. In humans, Epstein–Barr virus has been implicated in mononucleosis (which may resemble leukemia with atypical lymphocytes), nasopharangeal cancer, and Burkitt's lymphoma, a cancer seen not uncommonly in children in Africa but also less commonly in adult populations around the world. The well-known Rous sarcoma virus (RSV) was originally described in 1911 by Peyton Rous and is known to cause the leukemia-like diseases in chickens, cats, and mice. The human herpes viruses 16 and 18, among other strains, are known to be involved in the pathogenesis of cervical cancer, as well as papillomaviruses (Stoler, 1997).

In short, the cause of cancer lies in the loss of original DNA or substitution with new or altered genetic material. These mutations may be induced by environmental factors such as chemicals, viruses, or UV light and these mutations may accumulate over time with increasing age. An independent mutation, however, may also occur in a somatic cell without any influence from outside forces.

Host factors may influence the action of carcinogenic agents. Age and sex differences have been reported in certain cancers. For example, historically higher rates of lung cancer occur in men versus women. However, the prevalence of lung cancer in women has increased likely as a result of widespread smoking among women. Cancer of the gastrointestinal tract also involves more men than women. On the contrary, women are more prone to develop cancer of the breast and reproductive organs, as well as of the thyroid gland. Generally, older individuals have a higher incidence of cancer, although certain neoplastic diseases, such as neuroblastoma, are more prevalent in children.

# Drugs in the Treatment of Malignant Diseases

Chemotherapeutic agents have been introduced into medical practice after a painstaking search for useful compounds to stop malignant growth. As has been the case for much of the development of pharmaceutical agents of all kinds, the original active ingredients for some early, effective chemotherapeutic agents were discovered in plants. This text

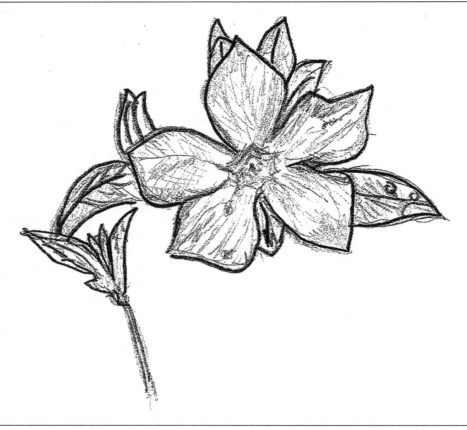

**The Periwinkle Plant** (*Vinca major*). Source of the vinca alkyloids, early chemotherapeutic agents, vinblastin, and vincristine.

focuses on the use of nutrients, herbs, and other complementary/integrative modalities in preventing and/or contributing to the care of people with cancer and in managing the side effects of chemotherapeutic agents. However, the plant world has also contributed to the discovery of chemotherapeutics agents themselves. For example, the flowering periwinkle (*Vinca minor*) was the source of the chemotherapeutic agents known as the vinca alkyloids, vinblastin and vincristin (see Figure 1.1). Likewise, the traditional Native American remedy May apple made its way into the herbal medicine chests of physicians during the colonial period. It was eventually developed as podophyllin, a topical treatment for skin tumors that is quite toxic if taken internally.

Active efforts continue today to search thousands of plants for compounds that have the ability to kill cancer cells (cytotoxicity). This approach assays for only one of the possible anticancer activites of plants, as herbs used for cancer in the Chinese (Chapter 15) and Ayurvedic (Chapter 16) traditions include those with activity to alter or redifferentiate cancer cells toward less malignant forms rather than killing the cancer cells outright. This approach appears to be less toxic to the patient as well.

Compounds used in the treatment of cancers fall into different chemical groups. Drugs may be effective or ineffective as anticancer agents in different individuals.

Prediction of clinical outcome is sometimes difficult for cancer and its treatment. Clinical trials are therefore extensive and therapy may be modified from time to time according to new information in the medical literature. Earlier cancer treatments were based on single-drug therapy. At present, chemotherapy regimens may include single drugs given in series or, in many cases, multiple-drug regimens. Cancer cell responsiveness to drug therapy varies from highly sensitive cells, such as Burkitt's lymphoma, choriocarcinoma, Wilms tumor, or Hodgkin's lymphoma, to cancer that is poorly responsive, such as hepatocellular or pancreatic carcinoma or malignant melanoma. Where there is known responsiveness to chemotherapy, prognosis and survival of the patient can usually be made within some margin of error. The optimal regimen or protocol, although specified exactly for each malignancy, may be changed according to individual response, health problems that independently accompany the disease, and side effects of the treatment.

Many drugs used in cancer chemotherapy are effective because of their interaction with cellular DNA. Some compounds, such as alkylating agents, attach to the chromosomes and prevent cross-linkage of DNA. Others cause formation of a faulty DNA molecule because of alteration in the DNA base sequence. The result of interaction with cellular DNA may be a decrease or a complete cessation of cellular proliferation. Many difficulties can be encountered in the treatment of cancer because of this mechanism of action.

The antineoplastic agents do not act specifically or selectively to inhibit cancer cells. The exact mechanism of carcinogenesis is not known and may be variable. Therefore, the therapeutic approach is that of an attack on the common final pathway and most prevalent feature of cancer, cellular proliferation, which relates to excessive DNA synthesis and mitosis. Although the drugs act on cancer cells, they also act on all cellular DNA at the same time, thus preventing proper synthesis. Antineoplastic drugs kill normal cells as well as cancer cells. The most sensitive normal cells are those present in rapidly growing tissues such as skin, hair follicles, gastrointestinal tract mucosa, bone marrow, and lymphatic tissues. These cells are also the most sensitive to radiation therapy for similar reasons. The toxic effects because of depression of normal cell proliferation are similar for all anticancer drugs.

Cancer cells may be susceptible for a period of time to the effect of anticancer drugs but eventually may develop resistance to the chemical agent. The promotion of cancer cell growth can be demonstrated with some cancer drugs, which themselves possess carcinogenic effects. For these reasons, treatment of malignant disease may be very difficult and frustrating. Changes in treatment are constantly made, effects evaluated, and new approaches to therapy sought.

However, extensive medical research in cancer chemotherapy has yielded results. Some cancers can be cured or placed into prolonged remission. Chemotherapy is not the only means available to treat these diseases. Radiation therapy and surgery have contributed to a positive outcome in many instances.

# Cancer Chemotherapy

The present-day approach to cancer chemotherapy is based on both single-agent and multiple drug therapy. A combination of compounds with slightly different mechanisms of action is used to cover all the vulnerable cellular periods of growth or synchronize the cells in the same growth phase. Because cancer cells are in different stages of the cell cycle at any one time, multiple drugs can stop proliferation much more effectively than can any one agent by acting on different periods of the cycle.

Cell growth is divided into four phases. The G1 phase refers to the time period after cell division has been accomplished. The G1 period is the phase of RNA and protein synthesis. The second phase, S, is the period of time during which DNA synthesis takes place. Drugs that produce damage to DNA will do so during this period of cell growth. The third phase, G2, represents a period before cell division. The fourth period, M, is the phase during which mitosis or cell division is taking place. Drugs that interfere with the mitotic apparatus will depress activity during this phase. During the generative cycle, the amount of DNA doubles and the cell becomes larger by accumulation of intracellular proteins and RNA. Differentiated cells are said to be in a resting period, or G0. In other cells, the G1 stage is prolonged.

Some drugs, such as methotrexate, inhibit the synthesis of chemical precursors needed for DNA synthesis. The therapeutic application of various anticancer drugs depends on their previous record of efficacy against certain types of malignant diseases. Beyond combination chemotherapy, the addition to chemotherapy of surgery and radiation may often be the best approach (O'Reilly, 2002).

Some cancers respond to specific drug therapy, even if the treatment is rather nonspecific (not only effective in killing cancer cells but also affecting all cells). Newer generations of chemotherapy are presently in development and have reached FDA approval in a few select malignancies. These anticancer drugs target specific and unique sites to the cancer cells and hold out promise. Many prospective and controlled trials are underway to evaluate the effectiveness of these new drugs; some show a significant improvement over standard chemotherapy regimens. However, the ideal anticancer drug is yet to be found.

# Summary

With the limitations of current therapies for cancer, there is natural interest in the possibility of alternative approaches. The cellular properties of cancer suggest the plausibility of cancer prevention and supportive care through the cellular actions of nutrients (Chapter 11), foods (Chapter 10), and certain herbs (Chapter 13), as well as traditional Chinese (Chapter 15) and Ayurvedic (Chapter 16) remedies and other alternatives.

## REFERENCES

Abeloff, M. D., Armitage, J. O., Lichter, A. S., & Niederhuber, J. E. (2000). *Clinical oncology* (2nd ed.). New York: Churchill Livingstone.

American Cancer Society. (2004). *Cancer facts and figures*. Atlanta, GA.

Bode, A. M., & Dong, Z. (2004). Targeting signal transduction pathways by chemopreventive agents. *Mutation Research/Fundamental and Molecular Mechanisms of Mutagenesis, 555*, 33–51.

DeClerck, Y. A. (2000). Interactions between tumor cell and stromal cells and proteolytic modifications of the extracellular matrix by metalloproteinases in cancer. *European Journal of Cancer, 36*, 1258–1269.

Deng, C. X., & Brodie, S. G. (2000). Roles of BRCA1 and its interacting proteins. *Bioessays, 22*, 728–732.

Greenlee, R. T., Murray, T., Bolden, S., & Wingo, P. A. (2000). Cancer statistics 2000. *CA: A Cancer Journal for Clinicians, 50*, 7–27.

Johnson, D. E. (2000). Programmed cell death regulation: Basic mechanisms and therapeutic opportunities. *Leukemia, 14*, 1340–1345.

O'Reilly, M. S. (2002). Targeting multiple biological pathways as a strategy to improve the treatment of cancer. *Clinical Cancer Research, 8*, 3309–3310.

Pazgal, I., Zimra, Y., Tzabar, C., Okon, E., Rabizadeh, E., Shaklai, M., et al. (2003). Combined therapy with direct and indirect angiogenesis inhibition results in enhanced antiangiogenic and antitumor effects. *Cancer Research, 63*, 8890–8898.

Stoler, M. (1997). The biology of human papillomaviruses. *Pathology Case Reviews, 2*, 8–20.

Talks, A. L., & Harris, A. L. (2000). Current status of antiangiogenic factors. *British Journal of Haematology, 109*, 477–481.

Taper, H. S., Keyeux, A., & Roberfroid, M. (1996). Potentiation of radiation therapy by nontoxic pretreatment with combined vitamins C and K3 in mice bearing solid transplantable tumors. *Anticancer Research, 16*, 499–503.

# Cancer as a Biologic Phenomenon

**2**

## Cancer and Human Biology

When cancer is viewed as a biologic phenomenon, it becomes apparent that this disease is part of the landscape of human experience and that the natural history of cancer can be viewed in an ecologic perspective. Cancer is also, however, a social phenomenon and psychologic event. To the physician, cancer is a problem to be treated and eradicated. To the patient,

Marc S. Micozzi

cancer is "bad." It may be viewed as punishment or as something unnatural placed on Earth to curse humankind. This personified perception or ethical conceptualization of cancer may in fact be productive in combating the disease, as with mental imagery (see Chapter 5).

To the scientist, cancer is viewed objectively and the same laws that govern the behavior of all processes in biologic systems are applied to cancer as well (Tannock & Hill, 1998). Thus the reason for the existence of cancer, its biologic basis, is sought within the realm of natural history and human biology. Cancer is ultimately a disease of organs (populations of cells) rather than of individual cells. Carcinogenic mechanisms operate on a population of cells. The responses of cells to their microenvironments may be likened to the response of human populations to the environment at large. Environmental influences cause adaptation of human populations through shifts in gene frequencies, which occur on the basis of differential reproduction in individual humans (natural selection). Environmental influences may cause "adaptation" of populations of cells by differential survival of individual cells (through clonal selection) (Nowell, 1976, 1993).

Highly specialized organisms may not have the adaptive flexibility to survive dramatic changes in environment because their adaptation is coded in their physical structures. Likewise, highly specialized, terminally differentiated cells may phenotypically manifest too much cellular sensitivity to survive changes in the microenvironment (they become too adapted to a few functions within a specialized environment to retain flexibility of response). However, relatively undifferentiated cells (unspecialized or generalized cells) may be relatively resistant to changes in the microenvironment, as these cells may experience differential survival, growth, and replication. End-stage terminally differentiated cells cannot grow or reproduce, but only die, in response to environmental stress. The undifferentiation, or dedifferentiation, of cells is regarded structurally and functionally as a cardinal sign of cancer.

The degree to which cells are sensitive or resistant to environmental stresses within a population of cells may be based on different expression of regulating genes (Vogelstein & Kinzler, 1998). Transformed tumor cells themselves manifest different degrees of malignancy, as selected by the microenvironment to which they must adapt. For example, if clones of cancer cells are isolated with differential degrees of malignancy, low malignant potential cells in a closed system can further dedifferentiate into high malignant potential cells, as might be expected (Nowell, 1993). However, high malignant potential cells can seemingly redifferentiate into low malignant cells, as can be seen in those at intermediate stages. Finally, if both low and high malignant potential cells are introduced into the same biologic system, they do not manifest intermediate levels of malignancy but maintain their original identities within the microenvironment.

# Models of Carcinogenesis

All cells must replicate themselves accurately through generations within individuals and between generations of individuals. During this process, it is important to maintain the fidelity of DNA replication for ongoing homeostatic functioning. Cancer involves alteration in the fidelity of DNA replication or in expression of the replicated DNA.

The somatic mutation hypothesis maintains that the basic alteration in cancer involves the fidelity of DNA replication. Somatic mutation implies any change in the sequence of DNA nucleotides or the structure of the genes themselves. A related alternative hypothesis is that alterations in regulation of gene expression influences cellular differentiation to cause development of cancer. The distinction between these two models is that the former implies acquisition of new properties by cancer cells (structural), whereas the latter involves selection of differently regulated cells (regulatory). These concepts of cancer may be related to genetic mechanisms in which distinctions are made between structural and regulatory genes.

In the somatic mutation model, genetic expression is changed by alterations in the structure of the genes themselves. In the gene expression model, alterations in regulatory gene activity influence differentiation of cells containing constant genetic material. There are important implications for cancer therapy in these two models. The goal of therapy in the somatic mutation model is to destroy cancer cells (because they are structurally abnormal), whereas in the gene expression model, the goal would be to make cancer cells normal (because there is only alteration in gene regulation). This latter model based on cell regulation appears to provide a mechanism by which observed modifications in cancer cells by Chinese (Chapter 15) and Ayurvedic (Chapter 16) herbal preparations may work.

The somatic mutation model is supported by a number of empirical observations. Nuclear DNA is a target of carcinogens in tissues and alteration in nucleotide sequence is the result of carcinogen action. Although inert particles such as certain asbestos fibers have been observed to cause cancer they contain soluble factors such as heavy-metal ions, such as iron (Stevens, Jones, Micozzi, & Taylor, 1988; Stevens, Graubard, Micozzi, Neriishi, & Blumberg, 1994), which may directly attack DNA. Many carcinogens are metabolized into products that have been shown to attack DNA directly. The observations of chromosomal aberrations that have been used to characterize malignancy are a direct result of this alteration of DNA. These properties of cells allow the pathologist to look under a microscope at a $4-\mu$ section of tissue (a vanishingly small sample of the total tumor tissue) and interpret events at the cellular, tissue, and organism levels (diagnosis), as well as predict with reasonable accuracy the course of events at these various levels of observation (prognosis) (Ackerman & del Regato, 1997).

These alterations in cellular DNA imply that cancer is heritable at the cellular level, and in fact, is heritable at the organism level. Many human diseases of DNA repair, which imply an inability to correct this damage to DNA, have been associated with cancer. In these genetic conditions, not all damage to DNA is repaired, and unrepaired damage may lead to malignancy.

A standard assay for carcinogenity is the ability of a substance to cause mutation in the genetic material. Although all carcinogens are mutagens, not all mutagens are carcinogens. There is a similar distinction between cell transformation (as with viral transformation) and mutagenesis. Factors in the environment that may cause infidelity of DNA replication include metal ions and intercalators. The ratio of correct nucleotides available to DNA replication, as well as damage to DNA by alkylation of the DNA template, have been associated with carcinogenesis in the somatic mutation model. Because the standard therapeutic agents for cancer also act by these mechanisms, the carcinogenicity of some anticancer drugs is well documented (Rubin & Williams, 2001).

## Cancer as Adaptation

The gene expression model of cancer implies that there is selection for "clones" of cells with different properties as determined by regulation of cellular DNA expression. This clonal selection for abnormal growth properties actually results in differential growth and survival of these cells. In this sense, cancer may be viewed as an adaptive phenomenon in that tumor cells grow, survive, and reproduce over all other cells. Thus, there is selection for dedifferentiated cells that experience differential reproductivity at the cellular level (somewhat similar to the mechanism of natural selection and differential reproduction in biologic evolution).

Dedifferentiation of cells may in fact be adaptive in given situations. A model of chemical carcinogenesis has been proposed for the liver (Stevens et al., 1988, 1994), which is based on adaptive dedifferentiation. All normal liver cells, which have exquisitely sensitive cellular mechanisms for metabolism, are susceptible to injury from a variety of toxins with which they come into contact through the gastrointestinal tract and bloodstream. These chemical toxins may cause the relatively sensitive liver cells to dedifferentiate into relatively resistant cells as an adaptive response to injury, which avoids cell death. This population of adapted, dedifferentiated cells may then redifferentiate to normally functioning liver cells (as is usually the case) or go on to cause cancer (a rare event).

For example, in a model for viral carcinogenesis in the liver, two populations of hepatocytes have been hypothesized—R cells for those resistant to infection and S cells for those that are sensitive. R cells are more primitive, undifferentiated or dedifferentiated cells that are resistant to injury (in this case by a virus). S cells are more mature, more differentiated cells that are susceptible to injury (again, in this case, infection by virus). The acquisition of the virus may occur in both the R and S cells, but cells of the resistant population tolerate the virus, whereas the sensitive cells are destroyed.

The acquisition of virus by the surviving R cells does not confer autonomy of growth, just alteration (such as the influence of chemical carcinogens). Stimulation for growth of R cells comes from the necessity to replace the destroyed S cells. Therefore, the virus transforms R cells (which do not become neoplastic directly as a result of viral infection) but kills S cells, and R cells are stimulated to grow on this basis.

Changes in the regulation of gene expression, or differentiation, defines which cells are R and which are S. These populations of cells then are clonally selected by environmental injury (virus or chemical) as an adaptive response. In a larger sense, genetic traits that are adaptive for the maintenance and reproduction of cells in early life may be just those traits that predispose to cancer in the postreproductive years during which most cancers occur but when a primary effect of natural selection can no longer operate at the individual level (see Chapter 8). Thus, those attributes of cells that are adaptive in the reproductive years may lead to cancer in the postreproductive period (as with breast cancer, for example; see Chapter 9).

This view of cancer as adaptation is given some credence by the identification of oncogenes—genetic sequences isolated from human cancer cells that may transform certain other normal cells to become malignant. Thus there is a "gene for malignancy" that may be uncovered through regulation of genetic expression by various carcinogenic influences (Vogelstein & Kinzler, 1998). This oncogene grants selective advantage to the cells that express it for growth, survival, and differential replication. The cellular growth effects of such a gene, when expressed, may be adaptive in situations not leading to cancer (or when a carcinogenic mechanism is not in effect).

Researchers have called this human genetic sequence, as isolated from human cancer tissues, an oncogene because of its ability to induce cancer in other biologic systems. However, the possibility of a role for such genetic material in normal development and differentiation may be explored in developmental biology. The adaptive significance of such a gene may lie in its structural presence and in the genetic regulation of its expression during developmental stages of human growth. The fact that growth and development are "channelized"—cellular growth responses occur in the proper series—implies a role for regulation in developmental expression of all genes. Although enzymes are present to catalyze a number of cellular metabolic reactions, the law of thermodynamics would preclude drawing from an infinite and random pool of precursors to produce this channelized growth. Rather, cellular growth mechanisms must be linked in a stepwise fashion to provide the recognizable sequence of growth and development (ontogeny), characteristic of animal species. The role of factors that stimulate cellular growth (hyperplasia and hypertropy) during development may have adaptive aspects. For example, although a virus may integrate itself into the nuclear DNA of a human cell, this process cannot induce the human cell to multiply per se. The cell is stimulated to proliferate by the necessity to replace other cells that are dying because of the viral infection. Control over all growth remains with the cell. It is in this role of growth regulation that the endogenous human oncogene may participate. Again, growth of cells is a normal, adaptive process that must be regulated at the cellular level by endogenous control. However, in this model, growth in a cell transformed by viral DNA may lead to cancer.

# Host Factors

Host factors are important in carcinogenesis. Age, sex, and genetic background have all been seen to cluster with cancer types epidemiologically. It is often difficult to separate genes from environment, as with ethnicity, which may imply a certain socioeconomic status, habitat, or geographic region of habitation, as well as defining a shared gene pool. The metabolism of carcinogens may vary within individuals. Although there are generally not qualitative differences in the metabolic pathways between individual humans or even between humans and some animals, there may be quantitative differences in the relative outcomes of these pathways. Such differences may be used to define the "hyper-susceptible" individual with increased risk to environmental carcinogens. The actions of various carcinogenic agents may be governed by host factors. Thus, metabolism of chemical carcinogens, initiation by infectious agents, promotion by hormones, and repair of DNA damage because of radiation induction (e.g., x ray and ultraviolet) are all under partial genetic regulation. For example, the development of a chronic carrier state with hepatitis B infection, which places the carrier at higher risk for liver cancer, appears to be genetically determined to some extent.

Genetic differences in the metabolism of therapeutic drugs (e.g., "fast acetylators" and "slow acetylators") may be related to the genetic differences involved in the metabolism of carcinogens, whose metabolic products may directly attack DNA. Extensive metabolizers receive one effective dose of carcinogen, whereas lesser metabolizers receive a different effective dose. Thus, genetic differences in carcinogen metabolism may again be related to quantitative rather than qualitative differences. Also, similar to drug metabolism, there may be environmental induction of metabolism. These acquired characteristics of cellular function may be separated from the primary genetic differences between individuals. Cells within the same individual may also manifest different pathways of cellular metabolism as determined by regulation of gene expression or hormonal stimulation in different cells within tissues or between different tissues of the body.

We may consider breast cancer as a prototype malignant condition (see Chapter 9) with significant public health implications, as well as social and psychologic implications. In the United States, breast cancer is responsible for more than 25% of all cancer deaths and over 10% of women die of breast cancer (American Cancer Society, 2004; Greenlee et al., 2000). It has been the number one cancer of women. The exact causes of breast cancer are not established, but the rates of this disease are much lower in Asia. In support of genetic influences, the ratios of the three major estrogens, estriol, estrone, and estradiol, are markedly different in Asian versus American women (Alison et al., 2003). However, in evidence of an environmental component, generations of immigrants to the United States show a dramatic shift upward in breast cancer rates (see Chapter 9).

# Chemotherapy and Chemosensitivity

Current principles of cancer chemotherapy, like those applied to infectious diseases in the past, are based on differential destruction of abnormal cells with relative preservation of normal host cells. In the preantibiotic era, agents used to treat infection were toxic to all cells but more toxic to bacterial cells while preserving the cells of the host. Thus, the use of arsenic compounds (themselves carcinogenic) in treating syphilis was successful for destruction of the bacteria but was also associated with severe, and anticipated, side effects in the human host. The development of antibiotics provided a "magic bullet" specific for bacterial cells. The development of drugs for fungi met with some resistance because fungi are more complex cells; they are more similar to human cells than are bacteria. For an extended time during the antibiotic era, there were no agents for viruses that were not also very toxic to human cells. Immunization for viral diseases was long used as an alternative to the necessity for treatment of viral infection. Because many viruses have been associated with cancer (Stoler, 1997), the successful immunization, prophylaxis, or treatment of viral infection may be a form of primary prevention for cancer as well.

Although the search is on for a true "magic bullet" for cancer, one that will destroy only abnormal human cells, it has yet to be developed. Thus, the state of the art in cancer chemotherapy remains differential destruction of abnormal over normal cells. Those normal cells that are most like the abnormal cancer cells (i.e., those normally having the fastest rate of growth) will be differentially affected by cancer therapy, thus causing the well-known side effects of chemotherapy.

However, a rational basis for selection of cancer chemotherapeutic agents may become available with the testing of tumor tissue for chemosensitivity. The principles involved are similar to those for testing the antibiotic sensitivity of bacteria, done routinely to ensure appropriate antibiotic therapy. Testing for tumor sensitivity to drugs may have a role in drug development and screening, as well as in individual clinical trials. This process is analogous to testing tumor sensitivity clinically, because there is a wide variation of response of a given tumor in a given individual. However, *in vitro* testing for tumor chemosensitivity allows prediction of the types of tumors (within individual variation) that are sensitive to a given drug prior to administration of uniformly toxic chemotherapeutic agents to the patient. By the same analysis, assays may be developed to predict the sensitivity of tumors to radiation therapy. Unfortunately, to date, any such assays that have been developed have not been able to predict clinical outcome (Abeloff et al., 2000).

Although we talk in terms of differential toxicity of chemotherapeutic agents to cancer cells, these agents may in fact be equally toxic to all cells. Thus, the observed therapeutic success of cancer chemotherapy may be based primarily on better survival of normal cells over cancer cells. Because there are more normal than cancer cells in the body, by sheer numbers, killing cells indiscriminately may eventually result in removal of most cancer cells from the host with survival of most normal cells. Chemotherapy is often more successful in young people because normal cells may replace themselves more rapidly at a given drug dose designed to kill cancer cells. In older adults, normal cells cannot replace themselves as quickly and the doses necessary to kill cancer cells may not be compatible with the patient.

# Conclusion

The biologic basis of cancer has led to the development of cancer chemotherapeutic agents that act by killing cancer cells. These agents are also toxic to normal cells, which results in many of the side effects associated with cancer therapy. Some complementary and alternative medical modalities are available for the alleviation of the known and accepted side effects of cancer therapy.

In addition, some observed actions of Chinese and Ayurvedic herbal preparations, for example, are consistent with a model of cancer involving the regulation of cell growth. Instead of killing cancer cells, as with cancer chemotherapy, these treatments appear to alter cancer cells to less abnormal forms through regulation. Finally, many herbs and nutrients contain constituents that may help prevent the early development of cancer, and may contribute to survival and quality of life in the cancer patient. These characteristics open the door to a role for complementary and alternative medicine in the prevention of cancer and in care of the patient with cancer.

## REFERENCES

Abeloff, M. D., Armitage, J. O., Lichter, A. S. (2000). *Clinical oncology* (2nd ed.). New York: Churchill Livingstone.

Ackerman, L. V., & del Regato, J. A. (1977). *Cancer: Diagnosis, treatment and prognosis*. St. Louis, MO: Mosby.

American Cancer Society. (2004). *Cancer facts and figures*. Atlanta, GA:

Duncan, A. M., Phipps, W. R., & Kurzer, M. S. (2003). Phytoestrogens: Best practice and research. *Clinical Endocrinology & Metabolism, 17*, 253–271.

Greenlee, R. T., Murray, T., Bolden, S., & Wingo, P. A. (2000). Cancer statistics 2000. *CA: A Cancer Journal for Clinicians, 50*, 7–27.

Nowell, P. C. (1976). The clonal evolution of tumor progression. *Science, 194*, 23–28.

Nowell, P. C. (1993). Chromosomes and cancer: Evolution of an idea. *Advances in Cancer Research, 6*, 1–17.

Rubin, P., & Williams, J. P. (2001). *Clinical oncology: A multidisciplinary approach for physicians and students* (8th ed.). Philadelphia: Saunders.

Stevens, R., Jones, D. Y., Micozzi, M. S., & Taylor, P. R. (1988). Body iron stores and the risk of cancer. *New England Journal of Medicine, 319*, 1047–1052.

Stevens, R. L., Graubard, B. R., Micozzi, M. S., Neriishi, K., & Blumberg, B. S. (1994). Moderate elevation of body iron level and increased risk of cancer occurrence and death. *International Journal of Cancer, 56*, 364–369.

Stoler, M. (1997). The biology of human papillomaviruses. *Pathology Case Reviews, 2*, 8–20.

Tannock, I. F., & Hill, R. P. (1998). *The basic science of oncology* (3rd ed.). New York: McGraw-Hill.

Vogelstein, B., & Kinzler, K. (1998). *The genetic basis of human cancer*. New York: McGraw-Hill.

# Antiquity and Ecology of Cancer

### Marc S. Micozzi

One of the premises of the standard textbook *Fundamentals of Complementary and Integrative Medicine* (Micozzi, 2006) is that traditional human cultures and societies may develop over time useful therapies for the medical problems that plague them. Such "alternative" therapies may then be studied by modern science for proof of efficacy.

As examined by this textbook, the investigation of evidence for true alternative cancer therapy is highly problematic. However, there are many approaches in the realm of complementary/alternative medicine that may help reduce the risk of cancer occurrence and that may help provide supportive therapy in the care of the cancer patient.

This chapter presents evidence and arguments that the cancers that are common in modern industrial societies were rare in antiquity and in traditional human societies. Because the modern pattern of cancer occurrence was rare in the past, traditional societies had few opportunities to develop alternative treatments for these cancers. However, cancer as a disease causes many metabolic, psychologic, and physiologic disruptions, and contemporary cancer treatment causes many side effects, for which complementary therapies may be helpful, although not necessarily in themselves providing treatment of the malignancy.

Likewise, if the picture of cancer today is not an inevitable consequence of the human condition (as is suggested by the apparent rarity of modern cancers in antiquity), then there should be effective ways of preventing the occurrence of cancer. The diet and lifestyle of traditional human societies, and of our human ancestors, may provide clues as to what a "cancer preventive" diet and lifestyle might be. This evidence is examined in the next section of this textbook.

Many medical textbooks begin with the statement that cancer has been known since earliest times. For example, *Closing in on Cancer: Solving a 5000-Year-Old Mystery*, published in 1987 by the National Cancer Institute, states, "Cancer is older than man, stalking dinosaurs long before the earliest written records document its ravages among humans." Statements are based, for example, on Egyptian medical papyruses that date from 3000 B.C. making reference to what has been translated by 19th-century Victorian Egyptologists (without medical training) as "tumors." Such statements refer to descriptions by the great 19th-century German pathologist Rudolph Virchow of cancer in bears from the Neanderthal period and earlier. However, modern medical texts and writings do not always address taphonomy (the study of postmortem change) or paleopathology (the study of diseases in antiquity). Modern translations of Egyptian papyruses, for example, often reveal not cancer but tumors in the traditional Latin sense of the word *swelling*, which can result from any of a number of causes; the Neanderthal cancer in bone described by Virchow was a healing bone fracture when subjected to modern analysis. There is little hard evidence of cancer in antiquity.

One could conclude on this basis that cancer in antiquity was not as common as it is today. A counterargument is that cancer is primarily a disease of old age (increasing age-specific rates observed for most cancers in modern populations), and because in antiquity people did not live to old age, they did not live long enough to get cancer. Yet, the most and best preserved human remains from antiquity are primarily in the form of bone, and primary bone cancer is more common in the young than in the old. If bone neoplasia were common in antiquity, we could observe it in ancient bones in younger age groups. Regarding soft-tissue cancers, Egyptian mummies provide an abundant source of preserved soft tissues. Wealthier ancient Egyptians had better, and more expensive, funerary preparations, and they are differentially represented among ancient mummified remains. Many wealthy Egyptians also lived to advanced old age, consistent with their better economic status. If cancer were common in antiquity, we should be able to detect it in ancient (and older) mummies. Postmortem transformations also influence what is available today to study in attempts to render a diagnosis of cancer or other disease in antiquity.

# Why Study Cancer in Antiquity?

Recent epidemiologic observations are consistent with the possibility that 80% to 90% of human cancer may be because of environmental exposures and that 30% to 40% of cancer can be explained by human diet and nutrition.

In light of current observations on variations in lifestyle, diet, and cancer patterns in human populations around the world, there has long been interest in establishing relations between adaptational changes in nutritional patterns and changes in the rates of certain cancers that accompany modernization and the influence of Western culture among human populations (Oiso, 1975). Numerous migrant studies suggest that acculturation of diet and lifestyle among various migrant groups to the United States, coming from home populations with low incidence rates of certain cancers, is accompanied by increases in the rates of these cancers toward those of the host country (Albanes, Schatzkin, & Micozzi, 1987). Acculturation is the process by which the dietary and other behaviors of migrant populations become similar to those of the host country (see Chapters 7–9).

Dietary and lifestyle patterns of human populations that have changed through time are also thought to have significant implications for the health of human populations (Eaton, Shostak, & Konner, 1988). Development of a long-term perspective on the antiquity of cancer in human populations undergoing demographic transition provides additional descriptive information about the possible influences of diet, lifestyle, and other environmental factors on cancer through time.

# How to Study the Antiquity of Cancer

Three types of descriptive observations are available to help build a diachronic perspective on the antiquity of cancer. The first category of evidence comes from human and animal remains, consisting primarily of skeletal remains that may or may not have undergone diagenesis (fossilization), as well as significant accumulations of soft-tissue remains preserved through artificial or natural means or combinations of the two. Selective preservation of such remains, as well as postmortem taphonomic transformations, and the morphologic appearance of such materials, are important methodologic considerations. Some of the fossil evidence of ancient cancers, reported by luminaries in the new field of anatomic pathology in the 19th century, has not been borne out as representing examples of malignant neoplasms when reexamined with the use of techniques of diagnosis in the 20th century and interpreted in light of postmortem transformations. However, the 19th-century reports of "ancient cancers" have made their way into the modern textbooks, whereas the results of 20th-century analyses have been less visible in the secondary scientific literature.

Modern and early 20th-century populations around the world that had not undergone transition to a modern diet and lifestyle also provide a window on the relations of diet and health, as do modern primate populations, as well as other animal species, in their natural habitats.

A second category of evidence comes from ancient clay tablets, papyruses, texts, and other documents that purportedly "report" ancient cases of cancer. Many of these texts, initially preserved from antiquity by the Islamic civilizations of the late 1st and early 2nd millennia A.D., came under serious scrutiny in Europe in the late 1800s. These documents were often acquired by Victorian gentlemen who either translated them or had them translated by scholars of antiquity with little or no medical or scientific background or training. The result is often scientifically uninformed (by then current standards) translations that are difficult to place into modern diagnostic or interpretive contexts.

Other literary and artistic depictions of disease have also led to speculation as to providing documentary evidence of cancers. Artistic and cultural representations from ancient civilizations have been interpreted as providing evidence for benign tumors and disorders, such as osteomas, osteitis, osteochondroma, and cranial meningioma, and possibly the malignant conditions of chondrosarcoma of the pelvis and nasopharyngeal carcinoma.

The third category of evidence comes from early demographic and statistical information in populations when and where coincidentally (1) such data began to be collected, (2) cancer became recognized as a clinicopathologic entity, and (3) cancer rates were observed to increase in human populations. Such medical and vital statistics, collected by the state for official purposes, may or may not have been accompanied by data on employment, housing, lifestyle, nutrition, and so on. Because increasing age is the greatest relative risk factor for most cancers, data on average life span and longevity are important to estimating age-specific rates of cancer in different historic populations.

# Preservation of Human and Animal Remains

Skeletal remains of biologic organisms, consisting of mineralized organic matrix, may be preserved postmortem under a variety of circumstances. The study of skeletal remains provides information on diseases of bone, as well as other diseases, provided they leave the slightest traces on the skeleton (Dastugue, 1980). Common examples are skeletal morphologic changes associated with hematologic disorders and reactive processes to meningioma, trauma of soft tissues, hemangiomas, aneurysms, and neurologic disorders. Skeletal remains also provide a permanent record of primary bone neoplasms, as well as metastatic cancers from other primary sites. This type of analysis does not permit consideration either of diseases that leave no traces on bone or of hypothetical diseases that are limited only to ancient populations, leaving noncomparable or undecipherable traces in skeletons.

However, the geologic law of uniformitarianism (Lyell, 1867) appears to apply to these studies as well. In any case of unequivocal diagnosis, all ancient diseases have appeared to be morphologically similar to their modern forms throughout 30 years of paleopathologic studies. In cases of suspected or doubtful diagnoses, the uncertainty generally can be attributed to known variability within the manifestations of modern disease (Kelley & Micozzi, 1984). It seems reasonable to assume that if cancer exists in ancient skeletal remains, we should know what it looks like when subjected to modern analysis. Such remains can be subjected to modern techniques of clinical diagnosis, including roentgenography and other imaging studies, as well as gross, microscopic, and ultrastructural pathologic analysis and trace element studies. In fact, the x-ray film appearance of pathologic findings in dry bone remains may be even more sensitive and specific than are x-ray film studies on living humans (Kelley & Micozzi, 1984; Micozzi, 1982; Ortner & Utermohle, 1981).

In addition to the relatively commonplace preservation of human and animal skeletal remains, there are certain conditions under which soft tissues may also be preserved after death. Postmortem decay (aerobic) and decomposition (anaerobic) occurs in most environments because of chemical changes and microbial actions (Micozzi, 1986). However, if dehydration (desiccation) occurs rapidly before the onset of decay and decomposition, these chemical and biologic changes can be arrested or indefinitely slowed. Postmortem preservation of tissue is essentially a competition between decomposition and desiccation. Desiccation occurs naturally because of environmental conditions that commonly exist in the deserts of North Africa, Australia, the western coasts of Chile and Peru, the southwestern United States, and northern Mexico. Desiccation can also be facilitated by freezing, as in the Artic, and by cultural processes of evisceration and chemical treatment that are practiced by various populations throughout the world.

Preservation of soft tissues also may occur under natural conditions, where tissues remain in which the diagnosis of cancer could be readily made if present. Zimmerman (1977) showed that malignant tumors from modern humans are well preserved and recognizable in tissues that are experimentally subjected to processes that accurately reproduce environmental desiccation and tissue preservation. This experimental approach reproduces changes in nonmalignant tissues that are identical to those observed in the preserved nonmalignant remains of ancient individuals from a variety of sources, including the Artic and Egypt. Also, experimental malignant tissues appear to be better preserved after desiccation than are nonmalignant tissues. Metastatic tumors are also preserved and remain recognizable. Therefore, if physical evidence of cancer exists in ancient human and animal remains, it should be preserved and relatively recognizable within the bone or soft tissue that remains.

# Paleopathologic Evidence From Human and Animal Remains

## Paleozoic and Mesozoic Eras

Primary malignancies of bone have not been positively identified among extinct animals (Brothwell & Sandison, 1967). The apparent absence of any recognizable diseases among animals of the early Paleozoic era (195 to 520 million years ago) has also been noted. The earliest example of a suspected neoplasm came from the fossilized remains of a large dinosaur (genus *Apatosaurus*) from the Comanchean period of the Mesozoic era (70 to 195 million years ago by recent estimate), showing evidence of a benign hemangioma between two caudal vertebrae; that is, a location that shows similar predilections in modern humans (Coley, 1960; Swinton, 1983). This specimen was collected from the Como beds of Wyoming by S. W. Williston at the time when these deposits were at the height of their fame as dinosaur quarries (Moodie, 1923).

The next oldest example is a benign osteoma that involved the dorsal vertebra of a mosasaur (genus *Mosasaurus*) from the later Cretaceous period of the Mesozoic era (Abel, 1924). Moodie (1923) and Lull (1933) also reported suspected cases of "multiple myeloma" that involved squamous bones and adjunct maxillas in horned dinosaurs (torosaurus) of the genus *Ceratopsia*. Swinton (1983) later reinterpreted the incorrect diagnosis of multiple myeloma in skulls of the *Ceratopsia*, writing that these lesions recalled the fenestrae that were seen in later mammal and early human skulls that may have been caused by a number of benign osteolytic processes. Finally, a dinosaur bone from Transylvania from 70 million years ago that originally was identified in a London hospital as "periosteal sarcoma" was diagnosed by Campbell (Brothwell & Sandison, 1967) as osteopetrosis.

## Cenozoic Era

The Cenozoic era comprises the Tertiary period (age of mammals) and the Quaternary period (age of humans), covering the past 70 million years to the present. As early as the mid–18th century, E. J. C. Esper (1774), in Erlangen, Germany, described what he thought was an osteosarcoma in the distal femur of a cave bear (*Ursus spelaeus*) from the Pleistocene epoch, as cited by Goldfuss in 1810 (Brothwell & Sandison, 1967). However, this lesion was later described as a healing fracture callus with necrosis by Mayer (1854). Virchow's studies (1870, 1895, and 1896) of the cave bears of Europe since the Middle Tertiary period were also well known historically but provided no evidence of cancer in antiquity.

Perhaps the earliest example of a suspected malignant tumor in a hominid was described in the Kanam mandibular fragment from East Africa by Lawrence (1935), probably of the Lower or Middle Pleistocene (Brothwell, 1967). The details of the tumor are somewhat obscured by extensive diagenesis. The interpretation of this lesion by Tobias as a subperiosteal ossifying sarcoma was accepted by Brothwell (1967), although there was some difference of opinion on this diagnosis. Goldstein (1969) also believed the lesion to be a "sarcomatous overgrowth." Finally, Stathopoulos (1975) suggested that the lesion in question could have been the site of a Burkitt's lymphoma (see Chapters 1 and 2). Wells (1964) and Sandison (1970, 1975), however, expressed serious reservations about a malignant diagnosis, favoring the possibility of trauma and low-grade inflammation in causing formation of subperiosteal new bone. Sandison (1975) concluded that it was by no means proven that this lesion represented Burkitt's lymphoma or was even neoplastic.

## Neolithic Period and Iron and Bronze Ages

Osteomas found in two femora from the Neolithic period were clearly benign (Pales, 1930). Beyond Pales, an osteosarcoma was diagnosed in the right ulna of an adult man from the Neolithic period that had been found in Bassa Padana, Italy (Novello, 1981). A lesion in the neck of a humerus from West Kennet, Wiltshire, England, described as a possible neoplasm by Brothwell (1961), was later thought by Wells to be an abscess (1962). Several reports cited by Ackerknecht (1953) relate to possible multiple myeloma in late Neolithic crania from Norregard, Denmark (Brothwell & Sandison, 1967, p. 342), and from the Pyrenees (Fuste, 1955); however, insufficient description is given to render independent diagnosis. The Norregard skull, and an additional skull with lesions from Grossbremach, Germany, were considered to be very improbable for cancer (Soulie, 1980). The bone destruction of the Norregard skull may also be taken as evidence of postmortem bone erosion (Brothwell, 1967).

Soulie (1980) described a female skull (age range, 50–70 years) from the European Bronze Age at Mokrin, Yugoslavia, that showed perforated lesions. The inner table of bone showed clear traces of neovascularization. Two lesions were centered on the course of meningeal vessels. The author suggested neoplastic diffusion of carcinoma through the external carotid system. The malignant character of two lesions of a skull from the Grotte de Terrevaine at La Ciotat, Bouches du Rhone, France, was questioned, based on gross and radiographic observation (Soulie 1980), in favor of pseudopathology caused by taphonomic transformation.

"Carcinomatous" destruction of bone in the temporal area of a skull from a Winchester (England) Saxon burial, in the frontal area from an Iron Age skull from the Bernese Oberland, as well as multiple myeloma in a medieval youth from Scarborough, England, have all been attributed to postmortem taphonomic changes (Brothwell, 1967). Insect destruction, as in the femur from a burial site on the island of Socotra (Brothwell, 1963), may simulate neoplastic destruction of bone. Conversely, what has been described by Hug (1959) as postmortem soil erosion in an Iron Age skull from Switzerland may have been a destructive tumor of the frontal sinuses (Brothwell, 1963). Hug (1956) had elsewhere described an osteosarcoma that involved the left humeral head and extended along the proximal one-third of the shaft in another Swiss Iron Age skull from Munsingen. Postmortem erosion appeared to have caused some irregularity in the appearance of the tumor (Brothwell, 1967). However, Jaffe (1958) pointed out that other tumors may simulate the appearance of osteosarcoma.

## Ancient Egypt and Nubia

In the early part of the 20th century Ruffer (1921) examined hundreds of Egyptian mummies. Many adult mummies from Egypt in the age group older than 50 years have also been examined more recently (Sandison, 1970; Zimmerman, 1976). Extensive radiologic surveys of the large collections of mummies in European museums (Gray 1967) and in the Cairo Museum (Harris & Weeks, 1973) have also been undertaken. Even so, meaningful occurrences of neoplasms in ancient Egypt have not been established (Sandison, 1970, 1975).

Initial diagnosis of an osteosarcoma in a femur from the cemetery of the Gizeh Pyramids (Vth Dynasty) by Elliot-Smith and Dawson (1924) has been more recently reinterpreted as benign (Rowling, 1961). Likewise, Elliot-Smith and Dawson (1924) referred to two cases of "sarcoma" in proximal humeri from Vth Dynasty graves in Gizeh. However, no illustrations or morphologic descriptions were provided, and it is likely that these neoplasms may have represented cases of mistaken diagnoses as well (Brothwell, 1967; Rowling, 1961). A pelvic tumor from an individual found in the catacombs of Kom el-Shougafa in Alexandria, from Roman Egypt (250 to 300 A.D.), was originally described by Ruffer and Willmore (1914) as an atypical osteosarcoma but more likely represented a benign chondromatous process of long duration (Brothwell 1967).

Rowling (1961) noted the relative lack of malignant epithelial tumors in ancient Egyptian mummies. Granville (1825) had described a large cyst of the right ovary and broad ligament in an Egyptian mummy, which may have represented a malignant cystadenocarcinoma of the ovary (Rowling, 1961) but was more likely a benign cystadenoma (Strouhal, 1976). In the relatively recent Byzantine Period, cases of malignant disease that involved the nasopharynx and rectum, respectively, were suggested by Elliot-Smith and Dawson (1924) on the basis of destructive lesions in the base of the skull and sacrum. Wells (1963) also observed a primary lesion of a skull from the IIIth–Vth Dynasties with 26 secondary deposits and destruction of the left maxilloalveolar region that may have represented carcinoma. Strouhal (1978) reported another case of nasopharyngeal carcinoma in a skull from the Vth Dynasty to the XIIth Dynasty in Upper Egypt. Derry (1909) had reported a similar case that involved the cranial base of a pre-Christian Nubian (300 to 500 A.D.), and Elliot-Smith and Derry (1910) described a Middle Nubian male skeleton with erosion of the sacrum, possibly the result of rectal cancer. However, these findings may also be the result of chordoma (Brothwell, 1967).

Changes in disease patterns were observed in ancient Nubia from 350 B.C. to 1400 A.D., with up to 12 malignant neoplasms reported for this later period. Marrocco (1969) and Marracco and Armelagos (1984) also reported two malignant tumors in the remains of 223 individuals from a cemetery in lower Nubia, dating from 350 B.C. to 500 A.D. Among 222 skulls that were collected from a vast Coptic cemetery near El Barsha from the early Christian period in Egypt (400 to 600 A.D.), five lesions were observed that possibly were consistent with nasal, oral, and other carcinomas (El-Rakhawy, El-Eishi, El-Nofely, & Gaballah, 1971).

## Ancient Middle East

A skull from the Tepe Hessar site of Iran (3500 to 3000 B.C.) showed destruction of the left maxillary alveolus and antral wall and was cited by Krogman (1940) as an example of primary carcinoma.

Wada, Ikeda, and Suzuki (1987) described multiple lytic lesions in bones of a 25- to 30-year-old woman from the Islamic period of Iraq. However, the relatively young age made eosinophilic granuloma (histiocytosis X) a more likely diagnosis than metastatic carcinoma or multiple myeloma (Steinbock, 1988).

## The New World

Human populations in the New World may be considered "prehistoric," in a technical sense, before the arrival of Christopher Columbus in 1492. For practical purposes, the search for cancer in antiquity may be limited to the pre-Columbian period in the New World, because the arrival of Columbus was associated with dramatic changes in lifestyle and marked the beginning of an evolution into disease patterns that are associated with the modern world.

MacCurdy (1923) attributed a tumor on a pre-Columbian skull from Peru to osteosarcoma. Brothwell (1963) reconsidered this tumor as a possible meningioma or angioma. Two cases of multiple myeloma have also been reported in skeletal remains of an adult male (Ritchie & Warren, 1932) and of a 10-year-old child (Williams, Ritchie, & Titterington, 1941). It is more likely that the lesions of the child represented secondary neuroblastoma or another childhood disease. Hooton (1930) recorded metastatic tumor of vertebrae, right radius and ulna, and left radius in an Indian from Pecos Pueblo (United States) (early level). However, he did not describe the lesions in detail and provided no illustrations for comparative purposes. Steinbock (1976) reexamined this specimen at the Peabody Museum at Harvard University (Cambridge, MA) and indicated that many of the skeletal findings were probably the result of erosion and postmortem taphonomic transformation. Findings in a second skeleton cited by Hooton (1930) may also be explained on the basis of processes other than metastatic carcinoma.

A pre-Columbian skull from a Peruvian collection was also reported to perhaps show evidence of metastatic carcinoma (Grana, Rocca, & Grana, 1954), although multiple trephinations also appeared in the skulls of this collection (Brothwell, 1967).

In a survey of the mummies of Ica, Peru, representing five different pre-Columbian cultures that dated from 600 B.C., no evidence of malignant neoplasms was found (Allison, Gerszten, & Dalton, 1974). However, the same group of investigators recorded metastatic tumor in the skeleton of a female from the Tiahuanco period of Chile (Allison, Gerszten, Munizaga, & Santoro, 1980).

Two ancient Peruvians (before 1500 A.D.) presented evidence of metastatic carcinoma in the view of Steinbock (1976), that is, a solitary skull from Llactashica and a skeleton from Huacho. The skeletons of several pre-Columbian mummies from Chancay, and Chongos, Ica, Peru, were thought to show evidence of malignant melanoma metastatic to bone (Urteaga & Pack, 1966), perhaps related to the high altitude of these sites in the Andes Mountains and increased exposure to solar radiation.

In Canada, the earliest known human remains (at least 7,500 years ago) showed no evidence of primary or secondary bone tumors (Cybulski, 1984). During the archaic or equivalent cultural periods (3,000 to 7,500 years ago), two tumorlike bone conditions were reported, one of which was a probable case of histiocytosis X in a child (Cybulski, 1984).

A Paleo–Eskimo skull (400 to 1300 A.D.) found in the Kitnepaluk necropolis in northwest St. Lawrence Island, Alaska, was reported to show evidence of malignant tumor or infection (Lagier, Baud, Arnaud, Arnaud, & Menk, 1982). The skeleton of a prehistoric Eskimo from Kachemak Bay, Cook Inlet, Alaska, was also thought to show evidence of advanced malignant hemangioepithelioma (Lobdell, 1981). However, Gregg (1981) disagreed with this diagnosis for several reasons that involved the epidemiology and pathology of this case. The findings could also be consistent with a benign process (Lobdell, 1981). Steinbock (1976) found evidence for metastatic carcinoma in two Alaskan Eskimo skulls (500 to 1500 A.D.) held in the Smithsonian Institution (Washington, DC), and Cassidy (1977) observed a probable malignant neoplasm in the mandible of a Sadlermiut Eskimo from the historic (post-Columbian) period.

# Documentary Evidence for Cancer in Antiquity

Zammit and Singer (1924) described two Neolithic human representations from Malta with artistic presentations of swelling in the abdomen and the groin. Two additional Neolithic figures from Sesklo, Greece, and Vinca, Yugoslavia, also showed swelling in the region of the throat (Brothwell 1967). The Neolithic art style was such that modern interpretations must remain tentative.

The Edwin Smith papyrus (approximately 1800 B.C.), Ebers papyrus (approximately 1550 B.C.), and Kahun papyrus (approximately 1750 B.C.) are representative of Egyptian medical papyruses. Early translations of these Egyptian texts were limited, in terms of both Egyptology (Dawson, 1953) and medical history (Ghalioungui, 1963). In light of their contents, the Ebers papyrus is thought of as a medical text, the Edwin Smith papyrus is thought of as a surgical text, and the Kahun papyrus is thought of as a gynecologic text. The Ebers papyrus has a series of prescriptions that are believed to be the remains of a "book on tumors," which deals with tumors and swellings. These tumors appear to have consisted of benign ganglionic masses, polyps, sebaceous cysts, varicose veins, and aneurysms. There is a reference to the "tumors of Chon" in which Brothwell (1967) found possible evidence of malignancy but which Ghalioungui (1963) cited as a "model clinical description" of leprosy. Elsewhere, "tumors of Chon" were originally translated as tubercular leprosy, but Ghalioungui (1963) believed that the description better represented gas gangrene, or possibly cancer. Esmond R. Long (1928), in *A History of Pathology*, described "ulcerating lumps" in the Ebers and Edwin Smith papyruses "that might be construed as cancer." In this case, the interpretation was more conservative than in some of those that followed. The word *tumor* appears frequently but always in the sense of swelling. The legendary rumor that malignant melanoma was described in the Ebers papyrus is apparently apocryphal (Urteaga & Pack, 1966).

Long (1928) also recounted Herodotus's story (111: 33) that Democedes of Crotona (520 B.C.), founder of the medical school in Athens, healed the Persian Darius's wife Athossa (daughter of Cyrus the Great) of a cancer of the breast. Herbal remedies for "cancers" or tumors have been described for ancient time periods (Riddle, 1985). However, the disease appeared actually to have been inflammatory mastitis.

The Greek Dioscorides, in the 1st century A.D. used a drug made from autumn crocus (*Colchicum autumnale* L.) and wrote that "the plant (kolchikon) should be soaked in wine and administered to dissolve tumors (oidemata) and growths (phumata) not yet making pus." Dioscorides terms *oidemata* and *phumata* may have included malignant neoplasms, but their use clearly was not restricted to malignant conditions (Long, 1928). Galen (129 to 210 A.D.) and the Byzantine physicians used the term *onkos* to cover all types of swellings, tumors, and lesions. Galen's Greek term *karkinos* (or *karkinoma*; Latin, *cancer*) could not have exclusively been applied to malignant neoplasms (Long, 1928).

In ancient India, medical conditions were described in the *Rigveda* (3000 B.C.), *Ayurveda*, *Ramayana*, and other texts (see Chapter 16). Human remains from prehistoric India and the Indus River Valley civilization have been unearthed at Harappa in Punjab, Lothul in Gujarat, and Inamgoen in Maharashtra. The state of decomposition in these tropical climates often precluded complete assessment of health status, and the writings in the ancient texts had not been confirmed in comparison to material remains (Suraiya, 1973).

Neck tumors, mentioned in the *Vedas*, were probably endemic goiter, as commonly encountered in some highland Aryan tribes that lived in the Himalayas, although a fatal tumor of the throat is described in the *Atharvaveda* (Suraiya, 1973). The physician Sushruta (approximately 600 B.C.) compiled a surgical treatise in which a chapter is devoted to *arbuda*, that is, glands and tumors. Here, *arbuda* is a swelling with characteristics that may implicate a malignant process. Overindulgence in eating meat is listed as one of the causes of *arbuda*. One description of *arbuda* is consistent with ulceration.

Tumors arising from other specific sites are not treated on the chapter on *arbuda* but described separately under different names. The practice of chewing betel nut is very ancient in India, and Sushruta described cancers of the lip, alveolus, tongue, palate, and pharynx, manifesting "lotus-like" growths. Tumors described in the gastrointestinal tract appeared to be benign. Approximately 20 diseases of the female breast and genital organs are described, but none are consistent with cancer of the uterus, ovaries, or breast. Part of the criteria used to assign a described disease to the category of malignancy is whether the disease is considered by the ancient author to be fatal (Suraiya, 1973). However, not all fatal diseases associated with swellings were cancers in the preantibiotic era.

# Cancer in Contemporary Societies

Modern primate populations and contemporary societies around the world that follow a traditional lifestyle may also provide insights into the origins of human cancer. No cancer was observed among diseases of wild apes (Schultz, 1967), for example. Several diseases are also characteristically uncommon among populations following a traditional lifestyle, including myocardial infarction and carcinoma of the lung (Polunin, 1967). Adenocarcinoma (glandular cancer of epithelial origin) that involves the breast, colon, pancreas, and prostate also appears to be rare in traditional societies (Micozzi, 1985).

However, as reliable 20th-century data were collected, it was recognized that oral and nasopharyngeal cancers are relatively common in parts of Africa (Clifford, 1961) and China (Kaplan & Jones, 1978). These patterns in contemporary Asian and African populations may be related to evidence for oral and nasopharyngeal cancers in ancient Egypt and India as documented in human remains and medical texts. However, ancient evidence for the contemporary pattern of cancers of civilization (Micozzi, 1985) remains elusive or simply nonexistent in examinations conducted around the world during the past century.

Understanding postmortem preservation and transformation of human and animal remains is important in interpreting cancer in antiquity. When historically suspected "cancer cases" are interpreted in light of current knowledge of postmortem artifacts, and utilizing modern diagnostic criteria, little evidence for malignant neoplasms in antiquity exists. Those cases of suspected malignancy are consistent with nasopharyngeal carcinoma or other cancers that remain common throughout the Third World today. Those cancers common in the modern industrialized world have left few traces of their existence in prehistory and early human civilizations.

Understanding changes in the occurrence and rates of diseases over time through history is important for a fuller understanding of whether cancer is truly a disease of modern society or whether it may be regarded as part of human heritage from earliest times.

# REFERENCES

Abel, O. (1924). Nuere Studien uber Krankheiten fossiler Wirbeltiere. Verh Zool Bolan Ges., *73*, 104.

Ackerknecht, E. H. (1953). *Paleopathology: A survey* (pp. 120–127). Chicago, IL: University of Chicago Press.

Albanes, D. A., Schatzkin, A. G., & Micozzi, M. S. (1987). A survey of time-related factors in research on diet and cancer. *The Journal of Chronic Diseases, 40* (Suppl. 2), 39S–44S.

Allison, M. J., Gerszten, E., & Dalton, H. P. (1974). Paleopathology in pre-Columbian Americans. *Laboratory Investigation, 30*, 407–408.

Allison, M. J., Gerszten, E., Munizaga, J., & Santoro, C. (1980). Metastatic tumor of bone in a Tiahuanaco female. *Bulletin of the New York Academy of Medicine, 56*, 581–587.

Armelagos, G. J. (1969). Disease in ancient Nubia: Changes in disease patterns from 350 BC to AD to 1400 demonstrate the interaction of biology and culture. *Science, 163*, 255–259.

Brothwell, D. (1967). The evidence for neoplasms. In D. Brothwell, A. T. Sandison, et al. (eds.), *Disease in antiquity: A survey of the diseases, injuries and surgery of early populations* (pp. 320–345). Springfield, IL: Charles C Thomas.

Brothwell, D., & Sandison, A. T. (Eds.). (1967). *Diseases in antiquity: A survey of the diseases, injuries and surgery of early populations.* Springfield, IL: Charles C Thomas.

Brothwell, D. R. (1961). The paleopathology of early British man: An essay on the problems of diagnosis and analysis. *Journal of the Royal Anthropological Institute, 91*, 318.

Brothwell, D. R. (1963). *Digging up bones.* London: British Museum.

Cassidy, C. M. (1977). Probable malignancy in a Sadlermiut Eskimo mandible. *American Journal of Physical Anthropology, 46*, 291–296.

Clifford, P. (1961). Malignant disease of the nose, paranalasl sinuses and post-nasal space in East Africia. *Journal of Laryngology and Otology, 75*, 707–733.

Coley, B. L. (1960). *Neoplasms of bone* (pp. 8–13). New York: Hoeber.

Cybulski, J. S. (1984). Tumors in antiquity in Canada: A preliminary survey. Presented at the 11th Annual Meeting of the Paleopathology Association. *Paleopathology Newsletter*, 3–4.

Dastugue, J. (1980). Possibilities, limits and prospects in paleopathology of the human skeleton. *Journal of Human Evol.ution, 9,* 3–8.

Dawson, W. R. (1953). The Egyptian medical papyri. In E. A. Underwood (Ed.), *Science, medicine and history.* New York: Oxford University Press.

Derry, D. E. (1909). Anatomical report. *The Archeological Survey of Nubia Bulletin, 3,* 29–52.

Eaton, S. B., Shostak, M., & Konner, M. (1988). *The Paleolithic prescription.* New York: Harper & Row.

Elliot-Smith, G., & Dawson, W. R. (1924). Mummification in relation to medicine and pathology. In G. Elliot-Smith, & W. R. Dawson, (Eds.), *Egyptian mummies* (pp. 54–162). New York: Dial.

Elliot-Smith, G., & Derry, D. E. (1910). Anatomical report. *The Archeological Survey of Nubia Bulletin, 5,* 11–25.

El-Rakhawy, M. T., El-Eishi, H. E., El-Nofely, A., & Gaballah, M. F. (1971). A contribution to pathology of ancient Egyptian skulls. *Anthropologie, 9, 59,* 71–78.

Esper, E. J. C. (1774). *Ausfuhrliche Nachrichten con neuendeckten zoolithen unbekannter vierfussiger Thiere.* Nuremberg, Germany.

Fuste, M. (1955). Antropologia de las poblaciones pirenaicas durante el periodo neo-eneolitico. Trab. Inst. "Bernardino de Sahagun" *Antropologica Ethnologia, 14,* 109.

Ghalioungui, P. (1963). *Magic and medical science in ancient Egypt* (pp. 84–91). London: Hodder & Stoughton.

Goldstein, M. S. (1969). The Kanam Mandible. In D. Brothwell & E. Higgs (Eds.), *Science and archaeology.* London: British Museum.

Grana, F., Rocca, E. D., & Grana, L. (1954). *Las trepanaciones craneanas en el Peru en la Epoca pre-Hispanica.* Lima, Peru: Maria.

Granville, A. B. (1825). An essay on Egyptian mummies with observations on the art of embalming among the ancient Egyptians XIII. *Philosophical Transactions of the Royal Society of London B: Biological Sciences, 115,* 269–316.

Gray, P. H. K. (1967). Radiography of ancient Egyptian mummies. *Medical Radiography and Photography, 43,* 3444.

Gregg, J. B. (1981). Annotated bibliography. *Paleopathology Newsletter,* 15–16.

Harris, J. E., & Weeks, K. R. (1973). *X-raying the Pharoahs.* New York: Charles Scribner's Sons.

Hooton, E. A. (1930). *The Indians of Pecos Pueblo: A study of their skeletal remains.* New Haven, CT: Yale University Press.

Hug, E. (1956). *Die Anthropologische Sammlung in Naturhistorischen Museum Bern.* Bern, Switzerland: Natural History Museum.

Hug, E. (1959). *Die Anthropologische Sammlung in Kantonsmuseum Baselland.* Liestal, Switzerland: Kantonsmuseum Baselland.

Jaffe, H. L. (1958). *Tumors and tumourous conditions of the bones and joints.* London: Kimpton.

Kaplan, H. S., & Jones, E. (1978). *Cancer in China.* New York: Alan R. Liss.

Kelley, M. A., & Micozzi, M. S. (1984). Rib lesions in chronic pulmonary tuberculosis. *American Journal of Physical Anthropology, 65,* 381–386.

Krogman, W. M. (1940). The skeletal and dental pathology of an early Iranian site. *Bulletin of the History of Medicine, 8,* 28.

Lagier, R., Baud, C. A., Arnaud, G., Arnaud, S., & Menk, R. (1982). Lesions, characteristic of infection or malignant tumor in Paleo-Eskimo skulls. *Virchows Archives A, 395,* 237–243.

Lawrence, J. E. P. (1935). Appendix A. In L. S. Leakey (Ed.), *Stone Age races of Kenya* (p. 139). New York: Oxford University Press.

Lobdell, J. E. (1981). The occurrence of a rare cancer in a prehistoric Eskimo skeleton from Kachemak Bay, Cook Inlet, Alaska. In J. S. Cybulski (Ed.), *National Museum of Man Mercury Series: Contributions to Physical Anthropology 1978–1980.* Ottawa: National Museum of Canada.

Long, E. R. (1928). *A history of pathology.* Baltimore, MD: Williams & Wilkins.

Lull, R. S. (1933). *A revision of the Ceratopsia: Memoirs of the Peabody Museum of Natural History* (Vol. 3, p. 131). New Haven, CT: Peabody Museum.

Lyell, C. (1867). *Principles of geology, 2 vols.* (10th ed.). London.

MacCurdy, G. G. (1923). Human skeletal remains from the highlands of Peru. *American Journal of Physical Anthropology, 6,* 217.

Marrocco, G. R., & Armelagos, G. J. (1984). Tumors in a Nubian population. Symposium of tumors in antiquity, the 11th Annual Meeting of the Paleopathology Association. *Paleopathology Newsletter,* 1–3.

Mayer, D. R. (1854). Uber krankhafter Knochen vorweltlicher Thiere. *In Nova Acta Leopoldina (Novorum Actorum Academia Caesareae Leopoldino-Carolinae Naturae)* (pp. xxiv, 673–689).

Micozzi, M. S. (1982). Skeletal tuberculosis, pelvic contraction and parturition. *American Journal of Physical Anthropology, 58*, 441–445.

Micozzi, M. S. (1985). Nutrition, body size and breast cancer. *Yearbook of Physical Anthropology, 28*, 175–206.

Micozzi, M. S. (1986). Experimental study of immediate postmortem change under field conditions: Effects of freezing, thawing and mechanical injury. *Journal of Forensic Science, 31*, 953–961.

Micozzi, M. S. (2006). *Fundamentals of complementary and integrative medicine* (3rd ed.) (p. 606). Philadelphia: Elsevier-Saunders.

Moodie, R. L. (1923). *Paleopathology: An introduction to the study of ancient evidences of disease* (pp. 38–39, 46–47, 61–78, 80–87, 91–97, 370–371, 402–403, 411, 434–435, 545–557). Urbana, IL: University of Illinois Press.

National Cancer Institute (1997). *Closing in on cancer: Solving a 5000 year old mystery*. Bethesda, MD.

Novello, A. (1981). Rilievi di paleopatologia sullo scheletro della Tomba 5 di San Cesario. In *II Neolithic e l'Eta del Rame-Ricerca a Spiamberto* (pp. 187–188). Bologna: Cassa di Risparmio di Vignola.

Oiso, T. (1975). Incidence of stomach cancer and its relation to dietary habits and nutrition in Japan between 1900 and 1975. *Cancer Research, 35*, 3254–3258.

Ortner, D. J., & Utermohle, C. J. (1981). Polyarticular inflammatory arthritis in a pre-Columbian skeleton from Kodiak Island, Alaska, USA. *American Journal of Physical Anthropology, 56*, 23–32.

Pales, L. (1930). *Paleopathologie et pathologie comparative*. Paris, France: Masson & Co.

Polunin, I. V. (1967). Health and disease in contemporary primitive societies. In D. Brothwell & A. T. Sandison (Eds.), *Disease in antiquity: A survey of the diseases, injuries and surgery of early populations* (pp. 69–94). Springfield, IL: Charles C Thomas.

Riddle, J. M. (1985). Ancient and medieval chemotherapy for cancer. *Isis, 75*, 319–330.

Ritchie, W. A., & Warren, S. L. (1932). The occurrence of multiple bony lesions suggesting myeloma in the skeleton of a pre-Columbian Indian. *American Journal of Roentgenology, 28*, 622.

Rowling, J. T. (1961). Pathological changes in mummies. *Proceedings of the Royal Society of Medicine, 54*, 409–415.

Ruffer, M. A. (1921). *Studies in the paleopathology of Egypt*. Chicago, IL: University of Chicago Press.

Ruffer, M. A., & Willmore, J. G. (1914). Studies in paleopathology: Note on a tumor of the pelvis dating from Roman times (250 AD) and found in Egypt. *Journal of Pathology, 18*, 480–484.

Sandison, A. T. (1970). The study of mummified and dried human tissues. In D. R. Brothwell & E. Higgs (Eds.), *Science in archaeology* (2nd ed.). New York: Praeger.

Sandison, A. T. (1975). Kanam mandible's tumour. *Lancet, 1*, 279.

Schultz, A. H. (1967). Notes on diseases and healed fractures of wild apes. In D. Brothwell, & A. T. Sandison (Eds.), *Disease in antiquity: A survey of the diseases, injuries and surgery of early populations* (p. 47). Springfield, IL: Charles C Thomas.

Soulie, R. (1980). New evidence for skull metastasis of malignant neoplasm. In *The European Bronze Age*. Papers on Paleopathology of the Third European Members Meeting of the Paleopathology Association, Caen, France.

Stathopoulos, E. (1975). Kanam mandible's tumour. *Lancet, 1*, 165.

Steinbock, R. T. (1976). *Paleopathological diagnosis and interpretation: Bone diseases in ancient human populations*. Springfield, IL: Charles C Thomas.

Steinbock, R. T. (1988). Annotated bibliography. *Paleopathology Newsletter, 62*, 11.

Strouhal, E. (1974). Tumours in the remains of ancient Egyptians. *American Journal of Physical Anthropology, 45*, 613–620.

Strouhal, E. (1978). Ancient Egyptian case of carcinoma (nasopharyngeal). *Bulletin of the New York Academy of Medicine, 54*, 290–302.

Suraiya, J. N. (1973). Medicine in ancient India with special reference to cancer. *Indian Journal of Cancer, 10*, 391–402.

Swinton, W. E. (1983). Animal paleopathology: Its relation to ancient human disease. In G. D. Hart (Ed.), *Disease in ancient man* (pp. 50–58). Toronto: Clarke, Irwin & Company.

Urteaga, O. B., & Pack, G. T. (1966). On the antiquity of melanoma. *Cancer, 19*, 607–610.

Virchow, R. (1870). Knochen wom Hohlenbaren mit krankhaften Veranderungen. *Zeitschrift für Ethnologie, 2*, 365.

Virchow, R. (1895). Ueber einen Besuch der westfallischen Knochenhohle. *Zeitschrift für Ethnologie, 27*, 706–708.

Virchow, R. (1896). Beitrag zur Geschichte der Lues. *Dermatologica, 3*, 4.

Wada, Y., Ikeda, J., & Suzuki, T. (1987). Tumor-like lesions in a human skeleton from the Himrin basin of Iraq. *Journal of the Anthropological Society of Nippon, 95*, 107–119.

Wells, C. (1963). Ancient Egyptian pathology. *Journal Laryngology and Otology, 77*, 261–265.

Wells, C. (1964). *Bones, bodies and disease* (pp. 70-76). London: Thames & Hudson Ltd.

Williams, G. D., Ritchie, W. A., & Titterington, D. F. (1941). Multiple bony lesions suggesting myeloma in preColumbian Indian aged ten years. *American Journal of Roentgenology, 46*, 351.

Zammit, T., & Singer, C. (1924). Neolithic representations of the human form from the Islands of Malta and Gozo. *Journal of the Royal Anthropological Institute, 54*, 67.

Zimmerman, M. R. (1976). *A paleopathologic and archaeologic investigation of the human remains of Dra Abuel-Naga Site, Egypt: Based on an experimental study of mummification.* Unpublished masters's thesis, University of Pennsylvania, Philadelphia.

Zimmerman, M. R. (1977). An experimental study of mummification pertinent to the antiquity of cancer. *Cancer, 40*, 1358–1362.

# 2

## Mind/Body Approaches

# Mind/Body Modalities

**4**

Carolyn Fang

## Introduction

The idea that thoughts and emotions can alter physical health has existed for thousands of years. Although ancient healers were convinced that the mind could influence the body, either by causing illness or curing disease, the concept fell into disrepute as medical advances discovered how infectious agents or chemical imbalances lead to illness. Over the past two decades, however, there has been growing interest in mind/body modalities, particularly as they relate to cancer care and the treatment of symptoms.

In our daily lives, we are often confronted with situations that create stress. Stress has been defined as a reaction to a potentially threatening (either psychologically, emotionally, or physically) situation. Stress occurs when we appraise events as harmful or challenging and as exceeding our ability to cope with the demands posed by these events or experiences (Cohen, Kessler, & Gordon 1995; Lazarus & Folkman, 1984). Walter Cannon was one of the first physiologists to study the powerful and long-lasting effects of stress on the human body (Cannon, 1932).

When an individual is confronted with a threat (either real or perceived), the sympathetic nervous system acts by preparing the body to flee or to confront the stressor. This response to stress is characterized by increased heart rate, blood pressure, and respiration. Circulation of blood to the skin is reduced, whereas circulation of blood to the muscles is increased. This physiological response is known as the fight-or-flight response (Cannon, 1932).

On the one hand, this physiological response is adaptive because it enables the individual to respond quickly to a threat. On the other hand, frequent or prolonged exposure to stress can be harmful over time because it disrupts normal physiological functioning and leads to *wear and tear* on various systems. Problems occur when we are frequently or continuously exposed to events that we perceive to be stressful. With chronic stress, the hormonal and physiological changes caused by the fight-or-flight response become damaging, making us more susceptible to illness.

Theoretically then, any method that alleviates or counteracts the effects of stress should lead to improvements in health. Mind/body modalities such as meditation, biofeedback, and hypnosis result in physiological and psychological effects that are consistent with decreased stress and increased relaxation. For example, the processes associated with meditation (i.e., brief periods of sitting still and concentrating on breathing) have been demonstrated to result in lowered blood pressure, decreased heart rate, and decreased galvanic skin response, which is a measure of stress. Biofeedback, which involves the use of a machine to monitor functions such as heart rate, muscle tension, or skin temperature, teaches individuals how to regulate physiologic activity. Hypnosis often involves physical relaxation coupled with imagery to facilitate the alteration of a subjective experience (e.g., pain). Therefore, these approaches have often been used to treat symptoms of illness and enhance health.

There is accumulating anecdotal and empirical evidence attesting to the physical and psychological health benefits of hypnosis, biofeedback, and meditation, especially for cancer patients. Cancer diagnosis and subsequent treatment are stressful events (Andersen, Kiecolt-Glaser, & Glaser, 1994) associated with disruptions in major life areas. For example, cancer patients report greater illness-related concerns and fears about death and dying, lowered motivation for interpersonal intimacy, and difficulty in returning to prediagnosis employment status (Cella & Tross, 1986). Many patients report increased fatigue and decreased physical stamina (Yellen, Cella, & Bonomi, 1993). Other disruptions range from sexual dysfunction or sterility (Andersen, 1986) to job discrimination (Winegard, Curbow, Baker, & Piantadosi, 1991).

In addition to the stress and anxiety that occurs with a diagnosis of cancer, patients often have to cope with treatment-related side effects as well. Common side effects associated with cancer chemotherapy include nausea, vomiting, fatigue, hair-loss, and dysphoria. After undergoing repeated chemotherapy treatments, some patients develop anticipatory or conditioned nausea, in which patients experience nausea in the context of specific cues that remind them of treatment (e.g., being in a particular hospital room). Although antiemetic medications have been fairly successful in treating nausea and vomiting that occur as a result of chemotherapy, they are not as effective for anticipatory nausea and vomiting. Antianxiety medicines such as benzodiazepines have been useful in this context and are fairly successful in countering anticipatory nausea.

For some individuals, nonpharmacologic methods for treating aversive side effects are needed or preferred. Various techniques have been used for this purpose, and each of these techniques has the potential to contribute to patients' psychological well-being and quality of life. The following sections review the efficacy of three mind/body modalities—hypnosis, meditation, and biofeedback—in reducing anxiety and distress, pain, and treatment side effects.

# Hypnosis

Hypnosis is a clinical technique used to bypass the conscious mind to achieve selective thought. Hypnosis has been defined as a "natural state of aroused, attentive focal

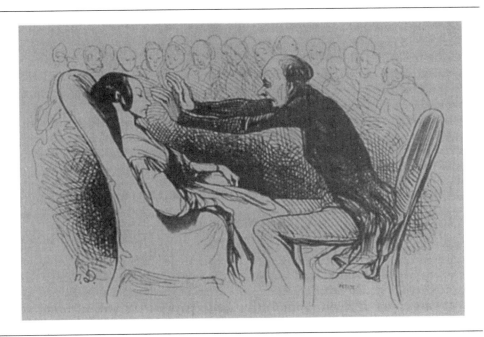

Mesmerism and hypnotism were the object of criticism during the nineteenth century.

concentration coupled with a relative suspension of peripheral awareness" (Spiegel & Moore, 1997) and as an "altered state of consciousness," which begins with relaxation and progresses to a cognitive state that involves changes in perceptions, cognition, and memory (Valente, 1991).

## Historical Perspective

Historic applications of hypnosis are attributed to Viennese doctor Franz Anton Mesmer (1734–1815), who believed that the imbalances of "animal magnetic" forces in the human body were responsible for causing illness. His therapy, called *mesmerism*, involved the use of tranquil gestures and soothing words to relax patients and restore balance in the patient's magnetic forces. Although some of his methods were later challenged, his practices laid the foundation for hypnosis by demonstrating that medical conditions could be affected by the power of suggestion.

Interest in mesmerism was revived by an English surgeon, James Esdaile, who performed hundreds of major operations in India on hypnotized patients. Another English doctor, James Braid, developed the eye-fixation technique and was credited with coining the term *hypnosis*, derived from the Greek *hypnos*, which means "sleep." Although Braid attempted to change the term when he realized that hypnotic trances weren't sleep, hypnosis remained the preferred name.

Twentieth-century research on hypnosis came to the forefront with Clark Hull's (1933) book on hypnosis and suggestibility. Although Hull eventually moved away from hypnosis research, his student, Milton Erickson, went on to develop a prolific program of research. Erickson proposed that hypnosis is an "altered state of mind" and that behavior is affected by the everyday trances that we all experience. Erickson was a proponent of a permissive and indirect approach to hypnosis that emphasized complex, individualized approaches (Erickson, 1980).

## Theoretical Perspectives

There are many theories as to what hypnosis is and how it works. During the 1960s and 1970s, hypnosis researchers and theorists could be categorized into two opposing camps: those who believed that hypnosis induces a unique state of consciousness that is fundamentally different from the waking state versus those who believed that the phenomenon of hypnosis is a product of social psychological factors, such as expectancies and attitudes (Kirsch & Lynn, 1995).

At one end of the continuum was the belief that a hypnotic state is fundamentally different from normal waking consciousness and from other states such as daydreaming and relaxation (Woody & Bowers, 1994). Based on evidence and theories reviewed by researchers at Macquerie University, hypnosis was regarded as a unique state of consciousness, affecting an individual both psychologically and physically. It was considered to be the same level of consciousness that produces fantasy and other primary thought processes, not simply the result of role play or compliance with instruction (McCabe, Collins, & Burns, 1979).

At the other end of the continuum were theorists who rejected the concept of an "altered state" and suggested that the effects of hypnosis stem from social influence and expectancies (Kirsch, 1991; Spanos, 1991). This perspective conceptualized the hypnotic state as continuous with other types of complex social behavior. Within this view, hypnotic response can be accounted for by social and cognitive constructs regularly employed to explain other forms of social behavior, including expectations, interpretations, and self-efficacy. Hypnotic subjects are seen as performing goal-directed actions based on their understanding of the demands of the situation. The hypnotic state is the result of active engagement of cognitive activities to reduce the negative aspects of a difficult situation. Within this perspective, individuals not easily hypnotized can be induced to reduce symptoms to the same extent as highly hypnotizable individuals (Spanos & Chaves, 1989).

A third perspective is that a hypnotic state is a naturally occurring phenomenon, similar to daydreaming or intense concentration (Spiegel & Spiegel, 1978). For example, daydreaming can be thought of as a form of hypnosis, perhaps light, sometimes deep. Almost anyone who has driven a car can recall situations that are conducive to hypnosis—out on the open road, relaxed at the wheel, eyes fixed on the white line of the road, the monotonous hum of the motor . . . and suddenly you realize you have passed through some town with no memory of having gone through it. Other situations involving intense concentration, such as reading a book or watching a movie, can also be viewed as engendering a state similar to that of a hypnotic trance. Therefore, it has been postulated that a hypnotic state is a common, normal phenomenon.

The American Psychological Association created a division (Division 30, Society of Psychological Hypnosis) devoted to the study of hypnosis. The Executive Committee of Division 30 presented a definition of hypnosis as a procedure in which "one person (the subject) is guided by another (the hypnotist) to respond to suggestions for changes in subjective experience, alterations in perception, sensation, emotion, thought or behavior"

(American Psychological Association, 2005). Two national societies, the Society for Clinical and Experimental Hypnosis and the American Society of Clinical Hypnosis, were formed to emphasize and promote research in this field. The American Medical Association recognized hypnosis as a legitimate therapeutic procedure in 1958.

## How Is It Done?

The method usually used to induce hypnosis involves induction of total body relaxation, followed by the presentation of relaxing and soothing imagery. Although hypnosis techniques are not standardized and induction techniques may differ from therapist to therapist, key components of hypnosis include muscle relaxation and guided imagery.

To induce a hypnotic state, the therapist leads the patient through relaxation exercises, mental imagery, and suggestions. Typically, a hypnotic induction contains suggestions for entering a hypnotic trance and for relaxation. Techniques for induction vary. Some inductions involve progressive neuromuscular relaxation, which is a method for contracting and relaxing muscles that calms the individual and induces relaxation. Progressive relaxation techniques can be preceded by visualization (imagining a calm and peaceful environment, such as being at the beach or in the woods). Other types of induction involve counting, such as counting backward from 10 to 1. Suggestions for hypnotic relaxation deepening are given in between the numbers. A confusion induction involves having the hypnotherapist count from 9 to 1 while the patient counts A, B, C (three numbers per each letter). The objective of this type of induction is to distract the conscious mind from thought.

Many inductions have a visual component. For example, one such induction involves having the patient imagine taking a shower with the perfect water temperature and pressure for relaxing. Patients are instructed to imagine the tension and stress being washed away. Or, patients may be asked to imagine moving an arrow vertically down a yardstick from 36 to 1. Each number deepens hypnosis. Similarly, hypnosis may be induced by telling patients to imagine walking down a flight of stairs to a safe and beautiful destination.

During a hypnotic trance, individuals may report feeling a comfortable heaviness or a sense of inertia. A sense of relaxation and peacefulness are also commonly reported. Physiologic changes associated with hypnosis may include a slowing of cardiac rhythm and respiration and changes in body temperature (depending on the suggestion presented). People in a hypnotic trance may appear to be asleep, but they are actually in an altered state of concentration and can focus intently when asked to do so by the hypnotherapist.

The depth of a hypnotic trance is usually categorized as a light state, a medium state, or a deep state. In a light state, the following phenomena may be observed: relaxation with a tendency not to move, an inability to open eyes when presented with suggestions to that effect, listlessness, a feeling of heaviness particularly in the arms and legs, and limb catalepsy (i.e., extreme rigidity or looseness of the muscles of the limbs, with a tendency for them to stay in any position in which they are placed).

Individuals who are in a medium depth trance may show complete body catalepsy, anesthesia of any part of the body (either partial or complete), partial amnesia on awakening if suggested, and even greater lassitude than in a light state. Individuals in a deep trance may experience age regression, complete anesthesia, complete amnesia, positive or negative hallucinations of all five senses, and time distortion.

Posthypnotic suggestions can be effective when presented at any depth, although the deeper the trance, the more likely that suggestions will be carried out. A posthypnotic suggestion is one that is given during hypnosis to be executed after awakening. For example, a hypnotherapist may suggest particular goals for a hypnotized individual, such as pain control, stress or anxiety reduction, or smoking cessation.

A person's ability to be hypnotized falls along a continuum from being easily hypnotized to experiencing much difficulty in entering a trance. About 5%–10% of the population are believed to be very susceptible to hypnosis, and 25%–30% are only minimally so. Individuals can also learn to hypnotize themselves (i.e., self-hypnosis). Prior to beginning hypnotherapy with a new patient, hypnotic susceptibility may be assessed using a scale, such as the *hypnotic induction profile* (Spiegel & Spiegel, 1978). Determining hypnotic susceptibility may be useful for several reasons. Classification of an individual's responsiveness to hypnosis can provide practical information regarding which hypnotic inductions and styles of suggestions are most suitable for use with that person. In addition, testing for hypnotic susceptibility can act as a preconditioning tool by helping the individual relax and preparing him or her for hypnosis.

## Myths and Misconceptions

There are some popular misconceptions of hypnosis. One misconception is that the hypnotized individual will carry out *any* suggestion presented to him or her. However, contrary to what many people believe, hypnotized individuals cannot be made to do something they do not want to do. An individual would not do anything under hypnosis that would be against his or her principles. Related to this is the belief that the patient will be under the "control" of the hypnotherapist. In fact, people under hypnosis are not under the control of the hypnotherapist, and people cannot be hypnotized involuntarily. A patient must be willing to accept a suggestion and will not accept any task or concept that is against his or her value system or moral judgment.

Another misconception is that a hypnotized person might reveal or disclose personal information that he or she did not want to disclose. However, under hypnosis, individuals normally discuss only those subjects they regard as safe and cannot be made to reveal anything they choose to remain confidential. Similarly, people hold the mistaken belief that a person is unable to lie or give misinformation under hypnosis. Yet, if a person wished to be untruthful while hypnotized, he or she could do so. In fact, people have been known to fabricate information during hypnosis because of their desire to please the hypnotherapist. This may be more likely to occur if the hypnotherapist queries the individual with "leading" questions (i.e., questions that are worded in such a manner as to lead to a particular response). Leading questions are therefore considered inappropriate.

Finally, the belief that an individual will not be able to come out of hypnosis is untrue. Each person is in control of his or her level of comfort during hypnosis and would either wake up or fall asleep if the hypnotherapist left the room during a session, depending on his or preferences. Individuals do not remain in a hypnotized state for an indefinite and prolonged period of time.

In summary, hypnosis involves bypassing the conscious mind, thereby suspending critical or judgmental thought, to achieve selective thinking. A hypnotherapist may act as a guide who helps an individual to relax and focus to achieve a hypnotic state. With the conscious mind distracted, appropriate suggestions are more readily accepted into the individual's subconscious mind, which stores information in a noncritical, nonjudgmental manner.

## Applications in the Cancer Context

The stress associated with cancer diagnosis and treatment may lead to considerable anxiety and depression for many cancer patients. In addition, patients may be experiencing pain and physical discomfort as a result of treatment-related side effects. Hypnosis has been proposed to be useful for helping patients to manage their illness-related stress or reduce aversive side effects. Since the early 1980s, a substantial amount of literature has accumulated documenting the efficacy of hypnosis in reducing anxiety, pain, and treatment side effects (e.g., nausea and emesis) in both adult and pediatric cancer populations. These studies are reviewed below.

### Anxiety and Distress

A variety of studies have examined the utility of hypnosis in reducing anxiety and distress among cancer patients (Burish, Carey, Redd, & Krozely, 1983; Genius, 1995; Jacobsen & Hann, 1998). The majority of these studies have incorporated hypnosis as one component within a larger combination of strategies (often including relaxation training and cognitive/attentional distraction). For example, Kaye and Schindler (1990) found that, when hospitalized cancer patients were provided with autohypnosis tapes as an adjuvant treatment method, 68% of patients reported a significant reduction in their feelings of depression and anxiety. Similarly, in a randomized controlled study, cancer patients who received hypnotherapy reported significant reductions in their level of anxiety and perceived stress compared to control subjects who received standard medical care only (Ali, 1990).

Hypnosis has also been used in the palliative cancer care setting to reduce distress and enhance coping skills. In one study, patients who had received hypnosis were asked to rate their coping with illness (Finlay & Jones, 1996). The majority of respondents reported that coping with their illness was easier following hypnosis. Several respondents noted that they were better able to cope with panic attacks and had a more positive attitude, less anxiety, and fewer negative thoughts (Finlay & Jones, 1996).

Given that children are more receptive to hypnosis and generally more hypnotizable than adults, hypnosis may be particularly useful for pediatric cancer patients. With children, hypnosis usually involves a combination of imagery and relaxation or imagery alone to distract children while they are undergoing medical procedures or receiving chemotherapeutic treatment. Results from studies of pediatric cancer patients indicate that hypnosis is effective in alleviating anxiety and distress associated with painful medical procedures, such as bone marrow aspiration (Hilgard & LeBaron, 1984; Kuttner, Bowman, & Teasdale, 1988). Further, the efficacy of hypnosis in reducing anxiety varied according to patients' levels of hypnotizability, with more hypnotizable patients reporting greater reductions in anxiety (Hilgard & LeBaron, 1984).

In summary, hypnosis has been found to be effective in reducing anxiety and distress in adult and pediatric cancer patient populations. Although some of these studies incorporated multiple behavioral methods (e.g., relaxation and distraction) within the intervention, hypnotic procedures were proposed to be the critical component of the intervention, especially for younger children (Kuttner et al., 1988).

## Pain

In cancer patients, acute pain responses are typically associated with cancer treatment, whereas chronic pain responses are associated with disease stage. Oncology treatments that evoke acute pain include invasive procedures, such as bone marrow aspirations (BMA) and lumbar punctures (LP). Although most patients understand that the discomfort caused by these treatments is temporary, high levels of anxiety can exacerbate the pain experienced by patients undergoing such treatments. Thus, hypnosis may be an effective adjunctive intervention for acute pain resulting from medical procedures.

Hypnosis-induced analgesia has been proposed to result from two processes: physical relaxation and attention control (Spiegel & Moore, 1997). Patients experiencing pain often tense up, and this results in greater sensations of pain. By increasing relaxation and replacing one's focus on pain with a competing sensation (such as the sensation of tingling in another part of the body), the perception of pain may be diminished.

A sizable literature documents the use of hypnosis for reducing acute pain associated with a wide variety of medical procedures, including surgery (Bowen, 1973; Evans & Richardson, 1988; Levitan & Harbaugh, 1989). Surprisingly, hypnosis has a long history of use in the management of patients undergoing surgery, dating back to the 19th-century work of Esdaile (1850), when hypnosis was used as a method of surgical anesthesia.

In the cancer context, studies have examined the utility of hypnosis in reducing treatment-related pain. In one well-controlled study (Syrjala, Cummings, & Donaldson, 1992), patients undergoing bone marrow transplant (BMT) were randomized to receive one of the following four treatment conditions: (1) hypnosis training, (2) cognitive behavioral coping skills training, (3) therapist contact only, or (4) usual care. Patients who received hypnosis training reported lower levels of post-BMT oral mucositis pain. However, nausea, emesis, and opioid use did not differ among the four treatment groups. Similarly, in a randomized prospective study (Spiegel & Bloom, 1983), metastatic breast cancer patients were assigned to one of three conditions: (1) a group therapy condition, (2) a group therapy plus hypnosis condition, or (3) a control group receiving standard care. Patients who received a combination of group therapy and hypnosis reported significantly lower levels of treatment-related pain than patients in the other conditions.

In pediatric cancer populations, the efficacy of hypnosis in alleviating pain associated with treatment procedures, such as BMA and lumbar puncture LP, has been demonstrated in numerous studies (e.g., Hilgard & LeBaron, 1984; Kellerman, Zeltzer, Ellenberg, & Dash, 1983; Kuttner et al., 1988). Moreover, the efficacy of hypnosis in relieving treatment-related pain appears to be related to hypnotizability (Hilgard & LeBaron, 1982). Among 24 children and adolescents with cancer, significantly lower levels of pain were reported by those patients who were high in hypnotizability compared to patients low in hypnotizability. In addition, the majority of highly hypnotizable patients were successful in reducing pain with hypnosis in the first session, demonstrating that for some individuals this type of intervention does not require extensive training to be effective.

The efficacy of hypnotic techniques in reducing anxiety and pain during procedures has also been compared to other, nonhypnotic behavioral techniques (e.g., deep breathing and distraction exercises). The data indicate that greater decreases in pain and anxiety associated with BMAs and LPs were observed with hypnosis compared to nonhypnotic techniques (Zeltzer & LeBaron, 1982). Similarly, a randomized trial compared hypnosis with cognitive-behavioral techniques in reducing pain and anxiety among pediatric patients undergoing BMA (Liossi & Hatira, 1999). Although both hypnosis and cognitive-behavioral training were effective in reducing pain, only hypnosis led to reductions in treatment-related anxiety.

In contrast, a few studies have reported that hypnosis did lead to lower levels of self-reported pain in comparison to other techniques. Wall and Womack (1989) compared the effects of hypnosis to active cognitive distraction in reducing anxiety and pain during BMA or LP among 20 pediatric oncology outpatients. In the active cognitive condition, patients were trained to use their own chosen distraction strategy during medical procedures. Both intervention conditions involved group practice sessions. The findings indicated that both treatment conditions resulted in significant decreases in self-reported and observed pain (Wall & Womack, 1989). Similarly, in a study of 36 children with acute lymphoblastic leukemia, patients were randomly assigned to either a hypnosis intervention or nondirected play (to control for time and attention). Children were followed for 6 months following the intervention. Children who responded to hypnosis reported less pain and anxiety during BMA (Katz, Kellerman, & Ellenberg, 1987) than children who were not easily hypnotizable. However, hypnosis did not reduce levels of anxiety and pain significantly more than the play comparison group (Katz et al., 1987).

As these studies demonstrate, level of hypnotizability may be an important factor in determining patient response. In a prospective controlled trial of 80 pediatric cancer patients undergoing LPs, patients were randomly assigned to one of four conditions: (1) direct hypnosis, (2) indirect hypnosis, (3) an attention control, or (4) standard care. Patients in both hypnosis conditions had lower levels of self-reported pain and observer-rated behavioral distress than patients in the two control conditions (Liossi & Hatira, 2003). As before, level of hypnotizability was significantly associated with patient outcomes. However, the observed benefits of hypnosis were diminished when patients were switched to self-hypnosis, thereby suggesting that other factors, such as therapist presence (or the presence of other supportive individuals) may be a critical component for achieving positive effects.

Although the bulk of the literature on hypnosis and treatment-related pain in pediatric patients has revolved around BMA and LP procedures, several case studies have reported the successful use of hypnosis in place of general anesthesia for pediatric patients undergoing radiotherapy (Bertoni et al., 1999). Because of the potential adverse effects associated with sedatives and analgesics, hypnosis has been proposed as a safe and effective alternative to general anesthesia for pediatric patients undergoing radiotherapy.

Given the abundance of evidence, a panel of experts concluded that the "evidence supporting the effectiveness of hypnosis in alleviating pain associated with cancer seems strong" (National Institutes of Health, 1996). In sum, it may be beneficial to consider using hypnosis in complement with standard pharmacologic approaches for reducing treatment-related pain (Richardson, Smith, McCall, & Pilkington, 2006). However, it is important to understand the parameters that lead to maximizing patient outcomes, as these factors (e.g., level of hypnotizability) can otherwise limit the practical use and benefits of hypnosis in this context.

## Nausea and Vomiting

Despite improvements in the efficacy of antiemetic medication, nausea and vomiting resulting from chemotherapy are common side effects reported by cancer patients. In addition to these aftereffects of treatment, patients may develop *anticipatory* nausea and vomiting; that is, some patients begin feeling nauseated when exposed to certain cues or stimuli (e.g., entering the infusion room or the sound of the nurse's voice) that have been previously associated with treatment side effects. There are considerable clinical data indicating that anticipatory nausea and vomiting results from "classical conditioning" and is a conditioned response to chemotherapy. Because anxiolytic drugs may at times be inadequate for treating anticipatory nausea, nonpharmacologic methods for reducing nausea have been sought.

Several studies have demonstrated the effectiveness of hypnosis in controlling anticipatory vomiting in adult chemotherapy patients. Most of these studies included hypnosis within a behavioral intervention that included other components as well, including relaxation and cognitive or attentional distraction. When hypnosis was used during chemotherapy treatments, anticipatory vomiting was eliminated completely. In contrast, anticipatory vomiting occurred among patients who received chemotherapy treatments without intervention (Redd, Andresen, & Minagawa, 1982; Redd et al., 1987).

In other clinical trials with adult patients who suffered severe side effects from chemotherapy, hypnosis resulted in improvements not only in conditioned nausea and vomiting but also for nausea and vomiting in the days following chemotherapy (Walker, Dawson, Pollet, & Ratcliffe, 1988). Other studies have also found that interventions incorporating progressive muscle relaxation and guided imagery tend to result in significantly less nausea during treatment and following treatment (Mastenbroek & McGovern, 1991).

Hypnosis is also effective in reducing chemotherapy-related nausea and vomiting among pediatric cancer patients (Zeltzer, Kellerman, Ellenberg, & Dash, 1983). In comparison to two other conditions (i.e. a cognitive distraction and relaxation condition and an attention–only control group), the hypnosis intervention resulted in significantly shorter duration of nausea and vomiting (Zeltzer, Dolgin, LeBaron, & LeBaron, 1991). Over time, somatic symptoms and side effects appeared to improve among children in the hypnosis group, whereas side effects either improved slightly or did not change for children in the distraction/relaxation group and worsened among children in the control group (Zeltzer et al., 1991). Thus, these studies consistently demonstrate the benefits of hypnosis in reducing chemotherapy-related nausea and vomiting for both adult and pediatric cancer patients.

## Cancer Progression and Management

Accumulating data from studies of cancer patients provide support for the role of psychological, behavioral, and biological influences on cancer progression (Goodkin, Antoni, Sevin, & Fox, 1993; Levy, Herberman, Lippman, D'Angelo, & Lee, 1991; Spiegel, Bloom, Kraemer, & Gottheil, 1989). It has been suggested that the effects of psychological factors on cancer growth and progression may be mediated by the immune system (Garssen & Goodkin, 1999). Data from both animal and human models suggest that natural killer (NK) cells play an important role in the elimination of metastatic tumor cells (Brittenden, Heys, Ross, & Eremin, 1996). Although natural killer cells may be limited in their ability to reduce solid tumor growth, it has been proposed that they are responsible for eliminating small tumor cell masses and monitoring metastatic cells (Garssen & Goodkin, 1999).

Several studies have shown that immune function can be altered through hypnotic techniques. In early studies, this phenomenon was demonstrated using the "double arm" approach (Black, 1963; Black & Friedman, 1965). Specifically, individuals were injected with an antigen (e.g., histamine) in both arms. Suggestions would then be given for one arm (e.g., left arm) that would be consistent with the inhibition of an allergic response but not for the other arm (i.e., right arm). As a result, the right arm was more likely to exhibit changes characteristic of hypersensitivity (e.g., itching and swelling), whereas the left arm did not.

Several studies have reported immune-enhancing effects of hypnosis in healthy populations, notably medical students (Kiecolt-Glaser et al., 1986; Whitehouse et al., 1996). However, to date, this relationship has not been comprehensively evaluated in cancer patients. One study of early stage breast cancer patients did find significant increases in absolute number of NK cells following an 8-week hypnotic-guided imagery intervention, but these changes were not maintained at 3-month follow-up (Bakke, Purtzer, & Newton, 2002).

Taken together, hypnosis can be an effective mind/body modality for reducing emotional distress and various treatment-related symptoms, such as pain, nausea, and emesis (Genuis, 1995; Meyer & Mark, 1995; Steggles, Damore-Petingola, Maxwell, & Lightfoot, 1997; Steggles, Maxwell, Lightfoot, Damore-Petingola, & Mayer, 1997; Trijsburg, van Knippenberg, & Rijpma, 1992). Although in certain instances there has been variability in findings, this can be attributed to several factors. One factor involves the hypnotizability of patients. In many studies, this variable was not assessed. Yet, it appears that level of hypnotizability may be an important predictor of whether hypnosis will be successful in bringing about the desired outcome. A second potential factor that may be contributing to discrepant findings is the delivery of the hypnotic intervention. In some studies, hypnosis was taught in group sessions, whereas in other studies, hypnosis was administered in an individualized format. A third factor involves key demographic differences between samples (e.g., patient age and gender) and lack of patient experience in using the intervention during medical treatment that may have also influenced outcomes (Wall & Womack, 1989).

## Potential Mechanisms of Hypnosis

The mechanism by which hypnosis affects cancer treatment side effects has yet to be completely understood. However, a number of studies and several theoretical models in clinical, health, and social psychology suggest that an individual's perception of control may be an important psychological process variable that mediates the therapeutic effects of hypnosis on psychological and physical health outcomes. Several lines of research support this notion.

First, several well-supported theories in the area of stress and coping argue that perceived control is a central determinant of emotional responses to health-relevant threats, such as cancer risk, diagnosis, and treatment (Rotter, 1966; Seligman, 1975; Taylor, 1983). A number of studies have consistently demonstrated that when individuals believe that they can alter, terminate, or influence stressful life events, their perceptions of the event are characterized as being less stressful and more positive (Suls & Mullen, 1981; Thompson, 1981).

Second, a number of studies have directly linked perceptions of control with lower psychological distress (e.g., anxiety and depression) among populations of cancer patients. A greater level of perceived control has been associated with healthier affective responses

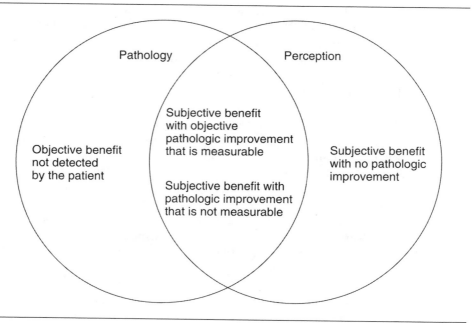

**Overlap of objective and subjective therapeutic benefits.**

among newly diagnosed breast cancer patients (Lowery, Jacobsen, & DuCette, 1993; Penman et al., 1987; Taylor, Lichtman, & Wood, 1984) and among heterogeneous samples of cancer patients (Ell, Mantell, Hamovitch, & Nishimoto, 1989; Newsom, Knapp, & Schulz, 1996; Taylor, Helgeson, Reed, & Skokan, 1991; Thompson, Sobolew-Shubin, Galbraith, Schwankovsky, & Cruzen, 1993). In particular, among newly diagnosed cancer patients, individuals who reported greater levels of perceived control also reported lower levels of depression associated with their diagnosis and its treatment (Marks, Richardson, Graham, & Levine 1986).

Third, research suggests that perceptions of control affect treatment-induced side effects, including pain. Studies have shown that chronic pain patients who view themselves as having more control over their pain reported lower levels of pain (Toomey, Mann, Abashian, & Thompson-Pope, 1991). In addition, perceptions of control also influenced pain relief. Among cancer patients undergoing BMT, those who had the ability to exert control over the administration of their pain medication needed approximately one-third of the amount of morphine requested by patients who received their medication by means of nurse-administered injection to achieve comparable levels of pain relief (Hill, Saeger, & Chapman, 1986).

# Meditation

Meditation has existed in many cultures around the world. In the late 1960s, Dr. Herbert Benson initiated a study of the physiologic effects associated with meditation. He reported that through meditation, individuals can enter into a state that is characterized by lowered heart rate, decreased rate of breathing, lowered blood pressure, slower brain waves, and an overall reduction in metabolism (Benson, Greenwood, & Klemchuk, 1975; Benson, Rosner, Marzetta, & Klemchuk, 1974). These changes counteract the physiological responses induced by stress and have been labeled as the *relaxation response* (Benson, Beary, & Carol, 1974).

There are two primary approaches to meditation: concentrative meditation and mindful meditation. Concentrative meditation involves focusing on an image, a sound (called a mantra), or one's own breathing. One form of concentrative meditation is transcendental meditation (TM), which was popularized in the United States in the 1970s by Maharishi Mahesh Yogi. Transcendental Meditation emphasizes the mind/body connection to create a state of deep rest, which along with heightened awareness, is experienced as "restful alertness." With attention centered on a single image or a mantra, usually one word or a short phrase, individuals can reach profound states of calmness and steadiness of attention.

The TM technique is a simple procedure practiced while sitting comfortably with the eyes closed. As the body becomes deeply relaxed, the mind transcends all mental activity to experience the simplest form of awareness, Transcendental Consciousness. The experience of Transcendental Consciousness develops the individual's latent creative potential while dissolving accumulated stress and fatigue through the deep rest gained during meditative practice. This experience enlivens the individual's creativity, dynamism, and organization, which is proposed to lead to greater effectiveness and success in daily life.

The second approach to meditation, mindfulness meditation, employs a different technique. Instead of focusing on a single sensation or sound, the objective of mindfulness meditation is to develop a heightened awareness of the present moment. Attention to one's breathing is used to focus attention and enhance concentration. From this foundation, the meditator cultivates the ability to note thoughts, feelings, and sensations as they occur and to observe them nonjudgmentally as they unfold in the field of awareness. As this practice matures, one is able to explore whatever emerges in the consciousness as it occurs moment by moment. As mindfulness of what is occurring in the present further unfolds, one is able to identify reflexive and habitual thoughts and perceptions. The goal is a calmer, clearer, nonreactive state of mind. This approach leads to reduction of stress and anxiety as one becomes able to identify the automatic reactions to external and internal events. The goal of mindfulness meditation is being in touch with, and aware of, exactly what is happening at the time it is happening (Kabat-Zinn, 1994).

## How Is It Done?

Meditation is usually performed while sitting, but moving forms of meditation include tai chi, Zen Buddhist walking, and the Japanese martial art aikido. Meditation can be self-directed or guided by doctors, psychiatrists, other mental health professionals, or yoga masters. Self-directed meditation is done by selecting a quiet place free from noise and distraction, sitting or resting quietly with eyes closed, and trying to achieve a feeling of peace. Certain meditative instructions can be used to elicit this type of response. One simple technique involves a four-step process that includes the following: (1) finding a quiet environment, (2) consciously relaxing the body's muscles, (3) focusing for 10 to 20 minutes on one's breathing, and (4) assuming a nonjudgmental perspective toward intrusive thoughts.

## Applications in the Cancer Context

For cancer patients, meditation can be helpful in facing and reducing the anxiety and stress that accompany cancer diagnosis and treatment. Indeed, there have been several studies demonstrating the benefits of mindfulness meditation. For example, among breast and prostate cancer patients who participated in a group-based mindfulness-based stress reduction (MBSR) program, significant improvements were reported in overall quality of life, symptoms of stress, and sleep quality from preintervention to postintervention (Carlson, Speca, Patel, & Goodey, 2004; Carlson & Garland, 2005). Similarly, among a mixed sample of cancer patients who were randomly assigned to either a MBSR intervention or a wait-list control condition, patients receiving MBSR reported significantly lower total mood disturbance, as well as lower levels of depression, anxiety, anger, and confusion, compared to control subjects (Speca, Carlson, Goodey, & Angen, 2000). In addition, there was a linear relationship between meditation and outcomes: those who attended more sessions and meditated more had better adjustment compared to those who participated less. Importantly, these improvements in psychological well-being were maintained 6 months following the intervention (Carlson, Ursuliak, Goodey, Angen, & Speca, 2001).

There is a growing body of research that suggests that meditation has beneficial effects on physical health outcomes as well. Initial interest in the health effects of meditation for cancer patients became widespread in the 1970s and 1980s when an Australian psychiatrist, Ainslie Meares, reported that intensive meditation was associated with cancer regression and reductions in tumor size (Meares, 1983). Since then, meditation has been reported to be associated with lower blood pressure among hypertensive adults (Benson, Rosner, et al., 1974), lower cholesterol among adults at high risk for cardiovascular disease (Patel et al., 1985), lower levels of cortisol (Sudsuang, Chentanez & Veluvan, 1991), and higher levels of melatonin (Massion, Teas, Hebert, Wertheimer & Kabat-Zinn, 1995). In addition, participation in a MBSR intervention was associated with an increased rate of resolution of lesions in patients with psoriasis, which is an immune-mediated disorder (Kabat-Zinn et al., 1998).

However, few published studies have examined effects of MBSR on physical outcomes in cancer patients. One study of breast and prostate cancer patients reported that MBSR participation was associated with changes in lymphocyte numbers and cytokine production (Carlson, Speca, Patel, & Goodey, 2003). Specifically, decreases in T-cell production of IFN-$\gamma$ were observed from pre- to postintervention, whereas IL-4 production increased. NK cell production of IL-10 decreased over the course of the intervention. The overall pattern of immune changes observed were consistent with a shift away from a proinflammatory (or Th1) response to an anti-inflammatory- (Th2) type response, which the authors postulated to be more beneficial in terms of cancer-fighting activities. The changes in immune profiles observed in these cancer patients are proposed to be a result of MBSR-related modulation of cortisol secretion patterns, which may represent a "normalization" of HPA axis functioning (Carlson et al., 2004).

Finally, one preliminary study found that the practice of self-regulation was associated with longer survival in patients with metastatic cancer (Cunningham, Phillips, Lockwood, Hedley, & Edmonds, 2000). Specifically, in a prospective, longitudinal study, 22 patients received a year of professionally led weekly group support and therapy sessions, which included a component on meditation. Through qualitative analysis, patients received a rating of their involvement in self-regulation. Strong personal involvement in self-regulation strategies (including meditation) was associated with longer survival duration (Cunningham et al., 2000).

Thus, meditation can be an effective mind/body modality for improving emotional health and well-being and eliciting positive physiologic changes. However, the underlying mechanisms associated with the reported changes in physical and mental health in response to mindfulness training are not well understood.

## Potential Mechanisms of Meditation

It has been proposed that meditation may operate to influence psychological and physical health outcomes via several pathways, including self-regulation, acceptance, and positive expectancies (Shapiro, Carlson, Astin, & Freedman, 2005). Mindfulness meditation training teaches individuals to be better able to attend to the information contained in each moment, without judgment. By developing this ability to recognize, and then eliminate, automatic and reflexive thoughts and behaviors, individuals learn key self-regulatory strategies that enable them to use adaptive coping skills in one's daily life.

Mindfulness meditation may also function as an exposure procedure in which sustained observation of aversive thoughts and feelings leads to reduced emotional reactivity to these stimuli (Baer, 2003). Through this direct exposure and acceptance, one learns that his or her emotions, thoughts, or bodily sensations are not so frightening and that thoughts are "just thoughts" and do not necessitate specific behaviors. Over time, this training would eventually lead to the extinction of fear responses and negative emotional reactivity.

Finally, it has been observed that patients' pretreatment beliefs in the efficacy of a treatment are often one of the strongest predictors of treatment outcome (Kirsch, 1985). Treatment expectancies can be considered as varying on a continuous scale from very negative ("This is never going to work") to very positive ("This is exactly what I need"). Thus, patients' expectancies regarding the efficacy of meditation may be one potential mechanism underlying its observed effects.

# Biofeedback

Biofeedback is a tool for helping patients learn how to control various physiologic processes that were previously believed to be beyond voluntary control (such as blood pressure and heart rate) with the help of electronic monitors that provide immediate feedback about physiologic changes that are occurring. Although the concept of being able to voluntarily control bodily processes has been accepted in many cultures for thousands of years, the origins of biofeedback date back only to the 1950s. Until then, existing equipment was not sensitive enough to measure the body's faint electrical impulses very accurately. As a result of World War II, however, electrical instrumentation became increasingly more sophisticated. In the early 1960s, Neil Miller, an experimental psychologist, demonstrated that patients could learn how to control various physiological processes (Miller, 1974). Biofeedback was promoted in the late 1960s and early 1970s as a method of alleviating migraine headaches when researchers discovered that elevating the temperature of the hands resulted in symptom improvement (Miller & Dworkin, 1977; Shapiro & Schwartz, 1972).

Since then, biofeedback has been used to treat numerous medical conditions. Biofeedback has been effective in reducing chronic pain as well as the pain associated with migraine headaches (Kaushik, Kaushik, Mahajan, & Rajesh, 2005). It has also been used for retraining, reconditioning, and strengthening muscles after an accident or surgery and overcoming urinary or fecal incontinence (Burgio et al., 2006). Individuals with Raynaud's disease (which involves a periodic loss of circulation in the fingers) have been able to rectify the problem through biofeedback (Kranitz & Lehrer, 2004). Biofeedback is under study as a potential aid in the treatment of a number of other ailments as well, although results have been more mixed.

## How Is It Done?

Since the early 1970s, biofeedback researchers have developed a set of tools to measure stress in different parts of the body. One of the primary tools for traditional biofeedback involves the electromyograph (EMG), which provides a graphical recording of muscle activity using surface electrodes. The underlying rationale for this is that people tense certain muscles when they experience stress. Because tense muscles have a higher electrical reading than relaxed ones, small sensing electrodes that are attached to these muscles are able to detect any changes that occur. The frontalis, or the forehead muscle, for example, is a primary target for EMG, because when people concentrate very hard or experience stress, this is one of the muscles that becomes tense.

Biofeedback training involves using this instrumentation to quantify and present information regarding subtle physiologic changes back to an individual. In a typical biofeedback session, electrodes are attached to a specific part of the body (such as the hands, fingers, or head). The monitoring device produces a variable-pitch tone or visual display to reflect activity detected by the electrodes. During training sessions, patients work with a therapist who guides the patient through physical and mental exercises designed to produce physiologic changes. These changes are detected by the electrodes, and the monitoring device then indicates that the desired physiologic change has occurred. Through the provision of immediate feedback, patients learn to connect changes in thought, breathing, and muscle tension with the desired alterations in physiologic function.

Thermal feedback (assessing skin temperature), often measured using the hand or finger, is another biofeedback tool. Skin temperature gauges show changes in the amount of heat given off by the skin, which is a measure of changes in blood flow. Below-normal temperatures usually occur in people with anxiety, migraines, and stomach disorders. This feedback is useful in the treatment of Raynaud's disease, high blood pressure, anxiety, and migraines. Another common type of feedback is galvanic skin response (GSR). Stress causes increased perspiration, which has a high salt concentration and therefore conducts electrical signals better. GSR, which is also called electrodermal feedback, is often used as a biofeedback tool for the reduction of anxiety.

Electroencephalographs (EEGs) measure brain-wave activity. Recent work has examined the utility of brain-wave biofeedback, using EEG, in the treatment of various neurocognitive conditions, including depression, attention deficit/hyperactivity disorder (ADHD), epilepsy, and problems resulting from mild, closed head injuries (Robbins, 2000). Electrocardiographs monitor the heart rate and may be useful in relieving an overly rapid heartbeat and controlling high blood pressure. Finally, respiration feedback devices concentrate on the rate, rhythm, and type of breathing to help lessen symptoms of asthma, anxiety, and hyperventilation and promote relaxation.

Along with training in the use of these specific biofeedback tools, the therapist may also provide instruction in deep breathing, meditation, visualization, and muscle relaxation exercises—each of which is helpful in relieving stress-related symptoms. In most cases, people can learn to raise or lower their heart rate, relax specific muscles, lower blood pressure, and control other functions within 8 to 10 training sessions. Some problems, such as ADHD, require more sessions.

## Applications in the Cancer Context

Biofeedback has the potential to help remedy certain ailments by teaching individuals how to control specific, measurable physiological reactions that can be contributing to health problems. In the cancer context, biofeedback has been used to reduce the side effects of cancer treatment (i.e., chemotherapy), improve treatment outcomes, and reduce psychological stress. For example, biofeedback is often used to relieve pain (either disease-related or treatment-related pain) through alterations in pain behaviors, such as muscle tension.

### Nausea and Vomiting

Biofeedback has been used to help patients learn to control anticipatory nausea and vomiting associated with chemotherapy (Burish, Shartner, & Lyles, 1981). Skin temperature biofeedback was used to monitor changes in skin temperature to note the fall in skin temperature that precedes nausea and emesis (Morrow, 1992). Using a single case design, a female cancer patient received biofeedback in combination with progressive muscle relaxation and guided imagery during four chemotherapy treatment sessions. In addition, the patient was instructed to practice these techniques at home. After biofeedback training was terminated, the patient was instructed to continue to use these techniques during the next three chemotherapy sessions. The patient reported reductions in nausea during the intervention as well as following termination of biofeedback training (Burish et al., 1981). Several studies have also reported that reductions in nausea during therapist-directed sessions are maintained in patient-directed sessions (Burish & Lyles, 1981).

Another study reported that biofeedback was effective in reducing nausea among cancer patients receiving chemotherapy when this tool was used in conjunction with relaxation training (Burish & Jenkins, 1992). However, although EMG and skin-temperature biofeedback training by itself was most effective in reducing indices of physiological arousal, it was found to be less effective than progressive muscle relaxation training for reducing nausea. These findings suggest that some of the positive effects observed with biofeedback interventions may be attributed to the fact that biofeedback usually includes some component of relaxation training (Burish & Jenkins, 1992).

### Physical Functioning

Biofeedback has been a useful tool for helping cancer patients to regain physical functioning following treatment. Videoendoscopic biofeedback has been used with cancer patients after head and neck surgery to support conventional swallowing therapy (Denk

& Kaider, 1997). Surgical resection of head and neck tumors often cause alterations in anatomy and physiology that result in eating and swallowing difficulties. In a study of 33 cancer patients that compared conventional therapy to conventional therapy combined with videoendoscopic biofeedback training, biofeedback training increased the likelihood of successful rehabilitation of swallowing function during the early stage of therapy (Denk & Kaider, 1997).

Empirical data also attest to the effectiveness of biofeedback in restoring urinary control among cancer patients following surgical treatment (i.e., prostatectomy) for prostate cancer (Burgio et al., 2006; Matthewson-Chapman, 1997; van Kampen, de Weerdt, de Ridder, Feys, & Baert, 2000). Research suggests that pelvic muscle exercise can be easily taught using biofeedback to improve learning and reduce urinary incontinence. In one study, prostate cancer patients were randomly assigned to an education/biofeedback intervention or a control group following prostatectomy for localized prostate cancer (Matthewson-Chapman, 1997). Patients in the intervention group received pelvic muscle education and biofeedback. Biofeedback was provided through two separate channels. One channel measured EMG muscle activity using a rectal pressure probe. The other channel measured abdominal muscle activity with EMG abdominal surface electrodes. Patients in the control group received no training in pelvic muscle exercise or biofeedback. The results indicated that the intervention reduced the frequency and duration of incontinence compared to the control group, although this difference was not statistically significant (Matthewson-Chapman, 1997).

In a similar study, 102 patients were randomly assigned into a treatment or control group (van Kampen et al., 2000). Treatment consisted of education regarding the anatomy and function of the pelvic floor and bladder, pelvic floor muscle exercises, and biofeedback. Patients in the control group also received pelvic-floor education but placebo electrotherapy (in place of biofeedback). The placebo electrotherapy was administered via four skin electrodes (two placed on the abdomen and two placed on thighs). After 3 months, a significantly greater proportion of patients in the treatment group were continent and the duration of incontinence was significantly shorter compared to the control group (van Kampen et al., 2000). Thus, in both studies, biofeedback was successful in improving urinary continence after surgery.

One study evaluated the efficacy of biofeedback provided preoperatively (rather than postoperatively) in reducing postsurgical incontinence (Burgio et al., 2006). Prostate cancer patients were randomized to receive either one preoperative session of biofeedback assisted training or standard care. Preoperative training resulted in significantly shorter duration of incontinence as well as fewer self-reported problems with leakage (e.g., urine loss during coughing).

## Neuroendocrine and Immune Effects

Because biofeedback is effective in reducing physiological arousal, it is plausible that reductions in the physiologic stress response would be accompanied by corresponding changes in neuroendocrine and immune variables. Only a few studies have attempted to examine these postulated effects in cancer patients. In one study of early stage breast cancer patients, EMG biofeedback training was as effective as cognitive therapy in reducing anxiety (Davis, 1986). Moreover, patients who received biofeedback training displayed stable levels of urinary cortisol, a stress hormone, over a follow-up period of 8 months compared to control group patients who exhibited significant elevations in cortisol at the follow-up assessment (Davis, 1986). These findings suggest that biofeedback therapy can contribute to the stabilization or normalization of the pituitary-adrenal-cortical system, which would also have implications for immune functioning.

Effects of biofeedback on immune measures were examined among 10 men and women with metastatic cancer (Gruber, Hall, Hersh, & Dubois, 1988). All 10 patients received extensive relaxation training prior to beginning six sessions of EMG biofeedback training. Because of the fact that most of the patients were quite skilled at relaxation, little change in muscle tension was observed between baseline and posttraining assessments. However, individuals who showed the largest decreases in EMG levels (indicating lower levels of muscle tension) also experienced the largest changes in immune measures following training. Specifically, greater NK cell cytotoxicity and increased lymphocyte responsiveness to mitogens were observed following training (Gruber et al., 1993).

Thus, these studies demonstrate that biofeedback is helpful for relieving treatment-related side effects and improving functional outcomes following cancer treatment. In general, biofeedback is easy to learn and individuals tend to respond favorably to biofeedback training, making it a useful adjunct to other interventions in the cancer context.

## Mechanisms Underlying Mind/Body Modalities

The mechanisms by which mind/body therapies have their effects on emotional and physical health have yet to be completely understood. However, the approaches described above have the following in common: (1) they are systematic methods involving practice and discipline, (2) they have physiological attributes associated with decreased stress and arousal, and (3) they provide greater perceived control. These mechanisms may contribute to better health through the following pathways.

### Relaxation

The mind/body techniques described above all incorporate some form of relaxation. For example, progressive muscle relaxation involves relaxation of muscles over which one has conscious control. Deep muscle relaxation may directly act to decrease autonomic arousal. Relaxation techniques result in decreased oxygen consumption, heart and respiratory rates, blood pressure, and muscle tension. These physiologic changes are believed to offset the negative physiologic effects caused by stress.

### Cognitive/Attentional Distraction

Cognitive/attentional distraction procedures are designed to draw the individual's attention away from the stressful procedure or situation, which leads to a reduction in distress. By refocusing the patient's attention elsewhere (i.e., distraction), the patient's perception of pain may be lessened because she or he is not attending to it. These techniques are often successfully used with children. One method of cognitive or attentional distraction involves storytelling or fantasy in which the patient is completely "cognitively engaged" and not focused on the painful procedure that might be taking place. Being highly absorbed in a story or fantasy distracts the patient's attention from the stressful medical procedure and reduces distress behaviors (DuHamel, Redd, & Vickberg, 1999).

**Perceived Control.** A sizable number of studies and several theoretical models in psychology suggest that the individual's perceptions of control may be an important psychological variable that mediates the effects of mind/body therapies on various health outcomes. Perceived control appears to be a central determinant of emotional responses to health-relevant threats, such as cancer risk, diagnosis, and treatment (i.e., Miller, Combs, & Stoddard, 1989; Taylor; 1983). Spiegel and Moore (1997) argued that loss of control is a central consequence of encounters with cancer threats and that this loss adversely affects psychological well-being. The complementary use of therapies such as hypnosis, biofeedback, or meditation may then be a valuable approach for assisting patients to regain perceptions of control. Indeed, a number of studies have directly linked perceptions of control with lower psychological distress (e.g., anxiety and depression) among cancer patients (Peter, 1996) and among patients facing a variety of stressful medical procedures (Miller et al., 1989). Greater perceptions of self-efficacy and control that result from use of mind/body therapeutic techniques are also believed to contribute to pain reduction (VanDalfsen & Syrjala, 1990).

Perceptions of control have also been shown to influence physiological responses to stressful life events. In particular, lower catecholamine levels and circulating endogenous

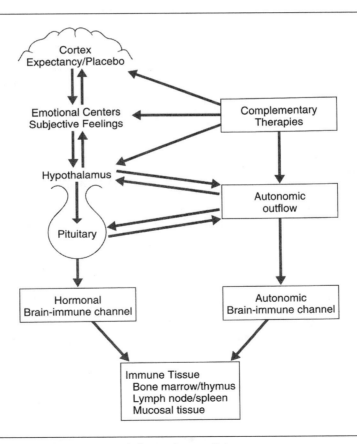

Brain-immune pathways of complementary and alternative medicine.

opioids have been shown to be associated with greater perceptions of control when individuals face stressful events (Miller & O'Leary, 1993). Further, there is evidence to suggest that perceptions of control have corresponding neuroendocrine and immune effects.

**Neuroimmune Correlates.** Although the relationship between immune functioning and cancer development or progression is widely debated, there are numerous immune mechanisms that may be responsible for combating tumor growth and metastasis. For example, T cells play an important role in rejection of solid tumors. Further, NK cells have the ability to kill tumor cells of many different types. When immune activity is suppressed, research with animal and human models suggests that this immunosuppression may affect cancer progression (Whiteside & Herberman, 1995).

In studies of cancer patients, psychological distress has been found to be associated with alterations in immune functioning. For example, among newly diagnosed, untreated cervical and endometrial cancer patients, higher levels of anxiety and depression significantly predicted decreased white blood cell counts after controlling for disease-relevant moderating factors (e.g., disease stage; Andersen & Turnquist, 1985). Likewise, among women with cervical and endometrial cancer who had not yet received treatment, measures of self-reported and interviewer-rated distress predicted a significant proportion of the variance in NK cell activity, controlling for relevant background and disease factors (Andersen et al., 1994). In a study of women with operable breast cancer (Tjemsland, Soreide, Matre, & Malt, 1997), preoperative levels of depression were associated with decreases in the numbers of circulating lymphocytes and NK cells (Tjemsland et al., 1997). Altogether, these findings suggest that psychological distress is associated with a variety of immunologic changes in cancer patients. Thus, given that mind/body approaches are effective in reducing anxiety and distress, they may also have indirect benefits for immune functioning and health outcomes.

# Conclusion

The above evidence suggests that mind/body modalities can confer considerable benefits for cancer patients. However, much of the existing evidence is preliminary or based on small samples or case studies. It has been a challenge to substantiate these claims because of the methodologic difficulties in conducting clinical trials of these strategies. Many of the variables of interest are difficult to define, quantify, or observe (Levin et al., 1997).

One challenge for conducting studies of mind/body approaches involves the fact that many therapeutic approaches use multiple strategies, which can vary considerably in substantive content and/or in application to particular individuals. For example, in hypnosis, different types of inductions (some involving progressive muscle relaxation and others involving focusing one's attention on an image) can be used to induce a hypnotic state, the depth of which may differ from individual to individual. Further, hypnotic suggestions are often individualized and tailored to be most appropriate for each individual. Therefore, a standardized approach and delivery is relatively uncommon.

It is also important to note that the delivery of a single mind/body intervention, whether based on meditation, biofeedback, or hypnosis, may elicit different responses when administered to different people. Depending on the outcome or goal that one is trying to achieve, individuals may find certain therapeutic approaches more beneficial and useful than others. Finally, these therapies are often delivered across an extended period of time, and the interval between initiation of treatment and observation of any effects may vary considerably among individuals.

It has been recognized that human health cannot be understood only in terms of isolated organs and systems as defined by conventional medicine. Thus, mind/body techniques, including hypnosis, meditation, and biofeedback, can provide benefits for cancer patients on several levels. They are useful methods for reducing anxiety and emotional distress, for ameliorating treatment-related side effects and pain, and for restoring physical functioning following treatment. Moreover, it is becoming clear that mind/body therapies can also improve quality of life by providing a strategy or tool for enhancing an individual's sense of personal control at a time when one is often experiencing a loss of control. Given that mind/body approaches have considerable potential to enhance psychologic and emotional well-being and to reduce suffering associated with cancer and its treatment, these approaches provide valuable tools for supporting the health of cancer patients.

## REFERENCES

Ali, F. F. (1990). The effects of individual hypnosis on stress, anxiety, and intractable pain experienced by Lebanese cancer patients. *Dissertation Abstracts International, 51,* 3111.

American Psychological Association. (2005). Society of Psychological Hypnosis, Division 30. *The Division 30 definition and description of hypnosis.* Retrieved January 2, 2005, from http://www.apa. org/divisions/div30/define_hypnosis.html

Andersen, B. L. (1986). *Women with cancer: Psychological perspectives.* New York: Springer-Verlag.

Andersen, B. L., Kiecolt-Glaser, J. K., & Glaser, R. (1994). A biobehavioral model of cancer stress and disease course. *American Psychology, 49*(5), 389–404.

Andersen, B. L., & Turnquist, D. (1985). *Emotions and immunity: Response to the diagnosis of cancer.* Paper presented at the meeting of the Midwestern Psychological Association, Chicago.

Baer, R. A. (2003). Mindfulness training as a clinical intervention: A conceptual and empirical review. *Clinical Psychology: Science and Practice, 10,* 125–143.

Bakke, A. C., Purtzer, M. Z., & Newton, P. (2002). The effect of hypnotic-guided imagery on psychological well-being and immune function in patients with prior breast cancer. *Journal of Psychosomatic Research, 53*(6), 1131–1137.

Benson, H., Beary, J. F., & Carol, M. P. (1974). The relaxation response. *Psychiatry, 37*(1), 37–46.

Benson, H., Greenwood, M. M., & Klemchuk, H. (1975). The relaxation response: Psychophysiologic aspects and clinical applications. *Internationa Journal of Psychiatry and Medicine, 6*(1-2), 87–98.

Benson, H., Rosner, B. A., Marzetta, B. R., & Klemchuk, H. M. (1974). Decreased blood-pressure in pharmacologically treated hypertensive patients who regularly elicited the relaxation response. *Lancet, 1*(7852), 289–291.

Bertoni, F., Bonardi, A., Magno, L., Mandracchia, S., Martinelli, L., Terraneo, F., et al. (1999). Hypnosis instead of general anaesthesia in paediatric radiotherapy: Report of three cases. *Radiotherapy and Oncology, 52*(2), 185–190.

Black, S. (1963). Inhibition of immediate-type hypersensitivity response by direct suggestion under hypnosis. *British Medical Journal, 5335,* 925–929.

Black, S., & Friedman, M. (1965). Adrenal function and the inhibition of allergic responses under hypnosis. *British Medical Journal, 5434,* 562–567.

Bowen, D. E. (1973). Transurethral resection under self-hypnosis. *American Journal of Clinical Hypnosis, 16*(2), 132–134.

Brittenden, J., Heys, S. D., Ross, J., & Eremin, O. (1996). Natural killer cells and cancer. *Cancer, 77*(7), 1226–1243.

Burgio, K. L., Goode, P. S., Urban, D. A., Umlauf, M. G., Locher, J. L., Bueschen, A., et al. (2006). Preoperative biofeedback assisted behavioral training to decrease post-prostatectomy incontinence: A randomized, controlled trial. *Journal of Urology, 175*(1), 196–201; discussion 201.

Burish, T. G., Carey, M. P., Redd, W. H., & Krozely, M. G. (1983). Behavioral relaxation techniques in reducing the distress of cancer chemotherapy patients. *Oncology Nursing Forum, 10*(3), 32–35.

Burish, T. G., & Jenkins, R. A. (1992). Effectiveness of biofeedback and relaxation training in reducing the side effects of cancer chemotherapy. *Health Psychology, 11*(1), 17–23.

Burish, T., & Lyles, J. (1981). Effectiveness of biofeedback and relaxation training in reducing adverse reactions to cancer chemotherapy. *Journal of Behavioral Medicine, 4*(1), 65–78.

Burish, T. G., Shartner, C. D., & Lyles, J. N. (1981). Effectiveness of multiple muscle-site EMG biofeedback and relaxation training in reducing the aversiveness of cancer chemotherapy. *Biofeedback and Self Regulation, 6*(4), 523–535.

Cannon, W. B. (1932). *The wisdom of the body*. New York: Norton.

Carlson, L., Ursuliak, Z., Goodey, E., Angen, M., & Speca, M. (2001). The effects of a mindfulness meditation-based stress reduction program on mood and symptoms of stress in cancer outpatients: 6-month folllow-up. *Support Care Cancer, 9*(2), 112–123.

Carlson, L. E., & Garland, S. N. (2005). Impact of mindfulness-based stress reduction (MBSR) on sleep, mood, stress and fatigue symptoms in cancer outpatients. *International Journal of Behavioral Medicine, 12*(4), 278–285.

Carlson, L. E., Speca, M., Patel, K. D., & Goodey, E. (2003). Mindfulness-based stress reduction in relation to quality of life, mood, symptoms of stress, and immune parameters in breast and prostate cancer outpatients. *Psychosomatic Medicine, 65*(4), 571–581.

Carlson, L. E., Speca, M., Patel, K. D., & Goodey, E. (2004). Mindfulness-based stress reduction in relation to quality of life, mood, symptoms of stress and levels of cortisol, dehydroepiandrosterone sulfate (DHEAS) and melatonin in breast and prostate cancer outpatients. *Psychoneuroendocrinology, 29*(4), 448–474.

Cella, D. F., & Tross, S. (1986). Psychological adjustment to survival from Hodgkin's disease. *Journal of the Consulting Clinical Psychologist, 54*(5), 616–622.

Cohen, S., Kessler, R. C., & Gordon, L. U. (1995). Strategies for measuring stress in studies of psychiatric and physical disorders. In S. Cohen, R. C. Kessler, & L. U. Gordon (Eds.), *Measuring stress: A guide for health and social scientists* (pp. 3–28). New York: Oxford University Press.

Cunningham, A. J., Phillips, C., Lockwood, G. A., Hedley, D. W., & Edmonds, C. V. (2000). Association of involvement in psychological self-regulation with longer survival in patients with metastatic cancer: an exploratory study. *Advances in Mind Body Medicine, 16*(4), 276–287.

Davis, H. T. (1986). Effects of biofeedback and cognitive therapy on stress in patients with breast cancer. *Psychology Rep, 59*(2 Pt 2), 967–974.

Denk, D. M., & Kaider, A. (1997). Videoendoscopic biofeedback: a simple method to improve the efficacy of swallowing rehabilitation of patients after head and neck surgery. *ORL: Journal for Oto-Rhino-Laryngology and Its Related Specialties, 59*(2), 100–105.

DuHamel, K. N., Redd, W. H., & Vickberg, S. M. (1999). Behavioral interventions in the diagnosis, treatment and rehabilitation of children with cancer. *Acta Oncology, 38*(6), 719–734.

Ell, K., Mantell, J., Hamovitch, M., & Nishimoto, R. (1989). Social support, sense of control, and coping among patients with breast, lung, or colorectal cancer. *Journal of Psychosocial Oncology, 7*, 63–89.

Erickson, M. H. (1980). Hypnosis: A general review. In E. L. Rossi (Ed.), *The collected papers of Milton H. Erickson on hypnosis* (Vol. 3, pp. 13–20). New York: Irvington.

Esdaile, J. (1850). *Mesmerism in India and its practical application in surgery and medicine*. London: Longmans Green.

Evans, C., & Richardson, P. H. (1988). Improved recovery and reduced postoperative stay after therapeutic suggestions during general anaesthesia. *Lancet, 2*(8609), 491–493.

Finlay, I. G., & Jones, O. L. (1996). Hypnotherapy in palliative care. *Journal of the Royal Society of Medicine, 89*(9), 493–496.

Garssen, B., & Goodkin, K. (1999). On the role of immunological factors as mediators between psychosocial factors and cancer progression. *Psychiatry Research, 85*(1), 51–61.

Genius, M. L. (1995). The use of hypnosis in helping cancer patients control anxiety, pain, and emesis: A review of recent empirical studies. *American Journal of Clinical Hypnosis, 37*, 316–325.

Goodkin, K., Antoni, M. H., Sevin, B., & Fox, B. H. (1993). A partially testable, predictive model of psychosocial factors in the etiology of cervical cancer II: Bioimmunological, psychneuroimmunological, and socioimmunological aspects, critique and prospective integration. *Psychooncology, 2,* 99–121.

Gruber, B., Hall, N., Hersh, S., & Dubois, P. (1988). Immune system and psychological changes in metastatic cancer patients using relaxation and guided imagery: A pilot study. *Scandanavian Journal of Behavioral Therapy, 17,* 25–46.

Gruber, B. L., Hersh, S. P., Hall, N. R., Waletzky, L. R., Kunz, J. F., Carpenter, J. K., et al. (1993). Immunological responses of breast cancer patients to behavioral interventions. *Biofeedback and Self Regulation, 18*(1), 1–22.

Hilgard, J. R., & LeBaron, S. (1982). Relief of anxiety and pain in children and adolescents with cancer: quantitative measures and clinical observations. *International Journal of Clinical and Experimental Hypnosis, 30*(4), 417–442.

Hilgard, J. R., & LeBaron, S. (1984). *Hypnotherapy of pain in children with cancer.* Los Altos, CA: William Kaufmann.

Hill, S., Saeger, L., & Chapman, C. (1986). Patient-controlled analgesia after bone marrow transplantation for cancer. *Postgrad Med, August,* 33–40.

Hull, C. L. (1933). *Hypnosis and suggestibility—An experimental approach.* New York: Appleton-Century-Crofts.

Jacobsen, P. B., & Hann, D. M. (1998). Cognitive-behavioral interventions. In J. C. Holland (Ed.), *Psyco-oncology.* New York: Oxford University Press.

Kabat-Zinn, J. (1994). *Wherever you go, there you are.* New York: Hyperion.

Kabat-Zinn, J., Wheeler, E., Light, T., Skillings, A., Scharf, M. J., Cropley, T. G., et al. (1998). Influence of a mindfulness meditation-based stress reduction intervention on rates of skin clearing in patients with moderate to severe psoriasis undergoing phototherapy (UVB) and photochemotherapy (PUVA). *Psychosomatic Medicine, 60*(5), 625–632.

Katz, E. R., Kellerman, J., & Ellenberg, L. (1987). Hypnosis in the reduction of acute pain and distress in children with cancer. *Journal of Pediatric Psychology, 12*(3), 379–394.

Kaushik, R., Kaushik, R. M., Mahajan, S. K., & Rajesh, V. (2005). Biofeedback assisted diaphragmatic breathing and systematic relaxation versus propranolol in long term prophylaxis of migraine. *Complementary Therapies in Medicine, 13*(3), 165–174.

Kaye, J. M., & Schindler, B. A. (1990). Hypnosis on a consultation-liaison service. *General Hospital Psychiatry, 12*(6), 379–383.

Kellerman, J., Zeltzer, L., Ellenberg, L., & Dash, J. (1983). Adolescents with cancer. Hypnosis for the reduction of the acute pain and anxiety associated with medical procedures. *Journal of Adolescent Health, 4*(2), 85–90.

Kirsch, I. (1985). Response expectancy as a determinant of experience and behavior. *American Psychology, 40,* 1189–1202.

Kirsch, I. (1991). The social learning theory of hypnosis. In S. J. Lynn & J. W. Rhue (Eds.), *Theories of hypnosis: Current models and perspectives* (pp. 439–466). New York: Guilford.

Kirsch, I., & Lynn, S. J. (1995). The altered state of hypnosis: Changes in the theoretical landscape. *American Psychology, 50,* 846–858.

Kiecolt-Glaser, J. K., Glaser, R., Strain, E. C., Stout, J. C., Tarr, K. L., Holliday, J. E., et al. (1986). Modulation of cellular immunity in medical students. *Journal of Behavioral Medicine, 9*(1), 5–21.

Kranitz, L., & Lehrer, P. (2004). Biofeedback applications in the treatment of cardiovascular diseases. *Cardiology in Review, 12*(3), 177–181.

Kuttner, L., Bowman, M., & Teasdale, M. (1988). Psychological treatment of distress, pain, and anxiety for young children with cancer. *Journal of Developmental and Behavioral Pediatrics, 9*(6), 374–381.

Lazarus, R. S., & Folkman, S. (1984). *Stress, appraisal and coping.* New York: Springer-Verlag.

Levin, J. S., Glass, T. A., Kushi, L. H., Schuck, J. R., Steele, L., & Jonas, W. B. (1997). Quantitative methods in research on complementary and alternative medicine. A methodological manifesto. NIH Office of Alternative Medicine. *Medical Care, 35*(11), 1079–1094.

Levitan, A. A., & Harbaugh, T. L. (1989). Hypnoanalgesia and hypnotizability. *Hypnosis, 16,* 140–148.

Levy, S. M., Herberman, R. B., Lippman, M., D'Angelo, T., & Lee, J. (1991). Immunological and psychosocial predictors of disease recurrence in patients with early-stage breast cancer. *Behavioral Medicine, 17*(2), 67–75.

Liossi, C., & Hatira, P. (1999). Clinical hypnosis versus cognitive behavioral training for pain management with pediatric cancer patients undergoing bone marrow aspirations. *International Journal of Clinical and Experimental Hypnosis, 47*(2), 104–116.

Liossi, C., & Hatira, P. (2003). Clinical hypnosis in the alleviation of procedure-related pain in pediatric oncology patients. *International Journal of Clinical and Experimental Hypnosis, 51*(1), 4–28.

Lowery, B., Jacobsen, B., & DuCette, J. (1993). Casual attribution, control, and adjustment to breast cancer. *Journal of Psychosocial Oncology, 10*(4), 37–53.

Marks, G., Richardson, J. L., Graham, J. W., & Levine, A. (1986). Role of health locus of control beliefs and expectations of treatment efficacy in adjustment to cancer. *Journal of Personal and Social Psychology, 51*(2), 443–450.

Massion, A. O., Teas, J., Hebert, J. R., Wertheimer, M. D., & Kabat-Zinn, J. (1995). Meditation, melatonin and breast/prostate cancer: hypothesis and preliminary data. *Medical Hypotheses, 44*(1), 39–46.

Mastenbroek, I., & McGovern, L. (1991). The effectiveness of relaxation techniques in controlling chemotherapy induced nausea: A literature review. *Austrian Occupational Therapy Journal, 38*(3), 137–142.

Matthewson-Chapman, M. (1997). Pelvic muscle exercise/biofeedback for urinary incontinence after prostatectomy. *Journal of Cancer Education, 12*, 218–223.

McCabe, M., Collins, J. K., & Burns, A. M. (1979). Hypnosis as an altered state of consciousness: A review of contemporary theories and empirical evidence. *The Australian Journal of Clinical & Experimental Hypnosis, 7*, 7–25.

Meares, A. (1983). A form of intensive meditation associated with the regression of cancer. *American Journal of Clinical Hypnosis, 25*(2-3), 114–121.

Meyer, T. J., & Mark, M. M. (1995). Effects of psychosocial interventions with adult cancer patients: A meta-analysis of randomized experiments. *Health Psychology, 14*(2), 101–108.

Miller, N. E. (1974). Editorial: Biofeedback: Evaluation of a new technic. *New England Journal of Medicine, 290*(12), 684–685.

Miller, N. E., & Dworkin, B. R. (1977). Effects of learning on visceral functions—Biofeedback. *New England Journal of Medicine, 296*(22), 1274–1278.

Miller, S., Combs, C., & Stoddard, E. (1989). Information, coping and control in patients undergoing surgery and stressful medical procedures. In A. Steptoe & A. Appels (Eds.), *Stress, personal control and health* (pp. 107–130). New York: Wiley.

Miller, S. M., & O'Leary, A. (1993). Cognition, stress and health. In *Psychopathology and cognition* (pp. 159–189). New York: Academic Press.

Morrow, G. (1992). Behavioural factors influencing the development and expression of chemotherapy induced side effects. *British Journal of Cancer, 66*(Suppl. 19), S54–S61.

National Institutes of Health. (1996). Integration of behavioral and relaxation approaches into the treatment of chronic pain and insomnia. NIH Technology Assessment Panel on Integration of Behavioral and Relaxation Approaches into the Treatment of Chronic Pain and Insomnia. *Journal of the American Medical Association, 276*(4), 313– 318.

Newsom, J. T., Knapp, J. E., & Schulz, R. (1996). Longitudinal analysis of specific domains of internal control and depressive symptoms in patients with recurrent cancer. *Health Psychology, 15*(5), 323–331.

Patel, C., Marmot, M. G., Terry, D. J., Carruthers, M., Hunt, B., & Patel, M. (1985). Trial of relaxation in reducing coronary risk: Four year follow up. *British Medical Journal (Clinical Research Edition), 290*(6475), 1103–1106.

Penman, D. T., Bloom, J. R., Fotopoulos, S., Cook, M. R., Holland, J. C., Gates, C., et al. (1986). The impact of mastectomy on self-concept and social function: a combined cross-sectional and longitudinal study with comparison groups. *Women Health, 11*(3–4), 101–130.

Peter, B. (1996). Hypnotherapy with cancer patients: On speaking about death and dying. *The Australian Journal of Clinical and Experimental Hypnosis, 24*(1), 29–35.

Redd, W. H., Andresen, G. V., & Minagawa, R. Y. (1982). Hypnotic control of anticipatory emesis in patients receiving cancer chemotherapy. *Journal of the Consulting Clinical Psychologist, 50*(1), 14–19.

Redd, W. H., Jacobsen, P. B., Die-Trill, M., Dermatis, H., McEvoy, M., & Holland, J. C. (1987). Cognitive/attentional distraction in the control of conditioned nausea in pediatric cancer patients receiving chemotherapy. *Journal of the Consulting Clinical Psychologist, 55*(3), 391–395.

Richardson, J., Smith, J. E., McCall, G., & Pilkington, K. (2006). Hypnosis for procedure-related pain and distress in pediatric cancer patients: A systematic review of effectiveness and methodology related to hypnosis interventions. *Journal of Pain Symptom Management, 31*(1), 70–84.

Robbins, J. (2000). *A symphony in the brain*. New York: Grove Press.

Rotter, J. B. (1966). Generalized expectancies for internal versus external control of reinforcement. *Psychology Monographs, 80*(1), 1–28.

Seligman, M. E. P. (1975). *Helplessness*. New York: W. H. Freeman.

Shapiro, S. L., Carlson, L. E., Astin, J. A., & Freedman, B. (2005). Mechanisms of mindfulness. *Journal of Clinical Psychology, 62*, 373-386.

Shapiro, D., & Schwartz, G. E. (1972). Biofeedback and visceral learning: clinical applications. *Seminars in Psychiatry, 4*(2), 171–184.

Spanos, N. P. (1991). A sociocognitive approach to hypnosis. In S. J. Lynn & J. W. Rhue (Eds.), *Theories of hypnosis: Current models and perspectives* (pp. 324–361). New York: Guilford.

Spanos, N. P., & Chaves, J. F. (1989). Hypnotic analgesia and surgery: In defense of the social-psychological position. *British Journal of Experimental and Clinical Hypnosis, 6*, 131–139.

Speca, M., Carlson, L. E., Goodey, E., & Angen, M. (2000). A randomized, wait-list controlled clinical trial: the effect of a mindfulness meditation-based stress reduction program on mood and symptoms of stress in cancer outpatients. *Psychosomatic Medicine, 62*(5), 613–622.

Spiegel, D., & Bloom, J. R. (1983). Group therapy and hypnosis reduce metastatic breast carcinoma pain. *Psychosomatic Medicine, 45*(4), 333–339.

Spiegel, D., Bloom, J. R., Kraemer, H. C., & Gottheil, E. (1989). Effect of psychosocial treatment on survival of patients with metastatic breast cancer. *Lancet, 2*(8668), 888–891.

Spiegel, D., & Moore, R. (1997). Imagery and hypnosis in the treatment of cancer patients. *Oncology (Huntingt), 11*(8), 1179–1189; discussion 1189–1195.

Spiegel, H., & Spiegel, D. (1978). *Trance and treatment: Clinical uses of hypnosis*. New York: Basic Books.

Steggles, S., Damore-Petingola, S., Maxwell, J., & Lightfoot, N. (1997). Hypnosis for children and adolescents with cancer: An annotated bibliography, 1985-1995. *Journal of Pediatric Oncology Nursing, 14*(1), 27–32.

Steggles, S., Maxwell, J., Lightfoot, N. E., Damore-Petingola, S., & Mayer, C. (1997). Hypnosis and cancer: An annotated bibliography 1985-1995. *American Journal of Clinical Hypnosis, 39*(3), 187–200.

Sudsuang, R., Chentanez, V., & Veluvan, K. (1991). Effect of Buddhist meditation on serum cortisol and total protein levels, blood pressure, pulse rate, lung volume and reaction time. *Physiology & Behavior, 50*(3), 543–548.

Suls, J., & Mullen, B. (1981). Life events, perceived control and illness: The role of uncertainty. *Journal of Human Stress, 7*(2), 30–34.

Syrjala, K. L., Cummings, C., & Donaldson, G. W. (1992). Hypnosis or cognitive behavioral training for the reduction of pain and nausea during cancer treatment: a controlled clinical trial. *Pain, 48*(2), 137–146.

Taylor, S. (1983). Adjustment to threatening events: A theory of cognitive adaptation. *American Psychology, 38*, 1161–1173.

Taylor, S., Helgeson, V., Reed, G., & Skokan, L. (1991). Self-generated feelings of control and adjustment to physical illness. *Journal of Social Issues, 47*(4), 91–109.

Taylor, S. E., Lichtman, R. R., & Wood, J. V. (1984). Attributions, beliefs about control, and adjustment to breast cancer. *Journal of Personal and Social Psychology, 46*(3), 489–502.

Thompson, S. C. (1981). Will it hurt less if I can control it? A complex answer to a simple question. *Psychology Bulletin, 90*(1), 89–101.

Thompson, S. C., Sobolew-Shubin, A., Galbraith, M. E., Schwankovsky, L., & Cruzen, D. (1993). Maintaining perceptions of control: finding perceived control in low-control circumstances. *Journal of Personal and Social Psychology, 64*(2), 293–304.

Tjemsland, L., Soreide, J. A., Matre, R., & Malt, U. F. (1997). Preoperative psychological variables predict immunological status in patients with operable breast cancer. *Psychooncology, 6*, 311–320.

Toomey, T., Mann, J., Abashian, S., & Thompson-Pope, S. (1991). Relationship between perceived self-control of pain, pain description, and functioning. *Pain, 45*, 129–133.

Trijsburg, R. W., van Knippenberg, F. C., & Rijpma, S. E. (1992). Effects of psychological treatment on cancer patients: a critical review. *Psychosomatic Medicine, 54*(4), 489–517.

Valente, S. M. (1991). Using hypnosis with children for pain management. *Oncology Nursing Forum, 18*(4), 699–704.

VanDalfsen, P. J., & Syrjala, K. L. (1990). Psychological strategies in acute pain management. *Critical Care Clinics, 6*(2), 421–431.

van Kampen, M., de Weerdt, W., de Ridder, D., Feys, H., & Baert, L. (2000). Effect of pelvic-floor re-education on duration and degree of incontinence after radical prostatectomy: A randomised controlled trial. *Lancet, 355*(9198), 98– 102.

Wall, V. J., & Womack, W. (1989). Hypnotic versus active cognitive strategies for alleviation of procedural distress in pediatric oncology patients. *American Journal of Clinical Hypnosis, 31*(3), 181–191.

Walker, L. G., Dawson, A. A., Pollet, S. M., & Ratcliffe, M. A. (1988). Hypnotherapy for chemotherapy side effects. *British Journal of Experimental and Clinical Hypnosis, 5*(2), 79–82.

Whitehouse, W. G., Dinges, D. F., Orne, E. C., Keller, S. E., Bates, B. L., Bauer, N. K., et al. (1996). Psychosocial and immune effects of self-hypnosis training for stress management throughout the first semester of medical school. *Psychosomatic Medicine, 58*(3), 249–263.

Whiteside, T. L., & Herberman, R. B. (1995). The role of natural killer cells in immune surveillance of cancer. *Current Opinion in Immunology, 7*(5), 704–710.

Winegard, J. R., Curbow, B., Baker, F., & Piantadosi, S. (1991). Health, functional status, and employment of adult survivors of bone marrow transplantation. *Annals of Internal Medicine, 114*, 113–118.

Woody, E. Z., & Bowers, K. S. (1994). A frontal assault on dissociated control. In S. J. Lynn & J. W. Rhue (Eds.), *Dissociation: Clinical, theoretical and research perspectives* (pp. 52–79). New York: Guilford.

Yellen, S. B., Cella, D. F., & Bonomi, A. (1993). Quality of life in people with Hodgkin's disease. *Oncology (Huntingt), 7*(8), 41-45; discussion 46, 50–42.

Zeltzer, L., Kellerman, J., Ellenberg, L., & Dash, J. (1983). Hypnosis for reduction of vomiting associated with chemotherapy and disease in adolescents with cancer. *Journal of Adolescent Health, 4*(2), 77–84.

Zeltzer, L., & LeBaron, S. (1982). Hypnosis and nonhypnotic techniques for reduction of pain and anxiety during painful procedures in children and adolescents with cancer. *Journal of Pediatrics, 101*(6), 1032–1035.

Zeltzer, L. K., Dolgin, M. J., LeBaron, S., & LeBaron, C. (1991). A randomized, controlled study of behavioral intervention for chemotherapy distress in children with cancer. *Pediatrics, 88*(1), 34–42.

# Guided Imagery

5

## Can Guided Imagery Treat Cancer Successfully?

Martin L. Rossman

The first thing most patients and doctors want to know is whether guided imagery is helpful in treating cancer. This is an understandable but somewhat naive question. There are no definitive studies on this and might not ever be. First, it would be unusual to find people who would be willing to treat cancer solely with guided imagery, and even if they were identified, it is unlikely that an Institutional Review Board would allow such a study. Second, such a cohort would likely be quite different from most people who would be unwilling to do the same and thus would be difficult, if not impossible, to match for controls. Third, you could neither randomize nor blind the process if you were willing to utilize imagery in all of its various forms to individualize treatments for individuals. Finally, there is the problem of assessing individual response, whereby even if it were shown that 76% of all cancer patients listening to guided imagery tapes twice a day had curative responses, we still would not know whether it would be helpful to any one individual asking the question.

What we can fairly say at this point is the following:

1 The evidence that people can stimulate an immune system component critical to fighting cancer seems convincing (Gruber et al., 1993). Hall, Minnes, and Olness (1993) found that 18 of 22 articles investigating the effects of imagery on immunity showed positive responses in numbers of circulating natural killer (NK) cells and their response to mitogen stimulation. Although NK cell activation is not equivalent to a survival end point, it is widely agreed to be a desirable effect in cancer treatments.

**2** There are four studies that seem to demonstrate favorable survival in patients utilizing various forms of psychosocial intervention, including imagery.

The first modern study that pointed to a potential survival benefit with cancer was reported in the early 1970s by radiation oncologist O. Carl Simonton and psychologist Stephanie Simonton. The Simontons presented a series of cases of cancer that had seemed to respond positively to mental imagery aimed at stimulating the immune system to destroy the cancer. Several of their patients had remarkable and unexpected responses to radiation therapy and they designed a pilot study looking at 59 patients employing their guided imagery method. The study looked at the compliance of patients as evidenced by number of times they practiced imagery and indicated a relatively direct association between participation in the process and enhanced survival. The study compared patient survival to historical controls. Of course, this study design is not definitive, but rather than triggering a series of follow-up studies in the cancer community, it stimulated a sometimes raging emotional debate that lasted over 20 years without any significant funds being made available either to the Simontons or other cancer researchers desiring to do more tightly designed studies.

While at Stanford, David Spiegel (1989) published his famous study showing that women with metastatic breast cancer had twice the longevity of a matched group of women who did not participate in support group and hypnosis for pain control. Spiegel's study was well designed and has survived rigorous analysis by both skeptics and supporters in the field. The major conclusion drawn from Spiegel's study is that group support is the "active ingredient" but these groups also taught women to utilize self-hypnosis (consisting of relaxation and imagery) to help reduce their anxiety and pain levels. Comparison studies of groups with and without hypnosis have not been done.

Psychiatrists Fawzy et al (2003), at UCLA, published the results of a prospective randomized study with patients newly diagnosed with malignant melanoma. Study subjects participated in a 6-week group, with groups lasting 90 min. They learned about the disease, active behavioral coping mechanisms, stress reduction, and relaxation/imagery techniques. Six years later they suffered less than one-third the mortality and one-half the recurrence rate of matched controls who did not participate in this 9-hr intervention. Their psychologic and immunologic function were significantly superior to control subjects Analysis of these effects after 10 years shows these survival benefits still hold.

Dean Shrock (1999), a psychologist who studied with Carl Simonton, published results of an 8-week cancer group teaching imagery healing skills in Stage 1 breast and prostate cancer patients. His results were congruent with the previous studies, showing a survival and recurrence free advantage of approximately twofold.

The most recent study of this type is reported by Cunningham et al. (2000), who showed that some participants in a mind/body support group have significantly enhanced survival. This study was aimed at identifying characteristics of individuals in such groups that have prolonged survival rather than being an intervention study. Six characteristics were found to have a relationship to extended survival: (1) ability to act and change, (2) willingness to initiate change, (3) application to self-help work, (4) relationships with others, (5) quality of experience, and (6) expectancy that psychologic efforts would affect the disease.

After carefully explaining the limitations of this observational study, Cunningham concludes that "it appears that there is a strong association between longer survival and psychologic factors related to the involvement of cancer patients in psychologic self-help activities. While causality cannot be inferred, reasons are given for believing that this is not a result of the disease influencing the patients' psychology, but rather the converse."

These studies taken together should at the very least rouse serious interest in studying the effect of support, meditation, imagery, and attitude in cancer survival. Many questions remain—is the support more important than the relaxation, stress reduction, or imagery? Are the techniques themselves simply a marker of intention and determination to survive or better care for the self, and is enhanced care a determinant in accounting for survival?

## Evidence for Treating the Patient

Whether someone believes that their mind can contribute to the cure of cancer, there is overwhelming evidence that imagery can be effective in improving the quality of a cancer patient's life. Imagery has been shown to be effective in reducing depression and anxiety (Baider, Peretz, Hadani, & Koch, 2000; Bisson, 1995; Caruso & Helge, 1999; McDonald & Hilgendorf, 1986), eliminating hopelessness (Covino & Frankel, 1993), reducing adverse effects of chemotherapy (Burish, 1987; Dahlquist, 1985; Troesh et al., 1993) and surgery (Bennet et al., 1986; Disbrow, Bennett, & Owings, 1993; Tusek, 1997), reducing pain and the need for pain medication (Krueger, 1987; National Institutes of Health, 1996; Syrjala et al., 1995), making difficult decisions and changing life-style habits (Agras, 1981; Barbasz & Spiegel, 1989; Cochrane & Friesen, 1986; Wynd, 1992), and finding meaning in the experience of cancer (Brown-Saltzman, 1997; Dahlquist, 1985; Krystal & Zweben, 1989; Richardson et al., 1997).

## What Is Imagery and Why Is It Important?

Imagery is essentially a way of thinking that uses sensory attributes in the absence of sensory input. It can be thought of as one of brain's two higher order encoding systems. The system we are most familiar with is the *sequential* information processing system that underlies linear, analytic, and conscious verbal thinking. Most health professionals are highly educated and highly rewarded for their abilities using this mode of information processing.

Imagery, however, is the language utilized by a *simultaneous* information processing mode, which underlies the holistic, synthetic, pattern thinking of the unconscious mind.

A brief clinical example may serve to bring the importance of this relational quality to life. A 60-year-old woman with metastatic melanoma was having difficulty imagining her immune system vigorously fighting her tumor. Her imagery consisted of a few relatively inert immune cells sitting on her image of the tumor, which she described as a "blob." Numerous therapeutic interventions failed to increase the activity she imagined until the author asked her to allow an image to form for anything standing in the way of her imagining her healing more actively. An image of a large chasm came to her mind and across the chasm she saw her husband and grown children waving for her to come over. She began to cry at this, the first evidence of emotion I had seen in our half dozen sessions. I asked about her tears and she told me that the one regret she had was that her family was emotionally distant and estranged from each other in varying degrees and she had not been able to change that. I asked her what she wanted to do in her imagery and she said she needed to build a bridge over to them (she was an engineer by training). She built a bridge and imagined walking across into the welcoming arms of her embracing family. When we discussed this, I asked her if there was anything she wanted to do differently in her outer life as a result of what she had experienced internally. She decided to ask her family to meet together with a family therapist, something they had never done. After a short series of deeply moving sessions the family had bonded together in a way it never had before. Subsequently her healing imagery became very vigorous and active, as did her participation in other aspects of her treatment, including nutrition, exercise, and an experimental clinical trial of monoclonal antibodies.

The imagery allowed her to access and experience an emotional barrier to being more participatory in her care, one that had not only cognitive but also emotional information and that brought that information to her in a nonlinear but meaningful way that led to action.

Imagery is the language of the arts and is also the language of emotions. Emotions show what is important to us and can be either potent motivators or barriers to changing lifestyle habits. Emotions motivate us to action, and they also produce characteristic physiologic changes in the body, including varying patterns of muscle tension, blood flow, respiration, metabolism, and neurologically and immunologically active peptide secretions. Modern research in psychoneuroimmunology points to the emotions as key modulators of neuroactive peptides secreted by the brain, gut, and immune systems (Sheikh, 1989). Because of these relations to cognition, emotion, and physiology, we might well consider imagery to be the "Rosetta stone" of mind/body interactions.

In addition to being a rapid route to insight and motivation, imagery has direct physiologic consequences and effects. In the absence of competing sensory cues, the body tends to respond to imagery as it would to a genuine external experience. Imagery has been shown in numerous research studies to be able to effect almost all major physiologic control systems of the body, including respiration, heart rate, blood pressure metabolic rates in cells, gastrointestinal mobility and secretion, sexual function, and even immune responsiveness (Sheikh, 1989).

# Treatment and Self-Care Options With Imagery

Because imagery is a natural way we think, and because it can almost always be helpful, there are virtually an unlimited number of situations where it can be helpful for people with cancer. For simplicity, it may be helpful to consider three major categories of use:

1  Relaxation and stress reduction, which is easy to teach, easy to learn, and almost universally helpful.

2 Visualization, or directed imagery, where the client/patient is encouraged to imagine desired outcomes in a relaxed state of mind. This affords the patient a sense of participation and control in their own healing, which itself is of significant value. In addition, it may well relieve or reduce symptoms, stimulate healing responses in the body or behaviors, and/or provide effective motivation for making positive life changes.

3 Receptive, or insight oriented imagery, where images are invited into awareness and explored to gather more information about a symptom, illness, mood, situation, or solution.

Variables to consider in choosing approaches include whether the client will be able to use imagery most effectively as a self-care technique in a group or class or as part of an individual counseling or therapy relationship. Self-help books and tapes are an inexpensive option for many clients who are capable of utilizing these techniques on their own, whereas dealing with highly charged emotional issues often requires the assistance of a competent professional imagery guide.

In practice, patients and practitioners often explore all of the above options and utilize the ones that suit a given client the best, given the unique nature of the issue, their coping responses, approach to healing, and the amount of time, energy, and funds they are willing or able to invest in the process.

# The Advantages of Interactive Guided Imagery

*Guided imagery* is a term variously used to describe a range of techniques from simple visualization and direct imagery-based suggestion to metaphor and storytelling. Guided imagery is used to help teach psychophysiologic relaxation, to relieve symptoms, to stimulate healing responses in the body, and to help people tolerate procedures and treatments more easily.

*Interactive Guided Imagery* is a service-marked term registered by the Academy for Guided Imagery to represent a particular approach to using therapeutic imagery. In this approach, imagery is evoked from the patient by a guide trained to do this without suggesting specific imagery. This gives patients ways to draw on their own inner resources to support healing, to make appropriate adaptations to changes in health, and to find creative solutions to challenges that they previously thought were insoluble. It encourages patients to access their own strengths and resources and tends to lead toward greater patient autonomy and self-efficacy.

The key to the extraordinary clinical effectiveness of Interactive Guided Imagery is the interactive communications component that it incorporates. By working interactively instead of just reading an imagery script, the Interactive Imagery guide ensures that the experience has personal meaning for the client and that it proceeds at a pace determined by the client's needs and abilities.

Because both the content and the direction are set by the client, it is the client who actually begins to guide the guide to the resources needed to support healing, change, and positive therapeutic results. We like to say that "the guide provides the setting while the client provides the jewel."

Whenever possible, the Interactive Imagery Guide uses nonjudgmental, content-free language because it encourages clients to tap their own inner resources to find solutions for solving their own problems. This sometimes leads to startling insights.

A 27-year-old patient with lymphoma was invited to allow an image to come to mind that could represent his disease. Rather than encountering a frightening image, a wraithlike spirit image appeared. The patient was encouraged to imagine that he could communicate with the image and it could communicate with him in a way he could understand. When he asked the image what it wanted from him, it said, to his surprise "You are a spiritual being but there is no room for me in your life. Make room for me to live or I will have to return with you to the world of the spirits." He cried and talked at length about his own spiritual seeking as an adolescent and young adult. He had become very involved in a lucrative business 5 years before his diagnosis and it consumed all his waking hours. He had already been divorced and lost many friends to his obsession with the business and now felt that what the image said was true. He changed his priorities and went through a chemotherapy regimen that worked beautifully. We cannot conclude that his treatment was successful because of his imagery, but we can observe that the development of a much more balanced life afterward, which included much more time with friends, a spiritual practice, and philanthropy, was initiated rather directly from that process. How many "imagery guides" would have suggested this particular imagery? And, more importantly, if they had, how likely would it have been to be perceived as meaningful by this patient? If you suggested this imagery to a hundred cancer patients, none of them might relate to it. Yet, by evoking the patient's own imagery, he was empowered to become aware of important unconscious needs that he related to his illness and healing.

There are important personal qualities that the Interactive Imagery Guide brings to the therapeutic experience, including a nonjudgmental attitude, patience, and trust in the client's own abilities. The consistent emphasis on resources and solutions, the repetitive inner focus as a source for solutions and strengths, and the modeling provided by the guide's belief that the client has within them more resources than they had imagined, leads to minimal transference, greater opportunities for effective client self-care, an enhanced sense of self-efficacy, and the rapid development of autonomy.

# Specific Uses of Interactive Guided Imagery in Cancer Care

A wide variety of Interactive Guided Imagery techniques can be useful with cancer patients. The more frequently used are outlined in the following.

## Imagery Relaxation and the Creation of a Safe or Healing Place

This is undoubtedly the most ubiquitous guided imagery technique used for any situation. Guiding the patient through some abdominal breathing, a simple body scan, or progressive muscle relaxation and then inviting them to imagine themselves in a "beautiful, safe place they love to be in" is a simple and relatively nonthreatening introduction to the effects of imagery. Depending on the patient and practitioner, this might be termed a "healing place" or "powerful place" rather than a "safe place," but safety is usually a good quality to begin with. It may be a place that the patient has been to before, either in real life or in their imagination, or a new place that comes to mind. If guided with an interactive approach, the patient is invited to describe the place they imagine themselves in, while staying there in their mind. The guide asks them what they see, hear, and feel there and allows them to respond. Questions such as "What time of day does it seem to be?" and "What's the temperature like?" help to focus the patient on their senses and deepen the subjective reality of the imagery.

As simple as this technique is, it illustrates the utility of the interactive approach. When I first started using guided imagery, I was taught to suggest that patients imagine themselves at a beautiful beach with warm sun and sand and blue-green waves breaking on the shore. This worked well for most people but once a young man sat straight up on the verge of panic when I mentioned this. It turned out he and his girlfriend had been brutally assaulted on a Lake Michigan beach a couple of years previously and this was *not* a relaxing image for him! The point is there is nothing to gain and something to lose by not guiding interactively and suggesting specific images, but when you invite a patient to go to place that is beautiful and safe and relaxing for them, they will unerringly pick a place that fulfills those criteria.

## Healing Imagery

This is what most people think of when they think about imagery and cancer: imagining a healing response, most often a vigorous immune response, symbolically or physiologically. This is an extremely useful practice for many people, both psychologically and physiologically. I find it especially useful early after diagnosis when people feel out of control and helpless. If nothing else, and there is evidence that it has greater effects than just this, it begins to relieve feelings of helplessness very quickly. People feel that there is something they can do while they are waiting for diagnostic tests and recommendations for medical treatment. The evidence that people do in fact enhance their natural killer cell response to mitogen stimulation is important for them to know and serves as a potent motivator in treatment.

There are several other components to creating personal and powerful healing imagery that I believe are clinically useful, though whether certain components are more effective than others has yet to be well studied. Clinically, it may well be that the most important factor is that the healing imagery is meaningful and engaging to the individual patient.

The first variable is that imagery consists of more than just visualization. Although vision is the most dominant sense for humans, it is one of five, and that is also true in imagery. For some people, there may be "sounds of healing" that they imagine, an odor that accompanies it, or body sensations of warmth, coolness, tingling, or others that accompany their healing imagery. I encourage patients to explore all the senses in creating and elaborating their personal healing imagery. Functional magnetic resonance imaging has shown that as people imagine in different senses, different area of the cerebral cortex are activated. Recruiting different senses and more cortical areas is likely to make the imagery more subjectively real to the patient and more powerfully stimulating of the subcortical responses that mediate healing and immune responsiveness.

I have found it useful to include, along with physiologic healing imagery, some imagery of the outcome that the patient desires. This is called Ideal Model imagery, which focuses on what it will be like when the patient is recovered. I encourage them to imagine doing what they love to do with the people they love to do it with and to imagine themselves enjoying significant landmark events and goals such as family weddings, births, graduations, and so on. Ideal Model imagery is not always easy for people and it may bring up significant barriers to investing their hopes in recovery. This allows us to work with those potential barriers in willing patients. Ideal Model imagery can bring up grief in some patients that can be simply acknowledged and processed as much or as little as needed until the patient can imagine their desired goal as an intended direction without the grief.

Another component of healing imagery that is often useful is what I call "medical counterweight" imagery. This is especially important if the patient has heard or experienced negative messages about prognosis from their doctors, whether communicated intentionally or unintentionally. Many patients will say something like "I will never forget the look on my doctor's face when he told me I had cancer," and they often do not. Patients waiting to hear a prognosis from an oncologist are frequently psychologically regressed and vulnerable to suggestion. In such a situation, we do not really want our doctors to be just plain people, we want them to be omnipotent and powerful, like an ideal parent. Verbal and nonverbal cues from doctors can create anxiety, depression, or an iatrogenic posttraumatic stress syndrome with intrusive thinking, sleep disturbance, excessive vigilance, and anxiety. This is an especially difficult condition to treat and often requires much attention to neutralize or negate. Imagery of being in the doctor's office, with a calendar on the wall, with a future date that is meaningful to the patient on the wall, imagining the doctor reviewing their tests and giving them good news and being pleased (or puzzled) often helps with this. It provides an image that the patient can substitute for the one they've unconsciously taken in and gives them a way to respond in an internally effective way.

We do not know the "dose response" of healing imagery even if we conclude that it has an effect. Most studies that have investigated the immune stimulation aspect of imagery have used protocols of 20 minutes two to three times a day. Studies such as those of Cunningham et al. (2000) and Simonton indicate that the more people do the practices, the more they benefit, whether that is because of the practice itself or because the intensive practice is a marker of intention, determination, and belief. We often encourage people to frequently think about their healing imagery, even for a few seconds, and especially whenever they do anything they hope or think will help their healing, like taking medications, vitamins, herbs, or other treatments. At the same time, I always encourage patients to take at least one time during the day to relax, shift their attention, and focus on nothing but their healing process, however they imagine it.

Using Interactive Imagery Dialogue processes can help people personalize their healing imagery and their practices in ways that are "custom fit" for them, which we believe is likely to be the most powerful healing imagery for each individual.

## Interactive Imagery Dialogue

This technique can be used with an image that represents anything the client or guide wants to know more about, and in many ways, it is the quintessential insight technique. With cancer patients, we can use it to explore an image of a symptom, whether physical, emotional, or behavioral; an image that represents the cancer; an image for resistance to healing that arises anywhere in the process; an image for an inner resource that can help the client deal with the current problem; or an image of healing. We use it, when appropriate for individual patients, to dialogue with the immune system, an image of the disease itself, an image of what they imagine to be eternal in them, or even to dialogue with an image of death. Obviously, the selection of focus is highly dependent on the clinical situation and orientation of the patient. None of these techniques should be forced on anyone but offered at appropriate times as possibilities.

When using Interactive Imagery, the point is not to analyze the images but to communicate with them as if they are alive, which of course, they are. This is not to say that they have an existence apart from the client but that the images represent complexes of thoughts, beliefs, attitudes, feelings, body sensations, and values that at times can function as relatively autonomous aspects of the personality. These constellations have been referred to as *subpersonalities* by Assagioli (1965) or *ego states* by Watkins and Watkins (1979).

**The Inner Advisor.** A very helpful specific imagery dialogue is the conversation with an imaginary figure that is both wise and loving. We call this figure the *Inner Advisor* but can also refer to it as the *Inner Guide*, the *Inner Healer*, the *Inner Wisdom*, *Inner Helper*, *Inner Physician*, *Higher Self*, or any other term that is meaningful and comfortable for the client.

The Advisor is defined and characterized by the two qualities of wisdom and compassion and can be characterized in analytic terms as an Ego Ideal. As the client is invited to imagine a figure that has these qualities, an exploration of whatever figure arises can be meaningful and helpful. The Advisor can provide a way for the client to access their own wisdom and compassion, useful qualities in most circumstances and especially in many situations that arise in the treatment of cancer.

**Evocative Imagery.** This state-dependent technique helps clients to shift moods and affective states at will, thus making new behaviors and insights more accessible. Through the structured use of memory, fantasy, and sensory recruitment, the client is encouraged to identify a personal quality or qualities that would serve them especially well in their current situation. For example, a patient of mine who had just suffered a recurrence of breast cancer was sobbing uncontrollably in my office. She kept repeating "I don't know if I can do it again, I just don't know if I can do it." I asked her what she felt she needed to go through the ordeals she was anticipating in treating her recurrence, and after a few minutes she said, "I don't think I have the courage or strength to do this." She was willing to do some imagery so I asked her to go back in her mind to some time when she did experience having the qualities she needed now. She imagined herself 20 years previously, comforting her mother, who had just been diagnosed with breast cancer. My patient, a nurse, was calm and strong, reassuring her mother that they would do whatever it took, and choose the best treatments, and that it would be OK. I asked her to imagine she was there again and to notice what she was seeing, hearing, and feeling. I also asked her to notice how it felt to be in touch with the strength and calmness she was manifesting at that time and to notice where she felt the strength in her body. I invited her to gradually allow the feelings of strength, calmness, and courage to grow larger and feel it throughout her body. At the end of about 10 minutes she opened her eyes, calmer, and said to me, "You know, I do have what I need. I just couldn't get to it." This is often true when people are terrified, as cancer patients often are. Evocative imagery helps people access the strengths they already have to help them make best use of their treatments and healing abilities.

Evocative imagery was researched by Dr. Sheldon Cohen at Carnegie-Mellon University and found to be highly effective in shifting affective states. Research aimed at assessing the effects of those altered affective states on subsequent behavior, problem solving, and self-efficacy remain to be done and offers a fertile field for future psychologic and behavioral research.

### Grounding: Moving From Insight to Action

This is the process by which the insights evoked by imagery are turned into actions, and the new awareness and motivation is focused into a specific plan for attitudinal, emotional, or behavioral change. This process of adding the will to the imagination involves clarification of insights, brainstorming, choosing the best option, affirmations, action planning, imagery rehearsal, and constant reformulation of the plan until it actually succeeds. It is often the "missing link" in imaginal therapy, connecting the new awareness to specific action. Imagery can be used to enhance this process, by providing creative options for action and allowing preaction troubleshooting and practice through imagery rehearsal. This is the process that can help patients actually change their dietary and exercise habits, quit smoking, and reduce stress by resolving problems they previously were unable to resolve.

# Precautions and Contraindications for Using Imagery With Cancer Patients

## Do Not Substitute Imagery for Necessary Medical or Surgical Interventions

The primary danger in using imagery to augment healing in medical situations is when it is used in lieu of appropriate medical diagnosis and/or treatment. We emphasize the necessity of an accurate diagnosis so that the patient can also be made aware of the medical options for treatment. At times, patients may decide they do not have good medical options available and will choose to use imagery and mind/body/spirit approaches as their first line of treatment. We believe there are situations in which this makes perfect sense, but each situation must be evaluated individually to ascertain the patient's ability to judge and make such choices. Consultation with the patient's oncologist to assess appropriate goals for therapy is recommended.

## Do Not Use Imagery Inappropriately With Patients With Psychopathology

There are several diagnostic categories of mental illness where the practitioner must use extreme care when utilizing exploratory receptive imagery techniques. In particular, patients who are psychotic or who are on the verge of psychotic breaks, patients with disassociative disorders, and patients with borderline personality disorders must be handled with care.

Although these diagnoses do not represent absolute contraindications for imagery work, they require health professionals to have expertise in these areas. Some clients with these diagnoses may in fact benefit from some uses of imagery (usually directed imagery scripts focusing on centering, calmness, self-control, safety, etc.), but great caution should be taken with potentially disorganizing receptive imagery techniques.

It is important to note that with clients who tend to pathologically disassociate, where there is a high incidence of survivors of traumatic abuse, imagery techniques can be one of the most effective ways to work. With these clients, too, the practitioner must be well versed both in working with survivors of abuse and in working with exploratory or Interactive Guided Imagery approaches.

## Do Not Confuse Responsibility With Blame

The fact that an illness can be helped through mental means does not necessarily mean it was caused by mental means. With exploratory techniques such as the Imagery Dialogue with symptoms, or with an Inner Advisor, there can be a tendency to confuse the ability to learn from illness with blame for causing the illness.

This issue needs to be handled with skill and sensitivity, and although the practitioner may not be able to prevent certain clients from self-blaming (this may be an important issue to address with them), they can help most people realize that using positive images to stimulate healing does not necessarily mean that their negative images *caused* their illness.

## Do Not Underestimate the Holotropic Principle and the Innate Resources of the Patient

Imagery is a potent form of communication and suggestion. Whenever possible, the Academy for Guided Imagery advocates utilization of the patient's own imagery and an interactive guiding style based on what has been termed the *holotropic principle*—the assumption that there is within all living organisms a drive toward wholeness and healing. Certainly the client has within them a great deal of information, experience, knowledge, and problem-solving abilities that IGI methods aim to access and utilize.

Although there are situations where a guide needs to supply suggestions and images, these are relatively rare and may rob the client of the opportunity to learn to help him- or herself. This helps to create or sustain a sense of dependency on the expertise of the guide rather than an attention to the inner abilities that have allowed them to help themselves.

# Training, Certification, and Issues of Quality Assurance

Many health professionals utilize guided imagery in their work, though they may have learned only to lead someone through noninteractive scripts. The quality of their training and competence with this intervention is quite variable. Because there is potential for doing harm when these techniques are used inappropriately or without adequate skills, standards of practice and quality control are important issues.

The Academy for Guided Imagery is a postgraduate training institution that was founded in 1989 to bring quality standards to the training and certification of imagery practitioners. Quality assurance is largely based on direct observation of clinical work in small group and individual supervision sessions during the training program. Each candidate is observed by four to six different faculty members during their 52 hr of supervision. We know of no other such standards of quality assurance established for imagery practitioners.

Information about the Academy's certification criteria and training programs can be obtained by using the contact information listed in the resources section.

## Reimbursement Status

Practitioners usually bill and are reimbursed for their work with imagery in the same way they are for other professional services. The work is usually identified as psychotherapy, counseling, stress reduction training, or medical hypnosis. When applied for medical purposes, medical practitioners may ethically bill for medical services, although insurance companies may challenge this if services are lengthy and repetitive. There are currently no separate billing codes for guided imagery or Interactive Guided Imagery.

Recently, however, insurance companies, including Blue Shield of California and American Specialty Health, nationally have been making guided imagery self-care tapes available to their insured members as a benefit. We anticipate that insurance for individual sessions with approved practitioners will soon follow.

## Relations With Conventional Medicine

Most physicians recognize the importance of attitude, stress, and mind/body effects in medicine but are not well trained to help patients with these issues. Imagery and visualization are increasingly accepted practices with both patients and physicians, and both have deeply penetrated our culture, especially in working with cancer patients. Although physicians continue to be wary about the promulgation of unrealistic expectations, and are rightly concerned that patients with potentially treatable serious disease do not substitute imagery for more definitive medical or surgical procedures, they are becoming increasingly more open to utilizing adjunctive mind/body approaches to healing.

Several studies have recently shown that almost 60% of physicians refer to the top five complementary approaches, with stress reduction, imagery, meditation, and hypnosis being the leading modalities. In addition, physicians utilize these services even more frequently for themselves and their families (Borkan, 1994).

## Summary

Imagery is a potent form of adjunctive treatment with a wide range of uses in cancer care. It is a simple yet profoundly effective, inexpensive, and safe form of care that allows patients to participate in their own process of healing. This attribute alone provides a benefit, although other significant benefits frequently accrue. Imagery is very rarely used as a sole form of treatment for cancer, yet it is almost always helpful in combination with nearly any other type of treatment.

When one examines almost every form of human therapeutic communication, imagery is centrally involved, simply because it is a fundamental language of the nervous system. All mind/body approaches rely heavily on imagery for their effects, whether for relaxation, meditation (which paradoxically teaches people to focus their minds so as to *not* be overwhelmed by negative imagery), biofeedback, hypnosis, or psychotherapy. The healing professions are learning more about the best ways to utilize these potent forms of thought to support good health and healing.

## REFERENCES AND RESOURCES

### Professional Training

Academy for Guided Imagery
    1-800-726-2070
    www.interactiveimagery.com
Mind Body Medicine Center, Washington, DC
    www.mbmc.org

### Guided Imagery Self-Care Books and Tapes

The Imagery Store
    415-389-9324
    www.interactiveimagery.com
American Specialty Health Guided Imagery Programs
    www.healthyroads.com
Belleruth Naparstek tapes
    www.healthjourneys.com

### Imagery Groups for People With Cancer

Simonton Cancer Center, Pacific Palisades, CA
    www.simontoncenter.com

Achterberg, J., Dossey, B., & Kolkmeier, L. (1994). *Rituals of healing: Using imagery for health and wellness*. New York: Bantam Doubleday Dell.

Agras, W. S. (1981). Behavioral approaches to the treatment of essential hypertension. *International Journal of Obesity, 5*(Suppl. 1), 173–181.

Assagioli, R. (1965). *Psychosynthesis*. New York: The Viking Press.

Baider, L., Peretz, T., Hadani, P. E., & Koch, U. (2000). Psychological intervention in cancer patients: A randomized study. *General Hospital Psychiatry, 23*(5), 272–277.

Barabasz, M., & Spiegel, D. (1989). Hypnotizability and weight loss in obese subjects. *International Journal of Eating Disorders, 8*(3), 335–341.

Barasch, M. I. (1995). *The healing path: A soul approach to illness*. New York: Penguin.

Bennet, H. L., Benson, D. R., & Kuiken, D. A. (1986). Preoperative instructions for decreased bleeding during spine surgery. *Anesthesiology, 65*, A245.

Bisson, J. I. (1995). Taped imaginal exposure as a treatment for post-traumatic stress reduction. *Journal of the Royal Army Medical Corps, 141*, 20–25.

Borkan, J. Neher, J. O., Anson, O., & Smoker, B. (1994). Referrals for alternative therapies. *Journal of Family Practice, 39*(6), 545–550.

Brown-Saltzman, K. (1997). Replenishing the spirit by meditative prayer and guided imagery. *Seminars in Oncology Nursing, 13*(4), 255–259.

Burish, T. G. (1987). Conditioned side effects induced by cancer chemotherapy: Prevention through behavioral treatment. *Journal of Consulting and Clinical Psychology, 55*(1), 42–48.

Caruso, P., & Helge, T. (1999). *Imagery in chemotherapy. Unpublished doctoral dissertation, CSPP, Alameda/Berkeley.*

Cochrane, G., & Friesen, J. (1986). Hypnotherapy in weight loss treatment. *Journal of Consulting and Clinical Psychology, 54*, 489–492.

Covino, N. A., & Frankel, F. H. (1993). Hypnosis and relaxation in the medically ill. *Psychotherapy and Psychosomatics, 60*(2), 75–90.

Cunningham, A. J., Edmonds, C. V., Phillips, C., Soots, K. I., Hedley, D., & Lockwood, G. A. (2000). A prospective, longitudinal study of the relationship of psychological work to duration of survival in patients with metastatic cancer. *Psychooncology, 9*(4), 323–339.

Dahlquist, L. M. (1985). Behavioral management of children is distress during chemotherapy. *Journal of Behavior Therapy & Experimental Psychiatry, 16*(4), 325–329.

Disbrow, E. A., Bennett, H. L., & Owings, J. T. (1993). Preoperative suggestion hastens the return of gastrointestinal mobility. *Western Journal of Medicine, XX*, 333–333.

Dossey, L. (1997). *Prayer is good medicine: How to reap the healing benefits of prayer.* New York: Harper-Collins.

Dossey, L. (1999). *Reinventing medicine: Beyond mind-body to a new era of healing.* New York: Harper-Collins.

Fawzy, F. I., Fawzy, N. W., Hyun, C. S., Elashoff, R., Guthrie, D., Fahey, J. L., & Morton, D. L. (2003). Malignant melanoma: Effects of an early structured psychiatric intervention, coping, and affective state on recurrence and survival 6 years later. *Archives of General Psychiatry, 50*(9), 681–689.

Gruber, B. L., Hersh, S. P., Hall, N. R., Waletzky, L. R., Kunz, J. F., Carpenter, et al. (1993). Immunological responses of breast cancer patients to behavioral interventions. *Biofeedback and Self Regulation, 18*(1), 1–22.

Hall, H., Minnes, L., & Olness, K. (1993). The psychophysiology of voluntary immunomodulation. *International Journal of Neuroscience, 69*(1–4), 221–234.

Krueger, L. C. (1987). Pediatric pain and imagery. *Journal of Child & Adolescent Psychiatry, 4*(1), 32–41.

Krystal, S., & Zweben, J. (1989). The use of visualization as a means of integrating the spiritual dimension into treatment. II. Working with emotions. *Journal of Substance Abuse Treatment, 6*(4), 223–228.

LeShan, L. (1999). *Cancer as a turning point: A handbook for people with cancer, their families, and health professionals.* New York: Touchstone.

McDonald, R. T., & Hilgendorf, W. A. (1986). Death imagery and death anxiety. *Journal of Clinical Psychology, 42*(1), 87–91.

Miller, E. (1997). *Deep healing: The essence of mind/body medicine.* Oceanside, CA: Hay House.

National Institutes of Health. (1996). Integration of behavioral and relaxation approaches into the treatment of chronic pain and insomnia. NIH Technology Assessment Panel on Integration of Behavioral and Relaxation Approaches into the Treatment of Chronic Pain and Insomnia. *Journal of the American Medical Association, 276*(4), 313–318.

Remen, R. N. (1997). *Kitchen table wisdom: Stories that heal.* New York: Riverhead Books.

Richardson, M. A., Post-White, J., Grimm, E. A., Moye, L. A., Singletary, S. E., & Justice, B. (1997). Coping, life attitudes, and immune responses to imagery and group support after breast cancer treatment. *Alternative Therapies in Health and Medicine, 3*(5), 62–70.

Rossi, E. (1999). *The psychobiology of mind-body healing: New concepts of therapeutic hypnosis* (rev. ed.). New York: W. W. Norton.

Rossman, M. (2000). *Guided imagery for self-healing.* New York: Kramer/New World Library.

Sheikh, A. A. (Ed.). (1989). The potential of fantasy and imagination. *Lancet, 2*(8668), 888–891.

Shinoda Boden, J. (1998). *Close to the bone: Life-threatening illness and the search for meaning.* New York: Touchstone Books.

Shrock, D. (1999). Group intervention in breast and prostate cancer patients. *Alternative Therapies in Health and Medicine, 4*, 333–444.

Simonton, O. C., Matthew-Simonton, S., & Creighton, J. L. (1992). *Getting well again*. New York: Bantam Books.

Siegel, B. S. (1990). *Peace, love and healing: Body-mind communication and the path to self-healing: An exploration*. New York: Harper Perennial Library.

Spiegel, D., Bloom, J. R., Kraemer, H. C., & Gottheil, E. (1989). Effect of psychosocial treatment on survival of patients with metastatic breast cancer. *Lancet, 2*(8668), 888–891.

Syrjala, K. L., Donaldson, G. W., Davis, M. W., Kippes, M. E., & Carr, J. E. (1995). Relaxation and imagery and cognitive-behavioral training reduce pain during cancer treatment: A controlled clinical trial. *Pain, 63*, 189–198.

Troesch, L. M., Rodehaver, C. B., Delaney, E. A., & Yanes, B. (1993). The influence of guided imagery on chemotherapy-related nausea and vomiting. *Oncology Nursing Forum, 20*(8), 1179–1185.

Tusek, D. L. (1997). Guided imagery: A significant advance in the care of patients undergoing elective colorectal surgery. *Diseases of the Colon and Rectum, 40*(2), 172–178.

Watkins, J. G., & Watkins, H. H. (1979). In H. Grayson (Ed.), *The theory and practice of ego-state therapy, in short-term approaches to psychotherapy*. New York: National Institute for the Psychotherapies and Human Sciences Press.

Wynd, C. A. (1992). Relaxation imagery used for stress reduction in the prevention of smoking relapse. *Journal of Advanced Nursing, 17*, 294–302.

6

Ilene Serlin

## Introduction

Expressive therapies are a powerful tool for mind/body healing, and their use as a complementary therapy can greatly enrich the range of those therapies. The intention of this chapter is to explain what expressive therapies are and demonstrate their role in an integrative treatment team and clinical setting and out in the community. Practitioners who are interested in bringing these practices into their own work are encouraged to explore further training. Although this chapter cannot provide that training, it can point out some of its underlying premises, processes, and applications. Additional resources for further study are provided at the end of the chapter.

Medicine has traditionally addressed issues of personal and community health but has also carried a 19th-century worldview of science and an image of the healer deity. However, a shift is happening in the way medicine is being viewed and practiced (Sperry, 1995). The popularity of Bill Moyer's show *Healing and the Mind* on alternative healing and the revelation in the January 28, 1993, issue of *The New England Journal of Medicine* that over one-third of Americans were then utilizing "unconventional medicine" signal a major shift in attitudes toward healing. This trend is growing (Dittman, 2004; Eisenberg et al., 1998; Gazella, 2004). At the National Institutes of Health, the U.S. Congress funded an Office of Alternative Medicine to support research into alternative approaches. Now called the National Center for Complementary and Alternative Medicine, its budget has been growing yearly. The new views of medicine are bringing about new imagery and metaphors for the healing professions. For example, a growing number of patients and health care practitioners see medicine with its roots in ancient healing practices and the physician as a wounded healer (Kabat-Zinn, 1994). Healing is distinguished from curing; whereas curing seeks to reduce symptoms or prolong life in a *quantitative* sense, healing is a process to improve the *quality* of life (Dossey, 1992). Healing brings an understanding of the meaning and full experience of symptoms (Dossey, 1991), the role of the mind in illness, and the centrality of imagery in the expression and relief of human suffering (Achterberg, 1985).

Western high-technology scientific medicine, in its effort to separate reason and science from religion, has excluded subjective experience and the "irrational." Expressive therapies bring this dimension back into the healing process. Understanding the meaning of the illness can bring acceptance, which relieves a good part of the suffering. Symbolic expression of the experience of living with illness is indirect and less threatening than direct expression. Therefore, patients can move beyond acceptance to a deeper confrontation with mortality and an awareness of the preciousness of life. The transformative power of the arts can be mobilized by recalling images of the healer as artist and shaman, connecting illness through meaning back to its roots in soul (McNiff, 1992).

The art therapies use a symbolic language of image, symbol, metaphor, myth, body, and ritual. They can convey images of both individual and collective ills, like the individual existential crisis portrayed in Munch's well-known figure of *The Scream,* or in the image of a whole society at war, as in Picasso's *Guernica.* Rollo May, the eminent American existential-analytic psychologist, understood the artist to be a prophet or a mirror of society. Expressing the soul of a culture takes courage. Facing death and still creating takes a leap of faith. Creating in the face of the void or the blank page or one's own mortality is a metaphor for the creative act in everyday life (May, 1975). The arts are both a modern and an ancient form of healing. As preventive health, art helped maintain the individual's balance among spirit, soul, and body, illustrating patterns of connection between the individual, the community, and nature.

The expressive therapies are especially useful to us today because they provide a cost-effective complement to traditional medicine. The creative force awakened in the healing arts is a powerful medicine when used in the service of healing. With this force, people are better equipped to face life with energy, flexibility, improvisational skills, an enriched inner life, and stronger resources. Through the arts, people can express their experience and meaning of having an illness, explore their own imagery and resources for healing, and decrease loneliness by sharing rhythmic and nonverbal connections with others (Goodill, 2005). In 1998, a survey showed that although 42% of Americans use alternative therapies, most do not inform their physicians of this use. To coordinate and maximize the different aspects of their patients' health care, therefore, it is helpful for physicians to know about their patients' use of complementary medical practices, such as expressive therapy (Eisenberg et al., 1998).

# What Is Expressive Therapy?

Expressive therapy is a psychotherapy that employs the arts and an indirect symbolic language to help patients deal with emotional, cognitive, and physical challenges. Expressive therapists often work with physicians in treating patients as diverse as those with breast cancer, cardiac illness, stress, and strokes. They are employed in all kinds of settings—in clinics, hospitals, special schools, and private practice. They work with individuals, groups, couples, and families. They work with adults, children, and geriatric patients. When they are part of a treatment team approach to medical care, expressive therapists can help ease some of the fears patients have about medical treatment, as well as their accompanying physical and psychologic issues. In particular, expressive therapists work with the debilitating depression and anxiety caused by life-threatening illness and treatment and help patients rebuild their lives.

Expressive therapy has been defined as follows:

> An orientation or an approach to therapy, rather than a series of techniques or tools. Underlying such an approach is a value system that believes in the inherent worth of creative expression and the importance in making the excitement and joy that originates in our innermost symbols find some expression in our outer behavior. (Robbins, 1986, p. 38)

Congruence between one's inner and outer realities is the primary goal of therapy, says Robbins. The process is improvisatory, with the therapist tracking, clarifying, and sometimes challenging the patient's images. These images are "verbal, visual, spatial, kinesthetic and aural" (Robbins, 1986, p. 17), to which the therapist responds with an equal "ability to see, hear, and experience his patients on a . . . visceral level" (Robbins, p. 20). Thus, many expressive therapies are multimodal, using either one primary modality or a mix of modalities to reflect the complex world of the patient. By containing the many levels and seeming contradictions of the patients' world, the expressive therapist helps the patient contain his or her own complexities.

For example, if a patient is experiencing extreme grief, he or she may not be verbal about it; in fact, prematurely verbalizing emotions can prevent or disguise the real experience of them. Symbolic or creative processes, however, are indirect forms of expression that provide some distance from the experience. Because of this relative safety, they allow patients to go deeper into their grief, understanding its meaning and feeling its full force. The symbolic expression helps to contain the enormous grief while giving it a form through which it can be resolved or transformed. This grief can be expressed in a drawing, a dance, lines of poetry, or in nuances of silence (Freud, 1959). The therapist picks up on it, using words or rhythms or images, and the experience is deeply shared. Through dialogue, the loneliness of carrying the illness alone is reduced. Through the connection with the warm and facilitative presence of the therapist, the patient can reexperience and release old memories and feelings, thus opening channels of deep healing.

# Origins of Expressive Therapies

What are the origins of expressive therapies? Images of healing appear in the early creation stories and in ancient healing practices (Bartenieff, 1972–1973). For example, the Ring Dance was basic to all mystery celebrations in the Mediterranean. The celebration of the Eleusian Mysteries "was combined with a ring dance which appears to have begun when the spirit emerged from its symbolic underworld journey and reached the splendid fields of the blessed" (Backman, 1972, p. 3). Midsummer dances, which are still performed in Scandinavia, originated in the 10th century with pagan dances in which dancers would go to the streams, dance in a circle around a fire, heap flowers, and leap through the flames, purging themselves with smoke and fire. This dance was intended to cure illness and also as preventive medicine to bring good health and harvests. The leader, or shaman, is an image for the expressive arts therapist as a wounded healer who is close to the sacred sources of healing. Combining art, ritual, diagnosis, and treatment, the expressive therapist helps restores the individual's courage to create life and find balance in relation to his or her community and world  (Serlin, 1993).

## Storytelling as Healing Art

The act of shaping raw material or emotion into symbol or image is healing, as it helps objectify the emotions, get some distance from them, and make active discriminations to portray them (Feinstein & Krippner, 1988; Jung, 1966; Serlin, 1999). The very act of telling a difficult story in the presence of empathetic others is at the heart of the  talking and narrative therapies, allowing the teller to experience him- or herself with respect and compassion. This shift transforms "affliction" . . . into "a powerful teacher" who brings "a turning point in one's life" (Kabat-Zinn, 1994, pp. xvi–xvii) so we feel ". . . like an important if not crucial participant in what is happening in our lives, with at least some degree of influence and control" (Kabat-Zinn, p. xvii).

Art has always healed, as the Greeks knew. As Aristotle explained, the function of art in Greek drama was to promote an identification with and working through emotional blocks via mimetic action and symbol. The working through was accompanied by *catharsis*, which cleansed the psyche. Art, therefore, functioned as a collective healing ritual.

## Applications of Expressive Therapy

Finally, movement rituals with roots in traditional religious practices have applications in everyday life today. For example, expressive therapy has been used successfully with patients with life-threatening illness to help them regain feelings of self-esteem and control over their lives. Studies show that expressive therapy can help patients cope with pain and ease depression, increase vitality, and improve body image  (Cohen & Walco, 1999; Serlin, Classen, Frances, & Angell, 2000).

Like other forms of psychotherapy, expressive therapy helps people control high blood pressure and manage migraine headaches. Breast cancer patients who participate in group psychotherapy are known to survive longer than those who do not (Spiegel et al., 1989). Studies show that psychotherapy can reduce risks for heart disease, cancer, and HIV, according to the American Psychological Association. Dean Ornish has shown that a diet plan, combined with stress-reducing yoga and stretching, may help reverse heart disease. Dance therapy draws on stretching and yogalike movements, integrating them with imagery and expression and a strong therapeutic relationship and building on these benefits. Stroke patients in expressive therapy classes attain needed exercise and build their coordination skills, as well as getting a boost in self-esteem.

In expressive therapy, the patient learns to transform illness or physical pain through the sheer joy of movement. In addition to cancer, stroke, and heart disease, expressive therapy may help with the following illnesses by providing exercise, emotional release and stress reduction: chronic fatigue, high blood pressure, fibromyalgia, and chronic pain.

# How Does Expression Affect Health?

Expressive therapies rest on the belief that mind and body are interrelated (Rossi, 1986). The work of Candace Pert has shown that the processing of emotions often affects physical illnesses and the ability to heal. Neuropeptide receptors in the brain and throughout the body are associated with emotional processing. They help regulate immunocyte trafficking and bolster the immune system. Research on healthy humans, as well as cancer and HIV-positive patients, has shown significant increases in immune function or positive health outcomes with emotional expression, such as that practiced in dance therapy (Pert, 1997). These findings suggest that emotional expression generates balance in the neuropeptide receptor network, which contributes to a functional healing system. Also, evidence that the expression of emotion is healthy was demonstrated by Pennebaker (1990), in his study of college students who kept a journal of their feelings and thoughts. Continuing the use of his experimental design, he collaborated with dance therapist Anne Krantz to explore the impact of dance therapy on health (Krantz & Pennebaker, 1993). Finally, neurological correlates of altered states have been investigated by Valerie Hunt in her laboratory at UCLA (Hunt, 1984).

Expressive therapy also addresses specifically psychologic functions. The physical and emotional expression of expressive therapy eases stress and increases healthy body image and self-esteem. Such treatments are vital in our society, where nearly half of Americans between the ages of 15 and 54 experience a psychologic disorder during their lifetime. As many as 75% of all patient visits in primary care practice, in fact, can be attributed to psychosocial problems that present through physical complaints, according to the American Psychological Association.

## Benefits of Expressive Therapy

The benefits of addressing these psychologic health problems are obvious. The economic burden of depression in our society is high. Statistics show that depression in the American workplace may cost as much as $43 billion, and depression is high in patients with cancer and other life-threatening illnesses. Expressive therapy, through the free expression of intense and preverbal emotions, is effective alone or with medications for some patients. The American Psychological Association supports the claim that cognitive and interpersonal psychotherapies, such as expressive therapy, have proven to be beneficial and effective treatments for depression.

Expressive therapy can also help address denial and resistance, fear and anxiety, grief and loss, isolation, and eating disorders. The ability to develop their own narratives helps patients regain their own voices, decrease depression and hopelessness, and increase psychologic well-being and life satisfaction, according to a study by researchers  Haight,

Michel, and Hendrix (2000) in the *International Journal of Human Development*. Because it also provides a physical outlet, expressive therapy can also improve skills such as coordination in stroke patients.

## Patients as Partners in Their Treatment Process

Expressive therapy may also help patients cope with their fear of medical treatments. Expressive therapists can work with physicians to teach patients how to listen to their own body wisdom and make confident choices about medical procedures. The therapists may create individualized audiotapes, for example, using the patients' own imagery to help them prepare for medical procedures.

Expressive therapy may ease anxiety reactions before examinations, mastectomy, reconstructive surgery, cosmetic surgery, general surgery, use of needles to give medications, and compliance with aftercare.

The arts can also be a powerful aid to counteract the adverse effects of the dehumanization of medicine. For example, one patient described her radiation treatments as follows:

> The simulation, which is the preparation for treatment where they take all the measurements, was . . . it was sort of like an acid trip really. It was so surreal. . . . You know, the room is very sterile and there's the big machine in there . . . and the whole thing involves four or five different people who come and go out of the room . . . you're alone in the room while they do an X-ray. They run out of the room. They'll make a mark on you. . . . Take an X-ray. Come back. Someone else will come in. They'll measure something. They make a little mark with a marking pen on your breast. And I felt almost like I was being sacrificed to some strange god. . . . Somehow I have been the one who was captured and I was being offered up, I guess, to the radiation machine.

Not only was the dehumanization distressing and disorienting, but it also kept her from functioning in her everyday life. A single mother with two children, she had to take care of herself while taking care of two children and a complicated life. With the shrinking resources of hospitals, patients have to do much of their own aftercare, which needs the kind of full energy and concentration unavailable to those undergoing debilitating treatments. This woman noted:

> But, you know, when I finished the simulation and I came out, I was in a semi-trance for about an hour. . . . We walked out of the clinic. I really wasn't sure where I was. That was the first time I got lost. This was the beginning of my getting lost.
>
> It all started with the simulation and then after that, every time I went in for a treatment, I would get lost. . . . And then I'd leave and I couldn't find my car and I lost my car every day for a week. . . . It was very upsetting, and I was afraid to stop and do any errands on the way home because I thought I'd forget where I left my car again. . . . I was really, really spaced out by the whole experience. I remember thinking maybe I was getting radiation to the brain.

Are these experiences inevitable? Can anything be done to counteract them? Yes, certain ways of moving and feeling can counteract feelings of dehumanization. Some practices, such as Authentic Movement (Adler, 1972), help people rediscover their core experiences and bodily memories. Changing dehumanizing hospital environments into healing spaces is even the focus of a new profession of health care architects and a group called the Society for the Arts in Healthcare. This is an interdisciplinary group, bringing their thinking about health from a variety of perspectives. One example of such a healing environment is the healing garden at Marin General Hospital. In this garden, a patient could sit in peace before a medical procedure, thus having a chance to reflect and ready him or herself in advance. Patients who have a voice in the design of their healing rituals generally report a better adaptation to it. A total treatment plan, therefore, optimizes emotional and physical healing by creating a healing environment in which patients feel free to discover their own healing movements and images.

For example, this patient noted:

> So the things that we did in the group were really helpful. We developed a ritual to help me back into my body. We did some movements on the floor that were sort of comforting and rocking and sort of womb-like. It relaxed me quite a bit to do those movements and, after that, whenever I felt anxious, I actually went home and I did movement, not necessarily on the floor, but some sort of dance movement, some repetitive rocking type of movement, and it helped a lot. It's important to get going again, to revive yourself, to begin to move and feel alive . . . that's where movement starts, the center of gravity, the center of the wave.

Another patient described her discovery that movement mobilized her life energy:

> Meaning like when I walk into the group sometimes I'm real constricted, my body is constricted, I'm stressed, I'm tensed, you know, and then all of a sudden we start with some of the conversation, the movement, the stories and I'm just a different human being. It gives spaciousness to my cells so it allows them to breathe and allows them to flow more freely and then it gives spaciousness to my spirit because all of a sudden I'm free, and joy or pain or whatever comes out. So that's where I find the healing in the work.

# Releasing Creative and Sexual Energy

The movement allowed her to access repressed parts of herself, explore herself as a *woman* and use the unleashed creativity for healing:

> . . . when we were dancing with the scarves. I was in there and what I got in touch with was how, when I was a young girl, I kind of shut down to my femininity . . . and really to the freedom that I felt. I went back and remembered that, even when I was in first grade, I loved to dance. . . . I remember my father saying that I was fat or something like that, and that I would never dance again. In the group I got in touch with that pain . . . and then I danced my dance. Out of that it freed up in me . . . the joy and the love that comes into my life from it. Also, the essential woman who has been in there was really afraid to

come out because, to me, it was always bad to be that way and bad to be interested in sensuality and sexuality.

*Self-care* is another benefit of healing practices that use group support. Through this support with others in a similar situation, patients learn to treat themselves with compassion and patience. The arts teach about pacing, space, and balance, elements needed to restore the experience of balance in life. Mary Catherine Bateson says: "Today, the materials and skills from which a life is composed are no longer clear. It is no longer possible to follow the paths of previous generations . . . A good meal, like a poem or a life, has a certain balance and diversity, a certain coherence and fit" (Bateson, 1989, pp. 2–4).

For example, one woman wrote:

And so I see that happening in the group where people are learning to take care of themselves . . . and therefore enhancing the creative process because, as I find as I take care of myself, all of a sudden I see what I'm willing to do and not willing to do and I have more space to do what I want to do.

She was able to translate this individual balance into a sense of balance within her group:

I will carry it as a renewed sense of who I am in a group . . . of being apart of a group of women and will carry over some of the artistic expressions . . . when I have something I need to express . . . rather than sit with it or not share it. . . .

Creativity teaches us this freedom and gives us resources and new alternatives. Hungarian psychoanalyst Susan Deri writes, "The creative side of life-enhancing good gestalts always implies a considerable plus on the side of Eros, of libido, which counteracts inertia and disintegration" (Deri, 1988, pp. 13–14).

# Cancer as a Metaphor

Expressive therapies help patients get in touch with that part of cancer that is symbolic and understand what it means. The meaning of the illness is expressed through imagery and metaphor.

One image that appeared with frequency was that of *speed*. Women in a support group at the Institute of Health and Healing at California Pacific Medical Center drew pictures of frenzied lines and talked of the overwhelming speed of modern life, of lacking time to rest, to digest, or to reflect. A cancer cell can be seen symbolically as a cell out of control, speeding and multiplying crazily. These pathologies of time, space, and composition, disorders of postmodernity, show up in the experience and symbolic representation of disconnection and speed in the body.

One woman, talking about this sense of speed, wrote:

What is cancer? Cancer is a cell that goes out of control. I think that's what's happening is that as a people we're out of control. We don't connect. It's a power kind of society and we need more support and more connections from each other. . . . With the technological revolution, we deplete our immune systems and therefore allow these opportunistic diseases to come in.

The meaning of the image of speed spoke to her perception of her daily life:

> So it's pretty lonely being an isolated woman in the 90's, I think. We think we've made it, but we haven't. I think we've lost it more than anything.

The symptom of *disconnection* was replaced by a new one of *connection*:

> I don't know what that means, art. . . . I know that in the group it's happened consistently that as we draw, all of a sudden people's drawings reflect each others' . . . sometimes I'm sitting next to a person I feel particularly connected to that day, and our drawings reflect the same kind of color or issue, or sometimes it's loneliness or sometimes it's anger and sometimes it's sadness or sometimes it's fire, sometimes it's isolation and the reds, the heat, or the green or the explosions of color when people feel energetic. It seems like there's very much an alignment going on in that particular process in the group. By opening it up, the creative process transforms life.

In today's postmodern world, we must ask ourselves how to live with the fragmentation and isolation. Much has been written about the problems of a postmodern society, but not much has been written about how to live with it. Do we surrender to despair? Or do we have enough existential freedom and resources to create a constructive alternative? Community healing rituals use practices from around the world "to enable the individual to help and sustain others" (His Holiness the Dalai Lama, 1999, p. 67).

# Healing the Family

Expressive therapy can involve the entire family as well. Friends and family members can participate in expressive therapy sessions and contribute to their loved one's emotional and physical health. Communication and emotional bonds within families can be strengthened by such participation. Improved communications helps family members deal with the illness of a member, so they can be more supportive in the healing process.

# Ecologic Body

The inability of the body to feel, to grieve its losses and the trauma of the Earth, has been related by contemporary theorists to our current ecologic crisis and the threat of extinction (Macy, 1991). We have become numb, inanimate. Susan Griffin makes a powerful case for the need to feel, to wake up, to bear witness to the suffering of human beings and of the planet when she says:

> . . . For perhaps we are like stones; our own history and the history of the world embedded in us, we hold a sorrow deep within and cannot weep until that history is sung. (Griffin, 1992, pp. 6–8)

The symptom of disconnection from self from others as a consequence of the Western, heroic, male myth of independence has often been described. In fact, the moment of self-consciousness, of separate identity, of the shift kinesthetic to visual perception, has been described by some as the beginning of alienation from the world (Berman, 1989). Singing, or telling the story, reminds us to bear witness to each other's stories and to the story of the Earth. Awakening to our own sense perceptions and embodied reactions of fear, grief, and compassion, we reconnect to the Earth. One image that came from a group dance is as follows:

> I liked a lot of the exercises where we would bend low and swoop up the earth and bring that energy up and then down through us. I think that is a movement I could continue to employ in my life. I think that whole sense of trying to stay grounded.... I look at in a different way, it is a beneficial thing to me to be rooted and grounded on the planet.

Drawing on the Gaia hypothesis (Lovelock, 1979), which suggests that the Earth is a living organism and our bodies and the Earth partake of the same elements, Roszak (1992, p. 93) reminds us that modern science and psychology have shifted our cosmologies away from the animistic worldview of "primitive" people who understood the whole world to be alive and who painted, sang, and danced about the forces animating their world. Some alternative and complementary medicine practices, however, such as acupuncture and a new area of medicine called "energy medicine," use a similar understanding of animating forces to facilitate the body's natural healing.

## Healing Rituals in the Community

Because they do not need expensive technological equipment, the arts can take the patient out of a clinical setting into his or her naturalistic setting. The integration back into community and movement away from an illness to a wellness model helps patients recover. The following are examples of community healing rituals that have pioneered this use of arts and healing.

## Movement Choirs

Rudolf von Laban (1879–1958) developed a system of space harmonics and dance, a highly sophisticated movement notation system used for diagnosis, research, and treatment. As a grandfather of modern dance, he developed a movement scale based on qualitative factors of movement. During the early 1900s, he created a series of large-scale events that involved whole villages moving in choirs together. Like singing together, this choir helped bring large groups of people into shared activities (Laban, 1980). In 1976, the form of movement choirs was introduced to the American Dance Therapy Association by Laban's student, Irmgard Bartenieff (Bartenieff, 1972–1973). In 1996, they were pioneered at the Race for the Cure to open the race. This race is an annual fundraiser, sponsored by the Susan G. Komen Foundation and other breast cancer associations, which gathers thousands of people together in Golden Gate Park, San Francisco. In the meadow, participants created circles of movement that, like a folk dance, brought people together and focused their energies. In 1997, the circles were expanded to include the annual Hike Against the Odds, sponsored by the Breast Cancer Fund, featuring a climb up Mount Tamalpais in Marin County.

# Conflict Resolution

Two expressive arts therapists from Lesley College and the Boston Arts Institute have developed a method of working directly with community healing projects through the arts. Calling it a "developmental approach," Marcow-Speiser and Speiser use a multimodal arts process to conflict resolution (personal communication, 2001). They describe their intention as follows:

> Working with the arts promotes the value of social relatedness among individuals of different backgrounds, through arts based activities which explore cultural differences and similarities. This approach is a cornerstone for developing conflict resolution and violence prevention strategies. These strategies emerge directly from the participants themselves and reflect their needs as related to their work places and communities.

Working directly with cultural symbols and narratives, the group leaders help participants recognize images of "common humanity" and "individual expression," mobilize and focus their energies, and use conflict for constructive change.

# Tamalpa Institute

Another example of a community-based healing arts project is the independent Tamalpa Institute, cofounded by Anna and Daria Halprin. Tamalpa takes support groups for cancer patients out into nature and sponsors a yearly healing dance called "Circle the Earth." In this dance, people who need healing are combined with families and other community members to celebrate Mount Tamalpais and draw from its healing energies.

# UCSF Cancer Support Group

Using movement and other art forms to amplify and work through themes also characterizes the work of Anne Krantz, a psychologist and movement therapist who started a support group for cancer patients in the winter/spring of 1996, as part of the program of the Cancer Resource Center of the UCSF Clinical Cancer Center (former UCSF/Mt. Zion Hospital). It meets weekly throughout the year, is open to both men and women with a variety of cancer diagnoses, and is an open group, free to the public. Based on the work of dance therapist pioneer Blanche Evans, it uses a semistructured format that flexibly follows the energy level and thematic material of the group and is based on improvisation. Krantz describes it as follows:

> Often the thematic content comes from the participants and focuses on dealing with cancer related health issues or on aspects of their psychophysical experiences of life.

such as dealing with loss, death, pain, trauma, the unknown, and change. We start with the body and what each person comes in with. The warm-up is both educative about the body's potential for movement, and oriented to self-directed movement, guided by subjective experience.

The goals of the group include the following healing skills: "the skill of listening to one's body, feeling more of what is there, interpreting the signals, such as pain or fatigue" . . . or "applications of their group work toward their life situations, what they will be facing today, this week, etc., so there is a reality focus as well" (personal communication, November 11, 2001). Psychologically and spiritually, the "group is very life-affirming and inspiring for all of us."

## Art for Recovery

Another healing arts project at the California Pacific Medical Center is "Art for Recovery," run by artist and cancer activist Cindy Perlis. Although Perlis and her students take their art to the patients' bedside, they are probably most known for their cancer quilt, which has become a traveling art show. Perlis and group take less of a clinical approach, and more of a community- and arts-based approach, to recovery.

## Art With Children

At Shands Hospital in Florida, John Graham-Poole, pediatric oncologist, poet, and clown, Mary Lane, nurse and artist, and their colleagues have created a beautiful environment that helps children with cancer cope. They have painted stars and clouds on the ceiling, hung the walls with only original patient art, and brought artists in from the community to create art with the patients. The hospital has become a gallery for their works, making it an environment devoted more to health than to illness (Rockwood & Graham-Pole, 1994).

## Summary

In conclusion, the arts are both a modern and an ancient form of healing. As preventive medicine, they have helped people maintain their balance among spirit, soul, and body and harmonize the patterns of connection among themselves, the community, and the cycles and forces of nature. Expressive therapy helps many kinds of patients express their emotions, and share and dissipate their fears. It provides a way for them to deal with chronic illnesses and live healthier lives. In today's health care environment, the expressive therapist offers holistic solutions for physicians and patients. The expressive therapist is, in essence, a healer who combines art, ritual, diagnosis, and treatment to restore patients' insight and well-being.

# REFERENCES AND RESOURCES

Achterberg, J. (1985). *Imagery in healing*. Boston: News Science Library.

Adler, J. (1972). Body and soul. *American Journal of Dance Therapy, 14*(2), 73–94.

Aldridge, D. (1998). Life as jazz: Hope, meaning, and music therapy in the treatment of life-threatening illness. *Advances in Mind/Body Medicine, 14*, 271–282.

American Art Therapy Association. 1202 Allanson Road, Mundelein, IL 60060; (847) 949-6064.

American Dance Therapy Association. 2000 Century Plaza, Columbia, MD 21044; (410) 997-4040. Retrieved from http://www.adta.org

*American Journal of Dance Therapy*. New York: Human Sciences Press.

Backman, L. (1972). *Religious dances*. London: Allen & Unwin, Ltd.

Bartenieff, I. (1972–1973). Dance therapy: A new profession or a rediscovery of an ancient role of the dance. *Dance Scope, 7*(1), 6–18.

Bateson, M. C. (1989). *Composing a life*. New York: The Atlantic Monthly Press.

Berman, M. (1989). *Coming to our senses*. New York: Simon & Schuster.

Berrol, C. (1997). Dance/movement therapy with older adults who have sustained neurological insult: A demonstration project. *American Journal of Dance Therapy, 19*(2), 135–160.

Butler, R. (1980–1981). The life review: An unrecognized bonanza. *International Journal of Aging and Human Development, 12*(1), 35–38.

Cohen, S., & Walco, G. A. (1999). Dance/movement therapy for children and adolescents with cancer. *Cancer Practice, 7*(1), 34–42.

Chaiklin, S. (1969). Dance therapy. In *American Dance Therapy Association Proceedings* (pp. 25–31).

Dalai Lama. (1999). The relevance of Tibetan medicine today. *Alternative Therapies. 5*(3), 67–69.

Deri, S. (1988). *Symbolization and creativity*. Madison, WI: International Universities Press.

Dittman, M. (2004). Alternative health care gains steam. *American Psychological Association Monitor, 35*(6), 42.

Dossey, L. (1991). *Meaning and medicine*. New York: Bantam.

Dossey, L. (1992). Era III medicine: The next frontier. *ReVision: A Journal of Consciousness and Transformation, 14*(3), 128–139.

Eisenberg, D., Davis, R., Ettner, S., Appel, S., Wilkey, S., Van Rompay, M., et al. (1998). Trends in alternative medicine use in the United States, 1990–1997: Results of a follow-up national survey. *Journal of the American Medical Association, 280*(18), 1569–1575.

Feinstein, D., & Krippner, S. (1988). *Personal mythology*. Los Angeles: Jeremy P. Tarcher.

Freud, S. (1959). On the relation of the poet to daydreaming. In *On creativity and the unconscious*. New York: Colophon Books.

Gazella, K. (2004). Practicing medicine for the future. *Alternative Therapies, 10*(4), 83–89.

Goodill, S. (2005). *An introduction to medical dance/movement therapy*. London: Jessica Kingsley.

Griffin, S. (1992). *A chorus of stones*. New York: Doubleday.

Haight, B., Michel, Y., & Hendrix S. (2000). The extended effects of the life review in nursing home residents. *International Journal of Aging and Human Development, 50*(2), 151–168.

Hospital Audiences, Inc. 220 W. 42nd. St., New York, NY 10036. http://www. hospitalaudiences.org

Hunt, V. (1984). A cognitive psychology of mystical and altered-state experience. *Perception and Motor Skills, 58*, 467–513.

*International Journal of Arts Medicine*. c/o MMB, *MMB Music, Inc.* (good resource for creative arts therapy materials). Contemporary Arts Building. 3526 Washington Ave., St. Louis, MO 63103-1019. Mmbmusic@mmbmusic.com

Jung., C. (1966). On the relation of analytic psychology to poetry. In *The spirit in man, art and literature* (pp. 131–193). Princeton, NJ: Bollingen.

Junge, M., & Asawa, P. (1995). *A history of art therapy in the United States*. London: Jessica Kingsley.

Kabat-Zinn, J. (1994). Foreword. In M. Lerner (Ed.), *Choices in healing* (pp. xi–xvii). Cambridge, MA: The MIT Press.

Krantz, A. M., & Pennebaker, J. W. (1993). *Expression of traumatic experience through dance and writing: Psychological and health effects*. Unpublished manuscript.

Laban, R. (1980). *The mastery of movement*. Estover, Plymouth, UK: Macdonald and Evans, Ltd. (Original work published 1950)

Levick, M. (1969). Art therapy. In *American Dance Therapy Association Proceedings* (pp. 19–20). Columbia, MD: American Dance Therapy Association.

Levin, H. (1969). Music in therapy. In *American Dance Therapy Association Proceedings* (pp. 16–18). Columbia, MD: American Dance Therapy Association.

Lovelock, J. (1979). *Gaia: A new look at life on earth.* New York: Oxford University Press.

Macy, J. (1991). *World as lover, world as self.* Berkeley: Parallax.

May, R. (1975). *The courage to create.* New York: Bantam.

McNiff, S. (1992). *Art as medicine.* Boston: Shambala.

Pennebaker, J. (1990). *Opening up: The healing power of expressing emotions.* New York: Guilford.

Pert, C. (1997). *Molecules of emotion: Why you feel the way you feel.* New York: Charles Scribner and Sons.

Pert, C., Dreher, H., & Ruff, M. (1998). The psychosomatic network: Foundations of mind-body medicine. *Alternative Therapies in Health and Medicine, 4*(4), 30–41.

Robbins, A. (1986). *Expressive therapy: A creative arts approach to depth-oriented treatment.* New York: Human Sciences Press.

Rockwood, M., & Graham-Pole, J. (1994). Development of an art program on a bone marrow transplant unit. *Cancer Nursing, 17*(3), 185–192.

Rossi, E. L. (1986). *The psychobiology of mind-body healing.* New York: W. W. Norton.

Roszak, T. (1992). *The voice of the earth.* New York: Simon & Schuster.

Runco, M., & Richards, R. (Eds.). (1997). *Eminent creativity, everyday creativity, and health.* Greenwich, CT: Ablex.

Schover, L. (1994). Sexuality and body image in younger women with breast cancer. *Monograph of the National Cancer Institute, 16,* 177–182.

Serlin, I. (1993). Root images of healing in dance therapy. *American Dance Therapy Journal, 15*(2), 65–75.

Serlin, I. (1996). Interview with Anna Halprin. *American Journal of Dance Therapy, 18*(2), 115–123.

Serlin, I. A. (1999). Imagery, movement and breast cancer. In C. Clark (Ed.), *The encyclopedia of complementary health practices* (pp. 408–410). New York: Springer-Verlag.

Serlin, I., Classen, C., Frances, B., & Angell, K. (2000). Support groups for women with breast cancer: Traditional and alternative expressive approaches. *The Arts in Psychotherapy, 27*(2), 123–138.

Spiegel, D., Bloom, J., Kraemer, H., & Gottheil, E. (1989). Effect of psychosocial treatment on survival of patients with metastatic breast cancer. *Lancet, 2,* 888–891.

Sperry, R. W. (1995). The riddle of consciousness and the changing scientific worldview. *Journal of Humanistic Psychology, 35*(2), 7–34.

Spintge, R., & Droth, R. (1992). *MusicMedicine.* St. Louis, MO: MMB Music, Inc.

Society for the Arts in Healthcare (publishes a newsletter listing events and resources and sponsors a yearly interdisciplinary conference). 45 Lyme Rd., Suite 304 Hanover, NH 03755-1223. (603) 643-2325. HealthArts@aol,com.

Stern's Book Service (they carry many creative arts therapy books). 2004 W. Roscoe St., Chicago, IL 60618. (773) 883-5100.

University of California Extension, Center for Media and Independent Learning (creative arts therapy videotapes for rent or purchase). 2000 Center Street, Fourth Floor, Berkeley, CA 94704. (510) 642–0460.

Wadeson, H. (1980). *Art psychotherapy.* New York: Wiley.

Web site on creative arts therapies: http://plaza.interport.net/cats/

Weishaar, K. (1999). The visual life review as a therapeutic framework with the terminally ill. *The Arts in Psychotherapy, 26*(3), 173–184.

# Religion and Spirituality

Kent C. Shih

David Larson

## Introduction

Although spirituality and religion are frequently used interchangeably, the two could also be viewed as unique but complementary entities. *Spirituality* could be seen as a search for something beyond oneself. Martin Buber, a Jewish philosopher, defined it as "[relating] beyond the reliable world of density and duration and to enter into a dialogical encounter with something beyond yourself" (Buber, 1970). For Buber, it is the transcendence of ordinary life experience into a journey for meaning, value, and purpose. Spiritual issues may include but are not limited to the following questions: Does life have any meaning? Does death have meaning? Why is there evil in this world? What is my purpose in being here? Why is there suffering? Is there a God?

In contrast, *religion* can be viewed as one type of infrastructure through which many may choose to address spiritual issues. For many, it is the practical outworking of their spirituality. Harold Koenig defined religion as an organized system of beliefs, practices, rituals, and symbols designed (1) to facilitate closeness to the sacred and (2) to foster an understanding of one's relationship and responsibility to others in living together in a community (Koenig, McCullough, & Larson, 2001). Thus for Western religious traditions religion involves God, who is the supreme being, and religious practices involve rituals, creeds, ceremonies, or participative communities that help mediate one's relationship or harmony with God.

Although this chapter deals with both religion and spirituality in the life of the cancer patient, much of the research in this field, especially the initial work that is highlighted here regards religion and the cancer patient. Therefore, as the field is emerging, we highlight these initial studies on cancer and religion. Future research is needed to look at spirituality separate from religion and how the two dimensions may conflict or support each other.

# Cancer in America

Cancer is of much concern to many Americans. It is not only the second leading cause of death in America but also the leading cause of death among Americans ages 25–64. According to the National Cancer SEER Registry (Survival, Epidemiology and End-Results), the incidence of cancer has been on a steady rise from 1973 to 2002, although cancer mortality has remained relatively stable, perhaps even declining somewhat from 1996 to 2001 (Howe et al., 2001). Nevertheless, over 550,000 people die each year, with 1.1 million cases diagnosed annually. In addition, over 8 million Americans are living with cancer or have previously received a diagnosis of cancer. Cases of cancer of the lung, breast, prostate, melanoma, and lymphoma have been increasing, whereas those of colorectal, endometrial, cervical, and stomach cancer have been decreasing. The age-adjusted mortality ratio for males to females in 2002 for all cancers was 1.1 and for incidence (i.e., initial diagnosis) was also 1.1. The mortality ratio for Blacks to Whites in this same year for all cancers was 1.25 and the incidence of newly diagnosed cancers in 2001 was 1.1. The risk for developing cancer for a newborn over a lifetime is estimated at 45%, somewhat surprisingly similar to the lifetime risk for persons aged 45 (i.e., 44%). By the age of 65, the risk decreases to 35%.

Lung cancer remains the greatest threat for cancer mortality risk, with an estimated 165,000 deaths in 2005 and accounts for 29% of all deaths related to cancer. In contrast, lung cancers are proportionally 13%, or about one-seventh, of all cancer diagnoses. Importantly, lung cancer's 1-year survival rate is up from 32% in 1973 to 41% in 1994, but the 5-year survival rate remains the same for both years at 14% (Howe et al., 2001). Not surprisingly, the strongest risk factor for lung cancer is smoking cigarettes.

Colon cancer is the second leading cause of death from cancer, with over 55,000 deaths a year, accounting for 10% of all deaths from cancer and a similar 11% of diagnoses (Howe et al., 2001). Survival rates for colon cancer vary based on spread of disease, age, symptoms at presentation, and history of perforation of the bowel. Ironically, the younger patient with colorectal cancer appears to have a lower rate of survival, as these patients tend to have more aggressive tumors. It has also been reported that patients who present with symptoms (rectal bleeding, abdominal pain, change of stool habits, etc.) and/or perforation of the bowel have a poorer prognosis, because of the advancement of their disease linked with these symptoms. Risk factors for colon cancer can also include genetic mutations leading to polyposis syndromes, inflammatory bowel disease, history of pelvic irradiation and other environmental mutagens such as fecal mutagens (substances either ingested or produced by bacteria that promote cancer), and consistent ingestion of red meat (see Chapter 8).

Breast cancer is the third leading cause of death, numbering over 40,000 per year and constituting 8% of deaths from cancer and a somewhat higher 16% of diagnoses (Howe et al., 2001). However, breast cancer is the leading cause of death among women ages 40–55. Over 210,000 new cases are diagnosed each year. Of these, Black women are equally at risk compared to White women; however, they are more likely to die of breast cancer. Risk factors for breast cancer include age, genetics (presence of the BRCA-1 or BRCA-2 gene), past history of breast cancer, nulliparity, or late parity. Dietary factors and oral contraceptives have also been discussed and debated as risk factors (Harris, Lippman, Morrow, & Hellman, 1996) (see Chapter 9).

# Spirituality and Religion in America

A Gallup poll done in 2000 revealed that 95% of Americans believe in God (Gallup, 2001). This number has remained relatively static since these polls were begun in 1944. During that period of time, a belief in the afterlife as well as acceptance in the divinity of Jesus have both remained virtually unchanged, at about 75%. In the same 2000 poll, 59% of respondents reported that religion played a very important role in their lives and 49% attended a worship service on a weekly basis. Americans are largely Protestant (56%) or Catholic (26%), with a smaller proportion of Jewish (2%), Muslim (2%), persons affiliating with other religious beliefs (5%), and no religious preference (9%). Since the mid-1950s, the number of Protestants has declined, except for Southern Baptists and Assemblies of God, two more conservative denominational groups. Over this same period of time, Catholic traditions, in contrast, have shown gradual growth, largely because of the immigration of Mexicans and Central and South Americans, among whom Catholicism is robust. Overall, however, since the mid-1960s, church attendance has surprisingly not changed measurably.

# Cancer Among Religious Groups

Initial research on cancer and religion classified cancer risk by religious denominational groups such as Jewish, Catholic, Protestant, and other smaller denominational groups (e.g., Seventh-Day Adventist, Latter-Day Saints, and Hutterite Christian groups). We highlight findings from these earlier cancer/religious denominational studies below.

## Jews

Early studies show a mixed prevalence rate of specific cancer in the Jewish population. Wolbarst (1932) looked at an ethnically diverse group of 40,709 patients across 205 hospitals in the United States, 1,628 of whom were Jewish (i.e., 4.4%), with 830 patients of the 40,709 diagnosed with penile cancer. Importantly, none of those with penile cancer were Jewish. The author also examined total number of cases of penile cancer reported in the United States, India, and Java and found that of the 2,517 cases of penile cancer, 2,484 (i.e., 98%) were found among uncircumcised men. The authors concluded that the ceremonial practice of circumcision probably afforded Jewish men a lower risk for penile cancer.

That same year, Hoffman (1932) reported a lower rate of uterine, stomach, laryngeal, and esophageal cancer among Jews, but they also found a higher rate of liver, gallbladder, rectal, ovarian, and breast cancer. Similarly, Wolff (1939) found that overall cancer rates in Berlin were nearly the same for Jews as for non-Jews but the distribution of cancer did vary. Again, esophageal, uterine, and stomach cancer rates were lower but those of colorectal, lung, ovarian and breast cancer were higher. It was later postulated that less frequent smoking, safer sexual practices, and lower intake of alcohol may have accounted for the lower rates of cancer for Jewish versus non-Jewish U.S. samples. In addition, genetic factors were postulated for and may contribute to higher ovarian and breast cancer rates in Jewish versus non-Jewish women.

Specifically, Egan et al. (1996) examined 6,611 women with breast cancer and compared them to 9,026 controls without breast cancer and found that Jewish women were at a slightly increased overall risk for breast cancer but had a significantly higher risk if a first-degree relative had breast cancer (RR 3.78, 95% CI, $p < .001$). Similarly, Toniolo and Kato (1996) found that Jewish women age 50 or younger with a family history of breast cancer had a higher risk (RR 2.33, 95% CI) than similarly aged women of other religious groups.

Steinberg and colleagues (1998) compared 471 women with ovarian cancer to 4,025 without ovarian cancer in a case-control study and found that Jewish women with a first-degree relative were more likely than non-Jewish women to have familial ovarian cancer (OR 8.8). We now believe that many of these Jewish women probably carry specific genetic mutations (BRCA-1 and -2) that increase their risk for breast and ovarian cancer. To summarize, it appears that Jewish persons are at a lower risk of uterine, cervical, and penile cancer (possibly related to behavioral factors such as sexual practice and circumcision status) as well as some gastrointestinal tumors (unknown reasons) but are at an increased risk for breast and ovarian cancers (possibly related to genetic factors and higher socioeconomic status).

## Seventh-Day Adventists

Seventh-Day Adventists (SDAs) are a Christian denominational group founded in the mid-19th century whose basic belief system is Christian but also includes a distinctive apocalyptic belief emphasis (i.e., *advent* referring to the conviction in the nearness of the return of Jesus Christ). Another distinctive belief is that unlike most Christian groups who worship on Sunday (the day of Christ's resurrection), SDAs worship on the seventh day or Saturday (i.e., Sabbath day). SDAs promote a close community of believers who foster healthy and protective lifestyle practice, including diet and sexual practices. Smoking and alcohol are expressly prohibited, as is pork and fish without fins and scales. In contrast, fruits, vegetables and plenty of fluids are encouraged. Although not mandatory, some practice lacto-ovo-vegetarianism, which is a strict vegetarianism, excluding animal products such as meat, eggs, and milk.

Wynder, Lemon, and Bross (1959) were the first to report that cancer and coronary artery disease rates were lower in California SDAs than in the general population. Phillips and colleagues later published a 17-year follow-up study concerning a cohort of 23,000 SDAs from California, 59 of whom had developed colorectal cancer, 24 of whom developed lung cancer, and 120 of whom developed breast cancer. The age- and sex-adjusted mortality ratios were significantly lower for SDA men and women with colorectal and lung cancer than the rest of the California sample. However, mortality ratios were also lower for SDAs of both sexes when compared to non-SDA nonsmokers with colorectal and lung cancer. The authors concluded that abstinence from smoking was a partial explanation for lower rates of colorectal and lung cancer but suggested that other aspects of the SDA lifestyle might also play a role (Phillips, Kuzma, Beeson, & Lotz, 1980).

Similarly, Berkel and deWaard (1983) found a 50% reduction in the likelihood of death from cancer in Dutch SDAs compared to the general Dutch population. Thus it appears, as in the Jewish population, that safer health practices promoted by religions such as smoking abstinence, healthier diets, and other yet unidentified practices or other roles of religion seem to promote a lower incidence and mortality from cancer.

## Latter-Day Saints

Mormons, also known as members of The Church of Jesus Christ of Latter-Day Saints, are a Christian group founded by Joseph Smith and his brother, Hyrum, in the early 19th century. In addition to the standard Christian canon of Scripture, Mormons believe in a subsequent revelation encompassed in the Book of Mormon. They are also a religious group whose religion forbids tobacco, alcohol, coffee, tea, and other "addictive" drugs; furthermore, they stress a well-balanced diet, a strong family life, and education. Enstrom (1975) was the first investigator to examine the relative cancer rates for Mormons as he examined 360,000 California Mormons from all across the state and compared them to the general California population. He found a lower mortality from lung, many gastrointestinal and genitourinary tumors for men, and for women lower mortality from breast and uterine cancers. Lyon et al. (1976) sampled 10,641 cancer deaths in Utah from 1966 to 1970 and found an overall lower incidence of cancer, especially breast, cervical, and ovarian cancer among Mormon women.

Enstrom (1989) published the most recent mortality study concerning Mormons and found that the 3,119 Mormons sampled had a lower death rate from cancer, especially from lung cancer. Interestingly, among the controls who attended weekly worship services (i.e., more Protestant and Catholic but some Jewish and Muslim as well) and engaged in three or more health-related practices (i.e., smoking abstinence, exercise, and at least 8 hr of sleep at night), the rates of cancer were comparable to those who were Mormon, implying that religiously active persons regardless of denomination appear to have the same low cancer risk as Mormons.

## Hutterites

Hutterites also are Christian in their beliefs but are quite small in number compared to Seventh-Day Adventists and Latter-Day Saints. They originated in Europe (Switzerland, Germany, Italy, and Austria) and now largely populate Canada and the midwestwern United States. Although their beliefs are close to those of the Baptist tradition, they stress communal living and are seen in essence to be an inbred social isolate (Steinberg, Bleibtreu, Kurczynski, & Kurczynski, 1967). Inbreeding increases the possibility of expression of otherwise rare genes and allows scientists opportunities to understand the role of genes in the development of cancer.

Martin et al. (1980) studied over 12,000 Hutterites to investigate the existence of recessive genes for various cancers. He found that although Hutterites had significantly fewer deaths from cancer and that most of the difference could be explained from fewer lung cancers (only 1 patient died from lung cancer where 13 were expected). The latter was attributed to the prohibition of smoking. Also, Martin noted that the low frequency of cervical cancer (only 1 patient developed cervical cancer) is consistent with evidence of an association between cervical cancer and infrequent promiscuity. He did note that there was an increased incidence of childhood leukemia and that the coefficient of inbreeding was twice as high in these patients than in the general Hutterite population, implying a possible genetic mutation that is passed down in leukemogenesis in these patients and could be true for other cancers as well.

# Religious Commitment and Cancer

In the earlier sections, we first briefly outlined the importance of cancer as a disease as it affects the morbidity and mortality of Americans. As well, we discussed the importance of religion or frequency of these beliefs and practices in the lives of Americans. In the next section, we examined the rates of cancer in several religious groups and seemed to find a consistent relation between religiously encouraged or even proscribed healthy lifestyles and a generally lower incidence of at least several key cancer groups. Also, in this next section, we take the religion/cancer connection a step further, examining the relations between the religiousness of U.S. samples and the development of cancer, as well as the subsequent diagnosis of cancer and how patients might utilize religious beliefs or practices to cope with their cancer.

## Development

To begin to examine the question of whether there exists a relation between religiousness or religious commitment and prevalence and mortality of cancer, researchers have most frequently assessed religiousness using single-item measures of worship attendance. Although a rather simplistic approach for measuring religious commitment, we review if there is a relationship between religiousness and cancer outcomes.

Monk, Lilienfield, and Mendeloff (1962) examined patients with colorectal cancer and in this age, gender, and race-matched population found that those with rectal cancer were less likely to associate with a worship congregation, whereas the authors did not find a similar relationship in the analogous colon cancer population.

Naguib, Lundin, and Davis (1966) examined close to 4,200 women 30–45 years of age from Washington County, Maryland, and reported an inverse relationship between frequency of their worship attendance and rates of abnormal Pap smears. Among the women who identified themselves as Christian (the authors did not delineate from which denominations), those who attended worship services less than twice a year were more than twice as likely to have a positive Pap smear than those who attended weekly. The authors note that there were "too few Jewish women in the study to justify conclusions." However, Comstock and Partridge (1972), in their prospective study of over 50,000 women also from Washington County, did not find a survival advantage for frequent church-goers when compared to infrequent attendees.

To further complicate the picture, two mortality studies were subsequently published and found somewhat conflicting results. Enstrom (1989) analyzed 5,231 Mormon high priests and 4,613 wives of the high priests and compared them to a representative sample of 3,119 adults in Alameda County, California. The standardized mortality ratios (SMR) for all cancers for the high priests were 47% and for the wives was 72%. The authors then defined a subgroup (whom they called "active Mormon-like persons") from among the 3,119 controls who were religious (those who attended worship services weekly) and did not smoke. The SMR for men in this group was 51% and for women was

54%, comparable to the Mormon high priests and wives. Furthermore, for those "active Mormon-like persons" who incorporated general health practices such as regular exercise and 7–8 hours of sleep, the SMR was 0% for males and 21% for females, considerably lower than the SMR for nonreligious nonsmokers, which was 58% for males and 59% for females. The authors report that in their sample, lifestyles that incorporate weekly worship attendance, not smoking and routine general health practices such as exercise and regular sleep, "could result in a major reduction in cancer mortality."

In contrast, Reynolds and Kaplan (1990) reported in a 17-year follow-up study of close to 7,000 patients from the same population pool as Enstrom used that although women who were socially isolated were at greater risk of cancer mortality (relative hazard, 2.2, and smoking-related cancers relative hazard, 5.7), no association was found between worship service attendance and rates of cancer or cancer mortality.

Finally, Hummer, Rogers, Nam, and Ellsion (1999) evaluated a nationally representative sample of 22,080 U.S. adults from the National Health Interview Survey and found that worship service attendance was associated with lower all-cause mortality in a graded fashion (i.e., people who never attended worship services exhibited a higher risk of death in the follow-up period than those who attended less than once a week, who in turn exhibited a higher risk of death in the follow-up period than those who attended church weekly). When subjected to multivariate analysis for cause-specific models for mortality, the authors reported that when controlled for age, gender, race, region, social ties, and health behaviors, the risk for mortality from cancer (hazards ratio 1.25, $p < .10$) and circulatory diseases (hazards ratio 1.32, $p < .10$) was not significantly different in subjects who never attended a worship service than for those who attended weekly. The greatest differences were observed in mortality from respiratory disease (hazards ratio 2.1, $p < .05$), diabetes (hazards ratio 2.1, $p < .05$), and infectious disease (hazards ratio 2.9, $p < .05$). The authors conclude "religious involvement is strongly associated with adult mortality in a graded fashion. Those who never attend services exhibit the highest risk of death, and those who attend more than once a week exhibit the lowest risk" but fail to show this strong association in the case of all-cause cancer mortality. However, as the authors did not examine mortality rates for individual cancers, it is possible that a significant difference might exist as shown in the above studies for various specific cancers.

Another method used to examine the relationship between religiousness or religious commitment and risk of cancer mortality is by assessing clergy or religious orders—the assumption being that these groups are in fact at least, if not more, religious than the general population would be intuitive. In an early study, Taylor, Carroll, and Lloyd (1959) examined cancer rates from three orders of nuns. He reported that the nuns experienced a lower rate of gynecological malignancies as well as lowered total cancer mortality for nuns ages 20–59 but the researchers also found that the nuns over 60 years of age had a higher rate of gastrointestinal and ovarian cancer when compared to age-matched controls. When combining all age groups 20 and older, the total overall mortality among all ages was unchanged. The conclusions observed are consistent with the notion that gynecological malignancies for younger women in part tend to be because of risky sexual habits (e.g., promiscuity and early intercourse). Furthermore, the authors' conclusion are also consistent with reports that married women are at a lower risk than single women of developing ovarian cancer and that multiparity affords a decreased risk compared to nulliparity (Chiaffarino et al., 2001).

King and Locke (1980) examined a sample of 28,000 clergy from Protestant churches over a 10-year period and examined cancer death rates from among the 5,200 deaths that occurred during that same 10-year period of time. They reported that the clergy were 46% less likely than the general population to die of cancer and 60% less likely to die from lung cancer.

Similarly, Ogata, Ideda, and Kuratsune (1984) looked at 4,300 Japanese male Zen-Buddhist priests and found that lung and other respiratory tract cancer rates were significantly reduced when compared to those of the general Japanese population, as were other medical conditions such as cardiovascular disease, peptic ulcers, and cirrhosis. A research also found that the priests smoked less, ate less red meat, and lived in less polluted areas while still drinking similar levels of alcohol as similarly aged Japanese males.

In summary, although addressing the question of whether there exists relations between religiousness or religious commitment and prevalence of and mortality from cancer, researchers have examined both worship attendance and clergy and religious orders. Conclusions from studies utilizing single item assessments of religion have tended to be mixed. However, studies examining clergy or religious orders and cancer mortality appear to show a relationship between clergy and religious commitment and mortality from cancer.

# Religion and Coping

Upon receiving a cancer diagnosis, the patient is faced with not only the physical manifestations of the disease but also the stress, fears, and anxiety concerning the future as well as coping with pain, discomfort, and fatigue and finally the nagging anxieties about death. To examine the question of how frequently patients use religion to cope with cancer, Johnson and Spilka (1991) surveyed 103 women from Colorado with breast cancer. Eighty percent of these women reported that religion was very helpful in their coping with cancer, whereas only 12% considered religion unimportant. The authors examined the relationship between intrinsic (IR) and extrinsic (ER) religiousness. IR is regarded as the search for God or a Higher Power or personal meaning through one's faith or religion, whereas ER is more utilitarian and instrumental, a faith or religion more motivated by external factors (e.g. family, friends, and job). The authors concluded that although extrinsic religiousness was found to be unrelated to religious coping, intrinsic religiousness was. Factors predicting these outcomes included (1) greater involvement with clergy, (2) their belief that God was concerned with their illness, and (3) a greater satisfaction from the use of religion as a coping behavior.

Similarly, Carver et al. (1993) also looked at a cohort of 59 women with breast cancer and concluded that religious coping, along with acceptance and positive reframing of the cancer diagnosis, were employed most readily as preoperative strategies to cope with psychological distress. The authors did note that use of religious coping became less frequent postoperatively through a 12-month follow-up.

Roberts, Brown, Elkins, and Larson (1997) at the University of Michigan surveyed 108 women with gynecological malignancies and found that a quite substantial 93% felt that religious commitment helped them sustain their hopes and 76% found their religious commitment important to them. Nearly half had become more religious since diagnosed with cancer. The authors concluded that women with gynecological cancer are dealing with fear as a primary problem and that they depend on their religious convictions and experiences as an important means to cope with their disease. It appears evident from these few studies that women who have cancer do seem to employ religion as a coping strategy.

Torbjornsen, Stifoss-Hanssen, Abrahamsen, and Hannisdal (2000) sampled a population of 107 roughly equal proportion male and female Norwegians with Hodgkin's lymphoma. At baseline, the patients' attitudes to religion differed little from that of the Norwegian population at large. In this study, 15% of the Norwegian patients defined themselves as atheists, 14% as agnostics, 23% as deists (defined by the authors as those who believe in "an impersonal supreme power"), and only 48% as theists (defined by the authors as those who believe in "a personal God"). However, the authors found that 40 of their patients (38%) changed their religious beliefs in part because of their illness, 33 becoming more religious, resulting in 58% of the respondents praying to God for a cure of their illness. The authors concluded that in their sample, cancer activated religiousness and seemed to help many patients cope with their illness.

The next question that logically follows would be how helpful is religion to patients who employ religion to cope with their cancers. Acklin, Brown, and Mauger (1983) examined 26 patients with a recent diagnosis of cancer (20 females and 6 males) and measured intrinsic religiousness (IR), church attendance as well as their coping strategies and their psychological well-being using the Grief Experience Inventory. The authors reported that IR and church attendance were related to greater transcendent meaning, less anger and hostility, and reduced social isolation.

Similarly, Jenkins and Pargament (1988) found that for 62 patients they studied with cancer perceived that God had some control over their disease. Their disease course was generally found to be linked with higher self-esteem and less maladjustment scores as rated by a group of nurses. Also, Pargament et al. (1988) found that positive mental health status related to a problem solving process involving active give-and-take between the individual and God.

Regarding anxiety, Kaczorowski (1989) reported that among the 114 cancer hospice patients they surveyed, religious well-being and anxiety were inversely related. Similarly regarding hope, Raleigh (1992) examined 90 chronically ill patients, half of whom had cancer and the authors concluded that the most common sources to support hopefulness were (1) family, (2) friends, and (3) religious beliefs.

We can conclude then that many but not all patients with cancer may use their personal religiousness to cope with their illnesses and that as a result many of them may seem to enjoy higher levels of psychological well-being, self-esteem, and general mental health as a result.

## Religious Patterns of Coping

A diagnosis of cancer presents a multitude of challenges to the patient. The cancer patient may use religion to cope with these threatening or difficult situations in a number of ways. According to Musick, Koenig, Larson, and Matthew (1998) at least four have been identified and include the following: (1) changing one's perceived locus of control from self to God, (2) relying on one's religious worldview, (3) employing religious practices, and (4) using religious social support. In the following, we discuss each of these.

Those faced with cancer have been found to struggle with loss of control, which in turn can lead to increased psychological distress (Folkman, 1988). Similarly, higher levels of perceived control can be associated with improved adjustment to a stressful context. In an effort to regain control, patients have, for example, options that include employing primary control ("things are under my control") or secondary control ("things are under the control of God, chance, nature, other people, etc. . . . "). Jenkins and Pargament (1988) showed that patients who use secondary God perceptions as a method of coping had higher levels of self-esteem and lower levels of psychological distress than those who employed primary control or other nonreligious means of secondary control. The authors observe that subjects tended to describe an active process of exchange with God rather than a passive submission to an external force. They conclude that those who coped most effectively tended to institute a "problem-solving" process involving an active give-and-take between the individual and God.

In 1999, Cole and Pargament (1999) report a pilot psychotherapy program where an intervention designed to redirect primary control to secondary control was instituted in 10 patients. Nine of the 10 reported preference for this support program over traditional nonspiritual approaches such as psychotherapy programs.

In addition to changing one's locus of control, patients may utilize a philosophical or theological interpretive framework, a worldview or a system of beliefs, through which to interpret their disease. For example, using a sample of 1,610 subjects, Brady and colleagues (Brady, Peterman, Fitchett, Mo, & Cella, 1999) assessed the relationship of transcendent meaning to quality of life in patients with cancer and HIV using questionnaires that evaluated functional status (level of fatigue and pain) and spiritual well-being. From these questionnaires, the authors were able to derive a "meaning–peace" score that correlated with the sense of meaning, harmony, and peacefulness in one's life. Similarly, the authors were able to derive a "faith" score that were related with one's strength and comfort in drawing from one's faith. Finally, the respondents were then asked a simple question: "Do you enjoy life right now?"

Of the group of patients that reported high levels of pain, 48% with higher Meaning/Peace scores answered that they enjoyed life compared to a much smaller 9% with low Meaning/Peace scores. Of those who reported no pain, 77% with high Meaning/Peace scores reported that they enjoyed life compared to only once again a much smaller 25% with low Meaning/Peace scores. Similar results to pain were observed for fatigue levels. Also, similar findings were found when looking at faith scores instead of meaning/peace scores. The authors conclude that patients need a metaphysical framework through which to interpret their disease and that despite symptoms, "spirituality might operate so as to help people continue to value themselves and their lives . . . as well as maintain strength to endure the symptom[s]."

Furthermore, Baider et al. (1999) surveyed a group of 100 malignant melanoma patients in Israel over a 6-month period and measured coping, psychological distress, and social support. They found that their patient sample used their system of beliefs to engage in an active-cognitive coping strategy and that strategy also was associated with lower levels of anxiety and depression. The authors conclude "a system of beliefs actually helps reduce the degree of psychological stress brought on by a life-threatening illness . . . they increase psychological health and serve as a source of effective coping." Their study supported previous research that had shown that religious beliefs were associated with lower levels of anxiety and greater activity and flexibility in dealing with illness (Baider et al., 1997).

A third method of coping with religion used by cancer patients could be viewed as utilizing personal religious practices. These religious practices have been referred to as "ways to encounter the God of transcendence, order and freedom—ways that are explicitly set aside, designated, and tried-and-true" (Underwood, 1985). Sodestrom and Martinson (1987) found that the most frequently cited coping strategies by hospitalized cancer patients were personal prayer and prayer of others. The second most common activity was reading religious literature such as the Bible and other religious books and listening to religious broadcasts. Furthermore, Halstead and Fernsler (1994) found that prayer was the most frequently cited coping strategy in their sample of patients diagnosed with cancer.

Quite similarly, Johnson and Spilka (1991), in the study noted earlier, evaluated the value of religion in 103 women with breast cancer by administering questionnaires before and after clergy visits. The authors found that on open-ended questions, "the words 'care' or 'caring' were repeatedly employed . . . and was repeatedly associated with prayer."

The fourth and final means cancer patients might use in coping with the diagnosis of cancer is the use of social support groups through the community or the religious community. Musick et al. (1998) note that community/social support may help the cancer patient by (1) allowing more contact with others of a similar fate bolster their own faith, (2) meeting with people and obtaining their promises to pray, (3) being part of a social group which may provide instrumental help or assistance, and (4) reminding the patient that she or he is part of a caring community.

Dunkel-Schetter, Fernstein, Taylor, and Falke (1992) examined 603 cancer patients to evaluate coping strategies and found that social support and focusing on the positive was associated with less emotional distress. The use of social support as a coping mechanism was more prevalent in patients with a greater perceived stress from cancer and those who more frequently worried about their disease. As the investigators followed the patients longitudinally through their disease course, coping through social support was associated with decreased emotional distress, whereas distancing (e.g., "making light of the disease" and "trying not to think about it"), though it was the most utilized coping strategy, was also found to be linked with more emotional distress.

In the first of two important interventional studies on social support, Spiegel and colleagues (Spiegel, Bloom, Kraemer, & Gottheil, 1989) examined 86 women with metastatic breast cancer and randomized them to weekly supportive group therapy meetings to discuss side effects of therapy and self-hypnosis for pain management versus a no intervention comparison group. The study time period was 1 year with multiyear follow-up. According to the authors, developing strong relations among members lessened the potential for social isolation. After 10 years, the average survival for the intervention group was 33.6 months compared with 18.9 months for women in the control group ($p < .0001$). As well, the authors reported that the time from first metastasis to death was also prolonged for the intervention group (58.4 months) compared to the control group (43.2 months, $p < .02$). The authors conclude that social support appears to be an important factor in survival of breast cancer patients. They suggest that the cancer support group "may have allowed patients to mobilize their resources better, perhaps by complying more vigorously with medical treatment or by improving appetite and diet through reduced depression. Treated patients learned about hypnosis for pain control and therefore may have been more able to maintain exercise and other routine activities." The authors furthermore conclude that neuroendocrine and immune systems may be a mediating link between emotional processes and cancer course. Critics of this study have cited sampling error as a problem (Fox, 1998) and have called for other studies to replicate Spiegel's work.

Subsequently, Fawzy et al. (1990, 1993) conducted a similar study in patients with melanoma and randomly assigned patients to weekly support groups to help patients better cope with illness or else to a comparison group of routine care (see also Chapter 4). The intervention group showed significant increases in large granular lymphocytes, natural killer (NK) cells, and NK cell activity compared with the control group. (These are cells that function in identifying and killing cancer cells.) As well, in a clinical follow-up study in 1993, the intervention group had a lower rate of cancer recurrence (21%–38%) and a lower rate of likelihood of death (9%–29%).

# Biological Mediating Factors

We have examined research revealing potential links between spirituality, particularly religion, and cancer. We now look at potential biological explanations for these links. Although much work remains to be done to elucidate the potential biological pathways and cascades, we describe some hypothetical examples. For example, it appears that psychological as well as the progression of cancer and survival are mediated at a biological level by neuroendocrine and inflammatory cytokine status. The neuroendocrine system is where the nervous system interacts with and helps regulate the release of hormones into the circulatory system. Inflammatory cytokines are proteins secreted by white blood cells that help signal for and mediate an immune response. Below we briefly discuss these relationships as well as the potential roles religion might have in such a relationship.

## Stress, Neuroendocrine, and Immune Status

Psychological stress in the form of anxiety and depression has been shown to increase the production of cortisol by the adrenal glands (Felten et al., 1987). This is accomplished by stimulating the production of corticotropic releasing factor (CRF) in the hypothalamus, which then stimulates the pituitary gland to produce adrenocorticotropic hormone (ACTH), which in turn signals the adrenal gland to produce cortisol.

Cortisol is the hormone that activates the sympathetic central nervous system and is important in an acute "fight-or-flight" response. It raises blood pressure, heart rate, mental awareness, and regulated glucose level and recirculates white blood cells, all of which are important in an acutely stressful event. However, chronic stress and activation of this CNS-mediated pathway has been shown to impair immunity. Repeated "hits" on this sympathetic nervous system may affect a compensatory hyperactivity of other mediators, including cytokines, which then down-regulate the immune system (McEwen et al., 1997).

Cacioppo et al. (1995) showed that brief psychological stressors elicit autonomic and neuroendocrine responses. This same study revealed that subjects who were characterized by high cardiac sympathetic reactivity to brief stressors also showed high stress-induced changes in plasma cortisol and ACTH levels, suggesting a relative activation of the hypothalamic-pituitary-adrenocortical system in these subjects. Kiecolt-Glaser et al.

(1993) observed that conflict and marital discord was strongly associated with fluctuation in cortisol, ACTH, and norepinephrine levels among female spouses.

As well, Rassnicke, Sved, and Rabin (1994) showed the in the locus coeruleus of awake rats the stimulation of the autonomic nervous system with CRH caused not only cortisol levels but also IL-6 levels to rise. The role of IL-6 is briefly discussed in the following. The authors also observed that T-lymphocyte responses were decreased. They conclude that the central nervous system/adrenal axis is involved in stressor-induced immune suppression.

Both "humoral" and "cell-mediated" immunity are part of an overall "adaptive" immune system that responds to cancer. The humoral system is the immune response mediated by antibodies, whereas the cell-mediated system is a specific lymphocyte-mediated immune response, not involving humoral antibodies. Specifically, the humoral system helps signal and trigger tumor-specific cytotoxic T lymphocytes (CTL), T helper cells (Th) as well as NK cells. Often, when a cell mutates into cancer, it is this adaptive system that can keep the cancer from growing and spreading and may eliminate the cancer altogether. The "innate" immune system also responds to cancer and is made up of NK cells that have cell-specific receptors that generate recognition of tumor cells and initiate cell signals that mediate cytotoxicity of tumor cells. Both the adaptive and innate immune systems appear to be depressed in the presence of psychological stressors, as stated previously possibly through a CNS-mediated pathway.

Early studies were performed in animals and focused on how stress affects the humoral immune system. Gisler (1974) reported that mice that were stressed by either restraint or crowding had blunted antibody responses over the first 3 days of exposure to the stressor. However, with repeated stimulus, the antibody responses eventually returned back to prestressor baseline. Similarly, Monjan and Collector (1977) exposed mice to auditory stress and measured antibody responses of lymphocytes to bacterial lipopolysaccharide, a protein on the surface of various bacteria and reported that in their mice the antibody responses were suppressed for up to 20 days.

Subsequent studies began to evaluate the role of stress on cell-mediated immunity. Reite, Harbeck, and Hoffman (1981) subjected pigtailed monkeys to maternal and peer separation for 2-week intervals and measured T-lymphocyte mitogen responses and reported, similarly to previous work, that these acute stressors elicited a degree of suppression of T-cell function that normalized only after reunion with peer monkeys. Maternal and peer separation represents an animal model for grief and loss-related depression (Reite, Short, Kaufman, Stynes, & Pauley, 1978). Similar studies have been performed demonstrating a relationship between the intensity of the stressor and the degree of suppression of T-lymphocyte function in rats. Keller, Weiss, Schleifer, Miller, and Stein (1981) reported that both number and function of T lymphocytes appear to be suppressed progressively more in rats as the level of electrical shock delivered to the rats increased.

In humans, Schleifer, Keller, Camerino, Thornton, and Stein (1983) showed the suppression of mitogen-induced lymphocyte proliferation (a process by which lymphocytes are activated to reproduce) after the loss of a spouse. The investigators measured lymphocyte function in 15 men before and after the death of their spouse to breast cancer and discovered markedly lowered immune responses during the first 2 months postbereavement. In a similar work on bereavement, Zisook et al. (1994) reported in their sample of 21 female widows who were evaluated for 13 months postbereavement that the subset of widows who met DSM-III-R criteria for major depressive disorders also demonstrated lower NK cell activity and lower mitogen stimulation compared to those who did not meet these criteria.

Furthermore, depression has been shown to correlate with increased oxidative damage to DNA, a process critical in tumor development and progression (Jackson and Loeb, 2001). Adachi, Kawamura, and Takemoto (1993) reported increased levels of a biomarker for cancer-related DNA damage in rats that had been subjected to multiple electrical shocks over control unshocked rats, the first evidence of such damage induced by psychological stress. This was replicated in human studies; Irie et al. (2001) reported that in their sample population of 376 health adults (276 males and 86 females) after adjusting for body mass index, cigarette smoking, and alcohol use, there were positive relationships of the biomarker for DNA damage to average working hours, a self-blame coping strategy, and recent loss of a close family member in male subjects.

Taken together, psychological stressors have been observed to result in (1) DNA damage thereby contributing to tumorigenesis; (2) suppressed humoral, cell-mediated immune responses; as well as (3) decreased NK cell number and function, all three of which may promote tumor growth and metastasis.

It is not surprising, then, that increased incidence and mortality of cancer has been theorized in populations with higher levels of psychological stressors. In fact, Shekelle et al. (1981) examined 2,000 men for 17 years and after controlling for sociodemographic and preexisting medical morbidities found that the likelihood of death from cancer was twice the rate in men who were depressed than in men who were not depressed.

In similar fashion, Levy, Herberman, Lippman, D'Angelo, and Lee (1991) reported that in their sample of 90 women with early-stage (Stage I or II) breast cancer who were followed for 5 years, fatigue/depression and lack of social support predicted not only levels of NK cell activity but also disease-free survival and rate of disease progression for those who relapsed. Mood as measured by the Profile of Mood States (POMS) and perceived familial social support both predicted rate of disease progression for the women who did eventually relapse.

## Religion, Stress, and the Immune System

Only a few studies have examined the relations among religion, stress, and immune function. Two studies discussed below assess the potential for religious factors to be linked with less stress and lower cortisol levels in cancer patients. For example, Katz, Weiner, Gallagher, and Hellman (1970) evaluated 30 women with known breast masses awaiting breast biopsies for possible cancer and assessed them for their approaches to coping and cortisol levels. The authors noted that the women employed one or more of five coping strategies (i.e., displacement, projection, denial, fatalism, and/or prayer/faith) They concluded that those who employed prayer and faith as coping mechanisms tended to have lower cortisol levels than other women ($p < .02$). Similarly, Schaal, Sephton, Thoreson, Koopman, and Spiegel (1998) evaluated 112 women with metastatic breast cancer and measured attendance at worship services, religious or spiritual expression, and diurnal salivary cortisol levels. The authors found that although overall salivary cortisol levels did not associate with worship service attendance, evening cortisol levels were significantly lower among women who scored higher on religious expression.

In an effort to examine the relationship among stress, religion, and immune function, cytokine markers such as IL-6 have been studied. IL-6 is a small protein that is involved in the acute inflammatory response but also is known to stimulate the growth and differentiation of B lymphocytes. Furthermore, it is elevated in cancer cachexia (i.e., cancer wasting syndromes). High levels of IL-6 have been found in various cancers, such as plasmacytomas, Hodgkin's lymphoma, and kidney and head and neck cancers (Blay, Schermann, & Favrot, 1994; Ershler, Sun, & Binkley, 1994; Ur, White, & Grossman, 1992). Some have suggested that IL-6 might serve as a marker for a "stable immune system" (Koenig et al., 2001).

Koenig et al. (1997) measured IL-6 levels in 1,718 elderly persons in North Carolina. The authors found that IL-6 levels correlated with frequency of religious attendance. Subjects who attended religious services were 49% less likely than nonattenders to have high IL-6 levels (>5 pg/ml). It is possible, however, that those who were healthier to begin with (lower IL-6 levels) were the individuals who were able to go to church, whereas those who were sicker (higher IL-6 levels) were not.

Lutgendorf (2001) examined the relationship between religious beliefs and behavior and IL-6 in 55 adults ages 65 to 89 in Iowa. Half of the subjects were moving from their homes to senior housing (considered in the study as a stressful event) and IL-6 levels as well as religious and spiritual coping were measured before, during, and after the key stressful event. The authors found that levels of IL-6 were inversely related to greater use of spiritual coping, independent of whether seniors were stressed.

Sephton, Koopman, and Schaal (2001) examined the effect of spirituality on the immune system of 112 patients with breast cancer and found that spirituality was associated with greater numbers of circulating white blood cells, total lymphocytes, helper T cells, and cytotoxic T cells.

There is also evidence to suggest that there are neurologic changes that occur during spiritual and religious activity. Newberg, D'Aquili, and Rause (2001) studied nuns and monks during meditation and prayer using single-photon emission computed tomography (SPECT), which images blood flow to various parts of the brain. They reported that both the Franciscan nuns and Buddhist monks experienced decreased brain activity in the left orientation association areas (posterior superior parietal lobes) during the height of meditation. Scientists tell us that the parietal lobe is important to establish our physical relationship to the outside world.

It could be that spirituality or in particular religiousness may, in essence, lead to lowered levels of stress and psychological distress and thereby may lower neurologic and/or neuroendocrine stimulation and normalize immune functioning (at least as represented by IL-6 levels). Although much further work remains to be done, preliminary data suggest a potential positive correlation between healthy immune systems to fight cancer (i.e., increased level and function of cytotoxic T lymphocytes and NK cells and lower IL-6, cortisol, and ACTH levels) and religious practice.

## Genetic Factors

Much is known about the role of genetic factors in breast cancer. Below we highlight some of the studies done in this area as it relates to religion. When a small religious group maintains over time similar family participants, there is increased chance for in essence intermarriage to occur and genetic factors to play an increased role. Therefore, similar groups from nearby locations with similar cultures and beliefs marry and may over time "intermarry." In this manner, genes are passed down, including unwanted mutant ones. Under this premise, the Hutterites, as previously highlighted, have been studied as a familial aggregate and deemed to be a human isolate. In Martin et al.'s study, the authors suggested that there was an association between inbreeding in these Hutterite populations and incidence of childhood leukemia, suggesting the existence of a gene or multiple genes responsible for the development of certain childhood leukemias.

Simpson, Martin, Elias, Sarto, and Dunn (1981) studied this same population of Hutterites and examined 177 cases of cancer, specifically addressing the relationship of inbreeding to incidence of breast cancer. The coefficient of inbreeding ($F$) can be seen as the proportion of alleles (genes) that are homozygous (paired together) by descent from a common ancestor. That is, it is the probability that a person with two identical genes received each individual gene from the same ancestor. The higher the $F$, the more likely that recessive gene(s) will be expressed. The authors conclude that a higher $F$ was present in women with early breast cancer (before the age of 45) when compared to age-matched controls and suggest the presence of recessive gene(s) that may cause a select subpopulation of breast cancer. Until recently, however, no specific gene(s) have been characterized.

## Genetic Factors in Breast Cancer

The cause of early familial breast cancer has now been in part elucidated. In 1990, Hall et al. (1990) reported that the genes responsible for this form of breast cancer, up to 10% of all cases, is located on chromosome 17q21 and was later named BRCA-1 and BRCA-2 (BReast CAncer). The presence of these mutations are a risk for early breast cancer and are thought to be histologically more aggressive in that they are highly proliferative, tend not to express hormone receptors (ER/PR), and are aneuploid—meaning they are chromosomally complicated (Bertwistle & Ashworth, 1999).

Jewish women appear at slightly higher risk for breast and ovarian cancer compared to the general population but significantly higher risk if a young, first-degree relative has breast cancer. Individuals who have Ashkenazi Jewish descent who bear the BRCA mutant gene usually carry one of three common mutations in either BRCA-1 or BRCA-2 (Beller et al., 1997). In Ashkenazi Jews the carrier rate is 1.2 and 1.5%, respectively, for these BRCA-1 and -2 mutations. Two of these BRCA-1 mutations can be found in 6.9% of Ashkenazi women with breast cancer (Robson et al., 1999). Thirteen percent of Ashkenazi women diagnosed by 65 years of age (Gershoni-Baruch, Dagan, Kepten, & Fried, 1997) and up to 24% of these same women diagnosed before 42 years of age have one of these mutations (Gershoni-Baruch et al., 1997; Offit et al., 1996).

It appears that these mutations can negatively affect survival in Ashkenazi women as Foulkes, Wong, Rozen, Brunet, and Narod (1998) identified a group of 117 Ashkenazi women and found that disease-free survival at 5 years was significantly higher in non-BRCA associated tumors than in BRCA mutated ones (88.7% vs. 68.2%). The overall survival was also significantly lower (95.7% vs. 64.3%). The mutation appears to affect the cells ability to heal itself (Bhattacharyya, Ear, Koller, Weichselbaum, & Baum, 2000). Specifically, the BRCA-1 protein binds with another protein, Rad51, which is involved in DNA repair. The cell harboring this complex (labeled BRCA-1:Rad51) has a decreased ability to repair DNA damage and ultimately leads to cell death.

This process of programmed cell death, or apoptosis, is mediated by a gene called p53 and is very important so as to disallow dysfunctional cells (cells with the BRCA mutation) to continue to proliferate. However, it has also been discovered that an inordinately high number of p53 mutations are found in the very same Ashkenazi Jews that go on to develop breast cancer, thus explaining why not all Ashkenazi Jews with a BRCA-1 or -2 mutation develop cancer and supporting a multistep process of oncogenesis (Hilakivi-Clarke, 2000). In other words, it appears that a series of mutations are necessary to originate and promulgate cancer and that BRCA-1 or -2 mutations are but a single step along the way. Genetic associations of cancer risk may be related to ethnicity and religion.

# Religion and Negative Health Outcomes

Thus far, with the exception of the preceding section, we have discussed what in essence are generally health enhancing or the health benefits of religious affiliation or commitment. However, the fact remains that the derivation of favorable health from religion is neither so simple nor straightforward and not always the case. There can be religious beliefs, practices, and coping strategies that have been found to negatively impact physical and mental health status.

The first method by which this may occur is by inculcating *unhealthy practices*. One example could be considered replacing religious healing practices for indicated medical treatment and care. For example, Lannan et al. (1998) reported in their study of over 500 women with newly diagnosed breast cancer who were compared with 400 demographically matched controls that cultural beliefs (including religious beliefs) and socioeconomic factors were both significant predictors of late-stage diagnosis. The authors viewed that faith played a problematic role. They concluded that, for a number of reasons, many in their study failed to seek early medical attention despite recognizing a breast lump and, although well-intended in their hopes and beliefs, believed "perhaps most importantly [that] prayer and a reliance on God [would] heal the disorder."

Other examples where religion might reduce use of appropriate medical care include the refusing of blood transfusions (Jehovah's Witnesses), childhood immunizations (various Amish groups, as well as "alternative medicine" adherents), prenatal care, medically assisted birthing (Faith Assembly), and traditional mental health care (more orthodox Protestant groups). Although the intent of these religious practices may be benevolent, overlooking appropriate and indicated medical treatments can lead to worse clinical outcomes. When the practice of traditional medical systems conflict with the theology and doctrines of the religious order these institutions and individuals may choose to reject medical care.

Another means by which religion can negatively influence health status is by using negative religious coping strategies. Koenig, Pargament, and Nielsen (1998) reported that coping strategies where God is viewed as benevolent or as a collaborative partner in coping with life's stresses tended to be associated with better mental health outcomes; in contrast, coping where God is viewed as a punishing or a rejecting deity were associated with poorer mental health outcomes. The authors note that because this was a cross-sectional study that preexistent psychological distress may have been responsible for such beliefs and further research in needed.

Recently, Pargament, Koenig, Tarakeshwar, and Hahn (2001) published a 2-year longitudinal study of 600 medical inpatients and concluded that these same forms of religious coping leading to religious struggle or conflict may actually increase the risk of earlier death. The patients who employed negative religious coping (e.g., "God has abandoned me because of a lack of devotion" and "God doesn't love me") had higher risk ratios for mortality than did patients who employed positive religious coping strategies. Even after controlling for demographics, illness severity, church attendance, depressed mood, and quality of life, these types of religious struggle continued to predict increased risk of mortality.

A third example of the negative effects of religion on health can be illustrated in "all or nothing" extremist cult groups. Dein and Littlewood (2000) report that violence and suicide among cult members are becoming somewhat more frequent, especially in light of a "divine millennium"—the end of the world or the return of God—not yet materializing. Upon this disappointment and because they may consider themselves immune to death, they often choose to attempt to exit their physical bodies and go to a better "spiritual" world. An example of these religious cults is the Heaven's Gate cult, who believed that aliens resided on the Hale–Bopp comet and committed mass suicide in an effort to be initiated into a higher existence. Likewise, the members of the Solar Temple, realizing that the New Age as promised by their leader did not come to pass, and believing that a spaceship would collect their souls and deliver them to another planet, committed mass suicide. Also, the Branch Davidians—a breakaway group from the Seventh-Day Adventists—believed that their leader, David Koresh, would usher in the end of the world and that the American government represented an evil enemy state.

Furthermore, the authors above report in their review of these extremist apocalyptic groups that commonalities exist among these various extremist cults; the commonalities are as follows: (1) they teach a strong dualistic philosophy (i.e., an evil physical world and a good spiritual world), (2) they have charismatic leaders with total control, and (3) they promote an isolationism among the members that makes it exceedingly difficult to object to the teachings or leave the group. The authors argue that health professionals need to understand the belief system and pattern of leadership before working with any members of these groups. They need to also understand that not all groups are so extremist. As well, they need to be sensitive to the fact that anyone leaving such a movement might also undergo stress, if not conflict, sometimes severe, in attempting to reconcile their past and present worldviews.

# Clinical Implications

Day-to-day care of cancer patients in helping to deal with the spiritual aspects of their care makes clinical sense. If not for supporting a patient's spirituality when it gives them hope or support, it even makes even greater sense when a patient has spiritual distress with the potential for such distress to worsen physical or psychological problems that may intercalate with depression, hopelessness, worthlessness, and/or meaninglessness. Furthermore, pain, fatigue, and the rigors and side effects of treatment may compound the anguish. Therefore it is important for the clinician to be aware of the potential for the spiritual distress or existential angst of their patient and to recognize the importance of questions such as: Where is God when I need him? Why has he abandoned me? Where am I going when I die? Is God punishing me? More importantly when there is such distress, it is very important to consult with a chaplain or an indicated health care consultant who can deal with such spiritual issues.

Toward this end, clinicians need to develop skills in addressing spiritual needs. Below we propose two necessary skills: (1) establishing rapport and a dialogue with patients about their needs and (2) recognizing the appropriate time for referrals to professional religious workers, particularly chaplains.

## Spiritual Dialogue

Addressing the importance of the role of dialogue in spiritual matters, Roberts et al. (1997) surveyed over 100 women with gynecological malignancies and found that a majority of these women placed greater emphasis on receiving "straight talk" (96%) from their physician, which was more important than compassion (64%). Over three-quarters of the women (76%) viewed religion as very important to them and of these, nearly half (49%) reported an increase in their religiousness after the diagnosis of cancer. Over 90% felt that religious commitment helped them sustain their hopes and 41% felt that it helped them sustain their worth. The authors concluded that women with gynecological cancer "depend on their religious convictions and experiences as they cope with disease" and that physicians should "aim to educate their patients sufficiently for them to exercise control over their experience, to allay fears and make personal decisions that further their aspirations."

Furthermore, King and Bushwick (1994) interviewed 203 medical inpatients and their religious and health behavior and found that 77% of the patients wanted their physicians to consider their spiritual needs. Somewhat surprisingly, 48% wanted their physicians to pray with them; however, 68% of their physicians had never discussed religious beliefs with patients.

Ehman, Ott, Short, Ciampa, and Hansen-Flaschen (1999) interviewed 177 pulmonary medicine patients and found that 51% described themselves as religious and 90% believed that prayer may sometimes influence recovery from an illness. Of those, 94% felt that physicians ought to ask them of their religious beliefs should they become gravely ill. Interestingly, of the 49% who did not describe themselves as religious, still about half felt that physicians ought to ask them of their religious beliefs should they become gravely ill.

Moadel et al. (1999) addressed what cancer patients desire from their physicians regarding spiritual care. They interviewed 268 ethnically diverse patients in an urban oncology center and found that 51% of patients wanted assistance in overcoming their fears in life (referring to existential fears about life), 42% wanted assistance in finding hope, 40% wanted help in finding meaning in life, and 39% looked to their physicians for spiritual resources.

Because patients are willing to discuss spiritual issues with their clinicians, the latter must be able to formulate relevant open-ended questions while communicating a nonjudgmental respect for that patient's beliefs and struggles (Post, Puchalski, & Larson, 2000). Puchalski (1999) offers one approach using the acronym FICA in obtaining a spiritual history from the patient. This tool incorporates questions dealing with the patients' faith (F), the importance or influence of this faith (I), the religious community they are in (C), and how it is the clinician can address (A) any needs.

Furthermore, the American College of Physicians–American Society of Internal Medicine Concensus Panel Statement on End-of-life Issues (Lo, Quill, & Tulsky, 1999) outlines an unassuming method to begin to open discussion, explore, and discuss spiritual and existential issues and answers objections to this approach. Open-ended questions such as "What are your hopes, your expectations, your fears for the future?" or "As you think about the future, what is most important for you?" Physicians and caretakers are encouraged to pursue an honest dialogue if patients appear available and willing.

Further questions such as "Is faith (religion, spirituality) important to you?" or "Do you have someone to talk to about religious matters?" More direct questions such as "What thoughts have you had about why you got this illness at this time?" or "What do you still want to accomplish during your life?" are also included. The consensus report authors note four important points for the caretakers to keep in mind: (1) uncovering painful emotions may increase short-term suffering but may lessen fear and anxiety in the long-term; (2) open and honest dialogue by both the physician and patient may lead to a connectedness between the two individuals; (3) caretakers can clarify their own roles, noting they are "fellow travelers" who may not have all the answers but who can listen and understand; and (4) caretakers do not have sole responsibilities for the patients suffering but can call on nurses, social workers, chaplains, psychologists, and psychiatrists for help.

## Referrals to Chaplains

The clinician should be thinking of referral for spiritual issues when (1) they are uncomfortable, (2) when there is spiritual distress, (3) the spiritual issues are complex, or (4) addressing these particular issues will take much more time than the allotted appointment time. The emergence of a spiritual distress in particular in the life of a patient may be the culmination of a lifetime of struggle, disappointment, or pain, and will not be adequately addressed with a few pat phrases. Opening a dialogue with the patient is important for the clinician as much to diagnose the spiritual problem as it is to begin treating it. Under these conditions it is best for the physician to refer to a chaplain or a spiritual care provider.

The clinician may want to invest some time in creating their network of support staff by establishing relationships through a local ministerium association, contract, volunteer arrangement, or pastoral care department of a local hospital or by working with students from local religious educational facility (Harris & Satterly, 1998). Because patients may have a diversity of cultural and religious backgrounds, clinicians need to keep in mind that one size may not fit all. That is, it is important for the clinician to be aware of a number of different spiritual or religious professionals with different backgrounds and different strengths so as to be able to refer patients with unique needs to the appropriate resource(s). More importantly, chaplains can often work with patients of different faith traditions and when needed make linkages to these traditions.

## Efficacy of Clinicians

Although it is becoming increasingly clear that patients desire their caretakers to address religious and spiritual issues, whether supportive or stressful, it appears that physicians and nurses may not integrate this level of care into their practice as frequently as they would like. Kristellar, Zumbrun, & Schilling, 1999) surveyed 94 oncologists and 267 oncology nurses regarding attitudes and practices regarding patient care, specifically spiritual distress. Of the oncologists and nurses surveyed, 37.5 and 47.5%, respectively, reported identifying themselves as the primary clinician responsible for addressing spiritual distress. However, only 11.8% and 8.5% of them, respectively, ranked spiritual distress as one of the top three psychosocial issues that they would actually address. Furthermore, although over 85% of these caretakers believed a chaplain to be the ideal person to address these issues, very few of them actually made a formal referral for spiritual distress (25% and 37% for MDs and nurses, respectively).

The Joint Commission on Accreditation and Health Care Organizations has now begun to address spiritual issues in health care settings. They require physicians to respond to spiritual issues in end–of–life care (RI.I.2), refer to pastoral counseling or chaplains when appropriate (RI.I.2.7), make an initial spiritual assessment to dying patients (PE.I.I), and address spiritual orientation when treating drug and alcohol dependency (PE.7). Toward this end, physicians are presently being better trained in taking a spiritual history as over 60 of the 126 medical schools presently have courses that specifically address this issue.

# Summary

Dealing with illness, particularly a serious illness such as cancer, can be an important aspect in the lives of Americans. Cancer is a leading cause of morbidity and mortality today as lung, colorectal, and breast cancer rank as the top three cancer-related causes of mortality each year. Overall, cancer is the second leading killer of Americans and since the early 1970s overall incidence has been on a steady rise. Religion is also an important aspect in the lives of Americans with levels of religious practices and beliefs remaining high and somewhat constant since the early 1950s. A majority of Americans believe in God and attend houses of worship on a regular basis.

Certain religious groups have been found to be of potential research interest given their differential prevalence and mortality rates from cancer. For example, Jews appear to have a lower incidence of penile cancer (i.e., from circumcision) and uterine and cervical cancer (i.e., from safer sexual habits) but slightly higher rates of breast and ovarian cancer (i.e., from genetic mutations). Seventh-Day Adventists have a lower rate of colorectal and lung cancer (i.e., from dietary and smoking-related practices) and Mormons similarly have lower rates of colorectal, lung, and genitourinary cancers (i.e., also from dietary, smoking, and possibly other health-related practices). Finally, Hutterites have been found to have lower lung cancer and cervical cancer rates (i.e., from smoking-related and safer sexual habits). Thus, it appears that various religious groups tend to promote safer and healthier lifestyles and these maybe translate into lower prevalence and mortality from cancer.

In addition to lifestyle modifications for certain religious groups, religious commitment also appears to provide health benefits as regular worship attendance has been found to protect against all-cause mortality in general, as well as cancer mortality specifically. Furthermore, in the few studies, it appears that clergy and religious professionals tend to have a lower cancer prevalence and mortality from cancer. Following the diagnosis of cancer, religion may provide additional health roles as it may be frequently employed successfully as a positive coping strategy to potentially reduce psychological distress and increase adjustment to serious illness. For example, cancer patients may employ secondary control, utilizing their system of beliefs, supported by their personal religious practices as well as access social support through their congregational settings.

The potential clinical benefits may be mediated by a psychoneuroimmunological model involving the stress response as well as the inflammatory cytokine cascades. Psychological stressors may induce DNA damage thereby contributing to tumorigenesis, suppressed humoral, cell-mediated immune responses, as well as decreased natural killer cell number and function, all of which may promote tumor growth and metastasis. Religion may reduce psychological distress, which may in turn mediate its beneficial effects by way of the immune system.

Religion may also, however, have a negative impact on health as it may promote unhealthy beliefs about oneself and God and in turn increase potential for psychological distress and negatively impact survival. Furthermore, religion may promulgate unhealthy practices such as avoiding or substituting religious ritual for traditional medical care, including surgery, antibiotics, chemotherapy, blood transfusion, and immunizations.

Considering all of the complicating issues surrounding religion and health, specifically regarding the diagnosis of cancer, patients appear to desire that their physicians address spiritual issues and their spiritual distress. Skills necessary in this process include asking a few questions, if not opening a dialogue with patients to ascertain the role of spiritual issues in their lives. When the physician has limited time, the issues are complex, or there is spiritual distress, subsequent appropriate referrals can be made to spiritual care providers such as chaplains. Although the numbers are growing, there is an increasing need in areas such as oncology for specialists to address these areas of concern and to educate and equip the clinician to be a genuine, capable provider of care to the whole person—mind, body, and spirit.

## REFERENCES

Acklin, M. W., Brown, E. C., & Mauger, P. A. (1983). The role of religious values and coping with cancer. *Journal of Religion and Health, 22,* 322–333.

Adachi, S., Kawamura, K., & Takemoto, K. (1993). Oxidative damage of nuclear DNA in liver of rats exposed to psychological stress. *Cancer Research, 53*(18), 4153–4155.

Baider, L., Perry, S., Sison, A., Holland, J., Uziely, B., & DeNour, A. K. (1997). The role of psychological variables in a group of melanoma patients. An Israeli sample. *Psychosomatics, 38*(1), 45–53.

Baider, L., Russak, S. M., Perry, S., Kash, K., Gronert, M., Fox, B., et al. (1999). The role of religious and spiritual beliefs in coping with malignant melanoma: an Israeli sample. *Psychooncology, 8*(1), 27–35.

Beller, U., Halle, D., Catane, R., Kaufman, B., Hornreich, G., & Levy-Lahad, E. (1997). High frequency of BRCA1 and BRCA2 germline mutations in Ashkenazi Jewish ovarian cancer patients, regardless of family history. *Gynecologic Oncology, 67*(2), 123–126.

Berkel, J., & deWaard, F. (1983). Mortality patterns and life expectancy of Seventh-Day Adventists in the Netherlands. *International Journal of Epidemiology, 12,* 455–459.

Bertwistle, D., & Ashworth, A. (1999). The pathology of familial breast cancer: How do the functions of BRCA1 and BRCA2 relate to breast tumour pathology. *Breast Cancer Research, 1*(1), 41–47.

Bhattacharyya, A., Ear, U. S., Koller, B. H., Weichselbaum, R. R., & Bishop, D. K. (2000). The breast cancer susceptibility gene BRCA1 is required for subnuclear assembly of Rad51 and survival following treatment with the DNA cross-linking agent cisplatin. *Journal of Biological Chemistry, 275*(31), 23899–23903.

Blay, J. Y., Schemann, S., & Favrot, M. C. (1994). Local production of interleukin 6 by renal adenocarcinoma in vivo. *Journal of the National Cancer Institute, 86*(3), 238.

Brady, M. J., Peterman, A. H., Fitchett, G., Mo, M., & Cella, D. (1999). A case for including spirituality in quality of life measurement in oncology. *Psychooncology, 8*(5), 417–428.

Buber, M. (1970). *I and thou.* New York: Charles Scribner's Sons.

Cacioppo, J. T., Malarkey, W. B., Kiecolt-Glaser, J. K., Uchino, B. N., Sgoutas-Emch, S. A., Sheridan, J. F., et al. (1995). Heterogeneity in neuroendocrine and immune responses to brief psychological stressors as a function of autonomic cardiac activation. *Psychosomatic Medicine, 57*(2), 154–164.

Carver, C. S., Pozo, C., Harris, S. D., Noriega, V., Scheier, M. F., Robinson, D. S., et al. (1993). How coping mediates the effect of optimism on distress: A study of women with early stage breast cancer. *Journal of Personality and Social Psychology, 65*(2), 375–390.

Chiaffarino, F., Pelucchi, C., Parazzini, F., Negri, E., Franceschi, S., Talamini, R., et al. (2001). Reproductive and hormonal factors and ovarian cancer. *Annals of Oncology, 12*(3), 337–341.

Cole, B., & Pargament, K. (1999). Re-creating your life: A spiritual/psychotherapeutic intervention for people diagnosed with cancer. *Psychooncology, 8*(5), 395–407.

Comstock, G. W., & Partridge, K. B. (1972). Church attendance and health. *Journal of Chronic Disease, 25*(12), 665–672.

Dein, S., & Littlewood, R. (2000). Apocalyptic suicide. *Mental Health, Religion and Culture, 3*(2), 109–114.

Dunkel-Schetter, C., Fernstein, L. G., Taylor, S. E., & Falke, R. L. (1992). Patterns of coping with cancer. *Health Psychology, 11*, 79–87.

Egan, K. M., Newcomb, P. A., Longnecker, M. P., Trentham-Dietz, A., Baron, J. A., Trichopoulos, D., et al. (1996). Jewish religion and risk of breast cancer. *Lancet, 347*(9016), 1645–1646.

Ehman, J. W., Ott, B. B., Short, T. H., Ciampa, R. C., & Hansen-Flaschen, J. (1999). Do patients want physicians to inquire about their spiritual or religious beliefs if they become gravely ill. *Archives of Internal Medicine, 159*(15), 1803–1806.

Enstrom, J. E. (1975). Cancer mortality among Mormons. *Cancer, 36*(3), 825–841.

Enstrom, J. E. (1989). Health practices and cancer mortality among active California Mormons. *Journal of the National Cancer Institute, 81*(23), 1807–1814.

Ershler, W. B., Sun, W. H., & Binkley, N. (1994). The role of interleukin-6 in certain age-related diseases. *Drugs Aging, 5*(5), 358–365.

Fahey, J. L. (1990). A structured psychiatric intervention for cancer patients. II. Changes over time in immunological measures. *Archives of General Psychiatry, 47*(8), 729–735.

Fawzy, F. I., Fawzy, N. W., Hyun, C. S., Elashoff, R., Guthrie, D., Fahey, J. L., & Morton, D. L. (1993). Malignant melanoma: Effects of an early structured psychiatric intervention, coping, and affective state on recurrence and survival 6 years later. *Archives of General Psychiatry, 50*(9), 681–689.

Fawzy, F. I., Kemeny, M. E., Fawzy, N. W., Elashoff, R., Morton, D., Cousins, N., et al. (1990). A structured psychiatric intervention for cancer patients. II. Changes over time in immunological measures. *Archives of General Psychiatry, 47*(8), 729–835.

Felten, D. L., Felten, S. Y., Bellinger, D. L., Carlson, S. L., Ackerman, K. D., Madden, K. S., et al. (1987). Noradrenergic sympathetic neural interactions with the immune system: Structure and function. *Immunology Review, 100*, 225–260.

Folkman, S. (1988). Personal control and stress and coping processes: A theoretical analysis. *Kango Kenkyu, 21*(3), 243–260.

Foulkes, W. D., Wong, N., Rozen, F., Brunet, J. S., & Narod, S. A. (1998). Survival of patients with breast cancer and BRCA1 mutations. *Lancet, 351*(9112), 1359–1360.

Fox, B. H. (1998). A hypothesis about Spiegel et al.'s 1989 paper on Psychosocial intervention and breast cancer survival. *Psychooncology, 7*(5), 361–370.

Gallup, G. (2001). Americans more religious now than ten years ago, but less so than in 1950s and 1960s. *Gallup News Service,* March.

Gershoni-Baruch, R., Dagan, E., Kepten, I., & Freid, G. (1997). Co-segregation of BRCA1 185delAG mutation and BRCA2 6174delT in one single family. *European Journal of Cancer, 33*(13), 2283–2284.

Gisler, R. H. (1974). Stress and the hormonal regulation of the immune response in mice. *Psychotherapy and Psychosomatics, 23*(1–6), 197–208.

Hall, J. M., Lee, M. K., Newman, B., Morrow, J. E., Anderson, L. A., Huey, B., et al. (1990). Linkage of early-onset familial breast cancer to chromosome 17q21. *Science, 250*(4988), 1684–1689.

Halstead, M. T., & Fernsler, J. I. (1994). Coping strategies of long-term cancer survivors. *Cancer Nursing, 17*(2), 94–100.

Harris, J. R., Lippman, M. E., Morrow, M., & Hellman, S. (1996). *Diseases of the breast.* Philadelphia, PA: Lippencott-Raven.

Harris, M. D., & Satterly, L. R. (1998). The chaplain as a member of the hospice team. *Home Health Nurse, 16*(9), 591–593.

Hilakivi-Clarke, L. (2000). Estrogens, BRCA1, and breast cancer. *Cancer Research, 60*(18), 4993–5001.

Hoffman, F. L. (1932). The cancer mortality of Amsterdam, Holland, by religious sects. *Amercian Journal of Cancer, 17*, 142–153.

Howe, H. L., Wingo, P. A., Thun, M. J., Ries, L. A. G., Rosenberg, H. M., Feigal, E. G., et al. (2001). The annual report to the nation on the status of cancer (1973 through 1998), featuring cancers with recent increasing trends. *Journal of the National Cancer Institute, 93*(11), 824–842.

Hummer, R. A., Rogers, R. G., Nam, C. B., & Ellison, C. G. (1999). Religious involvement and U.S. adult mortality. *Demography, 36*(2), 273–285.

Irie, M., Asami, S., Nagata, S., Ikeda, M., Miyata, M., & Kasai, H. (2001). Psychosocial factors as a potential trigger of oxidative DNA damage in human leukocytes. *Japanese Journal of Cancer Research, 92*(3), 367–376.

Jackson, A. L., & Loeb, L. A. (2001). The contribution of endogenous sources of DNA damage to the multiple mutations in cancer. *Mutation Research, 477*(1–2), 7–21.

Jenkins, R. A., & Pargament, K. I. (1988). Cognitive appraisals in cancer patients. *Social Science Medicine, 26*(6), 625–633.

Johnson, S. C., & Spilka, B. (1991). Coping with breast cancer: The roles of clergy and faith. *Journal of Religion and Health, 30*, 21–33.

Kaczorowski, J. M. (1989). Spiritual well-being and anxiety in adults diagnosed with cancer. *Hospital Journal, 5*(3–4), 105–116.

Katz, J. L., Weiner, H., Gallagher, T. F., & Hellman, L. (1970). Stress, distress, and ego defenses: Psychoendocrine response to impending breast tumor biopsy. *Archives of General Psychiatry, 23*(2), 131–142.

Keller, S. E., Weiss, J. M., Schleifer, S. J., Miller, N. E., & Stein, M. (1981). Suppression of immunity by stress: Effect of a graded series of stressors on lymphocyte stimulation in the rat. *Science, 213*(4514), 1397–1400.

Kiecolt-Glaser, J. K., Malarkey, W. B., Chee, M., Newton, T., Cacioppo, J. T., Mao, H. Y., et al. (1993). Negative behavior during marital conflict is associated with immunological down-regulation. *Psychosomatic Medicine, 55*(5), 395–409.

King, D. E., & Bushwick, B. (1994). Beliefs and attitudes of hospital inpatients about faith healing and prayer. *Journal of Family Practice, 39*(4), 349–352.

King, H., & Locke, F. B. (1980). American white Protestant clergy as a low-risk population for mortality research. *Journal of the National Cancer Institute, 65*(5), 1115–1124.

Koenig, H. G., Cohen, H. J., George, L. K., Hays, J. C., Larson, D. B., et al. (1997). Attendance at religious services, interleukin-6, and other biological parameters of immune function in older adults. *International Journal of Psychiatry and Medicine, 27*(3), 233–250.

Koenig, H. G., McCullough, M. E., & Larson, D. B. (2001). *Handbook of religion and health.* New York: Oxford University Press.

Koenig, H. G., Pargament, K. I., & Nielsen, J. (1998). Religious coping and health status in medically ill hospitalized older adults. *Journal of Nervous and Mental Disorders, 186*(9), 513–521.

Kristeller, J. L., Zumbrun, C. S., & Schilling, R. F. (1999). 'I would if I could': How oncologists and oncology nurses address spiritual distress in cancer patients. *Psychooncology, 8*(5), 451–458.

Lannin, D. R., Mathews, H. F., Mitchell, J., Swanson, M. S., Swanson, F. H., & Edwards, M. S. (1998). Influence of socioeconomic and cultural factors on racial differences in late-stage presentation of breast cancer. *Journal of the American Medical Association, 279*(22), 1801–1807.

Levy, S. M., Herberman, R. B., Lippman, M., D'Angelo, T., & Lee, J. (1991). Immunological and psychosocial predictors of disease recurrence in patients with early-stage breast cancer. *Behavioral Medicine, 17*(2), 67–75.

Lo, B., Quill, T., & Tulsky, J. (1999). Discussing palliative care with patients. ACP-ASIM End-of-Life Care Consensus Panel. American College of Physicians-American Society of Internal Medicine. *Annals of Internal Medicine, 130*(9), 744–749.

Lyon, J. L., Klauber, M. R., Gardner, J. W., & Smart, C. R. (1976). Cancer incidence in Mormons and non-Mormons in Utah, 1966–1970. *New England Journal Medicine, 294*(3), 129–133.

Lutgendorf, S. (2001). IL-6 level, stress and spiritual support in older adults: Personal communication. In H. G. Koenig M. E. McCullough, & D. B. Larson (Eds.), *Handbook of religion and health*. New York: Oxford University Press.

Marchbanks, P. A. (1998). Increased risk for familial ovarian cancer among Jewish women: A population-based case-control study. *Genetic Epidemiology, 15*(1), 51–59.

Martin, A. O., Dunn, J. K., Simpson, J. L., Olsen, C. L., Kemel, S., Grace, M., et al. (1980). Cancer mortality in a human isolate. *Journal of the National Cancer Institute, 65*(5), 1109–1113.

McEwen, B. S., Biron, C. A., Brunson, K. W., Bulloch. K., Chambers, W. H., Dhabhar, F. S., et al. (1997). The role of adrenocorticoids as modulators of immune function in health and disease: neural, endocrine and immune interactions. *Brain Research Reviews, 23*(1–2), 79–133.

Moadel, A., Morgan, C., Fatone, A., Grennan, J., Carter, J., Laruffa, G., et al. (1999). Seeking meaning and hope: Self-reported spiritual and existential needs among an ethnically diverse cancer patient population. *Psychooncology, 8*(5), 378–385.

Monjan, A. A., & Collector, M. I. (1977). Stress-induced modulation of the immune response. *Science, 196*(4287), 307–308.

Monk, M., Lilienfeld, A., & Mendeloff, A. (1962). *Preliminary report of an epidemiologic study of cancers of the colon and rectum.* Paper presented at the meeting of the epidemiologic section of the American Public Health Association Annual Meeting.

Musick, M. A., Koenig, H. G., Larson, D. B., & Matthews, D. (1998). *Religion, spiritual beliefs, and cancer* (pp. 780–789). In J. Holland (Ed.), *Textbook of psycho-oncology*. New York: Oxford University Press.

Naguib, S. M., Lundin, F. E., Jr., & Davis, H. J. (1966). Relation of various epidemiologic factors to cervical cancer as determined by a screening program. *Obstetrics and Gynecology, 28*(4), 451–459.

Newberg, A., D'Aquili, E., & Rause, V. (2001). *Why God won't go away: Brain science and the biology of belief.* New York: Ballantine.

Offit, K., Gilewski, T., McGuire, P., Schluger, A., Hampel. H., Brown, K., et al. (1996). Germline BRCA1 185delAG mutations in Jewish women with breast cancer. *Lancet, 347*(9016), 1643–1645.

Ogata, A., Ideda, M., & Kuratsune, M.b (1984). Mortality among Japanese Zen priests. *Journal of Epidemiology and Community Health, 38*, 161–166.

Pargament, K. I., Kennell, J., Hathaway, W., Grevengoad, N., Newman, J., & Jones, W. (1988). Religion and the problem solving process: three styles of coping. *Journal of the Scientific Study of Religion, 27*, 90–104.

Pargament, K. I., Koenig, H. G., Tarakeshwar, N., & Hahn, J. (2001). Religious struggle as a predictor of mortality among medically ill elderly patients: A 2-year longitudinal study. *Archives of Internal Medicine, 161*(15), 1881–1885.

Phillips, R. L., Kuzma, J. W., Beeson, W. L., & Lotz, T. (1980). Influence of selection versus lifestyle on risk of fatal cancer and cardiovascular disease among Seventh-day Adventists. *American Journal of Epidemiology, 112*(2), 296–314.

Post, S. G., Puchalski, C. M., & Larson, D. B. (2000). Physicians and patient spirituality: Professional boundaries, competency, and ethics. *Annals of Internal Medicine, 132*(7), 578–583.

Puchalski, C. M. (1999). Taking a spiritual history: FICA. *Spirituality and Medicine Connection, 3*(1): 17–23.

Raleigh, E. D. (1992). Sources of hope in chronic illness. *Oncology Nursing Forum, 19*(3), 443–448.

Rassnick, S., Sved, A. F., & Rabin, B. S. (1994). Locus coeruleus stimulation by corticotropin-releasing hormone suppresses in vitro cellular immune responses. *Journal of Neuroscience, 10*, 6033–6040.

Reite, M., Harbeck, R., & Hoffman, A. (1981). Altered cellular immune response following peer separation. *Life Science, 29*(11), 1133–1136.

Reite, M., Short, R., Kaufman, I. C., Stynes, A. J., & Pauley, J. D. (1978). Heart rate and body temperature in separated monkey infants. *Biological Psychiatry, 13*(1), 91–105.

Reynolds, P., & Kaplan, G. A. (1990). Social connections and risk for cancer: Prospective evidence from the Alameda County Study. *Behavioral Medicine, 16*(3), 101–110.

Roberts, J. A., Brown, D., Elkins, T., & Larson, D. B.(1997). Factors influencing views of patients with gynecologic cancer about end-of-life decisions. *American Journal of Obstetrics and Gynecology, 176*(1 Pt 1), 166–172.

Robson, M., Levin, D., Federici, M., Satagopan, J., Bogolminy, F., Heerdt, A., et al. (1999). Breast conservation therapy for invasive breast cancer in Ashkenazi women with BRCA gene founder mutations. *Journal of the National Cancer Institute*, *91*(24), 2112–2117.

Schaal, M. D., Sephton, S. E., Thoreson, C., Koopman, C., & Spiegel, D. (1998). *Religious expression and immune competence in women with advanced cancer*. Presented at the meeting of the American Psychological Association, San Francisco.

Schleifer, S. J., Keller, S. E., Camerino, M., Thornton, J. C., & Stein, M. (1983). Suppression of lymphocyte stimulation following bereavement. *Journal of the American Medical Association, 250*(3), 374–377.

Sephton, S. E., Koopman, C., & Schaal, M. (2001). Spiritual expression and immune status in women with metastatic breast cancer: An exploratory study. *Breast Journal, 7*, 345–353.

Shekelle, R. B., Raynor, W. J., Jr., Ostfeld, A. M., Garron, D. C., Bieliauskas, L. A., Liu, S. C., et al. (1981). Psychological depression and 17-year risk of death from cancer. *Psychosomatic Medicine, 43*(2), 117–125.

Simpson, J. L., Martin, A. O., Elias, S., Sarto, G. E., & Dunn, J. K. (1981). Cancers of the breast and female genital system: Search for recessive genetic factors through analysis of human isolate. *American Journal of Obstetrics and Gynecology, 141*(6), 629–636.

Sodestrom, K. E., & Martinson, I. M. (1987). Patients' spiritual coping strategies: A study of nurse and patient perspectives. *Oncology Nursing Forum, 14*(2), 41–46.

Spiegel, D., Bloom, J. R., Kraemer, H. C., & Gottheil, E. (1989). Effect of psychosocial treatment on survival of patients with metastatic breast cancer. *Lancet, 2*(8668), 888–891.

Steinberg, A. G., Bleibtreu, H. K., Kurczynski, T. W., Kurczynski, E. M. (1967). Genetic studies on an inbred human isolate. In J. F. Crow & J. V. Neel (Eds.), *Proceedings of the third national congress of human genetics*. Baltimore, MD: Johns Hopkins University Press.

Steinberg, K. K., Pernarelli, J. M., Marcus, M. J., Khoury, M. J., Schildkraut, J. M., & Marchbanks, P. A., (1998). Increased risk for familial ovarian cancer among Jewish women: A population-based case-control study. *Genetic Epidemiology, 15*(1), 51–59.

Taylor, R. S., Carroll, B. E., & Lloyd, J. W. (1959). Mortality among women in 3 Catholic religious orders with special reference to cancer. *Cancer, 12*, 1207–1225.

Toniolo, P. G., & Kato, I. (1996). Jewish religion and risk of breast cancer. *Lancet 348*(9029), 760.

Torbjornsen, T., Stifoss-Hanssen, H., Abrahamsen, A. F., & Hannisdal, E. (2000). Cancer and religiosity—A follow up of patients with Hodgkin's disease *Tidsskr Nor Laegeforen, 120*(3), 346–348.

Underwood, R. (1985). The presence of God in pastoral care ministry. *Austin Presbyterian Theological Seminary Bulletin, 61*(4), 7.

Ur, E., White, P. D., & Grossman, A. (1992). Hypothesis: Cytokines may be activated to cause depressive illness and chronic fatigue syndrome. *European Archives of Psychiatry and Clinical Neuroscience, 241*(5), 317–322.

Wolbarst, A. L. (1932). Circumcision and penile cancer in men. *Lancet, 1*, 150–153.

Wolff, G. (1939). Cancer and race with special reference to the Jews. *American Journal of Hygiene, 29*, 121–137.

Wynder, E. L., Lemon, F. R., & Bross, I. J. (1959). Cancer and coronary artery disease among Seventh-Day Adventists. *Cancer, 12*, 1016–1028.

Zisook, S., Shuchter, S. R., Irwin, M., Darko, D. F., Sledge, P., & Resovsky, K. (1994). Bereavement, depression, and immune function. *Psychiatry Research, 52*(1), 1–10.

# 3

## Diet, Nutrition, and Natural Products

# History of Diet and Cancer in Human Evolution

Marc S. Micozzi

## Introduction

Whether cancer in the United States can be significantly affected by diet remains an important question. It is now accepted on the basis of growing evidence that nutritional status, as well as individual nutrients, have an important role in the prevention and management of many diseases in the U.S. population (Fairfield & Fletcher, 2002; Fletcher & Fairfield, 2002). The ability to apply this information to individuals is based on present scientific information and understanding of (1) the person-to-person metabolic differences that influence nutritional status, (2) the relations among macronutrients (calories, fat, protein, and fiber), micronutrients (vitamins and minerals), and nutritional status, and (3) the time or times during carcinogenesis that nutrients exert their effects.

For example, in the micronutrient area, clinical trials of beta-carotene supplementation—an abundant dietary constituent—did not demonstrate a protective effect against cancer at the levels administered (Greenberg et al., 1990). However, studies on chronic beta-carotene intake from foods and capsule supplements indicate significant variations in individual response to a given dose of beta-carotene. It is also interesting to note that foods associated with a lower risk for cancer, although initially thought to be consistently high in beta-carotene (provitamin A) content (Peto, Doll, Buckley, & Sporn, 1981), are in fact much more consistently high in other carotenoids without vitamin A activity, low in fat and calories, high in fiber, and high in other micronutrients (Micozzi, Beecher, Taylor, & Khachik, 1990).

In the macronutrient area, there are relations among dietary modification, changes in nutritional status, and cancer prevention. The effect of dietary modification of macronutrients on cancer risk is being tested in large-scale clinical trials, particularly for breast, colon, and prostate cancer. Epidemiological and experimental evidence is not yet completely clear or consistent as to the "nutritional causes" of breast, colon, or prostate cancer.

Relative to breast cancer, evolutionary biology would suggest that for the majority of human history most women spent much of their adult lives pregnant or lactating, a status associated with lower rates of breast cancer (Chapter 9). Through prehistoric to modern times, human populations shifted from (1) high fertility/high mortality to (2) high fertility/low mortality to (3) low fertility/low mortality. The middle transition is held responsible for the tremendous world population growth of the past century, in which the state much of the world remains, whereas Europe and North America have made the final transition to Stage 3.

If the increasing rates of breast cancer, for example, in this country during this century are inevitable correlates of fundamental demographic shifts and changes in fertility (see Chapter 9), what is the role of diet and nutrition? The individual variations in how people absorb and metabolize dietary constituents ("nutritional individuality" in evolutionary biology terms) have received less emphasis by researchers. This is somewhat surprising when contrasted with cardiovascular disease (CVD), its association with dietary cholesterol, and the greatly improved preventive measures provided by the understanding of nutritional individuality as quantified by serum lipids and lipoproteins. For CVD, the association with dietary intake of foods high in fats was an important first step. The identification of serum lipids, lipid metabolism, and cholesterol receptors provided a greatly improved understanding of biological mechanisms.

# An Evolutionary Perspective on Diet and Cancer

If we come to view diet as an adaptation to the environment, and the epidemiology of diet and cancer as evidence of human maladaptation (Potter & Graves 1991), we may begin to consider dietary experience for the majority of human history as a clue to the type of diet to which human metabolism may be adapted (and that may help prevent cancer if followed or contribute to cancer if not). Prehistoric archaeologists can reconstruct some human dietary patterns from ancient remains (Eaton & Konner, 1985). Modern theories of human evolution and studies of primates and hunter-gatherer societies also provide some models. Until the development of agriculture and animal domestication approximately 10,000 years ago, omnivorous humans had available to eat only those plants and animals that appeared in the wild. Although we tend to have a concept of "man the hunter" as somehow characteristic of early human experience, "woman the gatherer" may be a more accurate account. Whereas big game hunting was a part of early human experience in some areas, most of the time its social significance may have been far greater than its nutritional significance. In any event, wild game (with 4%–6% body fat) is quite different nutritionally from modern domesticated animals (up to 40%–60% body fat), the latter largely a phenomenon of the 20th century.

Is cancer the result of leaving behind the heritage of our primitive diet and lifestyle? The actual evidence for cancer in animals and humans in antiquity in the Old World before Byzantium, and the New World before Columbus, is vanishingly small or nonexistent, even under many circumstances where cancer could be readily detected if present

(Chapter 3). Cancer research and prevention may be guided by greater understanding of human evolutionary biology or history.

Cancer is generally recognized as a sequence of steps resulting in increased molecular changes and increased numbers of abnormal cells (Chapters 1 and 2). Food constituents, macronutrients, or micronutrients may be recognized in the etiology of cancer by correspondence to the sequence of steps that lead to clinical cancer and specific abnormalities or variation in nutritional status. This section summarizes the role of nutrients in cancer and introduces the relations between macro- and micronutrients and other risk factors.

# Cancer and Biologic Adaptation

Humans have always had to eat and have always eaten the same basic nutrients—protein, fat, carbohydrates, vitamins, and minerals. Current research is investigating the relationship between specific dietary patterns and disease and has concluded that present patterns of diseases and changes in those patterns can be linked at least in part to food consumption. This relationship between diet and cancer may come from the intimate dependence of humans on their food supply. This dependence derives from long-standing adaptive patterns of dietary intake.

Humans are adapted to a seasonally variable diet, depending on intake of substances from the environment and of substances to which we have little or infrequent exposure. There are at least four broad ways in which aberrations in the dietary pattern of humans could produce disease such as cancer: (1) there may be an imbalance in energy intake and output; (2) there may be an alteration of the pattern of nutrients in the diet; (3) specific deficiencies may occur; (4) the food supply may contain substances to which the organism is almost never exposed, and therefore, for which there may not be a relevant metabolic response.

We cannot be certain as to what kind of diets humans are well adapted biologically (although the length and morphology of the gastrointestinal tract, dentition, and enzyme patterns provide some clues). However, it is possible to attempt to describe our early diet. Extensive variability in diets must have existed in the same way that we observe extensive geographic and temporal variability in contemporary diets. Some common features are as follows:

- a high intake of a wide variety of foods—leaves, nuts, seeds, fruit (domesticated grains could have only become a staple in the last 10,000–15,000 years but were probably gathered wild in season);
- sporadic intake of lean meat low in saturated fat (a more secure and regular supply of fish and seafood for costal dwellers);
- intake of insects, grubs (high in protein), and bone marrow and organ meats;
- very low intake of alcohol;
- little refining or fractioning of food;
- low and irregular intake of eggs and very little nonhuman milk (dairy domestication is probably only 10,000 years old);

- variability, by season, both of total amount of food available and of kinds of foods, resulting in variability in intake of particular nutrients.

Other variations in this overall intake pattern would have been defined by climate as it changed over time and from place to place, including the consumption of high-fat (but not high-saturated-fat) diets in extreme northern populations. In general, until very recently, saturated fat and alcohol intake would have been low, plant food (but not grain) intake high, and food sources highly diverse.

Adaptation is not just a list of taste preferences but a spectrum of human/environment dependencies. Deviation may have significant consequences for health.

One important argument in favor of human adaptation to specific kinds of foods and eating habits is that there are many substances for which the organism is known to be dependent on the environment. This well-established concept in nutrition has some important implications for cancer. Dietary deficiency disorders can arise if an organism cannot make a given nutrient. If there is no natural selection pressure for an ability to make certain nutrients, that is to argue that the essential substances are widely available in the environment. Therefore, because certain nutrients are widely available in nature, and humans cannot make them, deficiencies are possible. Essential amino acids, essential fatty acids, microelements, and vitamins are examples. What is essential varies among mammalian species and underscores the importance of the adaptation process. In sum, the essential nutrients—both energy bearing and micronutrients—are available to varying degrees in nature; they have important functions in growth, development, and reproduction; the organism is dependent on their ubiquity; and deficiencies or excess may impair growth, development, and reproduction.

The normal long-term function of cells is dependent on the presence of a variety of widespread dietary constituents, including those necessary for growth and development. In their absence, cells malfunction. This malfunctioning state may make the cells more susceptible to exposure to carcinogens or may impair some specific protective mechanisms. It may also be characterized by higher cell replication rates as somatic cells seek to adapt to the new conditions. Maintenance is a continuous function from birth but growth, development, and reproduction are time limited (Chapter 2).

For those dietary constituents that are rare in nature, intensive ingestion may have untoward consequences. This applies to rare exposures that produce acute toxicity and to unaccustomed intake levels that overwhelm the metabolic processes that normally can handle the exposure. Bacterial, plant, and fungal toxins are examples. Examples exist of other types of toxic dietary exposures, which increase risk of disease (Table 8.1; see also Chapter 14 on naturopathy)

An objection to an adaptation argument, in relation to cancer, is that natural selection influences reproductive success and that cancer is largely a disease of postreproductive years. There are four responses: first, humans have a long period of infant and juvenile dependence and survival of parents and grandparents in a healthy state (i.e., longevity) is likely to be selected for.

The second response requires some consideration of the unit of selection. If the issue is the survival of tribes or bands, then those bands would have survived better that had sufficient elders who knew how to respond to infrequently met hazards—food or water shortage, epidemic disease, and natural hazards such as fire or extreme weather.

**High Risk or "Toxic" Diets**

1. A high fat/calorie intake has consequences for cholesterol and insulin metabolism, adipose storage, and sex steroid hormone production
2. A high grain diet (such as that found in predominantly agricultural communities) is often associated with a reduced intake of other plant foods (and a lower intake of animal foods) and contains large amounts of abrasive material that may increase cell replication rates in the digestive tract
3. A high intake of alcohol, which together with a generally reduced range of foods, is associated with a wide variety of metabolic abnormalities

*Note:* There may be differing degrees of adaptation in long-exposed versus unexposed populations in each of these cases.

The tribal wisdom maintained by the old would have meant survival of the tribe. Tribes without elders and without knowledge would be more likely to perish. Therefore the tribes in which longevity was selected would, in turn, have survived other threats to pass on their wisdom, their adaptive eating habits, their adapted metabolisms, and their genes. Third, cancer is a phenomenon of older age. Conversely, cancer is not primarily a disease of younger ages. Therefore, some resistance to this biological phenomenon (at least to the point of postponing cancer to older ages) has been selected for.

Finally, a diet that reduces the risk of cancer may also coincidentally improve reproductive success. There are a wide variety of substances that may cause cancer and are also toxic in other ways. Selection for improved reproductive success may directly select for reduced risk of cancer.

Some of the relations that have been established among diet and cancer are explainable in relation to three kinds of aberrations in dietary behavior: (1) energy imbalance, (2) nutrient imbalance, and (3) specific nutrient deficiency. Each of these is considered.

# Energy Imbalance

Three measures relevant to energy balance have been explored in relation to cancer: (1) total intake, (2) energy output, and (3) measures of growth and overweight. No simple established relation exists between any of these measures and all cancers.

The present evidence suggests that higher physical activity is related to a lower risk of colon cancer. For endometrial cancer and postmenopausal breast cancer, obesity is a risk factor (de Waard, Baanders-van Halewijn, & Huizinga, 1964; de Waard & Trichopoulos, 1988). There is a general association between obesity and overall cancer risk (Lew & Garfinkel 1979). Body fat distribution (known to be related to diabetes and coronary artery disease) is increasingly under investigation as a cancer risk factor.

Three possible mechanisms are (1) hormonal, (2) mechanical, and (3) cellular replication. On the *hormonal* front, peripheral adipose tissue is the major source of postmenopausal estrogens. Excess body fat in older women is association with endometrial and breast cancer, both of which are thought to be associated with high (perhaps cumulative lifetime) estrogen exposure.

The role of physical activity in colon cancer is possibly a *mechanical* effect—higher activity results in shorter mouth-to-anus transit time. Because high energy intake and low physical energy output are risk factors for colon cancer, there may be metabolic differences in those who get colon cancer compared with those who do not. The total amount of food passing through the colon may represent a measure of total cellular activity (absorption, mucus and enzyme production, and detoxification) and therefore could cause higher *cellular replication* rates.

These complex relations among dietary intake, obesity, physical activity, and cancer risk may be explained by relevant metabolic intermediate steps, including effects on gut function, cell replication, and hormone production. The observation that aspects of energy imbalance are related to cancer is clearly established.

The human organism is adapted to a high degree of variability in food intake and is able to make rapid use of a sudden increase in food supply to better survive through lean periods. This is the essence of the thrifty gene hypothesis, originally proposed as an explanation for survival advantage for the predisposition to diabetes. A high intake of food on a regular, rather than sporadic, basis is also likely to "jam open" processes other than insulin response. Thus, as low intakes of food, (e.g., at the end of winter) gave way to a more plentiful supply, reproductive success might be higher in those females who gained sufficient body fat rapidly. Further, increasing colonic surface area would be particularly valuable in extracting energy via bacterial fermentation from relatively energy-poor food sources. Such changes may also increase peripheral adipose production of estrogen, a factor perhaps originally associated with reproductive success—sufficient body fat, plus hormonal support, to carry a child to term.

Animal data show that with low dietary intake, or in a fasting state, the structure of the colonic epithelium is much simpler and cell replication rates much lower. With refeeding, cell replication rates increase, as does the complexity of the epithelial surface and the total surface area. This appears to be a highly adaptive response to marked variability in food availability—high cell turnover and large absorptive area in times of abundance but low activity during shortage to conserve energy. In the presence of a high-intake diet on a regular basis, however, high cell turnover and colonic epithelial surface area provide a favorable environment for carcinogensis via (1) increased ingestion of carcinogenic substances, (2) maximal absorptive surface area, and (3) increased probability of a carcinogenic mutational "hit" in rapidly replicating tissue. An association between increased frequency of food consumption and risk of colon cancer has been confirmed.

Thus, although obesity itself was almost certainly uncommon in human ancestors, the capacity to assimilate food rapidly and store energy when it was available has probably been selected for. Inheritance of this metabolic profile in a society where food is widely available appears to have consequences for cancer risk at a number of sites.

High fat (Ip, Birt, Rogers, & Mettlin, 1986), high alcohol (Hiatt & Bawol, 1984; International Agency for Research on Cancer [IARC], 1988), or high grain consumption were not dietary patterns to which humans in their original state were *regularly exposed*. An intermittent high intake (in a feast/fast environment) produces rapid adaptive responses (increased gut epithelial proliferation, increased secretions of bile acids, and hormones), which, as an energy-conserving mechanism, then subsided when food became scarce. High metabolic activity and cellular turnover is a cost to the organism that is not a good investment in the presence of reduced food availability. The capacity for rapid response becomes nonadaptive in the presence of consistent high intake leading not only to alcoholism and obesity but also to chronic high gastrointestinal hormone levels and elevated cellular epithelial proliferation rates. High intakes of abrasive fibers result in elevated alimentary tract proliferation rates and increased risk of carcinogenesis.

Another aspect to the adaptive argument is related to the internal ecology of the colon. The large bowel can be considered a complex escosystem in which the colonic contents act as a culture medium for bacteria and colonic cells. The culture medium, in turn, is influenced extensively by host conditions, including hormones, and by ingested foods and alcohol. This ecosystem may be one of the most flexible parts of the human/environment adaptation relationship. However, there are limits to its flexibility with consequences for carcinogenesis.

## Specific Deficiencies

A diet to which humans are adapted should include protective factors. One obvious "macronutrient" that has been proposed as protective against cancer is dietary fiber (Aldercreutz, 1982; Jacobs, 1983).

Fiber and cereals, as potentially protective agents particularly in colon cancer, have attracted considerable attention. In 1971 Burkitt proposed that the reason Africans were at low risk of colon cancer was not (as his mentor and colleague, Cleave, believed) because their diets were low in sugar but rather because their diets were high in fiber. This hypothesis is attractive but problematic, and the evidence in its favor is equivocal. In brief, there is a wide variety of substances all referred to as "fiber" that have never been categorized in epidemiologic studies largely because the dietary databases used in such studies are incomplete (and even inconsistent). Further, these fibers vary extensively in their physicochemical properties, solubility, bile acid–binding capacity, fermentability, and water-holding capacity. Measurement problems complicate this classification issue.

The association between "dietary fiber" and colon cancer has produced mixed findings. However, there are data to show that a diet high in fiber may be relevant, not only in colon cancer but also in pancreas and other cancers. These effects may be consequences of other less well-understood dietary constituents that are found in foods such as vegetables, fruits, and nuts for which "dietary fiber" as a nutrient may be a proxy or marker.

Specific cereals may actually be associated with a higher risk of esophageal cancer. Of course, this argument relates to cereals as a food, not fiber as a nutrient. For colon cancer, some cereals (particularly rice) have been associated with increased, not decreased risk—despite the fact that, internationally, rice eating is associated with a reduced population risk of colon cancer.

The most obvious specific deficiencies after fiber are those of micronutrients. For beta-carotene, retinol, and vitamin C (ascorbate), higher risks of particular cancers have been reported in individuals with lower intakes or blood levels (Chapter 9). There are several cancers that have a probable relationship with micronutrient deficiencies—notably lung cancer and cervix cancer. Lower dietary ascorbate levels have been reported for rectal cancer and lower intakes of minerals such as calcium and trace elements such as selenium may be important.

The most consistent finding in the dietary etiology of cancer is the more general relation between a higher intake of vegetables and a lower risk of cancer of a wide variety of sites, including mouth and pharynx, lung, stomach, pancreas, colon, and rectum (Chapter 10). In general, over 100 studies looking at the role of vegetable and fruit intake in relation to cancer reveal a very consistent picture of lower risk in association with higher consumption of these foods (Micozzi et al., 1988, 1990).

It may be worthwhile considering vegetables or plant foods as adaptive packages of required intakes for humans. Vegetables contain a wide variety of substances that have been shown to have anticancer properties—phenols, isothiocyanates, flavonoids, indoles, lignans, for example, as well as vitamins, minerals, and trace elements. It is not possible to provide an estimate of the intakes of most of these "nonnutrient" substances that are biologically active. Food tables do not provide the data, most of the relevant food analyses have not been done, and it is likely that many important constituents remain to be identified.

Plant foods, conversely, are also an important source of carcinogens in the diet, including some of the compounds actually identified as "anticarcinogens." as listed prior. Varying conditions and doses may alter the likely carcinogenic outcome—a yin/yang phenomenon. The same substance may have different physiologic effects at markedly different doses, one of the key concepts of homeopathy (Chapter 17).

Some substances, including vitamins and trace elements, are known to be essential for the organism to grow, maintain integrity, and reproduce optimally. The consequences of low (dietary or tissue) levels of these substances may include carcinogenesis. Humans may be equally dependent on the environment to provide substances that have specific anticarcinogenic properties. In the absence of these substances, organisms are at a higher risk of cancer at a number of sites, particularly those where cellular epithelial surfaces are exposed to environmental agents—lung, digestive tract, and cervix. These diet supplied compounds may act to induce detoxifying enzymes, to block activation, and so on, and organisms may be reliant on them to do so. Host defenses can be enhanced by environmentally supplied nutrients that "tune" the system. In low doses (hence the yin/yang phenomenon) even carcinogens may be beneficial, inducing the system to metabolize higher doses. In high doses, even normally benign compounds may overwhelm the system and either produce toxic/carcinogenic effects themselves or allow other more potent compounds to do so (see Chapter 17 on homeopathy).

Adaptation relates to each of the dietary phenomena associated with increased cancer risk and specific micronutrient deficiencies (or specific exposures). However, there is no way to modify levels of energy intake or macronutrients without also modifying other nutrients: for example, any attempt to decrease fat will result in decreased calories or increases in other nutrients. Similarly, attempts to reduce obesity or change body mass results in changes of nutrient intake, energy intake, energy expenditure, or all three. However, addition of either specific compounds to the diet or modification of vegetable intake provides both a test of the protective effect and a test of possible health strategies.

# Diet and Cancer in Modern Perspective

Research associating nutritional elements with chronic diseases has been ongoing since the mid-1950s. In the meantime, progress has also been made in the underlying sciences regarding cellular mechanisms of action of nutrients, as well as the classification of carcinogens according to their individual modes of action. The early discoveries in the area of nutrition and health, and specifically nutrition and cancer, dealt with associations discovered in population and epidemiologic studies. Studies in experimental models, including human, through the techniques of metabolic and biochemical epidemiology are also relevant. Interpretation of the combined results in light of the underlying mechanisms provides some understanding of the role of specific dietary risk factors.

The current approach to uncovering causative factors is to consider each type of cancer as a specific disease entity with its own risk factors. In fact, in some instances, cancer in a given organ may have distinct risk factors affecting dissimilar targets within the organ. For example, it is not certain that breast cancer is a homogeneous disease, but rather that premenopausal breast cancer may involve causative elements distinct from those operating in postmenopausal breast cancer (Wynder & Cohen 1982; Wynder, Rose, & Cohen, 1986). Also, it is reasonably well established that large bowel or colorectal cancer actually represents three disease entities, (1) proximal, (2) distal colon cancer, and (3) rectal cancer, each with its own dietary risk factors. Studies on the association of nutrients and "large bowel cancer" are apt to have poor correlations, and even reach erroneous conclusions, because a given nutrient may not bear on all three types of large bowel cancer.

For each cancer, information has been sought on the causative factors. This factor may be a single chemical, as is often true in occupational-related cancers, or a mixture of related chemicals, such as the class of polycyclic aromatic hydrocarbons and nitrosamines, associated with lung cancer. It could also be a mixture of closely related aromatic amines produced during cooking, which may bear on the nutritionally linked cancers. Importantly, most types of cancer seen in humans also require the presence of promoting or enhancing factors. In the nutritionally linked cancers, for example, this role has often been assumed to be the total fat intake through specific metabolic mechanisms appropriate to each type of cancer. To understand where and when different factors may influence the development of cancer, consider the "two-stage" model.

## Two-Stage Model of Cancer

At least two distinct stages of carcinogenesis, an early stage and a late stage, related to "initiating" agents and "promoting" agents, have been recognized. Carcinogens that initiate cancers have been associated with cancers of environmental or occupational origin, or important types of cancer related to life-style, the use of tobacco products, and exposure to tobacco smoke. Such carcinogens may also be present in foods as a result of cooking, salting, or pickling.

Later sequences in the growth and development of cancer are subject to a different set of growth-controlling elements that operate through distinct mechanisms. This area of "promotion and progression" plays a key role in eventually leading to clinical, overt cancer.

Some micronutrients, such as vitamin A, can serve to decrease cancer-promoting actions (Wald, Idle, Boreham, & Bailey, 1980). A major role of dietary components such as fat, fiber, or micronutrients is thought to influence the growth and developmental aspects of cancer cells. These actions are highly dose dependent and are also reversible. Lowering the concentration of a growth-promoting substance by only 50% may exert growth retardation of cancer cells. Complete elimination of promoting substances can almost immediately and sharply decrease the development of cancer cells. Smoking cessation, for example, progressively lowers the risk of the development of bronchogenic carcinoma. Because it is possible to delay or abolish the growth of abnormal cells, there is a foundation for dietary recommendations for the prevention of diet-related cancer. In patients with appropriately treated diet-sensitive cancers, a decrease in promoting factors may be designed to prevent or delay recurrences, providing a sound means of supportive therapy.

# Specific Cancer Factors

Progress in documenting specific cancer factors has resulted from multidisciplinary approaches. In the field of occupational health, or in the study of smoking and health, much has been learned from comparing groups of people exposed to carcinogens, such as smokers, with people not exposed. In the area of nutrition and health, and specifically nutrition and cancer, the approach needs to be more refined, because everyone eats. Thus, studies in a country with a given traditional diet often show few clear-cut differences in dietary habits between those who develop cancer and those who do not. There may be certain differences, but within a given country, the group with the lowest compared with the highest intake of a nutrient may cover a fairly narrow range. Therefore, many studies in the area of nutrition and cancer examining the role of macronutrients such as fat or fiber, or micronutrients like vitamin A or calcium, have often yielded ambiguous results.

The most rewarding and relevant approach involves the study of populations with traditionally distinct nutritional habits and exposure to toxic (IARC, 1976) or high-risk diets (see, for example, Table 8.1). Foods customarily consumed in Japan used to be quite different from those in the West, specifically North America or the United Kingdom (Stocks 1957, 1970). In Japan, the major nutrient was carbohydrate (rice) with some protein from fish, and a limited amount of total fat, approximately 15% of calories. In contrast, the typical Western diet consisted of 40%–45% carbohydrates and 40%–45% total fat. These Japanese traditions were paralleled by a dramatically distinct lower incidence in mortality from cancer of the breast, colon, ovary, endometrium, pancreas, and prostate, as well as from myocardial infarction. Studies in migrants from China (Koo, 1988) or Japan to Hawaii and North America reveal a sharp increase in risk for colon cancer in migrants themselves and of breast or prostate cancer in the second generation (Kolonel, Hankin, Nomura, & Chu, 1981). Migrants progressively adopt the dietary traditions of their new host country (Hirayama, 1978; Hirayama, Eylenbosch, Van Larebeke, & Depoorter, 1988). A reason for the delayed increase for cancers such as breast and prostate may stem from the fact that residency in a lower risk environment during the important developmental stages at puberty protects these tissues from later development of cancer. However, cell turnover in the distal colon occurs at a relatively constant rate and may account for the sensitivity in the migrants themselves.

Current evidence of a major role for diet lies in the appreciable increase in cancer of the breast and the distal colon, but not the proximal colon, in Japan. The rise is particularly noteworthy in urban Japan, associated with the progressive introduction of Western dietary habits, essentially increasing fat and decreasing carbohydrate intake.

Other parts of the world provide supporting information. People in southern Italy had largely maintained the traditional Italian dietary pattern, whereas the diet of the industrial northern Italian population is similar to that of the rest of Western Europe or the United States. The southern Italian diet uses olive oil as the main lipid, and the total lipid intake is about 32% of calories. In northern Italy the fat intake also involves olive oil, but there is a more varied fat consumption, and the total linoleic acid intake is higher. Associated with this distinct dietary pattern is an appreciably lower rate of breast cancer in southern Italy compared to northern Italy or the United States.

Another exceptional population is in Finland, especially in rural areas. As a rule the Finnish people consume large amounts of total fat, mostly saturated fats from extensive use of dairy products, a habit typical of a region at high risk for coronary heart disease. Even so, Finnish people display a low incidence of distal colon cancer. Also, postmenopausal breast cancer mortality is lower than in neighboring Denmark or the United States. An explanation may rest on the fact that the Finnish people consume much higher amounts of foods rich in cereal fibers. The increased fiber intake yields a larger stool bulk, diluting promoters for colon cancer, bile and fatty acids. The lower breast cancer rate has not been fully clarified. Similar trends are apparent in studies of vegetarian populations.

As noted, Japanese with a low risk for the Western-type nutritional cancers consume a low-fat diet; moreover, a fair proportion of the fat in their diet comes from fish oils. Recent studies in several models of breast and colon cancer have observed that fish oil at any dose level is protective; parallel to the findings with atherosclerosis and heart disease, where regular intake of fish is also protective.

## Breast and Pancreas

Cancer of the pancreas may in part be related to exposure to nitrosamines. Some such amines are formed during cooking. In animal models exposed to high doses, these types of chemicals have specific target organs, including the breast, colon, and pancreas, where the effect is powerfully enhanced by fat. Other organs, such as liver or urinary bladder, are not subject to promotion by dietary fat. Under typical conditions of human consumption (usually a low but daily intake of such compounds beginning in childhood) target organs such as the liver would not likely be affected. However, in those tissues where dietary fat exerts a promoting effect, such as breast, there would be an increased risk of disease development (Petrakis et al., 1980). Much more is discussed in Chapter 9.

## Colon

Colon cancer can be induced specifically by a number of carcinogens that also cause cancer in the breast, pancreas, and prostate. Carcinogens belonging to a cancer-causing class of amines are formed during cooking and especially during browning of meat or fish. These chemicals may induce cancer in several tissues, including the colon, breast, and pancreas.

Irrespective of the carcinogen, it has been found that high dietary levels of most types of fat may have a promoting effect. Safflower and corn oil are stronger promoters than olive oil. Modulators such as vitamin A or carotenes may also reduce cancer to some extent.

The amount of total bile acids in the intestinal tract and in the stool is a function of the type and amount of fat consumed in animal models and in humans. Switching people from a high fat intake to a low fat intake lowers the amount of bile acids within days. On return to a high fat diet, the amount of stool bile acids returns to its former level. Because bile acids are promoters, the risk for colon cancer development may be sharply reduced within days by switching from a high-fat to a low-fat diet. The proposition that carcinogenesis is determined through early life events, and therefore would take decades for an alteration of risk, may not apply to situations where the essential controlling factor depends on a promoting effect (Bruce, 1987).

## Endometrium and Ovary

For these organs, the carcinogens have not been fully documented. However, it has been suggested that specific metabolic steps affecting estrogen in these organs may yield a carcinogenic intermediate. These types of cancer are more often seen in women who are obese, and therefore have higher levels of available estrogen, which could be thus modified in a specific way. The effect may be enhanced by dietary fat and by estrogen biosynthesized by fat cells.

## Oral and Esophagus

In the Western world, these types of cancer are seen mainly in individuals who chew tobacco or who smoke and drink alcoholic beverages and often have a poor nutritional intake, especially as regards essential micronutrients. In a broad area, beginning in eastern Iran through former Soviet Central Asia to parts of China, there is a high incidence of cancer of the esophagus, traced to generally poor nutritional status and probable formation of certain nitrosamines. Improvement in nutritional status would most likely lower the risk of this type of cancer.

## Stomach

This type of cancer has declined sharply in the United States since the mid-1950s and is beginning to decrease in northern Europe and Japan. It remains a major type of cancer in Eastern Europe, Latin America, Japan, and parts of China. The associated factors stem from a relatively low intake of essential micronutrients and especially the traditional use of salted, pickled foods or a geochemical environment with high soil, and therefore food, nitrate levels. Specific nitrogen-containing compounds may be the associated risk factors. Recommendations for prevention include lower intake of salted, pickled foods and better nutritional balance, including availability of foods containing micronutrients such as vitamins A, C, and E (Wattenberg, 1983, 1985).

# Modifying Factors

## Dietary Restriction

Investigators in the field of nutrition and cancer observe that significant dietary restriction yields fewer cancers (Willett et al., 1987). This situation may have prevailed in human populations when there was famine, such as in The Netherlands or Norway during World War II, where fat intake was especially depressed. This situation resulted in an apparent lowering of the nutritionally linked cancers, as well as delayed puberty. In breast cancer, dietary restriction may have an indirect explanation, based on altered hormonal balance. Several investigators have also reported that dietary restriction results in a dramatic decrease in DNA synthesis, mitosis, and cell cycling. Thus, dietary restriction may inhibit carcinogenesis through various mechanisms. A high-fat diet at restrictive calorie levels would not lead to promotion, because the dietary calorie restriction would have the opposite effect.

However, most human populations do not voluntarily undergo lifelong dietary restriction but rather eat freely, and indeed overeat, considering that modern humans are often sedentary and their caloric requirements are lower. Exceptional situations such as war and famine temporarily have restrictive effects, with consequent lower risk. Thus, experimental findings cannot be applied to a free-living population with reasonable access to a variety of foods, as is true in the developed world. For such populations, other means of lowering disease risk are needed. This includes the adoption of new dietary traditions or rediscovery of the older, healthier ones.

## Fiber and Calcium

People in rural Finland consume a high-saturated-fat diet and thus have an elevated incidence of heart disease. In sharp contrast, they display a low distal colon cancer risk. The underlying mechanism is a regular high wheat bran intake, leading to a large stool bulk, 200–280 g, in one or more passes. For that reason, fatty and bile acids, which are promoters in colon carcinogenesis, occur at a threefold lower concentration than what is found in high-risk populations. This situation has been reproduced in animal models where fiber has reduced colon cancer. Fat and fiber interact, the effect depending on the ratio. The rate of breast cancer in Finnish women is also lower than in Western women. Fibers appear to be protective. Also, food fibers contain complex chemicals, some with antiestrogenic activity. Estrogen, as is commonly known, can proliferate breast cancer cells. Fibers also affect the microflora, intestinal pH, and activity of bacterial enzymes, in turn altering the cycling of estrogen and yielding protective hormonal patterns (Aldercreutz, 1984).

Supplemental calcium salts and wheat bran lower the rate of cell cycling in the intestinal tract of high-risk patients. The rate of cellular DNA biosynthesis and mitosis controls the overall sequence of events leading to clinical cancer. Currently, the potential benefits of calcium and vitamin D in the fat-associated cancers is under active investigation in humans. Wheat bran also lowers cell replication rates in the rectum in high-risk patients, an indicator of beneficial effects.

## Exercise

People who have regular occupational or recreational exercise have lower risk of colon cancer than sedentary individuals. Women who were athletic in the first 25 years of their lives appear to have lower breast cancer rates later in life than women who were not (Frisch et al, 1974 1985). Thus, early lifestyle is carried as a benefit to a subsequent period of life (LeMarchand et al., 1988; Micozzi, 1985). These situations are mimicked in rats who had free access to a wheel cage. Some rats were active runners and others were less frequent users. Researchers found that even on a high-fat diet, the percentage of rats with mammary gland cancer was lower in rats that were moderate runners than in rats that were low and high runners. Similar results were obtained for colon cancer. The protective effect of exercise was not because of a lower food intake or a lower weight gain. The animals on the exercise wheel weighed as much or more than the sedentary controls, but their body contained less fat and more protein and especially more water.

## Total Diet

Cancer affecting certain target organs is clearly a multistep disease providing the opportunity to block or at least decrease carcinogenesis at a number of points and therefore lead to a lower overall risk, and thus incidence, of specific types of cancer. Directly linked with macronutrients, dietary fat, and fiber are cancers in the postmenopausal breast, ovary and endometrium, and prostate, pancreas, and distal colon. Cancers of the breast, colon, and pancreas, and perhaps others for which evidence remains to be acquired, may involve carcinogenic amines formed during cooking (United States Department of Health and Human Services, 1988). It is possible that cancer of the prostate likewise is caused by such chemicals. The events as regards cancer of the ovary and endometrium are ill defined, but it may be that estrogen can be converted through metabolism to DNA-reactive metabolities. Exposure to such cancer-causing agents occurs early in life, when rapid growth of tissues involving high levels of DNA synthesis and mitosis facilitates transformation of normal cells to early neoplastic cells.

Without promotion or enhancing effects, it is likely that these effects would not translate to clinically overt cancer. The common cancer of the prostate seen in older men represents such an early effect leading to dormant tumor cells. Control and prevention of the nutritionally linked types of cancer rests on proper definition of the maximal amounts of dietary factors that would not increase the risk of these cancers. For example, the National Academy of Sciences forwarded preliminary recommendations that the intake of total fat, traditionally about 38%–44% of calories consumed in populations in the United States and Western Europe, be lowered to about 30%. This decision was based on parallel recommendations of the American Heart Association and federal agencies concerned with heart disease risk, which had also adopted a recommendation of 30% of fat calories.

Data since the early 1980s in models for colon and breast cancer, and observations in humans, indicate that 30% is not likely to have a preventive effect. For example, a large prospective study on breast cancer incidence in nurses as a function of dietary fat indicated no effect. In the five subgroups, the one with the lowest fate intake consumed diets with about 32% fat calories, with the highest at 46%. Therefore, based on current knowledge, there is no difference in the effect of fat in breast cancer at intakes between 20% and

| Table 8.2 | Framework for an Original Human Diet |
|---|---|

There is a dietary pattern to which humans are well adapted—an "original diet." This original dietary pattern had specific features that included regular exposure to a variety of substances on which human metabolism is dependent but that have not, previously, been explicitly labeled as "essential nutrients."

The original dietary pattern was low in highly abrasive cereal products (consumption of large amounts of grains is a relatively recent phenomenon) with less resultant damage and less need for frequent cell repair to the gastrointestinal tract.

The diet involved variability in intake, which was accompanied by variability in cell replication rates, particularly in the gastrointestinal tract, and little risk of obesity.

There was little intake of alcohol and therefore little exposure to its solvent and chronic cell damage capacities.

Abandonment of each of these aspects of dietary adaptation has consequences for carcinogenesis. Most notable is the reduction of intake of vegetables and fruit with subsequent loss of enzyme "induction" and a generally increased rate of cancer at a number of sites. A high intake of fat, grains, and alcohol and increased obesity are each associated with an identifiable pattern of cancers. Increasing intake of vegetables and fruit may reduce the risk of colon cancer and perhaps of colonic adenomatous polyps, even in the presence of a high fat intake, and of esophageal cancer even with exposure to specific carcinogenic compounds. Testing will provide more definitive answers regarding the specific compounds and their sites and modes of action. Meanwhile, the data encourage us to eat more vegetables as well to reduce fat, alcohol, and obesity.

30% calories from fat. Hence, based on these facts and the underlying mechanisms, the promoting aspects of dietary fat in humans could be reduced only by a recommendation that the total fat consumption approach less than 20% of calories. Public education, especially as regards information on sources of fat, on foods high or low in fat, and likewise desirable substitutes such as bran cereal fibers, other carbohydrates, vegetables, and fruits, is important. Production and marketing of low-fat/high-fiber foods has been promoted as a more wholesome lifestyle, which is claimed also to reduce the risk of cardiovascular diseases (Table 8.2).

As discussed, micronuturients can modulate, sometimes quite appreciably, the effect of macronuturients. For example, vitamin A may help reduce the risk of breast cancer associated with dietary fat or of lung cancer in smokers. Therefore, it remains to define the optimal composition of the total diet as regards protein, fat, fiber, carbohydrate, and micronutrients to minimize cancer risks and chronic disease risks generally.

# Summary

There are areas of the world where cancer risk is related to reduced intakes of specific nutrients and to exposure to specific dietary carcinogens (e.g., China, where cancer is associated with $N$-nitroso compounds and low intakes and blood levels of a variety of vitamins and trace elements). Supplementation with the missing nutrients has been, to date, disappointing in reducing risk. It follows from the adaptation argument that what may be missing are not the obvious micronutrients (these may be markers for the real deficiencies) but specific plant compounds containing various detoxifying enzymes. What may actually be essential is to add either a variety of vegetables and fruits or perhaps various specific enzyme-inducers, blocking agents, and so on, to that diet. Similar arguments apply to the role of vegetables in the prevention of the recurrence of cancer.

There are a variety of ways in which diet may influence the development of human cancers. Previous views of this topic have largely been descriptive and mechanistic: exposure to a macronutrient such as fat is associated with increases in certain cancers; increased intake of a micronutrient appears to reduce the risk of certain cancers. A framework can be constructed as shown in Table 8.2, which provides an appropriate summary and conclusion for this chapter.

## REFERENCES AND RESOURCES

Adlercreutz, H. (1984). Does fiber-rich food containing animal lignan precursors protect against both colon and breast cancer?: An extension of the "fiber hypothesis." *Gastroenterology, 86*, 761–766.

Bruce, W. R. (1987). Recent hypotheses for the origin of colon cancer. *Cancer Research, 97*, 4237–4242.

Burkitt, D. P. (1971) Epidemiology of cancer of the colon and rectum. *Cancer, 28*, 3–13.

de Waard, F., Baanders-van Halewijn, E. A., & Huizinga, J. (1964). The bimodal age distribution of patients with mammary carcinoma: Evidence for the existence of 2 types of human breast cancer. *Cancer, 17*, 141–151.

de Waard, F., & Trichopoulos, D. (1988). Unifying concept of the aetiology of breast cancer. *International Journal of Cancer, 41*, 666–669.

Eaton, B. S., & Konner, M. (1985). Paleolithic nutrition. *New England Journal of Medicine, 312*, 283–289.

Fairfield, K. M., & Fletcher, R. H. (2002). Vitamins for chronic disease prevention in adults: Scientific review. *Journal of the American Medical Association, 287*, 3116–3126.

Fletcher, R. H., & Fairfield, K. M. (2002). Vitamins for chronic disease prevention in adults: Clinical applications. *Journal of the American Medical Association, 287*, 3127–3129.

Frisch, R. E., & McArthur, J. W. (1974). Menstrual cycles: Fatness as a determinant of the minimum weight for height necessary for their maintenance or onset. *Science, 1985*, 949–951.

Frisch, R. E., Wyshak, G., Albright, N. L., et al. (1985). Lower prevalence of breast cancer and cancers of the reproductive system among former college athletes compared to nonathletes. *British Journal of Cancer, 52*, 885–891.

Greenberg, E. R., Baron, J. A., Stukel, T. A., et al. (1990). A clinical trial of beta-carotene to prevent basal cell and squamous-cell cancers of the skin. *New England Journal of Medicine, 323*, 789–795.

Hiatt, R. A., & Bawol, R. D. (1984). Alcoholic beverage consumption and breast cancer incidence. *American Journal of Epidemiology, 120*, 676–683.

Hirayama, T. (1978). Epidemiology of breast cancer with special reference to the role of diet. *Preventive Medicine, 7*, 173–195.

Hirayama, T., Eylenbosch, W. J., Van Larebeke, N., & Depoorter, A. M. (Eds.). (1988). *Primary prevention of diet related cancers.* In *Primary prevention of cancer.* New York: Raven.

International Agency for Research on Cancer (IARC). (1976). *Some naturally occurring substances* (IARC Monographs, Vol. 10). Lyon: IARC.

International Agency for Research on Cancer (IARC). (1988). *Alcohol drinking* (IARC Monographs, Vol. 44). Lyon: IARC.

Ip, C., Birt, D. F., Rogers, A. E., & Mettlin, C. (Eds.). (1986). *Progress in Clinical Biological Research: Vol. 222. Dietary fat and cancer.* New York: Alan R. Liss.

Jacobs, L. R. (1983). Enhancement of rat colon carcinogenesis by wheat bran consumption during the stage of 1,2-dimethylhydrazine administration. *Cancer Research, 43*, 4057–4061.

Kolonel, L. N., Hankin, J. H., Nomura, A. M., & Chu, S. Y. (1981). Dietary fat intake and cancer incidence among five ethnic groups in Hawaii. *Cancer Research, 41*, 327–328.

Koo, L. C. (1988). Dietary habits and lung cancer risk among Chinese females in Hong Kong who never smoked. *Nutrition and Cancer, 11*, 155–172.

Le Marchand, L., Kolonel, L. N., Earle, M. E., et al. (1988). Body size at different periods of life and breast cancer risk. *American Journal of Epidemiology, 128*, 137–152.

Lew, E. A., & Garfinkel, L. (1979). Variations in mortality by weight among 750,000 men and women. *Journal of Chronic Diseases, 32*, 563–576.

Micozzi, M. S. (1985). Nutrition, body size, and breast cancer. *Yearbook of Physicial Anthropology, 28*, 175–206.

Micozzi, M. S., Beecher, G. R., Taylor, P. R., & Khachik, F. (1990). Carotenoid analyses of selected raw and cooked foods associated with a lower risk for cancer. *Journal of the National Cancer Institute, 82*, 282–285.

Micozzi, M. S., Brown, E. D., Edwards, B. K., Bieri, J. G., Taylor, P. R., Khachick, F., Beecher, G. R., & Smith, J. C. (1988). Plasma carotenoid response in men to chronic intake of selected foods beta-carotene supplements. *American Journal of Clinical Nutrition, 48*, 1061–1064.

Peto, R., Doll, R., Buckley, J. D., & Sporn, M. D. (1981). Can dietary beta-carotene materially reduce human cancer rates? *Nature, 290*, 201–208.

Petrakis, N. L., Mack, C. A., Lee, R. E., et al. (1980). Mutagenic activity in nipple aspirates of human breast fluid. *Cancer Research, 40*, 188–189.

Potter, J. D., & Graves, K. L. (1991). Diet and cancer: Evidence and mechanisms—An adaptation argument. In I. Rowland (Ed.), *Nutrition toxicity and cancer*. Boca Raton, FL: CRC Press.

Stocks, P. (1957). Cancer incidence in North Wales and Liverpool region in relation to habits and environment. In *British Empire Cancer Campaign 35th Annual Report, Supplement to Part 2, London* (pp. 1–127). London: British Empire

Stocks, P. (1970). Breast cancer anomalies. *British Journal of Cancer, 24*, 633–643.

United States Department of Health and Human Services. (1988). The Surgeon General's Report on Nutrition and health [Public Health Service, DHHS Publication No. (PHS) 88-50210]. Washington, DC: Author.

Wald, N., Idle, M., Boreham, J., & Bailey, A. (1980). Low serum-vitamin A and subsequent risk of cancer: Preliminary results of a prospective study. *Lancet, 2*, 813–815.

Wattenberg, L. W. (1983). Inhibition of neoplasia by minor dietary constituents. *Cancer Research, 43* (Suppl.), 2448s–2453s.

Wattenberg, L. W. (1985). Chemoprevention of cancer. *Cancer Research, 45*, 1–8.

Willett, W. C., Stampfer, M. J., Colditz, G. A., Rosner, B. A., Hennekens, C. H., & Speizer, F. E. (1987). Dietary fat and the risk of breast cancer. *New England Journal of Medicine, 316*. 22–28.

Wynder, E. L., & Cohen, L. A. (1982). A rationale for dietary intervention in the treatment of post-menopausal breast cancer patients. *Nutrition in Cancer, 3*(4), 195–199.

Wynder, E. L., Rose, D. P., & Cohen, L. A. (1986). Diet and breast cancer in causation and therapy. *Cancer, 58*, 1804–1813.

# Diet, Biology, and Breast Cancer

**9**

**C**ancer, when viewed as a process of human maladaptation, is well illustrated by the interrelationship among diet, reproductive biology, and breast cancer specifically. Overall breast cancer risk is associated with a very complex array of cultural and biologic factors. Breastfeeding, for example, appears to confer protection against breast cancer in two major ways: first, through being breastfed as an infant and, second, through breastfeeding as an

**Marc S. Micozzi**

adult. Dietary events relevant to breast cancer risk probably occur early in life. If a woman was not breastfed, there is a risk of overnutrition associated with bottle feeding and early supplementation. Overnutrition is associated with larger body size and early menarche, both of which are known risk factors for breast cancer. Animal studies have shown that increased dietary protein can lead to tumor production, and, in human studies, breast cancer has been related to high-protein diets, particularly those containing animal protein. Many infant formulas are based on cow's milk, which has several times more protein than human milk. Total caloric intake can also be a risk factor, and there is a greater possibility for formula-fed babies to consume excess calories. As well, breast cancer rates are related to consumption of milk and dairy products, based on the observation that lactase-deficient populations have lower levels of breast cancer, and most infant formulas are based on cow's milk. Another theory that has been put forth is that formula-fed infants have inferior immune systems, as they have missed out on the immunities conferred by breast milk, compared to those of breastfed infants, leading to a greater susceptibility to carcinoma.

If a woman breastfeeds her own children, she may experience protection against breast cancer on two levels, hormonal and microenvironmental. Nonpregnant, nonlactating women have higher levels of estrogens, which appear to be associated with breast cancer risk. Prolonged lactation produces a microenvironment that is less carcinogenic for breast tissue, and avoids conditions of stasis in the breast. The longer a woman breastfeeds, the more she will benefit in terms of reduced cancer risk. This is confirmed in studies on Asian women, who traditionally nurse their infants for long periods. Probably one of the reasons that breastfeeding has not yet been identified as a stronger protective factor in North American studies is that few women breastfeed in the "ancient pattern," that is, on demand, at night, and for periods longer than 1 year.

# The Problem of Breast Cancer

The epidemiological evidence is not yet clear or consistent as to all the major risk factors for breast cancer. To many women, and to those doing research in breast cancer, the reaction has been one of concern: "We still don't know what causes breast cancer," while incidence rates in the United States have continued to climb. During the past decades of studies on the epidemiology of breast cancer, incidence rates have increased from 1:11 to 1:9 U.S. women. Whether this represents a higher detection rate because of improvements in breast cancer screening, a genuine increase in cancer rates, or a combination of the two, remains a subject of debate. But to a considerable extent, we have had an idea about some of the correlates of breast cancer in modern populations for quite some time: the complex associations between early age at menarche, late age at first pregnancy, low parity, and lack of infant suckling.

Evolutionary biology (Chapter 8) would suggest that for the preponderance of human evolutionary history, most women spent much of their adult lives pregnant or lactating. This circumstance is not the case in the modern United States, where medical students hear surgeons routinely refer to the breast as a "premalignant organ." However, is the nonpregnant, nonlactating breast to be considered "premalignant" in attempts to prevent breast cancer (see Table 9.1).

If, for example, dietary modification to prevent breast cancer remains difficult and problematic, or proves to be inefficacious, are we justified in giving drugs (such as Tamoxifen) to prevent breast cancer (a kind of medical "prophylactic mastectomy")? The prevention of breast cancer with Tamoxifen, which requires individual administration of an expensive, potentially toxic drug under ongoing medical supervision, is an example of what I have called the "medicalization of prevention" in contrast to traditional population-based efforts at prevention, e. g., diet and life-style.

## Demographic Transition, Fertility, and Breast Cancer Rates

Demographic transition theory postulates that through time, populations shift from (1) high fertility/high mortality to (2) high fertility/low mortality to (3) low fertility/low mortality. The middle stage (2), where much of the world remains today, is seen to be responsible for the tremendous world population growth of the past century. Western Europe and North America have made the final transition of Stage (3). If increasing rates of breast cancer in this country during the past century are inevitable correlates of fundamental demographic shifts to lower fertility rates, what is the role of specific risk factors or dietary interventions?

If we come to view human behavior as an adaptation to the environment, and the epidemiology of breast cancer as evidence of human maladaptation, we may begin to consider human experience for the preponderance of human evolutionary history as a clue to the type of lifestyle to which human metabolism may be adapted (and that may help prevent cancer if followed or contribute to cancer if not).

For example, archaeologists can reconstruct some human lifestyle and dietary patterns from prehistoric remains (just as modern urban archaeologists can validate contemporary dietary surveys by looking through refuse). Modern theories of human evolution and studies of nonhuman primates and hunter-gatherer societies also provide some models. Certainly, until the development of agriculture and animal domestication approximately 10,000 years ago, omnivorous humans had available to eat only those plants and animals that appeared in the wild. Although we have tended toward a concept of "man the hunter" as somehow characteristic of early human experience, "woman the gatherer" may ultimately be a more accurate account. Whereas big game hunting was a part of early human experience in some areas, its social significance may have been as great or greater than its nutritional significance much of the time. Furthermore, in terms of nutrition, wild game, with 4%–6% body fat, differs substantially from modern domesticated animals, with up to 40%–60% body fat, largely a phenomenon of the 20th century in industrialized countries where cattle are grain fed in feed lots.

Evolutionary biology might tell us that a healthy lifestyle and diet are simply the lifestyle and diet that well-nourished humans had "in the wild" (before the advent of agriculture and animal domestication). Agriculture, especially irrigation agriculture, has been regarded traditionally as a central force in human settlement and the origin of complex civilization, as well as a strongly positive development in human nutritional and health status. However, paleopathologists have also uncovered evidence that sedentism and agriculture were associated with increased disease and malnutrition in human populations (Cohen, 1989). Some argue, however, that bioarchaeological evidence is equally consistent with improvements or declines in health and nutritional status with the advent of agriculture (Wood, Milner, Harpending, & Weiss, 1992). Some also argue that cancer is a relatively recent disease in human evolutionary history. Is cancer a result of leaving behind the heritage of our traditional hunter-gatherer diet and lifestyle? The actual evidence for cancer in animals and humans in the Old World before Byzantium, and the New World before Columbus, is weak or nonexistent, even in many circumstances where cancer should be readily identifiable paleopathologically if present (Chapter 3).

Better insights into modern human biology and culture in the context of epidemiologic observations are needed to help understand the causes (and to develop methods of prevention) of chronic diseases such as cancer. In this broad context, the relations between breast cancer and breast-feeding must be considered in at least two regards: (1) the influence of breast-feeding and other reproductive practices in the subsequent development of breast cancer in women (who do or do not breast-feed) and (2) the effects of breast-feeding or lack of breast-feeding in infancy and the long-term risk of breast cancer in adulthood (in individuals who were not breast-fed).

Historically, breast cancer has been the most frequent cancer in women and the leading cause of cancer death in women in the United States. The precise etiology of breast cancer is less understood than that of many other cancers (Chapter 10), and specific

| Table 9.2 | Major and Minor Risk Factors for Breast Cancer |
|---|---|

**Major risk factors for breast cancer**[a]
- Increasing age
- History of cancer in the opposite breast
- History of bilateral premenopausal breast cancer in a first-degree relative
- Residence from an early age in North America or Northern Europe (as compared to Africa or Asia)

**Minor risk factors**[b]

- Early age at menarche
- Single marital status
- Upper socioeconomic status
- Urban residence
- Obesity
- High-dose radiation to the chest (e.g., for prior treatment of other malignancies)
- Previous ovarian or endometrial cancer
- Whether the ovaries have been surgically removed
- White (as compared to Black) ethnicity

[a] Associated with significant relative risks, defined as a magnitude of risk differential greater than 4.0), that is, women who have the factor are more than four times more likely to develop breast cancer than those without the factor.
[b] Associated with small but significant relative risks (magnitude of risk differentials between 1.0 and 3.9).

major risk factors have been difficult to identify (Table 9.2). Although the identified risk factors distinguish women at increased risk of breast cancer, they do not entirely explain the rates of breast cancer among women around the world.

International differences in breast cancer morbidity and mortality, and studies on migrant populations, point to the importance of environmental and lifestyle factors in the etiology of breast cancer. Data on breast cancer can be obtained from national or regional cancer registries around the world, and two types of cancer data can be considered, based on either incidence or mortality rates. Incidence data are better linked to etiology but are probably less accurate because of difficulties in ascertaining diagnosis in many countries or populations.

Mortality data are more accurate (being based on death certification) but are less directly linked to etiology because of variations in screening, detection, diagnosis, treatment, and survival in different countries and among different populations. The use of age-specific data allows reasonable distinction between premenopausal and postmenopausal cancer rates in different populations.

Overall age-adjusted cancer rates allow comparison of breast cancer in populations of women with different age distribution, longevity, and risk. Comparison of age-adjusted breast cancer incidence and mortality rates among different populations around the world shows marked variation. For example, breast cancer rates are five times higher among women in the United States than in Japan. These differences cannot be explained solely on the basis of genetic factors, because there is a higher incidence of breast cancer in Japanese-American women than in Japanese women living in Japan. In fact, some of the strongest evidence for the role of environmental and lifestyle factors in breast

| Table 9.3 | Rates of Breast Cancer in Japanese-American Women Over Time |
|---|---|

1. 23 per 100,000 during 1960–1964 among Japanese–Hawaiian women
2. 44.2 per 100,000 during 1973–1977 among Japanese–Hawaiian women
3. 41.0 per 100,000 during 1969–1973 among premenopausal Japanese women in California
4. 55.7 per 100,000 during 1969–1973 among premenopausal Caucasian women

cancer comes from epidemiologic studies on Japanese migrants to the United States and Japanese living in Japan.

First- (Isei), second- (Nisei), and third- (Sansei) generation Japanese-American women are present in California and in Hawaii in sufficient numbers to allow meaningful comparisons of breast cancer rates with those of women living in Japan, where breast cancer rates have historically been low. In migrant studies, genetic factors may be considered relatively constant, although the extent to which migrant populations are a selected group, and the effects of inbreeding reduction and interbreeding on successive generations must be considered. Migrants experience rapid changes in environmental risk factors and lifestyle, and changes in health outcomes, through time and space. Migrant studies may be conducted synchronologically (cross-sectionally), at one point in time, or diachronically (longitudinally), through time, or in one or more places. Such descriptive studies have provided useful observations about environmental risk factors and breast cancer.

Breast cancer rates have increased in succeeding generations of Japanese migrants to the United States. Age-standardized breast cancer incidence rates have been relatively low in Japan and intermediate in Japanese Hawaiians compared to rates in Whites in the United States. There is also an effect of time on the breast cancer incidence rates in Japanese Hawaiians (Table 9.3).

In Japan itself, there have also been recent increases in breast cancer rates that correspond to "Westernization" of lifestyle. The annual number of breast cancer deaths in Japan doubled during the period between 1955 and 1975. Normalized to the increased population, the rate of death from breast cancer has steadily increased from 3.5 per 100,000 in 1955 to 5.8 per 100,000 in 1975. The increase has been greatest among women 45 to 59 years of age and among higher socioeconomic groups in urban areas.

In addition to ecologic and geochemical features, the environment includes cultural factors, such as health beliefs and behaviors, which also may be related to human health outcomes. With respect to cancer risk factors, breast cancer incidence rates in Japanese migrants appear to be related to the degree of acculturation to Western lifestyle and diet.

The Japan-Hawaii Cancer Study compared the diet of Japanese men whose wives had developed breast cancer with the diets of Japanese men whose wives did not. If it is assumed that the diets of husbands and wives are similar, the result indicated that the women who developed breast cancer followed a more western-style diet (more beef or other meat, butter/margarine/cheese, corn, and hot dogs and less Japanese foods) than the control group. Increasing incidence of breast cancer among Japanese-American women is associated with changes in lifestyle, including diet, in successive generations (cross-generational acculturation).

In a descriptive study of migrants, researchers found increasing incidence of breast cancer in successive generations of Japanese women in America compared to those in Japan. The increasing rates were attributed to acculturation of diet and to increased height and weight. However, year of migration and age at migration can be independently related to the year of acculturation and age at acculturation, respectively. Although the distribution of ages among migrants in a given year of migration can be determined, different times of acculturation among different age groups may result in an irregular distribution of acculturated migrants making acculturation a difficult parameter to utilize.

The increasing cancer rates in Japanese-American women are reflected in age-specific cancer rates in Los Angeles. Younger Japanese-American women have higher breast cancer rates (like those of U.S. White women) than do older Japanese-American women. Further, in San Francisco, the incidence of breast cancer among young Japanese-American women is almost as high as that among White women.

That young Japanese-American women have higher breast cancer rates than older Japanese-American women is consistent with a cohort effect. The cohort effect is also seen in the growth in stature of Japanese-American children born in 1940 compared to those born in 1955. The mean adult stature of Japanese-American women born in 1940 was 154 cm, whereas that of Japanese-American women born in 1955 was 158 cm. The generation of Japanese-American women with high breast cancer rates is the generation that had greater growth during childhood and was probably exposed to a more western-style diet from infancy.

Thus, the time in life when environmental changes occur appears to be important to the long-term risk of breast cancer in women. It has been reported that persons who emigrate during childhood and adolescence experience the greatest changes in patterns of breast cancer. Buell's (1973) descriptive study also indicated a relation between height and weight and breast cancer risk within Japanese-American migrant groups. It appears that only the Nisei (second generation) and those Isei (first generation) who migrated before puberty attain greater stature, which, together with increased body weight, seems to be associated with an increased incidence of breast cancer. The migrant studies therefore suggest that acculturation early in life may be a critical factor in breast cancer risk.

# Risk Factors for Breast Cancer: Early Nutrition and Breast-feeding

## Evidence for the Role of Nutrition

The dramatic environmental and temporal variations in cancer patterns and the changing rates of cancer in migrants suggest differential exposure of various populations to cancer risk factors. Although often it is not possible to pinpoint the environmental factors responsible for observed differences in cancer rates in the various ecologic and migrant studies, lifestyle, dietary, and nutritional factors appear to play a prominent role.

Evidence for the role of nutrition in breast cancer relates primarily to relative dietary deficiencies of certain micronutrients (which may act as cancer protective factors) and relative dietary excesses of certain macronutrients (which may act as cancer-promoting factors). The specific macronutrients of interest with respect to breast cancer risk are dietary fat, protein, and total calories, for which there are complex relationships with nutrition-mediated variables such as body size.

## Timing of Nutritional Experiences

The timing of nutritional experiences appears important in the relation between dietary intake and breast cancer. Dietary patterns early in life may be related to the long-term risk of breast cancer, whereas effects of adult nutrition on body fat may mediate later hormonal influences on breast cancer. The effects of nutrition may also be partitioned anthropometrically by differentiation according to various measurements of body size.

Anthropometry provides information on past nutritional history and growth in human populations. Overnutrition during childhood is associated with increased stature and lean body mass and accelerated rates of maturation. The former are reflected in increased height and body size in adults and the latter by early age of menarche in women. Overnutrition in childhood is also related to increased deposition of adipose tissue. Obese and lean individuals differ in specific ways from infancy through old age. In general, fatter children are taller, heavier, and developmentally more advanced than their leaner counterparts. The obese are more advanced than the lean in skeletal and muscle mass and in age at menarche by as much as 5 years. Obese children also tend to be tall at pubescence. It should be noted that these anthropometric observations are highly correlated with each other.

Despite these findings, research has not borne out much of an association among overnutrition, obesity, and risk of breast cancer. In fact, there appears to be an inverse relationship between obese women and premenopausal breast cancer risk (Huang et al., 1997; Van den Brandt et al., 2000). Authors have suggested that heavier premenopausal women have more irregular menstrual cycles and therefore have a lower ovarian hormonal milieu. In observational studies, the association between obesity and postmenopausal women is weak or nonexistent (Hunter & Willett, 1993; Van den Brandt et al., 2000), which is surprising given the fact that obese postmenopausal women have endogenous estrogen levels nearly double those of lean women. Other researchers have explained this phenomenon as opposing risks: the risk reduction of early weight gain and the increased risk postmenopausal cancel each other out. Thus, weight gain rather than attained weight in the postmenopausal women should pose a greater risk to breast cancer development. In fact, this appears to be true (Wenten, Gilliland, Baumgartner, & Samet, 2002).

## Breast-feeding and Influences in Early Life

Tendencies toward obesity begin early in postnatal life if nutritional intake is not properly balanced. Excessive protein intake during the neonatal period may stimulate increased muscle growth, fat deposition, or, most notably, both. An environmental stimulus of overabundant nutrition during early growth and development may eventually lead to an adult whose body size is close to the maximum for that genotype.

Effects in utero may also be important. For example, women born to young mothers have a significantly lower risk of breast cancer than women born to older mothers. Whether a maternal age effect is transmitted through the fetal environment in utero or through the neonatal environment through breast-feeding is not known; the older and younger mothers did not differ in breast-feeding practices. Alternatively, older mothers may be better established financially and can afford "better" nutrition, in this case, relative overnutrition.

A case-control study on over 200 children was undertaken to determine whether inadequate exposure to the immunologic benefits of human milk may affect infant response to infection and increase susceptibility to childhood cancers. An increased risk for cancer was found among children breastfed fewer than 6 months or not breast-fed at all, largely because of a six- to eightfold increased incidence of lymphoma.

Whether an infant is breastfed also has significant effects on neonatal nutrition and growth. Failure to breastfeed in early infancy may lead to overnutrition and overweight infants. Human breast milk has among the lowest levels of protein of any mammalian milk, characteristic of species that suckle their young almost continuously. There is a positive relationship between the species-specific protein content of mammalian milk and the rate of early growth in neonates of the species. The percentage of protein in cows' milk, for example, is three times higher than that in human milk. Early survival in most mammals demands rapid growth and maturation. However, humans are unlike most mammals in this respect. Cows' milk also differs from human milk in the type of protein present, as well as the concentration of total protein. That is, the casein content of cows' milk is six times higher than that of human milk. Calcium and phosphorus are also much more abundant in cows' milk than in human milk.

Protein intake is a major environmental factor determining growth rate, size at a given age, and ultimate adult height. Some evidence also suggests that dietary protein intake at the time of maturity is a major environmental factor determining normal variation in growth and height. Conversely, among a wide range of anthropometric variables, height gains provide a good degree of discrimination among different levels of protein intake. Additionally, age at menarche is closely related to higher animal protein intake, with early menarche in populations with high levels of protein intake. The common influence of increased nutrition early in life on both increased body size and early menarche is indicated by Malcolm's law, which states that "the later the average age at menarche, the smaller the average stature in the population." Increased body size and decreased age at menarche appear to share a common relation with nutritional patterns that may also place the individual at increased risk of breast cancer later in life. Because all these factors must be taken into account, it is important to examine the correlations among these risk factors and to reconcile their common relation with breast cancer in a consistent fashion. Therefore, the effects of age at menarche on body size must be considered.

Eveleth and Tanner (1976) originally reviewed the relation of maturation to body size and shape. From infancy to adolescence, the trunk grows more slowly than the legs; however, at adolescence, the growth spurt is greater in sitting height than in leg length. Individuals who mature early have shorter legs in relation to the trunk because their preadolescent period (when the legs are growing relatively faster) is shorter. In terms of body shape, later maturers usually present a more linear body physique with relatively low weight-for-height, which may also be reflected in lean body mass.

An early cancer study in women that used anthropometric dimensions beyond height and weight (or indices derived therefrom) showed greater sitting height and frame size in breast cancer cases compared to controls. Therefore, although increased nutrition goes hand in hand with greater height, larger body size, and earlier age at menarche, the conjunction of these factors (which are, in turn, risk factors for breast cancer) produces an anthropometric pattern that may be distinctive. Increased sitting height, frame size, and lean body mass are the anthropometric variables correlated with the early nutritional pattern that places women at greater risk of breast cancer in later life. An increased intake of macronutrients early in life may be a critical factor for breast cancer. These anthropometric indicators are consistent with other known risk factors and are consistent with available studies on breast cancer and body size.

# Dietary Fat Intake

There has been a popular scientific perception that excess dietary fat intake in modern as opposed to traditional human populations may be related to a number of negative health outcomes, including cancer. In fact, some early studies might have suggested such a trend. However, more recent studies have allowed us to conclude that, in fact, no relationship occurs.

Animal experimental evidence implicating dietary fat intake with breast cancer has been derived from studies of both spontaneous mammary tumors and chemically induced mammary tumors, as well as other site-specific tumors. Most of the data suggest that dietary fat promotes the growth of populations of cancer-initiated cells in the multistage process of carcinogenesis. The additional possibility that dietary fat plays an initiating role in carcinogenesis cannot be ruled out.

Human epidemiologic studies show high correlations between national levels of breast cancer and per capita consumption of total fat, animal fat, total protein, animal protein, and eggs. For example, in Japan, per capita fat intake (especially animal fat and pork) is positively correlated with breast cancer mortality rates by geographic prefecture. In Britain, breast cancer mortality is positively related to per capita intake of animal fat and protein during the decade prior to death. In the United States, age-adjusted cancer mortality is positively correlated with per capita intake of fat, protein, beef, milk, and total calories. When nutrition-mediated factors such as height, weight, and age at menarche are statistically controlled, per capita intake of animal fat and protein remains an independent correlation with breast cancer risk. Increased consumption of fat, measured as total fat, animal fat, saturated fat, or unsaturated fat, is correlated with increased incidence of breast cancer among different ethnic groups in Hawaii.

The first case-control study of diet and breast cancer among Seventh-Day Adventists showed a slightly positive association of lifestyle and dietary habits inhibits the growth of spontaneous and chemically induced tumors, whereas evidence supports a tumor-promoting role for protein in dietary carcinogenesis. Substantially lower rates of colon cancer, however, were observed.

A meta-analysis (Howe et al., 1990) of 12 case-controlled studies totaling 4,312 cases of breast cancer found a slightly increased overall pooled risk among postmenopausal women for a 100-g increase in daily fat intake but no association in premenopausal women.

However, the authors note that because the average fat consumption in U.S. women is about 70 g/day, a reduction of 100 g of total intake would not be feasible.

Ten prospective cohort studies have been published and not one study reported a significant positive association with total fat intake. A collaborative pooled analysis that included 337,819 women and a total of 4,980 women with breast cancer also failed to show an association between intake of total, saturated, monounsaturated, or polyunsaturated fat and risk for breast cancer. These prospective trials provide strong evidence that no major relation exists between total dietary fat intake over a wide range during midlife and breast cancer incidence (Holmes & Willett, 2004).

# Dietary Protein Intake

Ross and Bras (1983) observed an increasing incidence of spontaneous tumors, including mammary tumors, with increasing dietary protein intake in rats fed various isocaloric casein/sucrose ratios. This experiment was apparently testing the tumorigenic effect of protein. In animals with identical caloric intake, more tumors were found in groups with higher protein intake. Higher levels of protein intake early in life contributed to both a high tumor risk and a high mature weight in laboratory animals. This finding suggests that diet-mediated early-life processes involved in the regulation and duration of growth are also related to susceptibility to spontaneous tumor formation in rats.

In human epidemiologic studies, the possibility of a dietary effect of protein on cancer mortality or survival, as well as cancer incidence, has been suggested. With breast cancer specifically, there was a stronger association with animal protein than with total protein (possibly explained by the dietary association of animal protein consumption with fat consumption), but the correlation with total protein consumption was as strong as with total fat consumption. With other risk factors controlled, per capita intake of animal protein has also been related to breast cancer rates among different populations, including the United States. Although breast cancer mortality was correlated with level of per capita food intake (protein, fat, and animal products) from the prior decade, the time-trend in Britain indicated that fat consumption was somewhat better correlated with breast cancer mortality than was protein consumption. From both human and animal studies, an independent effect of protein consumption on breast cancer risk should thus be considered.

# Energy Intake

Although the precise composition of the diet appears to be important for breast cancer risk, the total amount of food consumed may also be an important variable. Total caloric intake is a less precise variable than dietary fat or protein intake because it is difficult to determine whether effects brought about by changing the quantity of the diet are because of resulting changes in the caloric intake or to changed distribution of specific nutrients. Further, the concept of excess dietary intake of calories requires knowledge of calories expended as well as calories consumed. Thus, the level of energy expenditure (i.e., physical activity in various forms) is necessary to determine the level of excess caloric intake in an individual or population. Some measurements of physical activity do not directly address total caloric expenditure and may be focused on determination of fitness relative to cardiovascular disease.

Much of the animal experimental evidence and human epidemiologic studies, previously reviewed in the sections on dietary fat and protein intake, have also considered the effects of total caloric intake on cancer risk. Variable results have been reported and appropriate controls have not always been used; thus, these results are difficult to evaluate. Ross and Bras (1983) found that caloric restriction early in life of the rat is associated with a decreased prevalence of spontaneous tumors later in life. Berg (1975) has suggested that the international pattern of distribution of some cancers appears to be related to socioeconomic status and affluent diets. Armstrong and Doll (1975) and Gaskill, McGuire, Osborne, & Stern (1979) also found that total caloric intake is related to cancer incidence and mortality, including breast cancer. The case-control study of breast cancer by Miller et al. (1978) found a higher mean intake of total calories in cases than in controls.

Excess intake of total calories, as well as fat and protein, may be reflected in measurements of body size. From this view, caloric intake may be related to anthropometric variables such as weight and fatness, absolute or relative. The level of caloric intake (together with protein intake) may also have an effect on height, lean body mass, and other variables mediated during growth.

# Lactose Intolerance

Lactose intolerance rates in various populations have also been related to the risk of breast cancer. In ecologic studies, populations that have no traditional or modern dairy industry and do not consume milk or milk products also have low rates of breast cancer, (e.g., China). Breast cancer mortality has been directly correlated with the proportions of various populations that continue to secrete lactase in adulthood. The biocultural corollary that breast cancer rates are related to per capita consumption of milk and dairy products among different human populations is suggested by a number of studies. Although Japanese populations have a high proportion of lactose intolerance, the recent increase in milk drinking in Japanese schools has been identified as a possible influence on the increased growth of Japanese children.

Societies with a high rate of lactose intolerance may exploit dairy food sources through consumption of yogurt rather than raw milk. Large quantities of yogurt are consumed by some lactase-deficient populations. Yogurt contains microorganisms, such as *Lactobacillus acidophilus*, that digest lactose and facilitate intestinal absorption, thus making yogurt more digestible to lactase-deficient populations. The organisms in yogurts may also prevent formation of carcinogenic substances from the diet in the gastrointestinal tract. Thus, lactase-deficient populations may be protected against some cancers by consumption of dairy products in the form of yogurt rather than milk. *Lactobacillus* has been shown to influence intestinal flora as well as fecal enzymes in animal models (Sreekumar & Hosono, 2000).

# Overview of Overnutrition

The evidence linking excess dietary intake of macronutrients and breast cancer in adult case-control studies has not been as strong as results from ecologic, descriptive, and correlation studies. Because the dietary relation with breast cancer appears stronger in correlation studies than in adult case-control studies, the important dietary events relevant to breast cancer risk may occur early in life. For example, dietary acculturation among Japanese migrants early in life appears central to the role of nutrition in the etiology of breast cancer. If nutrient intake in early life is a critical variable for long-term breast cancer risk, case-control studies on elderly women with breast cancer may not be the most appropriate manner of detecting a relation.

The pattern of human epidemiologic evidence of breast cancer in women appears consistent with a role for excess dietary fat, protein, and total caloric intake early in life. Events early in life, such as breastfeeding, that relate to diet, nutrition, and growth may have an impact on subsequent cancer incidence in human populations. Furthermore, given the limitations of accurate dietary assessment, nutrition-mediated factors that can be accurately measured (such as various indices of body size) may also be meaningful for comparisons of breast cancer rates in human populations. To the extent that breastfeeding and human breast milk provide a more appropriate species-specific diet in human infants (resulting in lower early dietary intake of calories, fats, and proteins and slower growth rates), nursing may serve as a protective factor against breast cancer in later life for individuals who were breastfed.

# Reproductive Biology and Breast-feeding

Reproductive variables and reproductive history have a marked effect of breast cancer risk. These factors are related to hormonal status, and increased estrogen levels (also decreased progestogen levels) have been hypothesized as contributing to increased breast cancer risk.

Early age at menarche and late age at menopause have relative risks for breast cancer in the range of 1.2 to 1.9, whereas late age at birth of the first child has a relative risk between 2.0 and 4.0 (Table 9.2). However, the effects of later maternal age at birth may be complex; among women who develop breast cancer, the earlier the first child, the earlier the age at the time of breast cancer diagnosis. The protective effects of high parity in breast cancer appear related to early age at birth of the first child.

Although the important influence of a woman's reproductive history on her risk of breast cancer is widely recognized, it has not been clear whether these observations are entirely explained by age at first full-term pregnancy or whether there are additional, independent influence of breastfeeding and parity. A logistic regression analysis of nearly 5,000 women in the U.S. Cancer and Steroid Hormone Study confirmed the strong influence of age at first full-term pregnancy while revealing that parity and duration of breastfeeding also had strong influences on the risk of breast cancer.

In a population-based, case-control study designed primarily to investigate the role of oral contraceptives in breast cancer, it was observed that the risk of breast cancer fell with increasing duration of breastfeeding and the increasing numbers of babies breastfed among young women. In Australia, a study of nearly 500 breast cancer cases indicated that lactation may play a modest direct or indirect role in reducing the risk of breast cancer. A case–control study in King County, Washington, showed that the risk of breast cancer decreases with increasing duration of lifetime lactational experience. Among women with breast cancer in Buffalo, New York, there was evidence of a negative association between length of nursing and breast cancer risk. It was not clear, however, whether this observation means that breastfeeding is protective or that some women who are unsuccessful at lactation are at increased risk for subsequent breast cancer.

In the Nurses Health Study the relation between lactation and the risk of breast cancer was specifically examined in a prospective cohort of nearly 90,000 women ages 30–55. However, there was no independent association found between lactation and breast cancer risk.

Although several epidemiologic studies conducted in Scandinavian countries have not individually confirmed an association between age at first full-term pregnancy (independent or parity) and breast cancer risk, a meta-analysis of eight studies involving over 5,500 breast cancer cases confirmed that both low parity and late age at first full-term pregnancy are independent and significant risk factors. These findings point out that risk factors with low relative risks (as are many of the reproductive factors including breastfeeding) may not always be detected in studies with relatively small numbers of cases and inadequate statistical power.

A review by Kvale (1992) confirmed that abundant epidemiologic evidence exists showing early menarche, late menopause, low parity, and late age at first full-term pregnancy to be related to increased risk of breast cancer. Kvale and Heuch (1988), in a study of over 50,000 parous women in Norway, concluded that breastfeeding is not strongly related to the risk of breast cancer or any other common cancer. Results reported from two large prospective studies also suggest that breastfeeding is not strongly related to the risk of breast cancer among Western populations. In a discussion of whether these epidemiologic findings provide a basis for primary prevention of breast cancer, Kvale and Jacobsen (1990) considered several known and suspected risk factors, including lactation, and concluded that it is difficult to suggest any feasible intervention strategy that would have a high probability of reducing the occurrence of breast cancer in the general population.

However, recent evidence exists for a relation between breastfeeding and breast cancer in non-Western populations. Various studies on small numbers of cases around the world have attempted to differentiate the effects of lactation on overall breast cancer risk. For example, in a study in Japan, lack of breastfeeding had a relative risk of 2.3 compared with a relative risk of 2.6 for prior benign breast disease; early age at menopause and early age at first full-term pregnancy were associated with lower risk of breast cancer. In a self-reported study of breast cancer cases in Beijing, high parity and long duration of lactation were protective factors against breast cancer. In Shanghai, long duration of breastfeeding was associated with lower breast cancer risk. This study demonstrated a clear and independent effect on breast cancer risk of breastfeeding in the majority of women in a population characterized by a long cumulative duration of nursing.

Ing, Petrakis, and Ho (1977) studied women in fishing villages in Hong Kong, who by custom breastfeed only from the right breast. Although in the general population the ratio of cancer in the left/right breast is essentially 1, women who have consistently breast-fed from only one breast show a significantly lower risk for development of cancer in the suckled breast. The actual physical process of breast-feeding may help to protect the suckled breast against cancer. This remarkable research provides the ultimate example of a controlled study in that both breasts of each of the women had been exposed to identical reproductive history and environmental (including systemic hormonal) influences, with the only difference being presence or absence of breast-feeding in one breast versus the other.

The relatively short periods of lactation seen in women in western countries generally do not appear to be associated with a significantly lower risk of breast cancer. However, more intensive and longer durations of breast-feeding as observed in China, Hong Kong, and elsewhere appear to reduce the subsequent risk of breast cancer.

Finally, a study in Maine, Massachusetts, New Hampshire, and Wisconsin showed a distinction between women with premenopausal versus postmenopausal breast cancer. Overall, lactation was not associated with the risk of postmenopausal breast cancer. However, among premenopausal women, a slight inverse association was observed, and lactation at early maternal ages and for long duration was associated with more substantial reductions in risk.

This study indicates that even in Western populations, those mothers that do breast-feed at young ages and for long durations show a significant reduction in the risk of premenopausal breast cancer. The authors suggest that a 25% reduction in breast cancer incidence could be achieved if all women with children lactated for 24 months or more. Menopausal status may influence the effects of breast-feeding on breast cancer, as it appears to do for certain other risk factors.

Breast-feeding may not hitherto have been clearly identified as a protective factor against breast cancer in women who breastfeed in Western societies because in these societies women do not breast-feed in the ancient or traditional pattern (i.e., on demand, throughout the night, and for a duration of at least 1 year). Sporadic breast-feeding, or breast-feeding on the same time schedule as bottle feeding, probably does not have the same physiologic effect. The application of more rigorous epidemiologic methods in larger, nonwestern cohorts and better definition of breastfeeding patterns in epidemiologic studies should help resolve this question in the future.

# Endogenous and Exogenous Hormones

Various hormonal mechanisms have been investigated in an attempt to explain the observation that early age at menarche, late age at birth of first child, lack of breast-feeding, and late age at menopause are associated with increased breast cancer risk. All of these factors would result in prolonged, unopposed estrogen stimulation of breast tissue. Moolgavkar, Day, and Stevens (1980) and Thomas (1983) have argued, however, that hormones per se are unlikely to be of primary importance in determining overall risk in populations, although they may influence the epidemiology of breast cancer through their actions on the growth of nonneoplastic breast tissue.

No difference is total estrogen levels have been observed between groups of women with high rates of breast cancer in England compared to those with low rates in Japan and in populations elsewhere. Hormonal status in British, Japanese, and Japanese-Hawaiian women showed no differences in estrogen levels among populations with different rates of breast cancer. However, there was an association between increased levels of estrogens and breast cancer in a study in Greece. Although most studies on total endogenous estrogens and breast cancer have been negative, endogenous estrogen fractions have been studied in association with body fatness (see below).

Exogenous hormones have been studied in the form of oral contraceptives in premenopausal women. Studies have presented conflicting results on the risk for breast cancer of oral contraceptive use in young women. A large, population-based case-control study showed no association between oral contraceptive use and the risk of breast cancer (Centers for Disease Control Cancer and Steroid Hormone Study, 1983), but subsequent studies showed an association between high-progestogen combination-type oral contraceptives and breast cancer in women before the age of 37 years and an association between oral contraceptives use prior to the first full-term birth and increased risk of breast cancer prior to age 45 years. Reanalysis of the CDC (1983) data showed no effect on breast cancer risk of high-progestogen oral contraceptives or of oral contraceptive use before the first full-term pregnancy.

Studies of replacement doses of estrogens given to postmenopausal women have also yielded inconsistent results with respect to the risk of breast cancer. A large, case-control study in a hospital-based population indicated that exogenous estrogens did not appear to influence the risk of breast cancer, even when taken for many years and even in subgroups of women with other defined risk factors. More epidemiological studies on exogenous hormones and breast cancer are unlikely to produce more definitive results.

There is substantial evidence that alcohol consumption increases breast cancer risk and that it does so by increasing estrogen levels. In a pooled analysis of six of the largest cohort studies with data on alcohol, the risk of breast cancer increased significantly with increasing intake of alcohol (Smith-Warner, Spiegelman, & Yuan, 1998). Adjustments for other breast cancer risk factors had little impact. Beer, wine, and liquor all contribute to the positive association, suggesting that it is alcohol itself that increases breast cancer risk, not components of alcoholic drinks. Furthermore, consumption of one to two alcoholic beverages per day increases estrogen levels in both pre- and postmenopausal women, suggesting a mechanistic link between alcohol and breast cancer risk. Interestingly, several large prospective studies have shown that intake of high levels of folic acid appears to mitigate the risk of alcohol and breast cancer development.

## Body Fat and Hormones

Estrogen hormones are thought to influence the risk of breast cancer (Muti et al., 2000) and regulation of endogenous hormones may be influenced by diet and body fat (Lord et al., 2002). Dietary fat intake may influence overall levels of endogenous hormones, whereas body fat content may influence endogenous metabolism of estrogens, especially in postmenopausal women. Conversion of androstenedione to estrone in adipose tissue is an important determinant of endogenous estrogen levels in postmenopausal women. Dietary fat may contribute to increased body fat stores through excess caloric intake.

Diet also influences the excretion of estrogens in both premenopausal and postmenopausal women. Omnivores have higher plasma estrone and estradiol levels than do vegetarians and premenopausal women. South African women fed a high-fat (western-style) diet have an apparent increase in estradiol levels. Postmenopausal vegetarian women have lower urinary excretion of estriol and total estrogens than nonvegetarian women. In postmenopausal women especially, endogenous estrogen balance is influenced by interconversion of hormones in adipose tissue. Thus, the total body fat may also be an important variable for breast cancer among women, based on hormonal mechanisms. In addition to endogenous estrogens, phtyoestrogens, or estrogen hormones from plants are also thought to influence the risk of breast cancer (Duncan et al., 2003; Ziegler 2004; see also Chapter 13).

# Breast Biology and Apocrine Gland Function

Breast secretory activity has been related to the risk of breast cancer. Breast secretory activity may be influenced both by nutritional patterns and endogenous hormone activity. Although difficult to measure reliably, studies on the relation of estrogens to breast endothelial activity and breast fluid secretion shed light on the role of diet and endogenous estrogens in breast cancer. Although estrogen levels in plasma and urine have been studied in relation to the risk of breast cancer, levels of estrogen in breast fluid should be a critical observation relative to breast cancer, because it reflects most directly the microenvironment of breast tissue.

Early menarche is associated with early breast secretory activity, and increased nutrition may lead to increased breast secretory activity. In turn, breast biology is influenced by dietary protein levels. Based on an observed relation between higher socioeconomic status and increased breast secretory activity, Petrakis et al. (1982) hypothesized a relation between increased dietary intake ("improved" nutrition) and increased breast secretory activity, as assessed by measuring the quantity of breast fluid aspirated from the nipple in the nonlactating breast.

The amount of breast fluid has also been related to the type of cerumen secreted from related apocrine glands, which is, in turn, correlated with breast cancer mortality rates. The association between secretory activity of the nonlactating breast and related apocrine glands (cerumen-type) may have significance for breast cancer risk because exogeneously derived substances that may act as carcinogens are secreted into breast fluid. The turnover rate of substances secreted in the breast fluid may be a primary determinant of exposure of the breast epithelium to environmental and endogenous carcinogens and promoters. Breast-feeding, in turn, has a strong influence over the turnover rate of substances secreted in the breast fluid and prolonged lactation should minimize the exposure of breast epithelium to carcinogens.

## Apocrine Gland Function

Observations on apocrine gland function at the population level have been related to susceptibility to breast cancer. Physiologically, female breast secretory glands, certain axillary sweat glands, and ceruminous (ear wax) glands compose the apocrine glandular system of the human body. Matsunaga (1962) illustrated that human cerumen occurs in two phenotypic forms, wet (sticky) and dry (hard). These phenotypic forms are governed by a single gene with two alleles, wet or dry. The allele for the wet type is dominant over that for the dry type. The recessive dry type is predominant among Native American and Asian women, and the wet type is predominant among African and European women. Petrakis (1977) observed that the frequency of the allele for the wet type of wax is high in populations at high risk for breast cancer and low in populations at low risk for breast cancer. Petrakis et al. (1975) determined that the frequency of the wet-type gene is related to frequency of breast fluid secretor status in nonlactating women among different populations. Studying women from African-American, White, Chinese, Filipino, Japanese, and Mexican-American populations in San Francisco, these investigators found the highest rates of breast fluid secretor status among White women and the lowest rates among Chinese women. Breast secretory fluids could be obtained by nipple aspiration in 81% of premenopausal White women but only in 30% of premenopausal Chinese women.

Age and menopausal status also have an effect on secretor status among women: 60% of postmenopausal Whites were secretors and only 4% of postmenopausal Chinese were secretors. This pattern appears to parallel the decline in estrogen production associated with menopause and the decrease in breast secretory activity associated with advancing age. It would be important to determine if the estrogen profiles of women who are genetically susceptible to breast cancer might be correlated with breast secretory activity or cerumen characteristics. The hormonal basis of breast cancer risk, including the relevancy of maternal age at birth of first offspring for breast cancer risk in both mother and offspring, was covered earlier in this chapter.

Wynder, Laht, and Laakso (1985) found no statistically significant influence of menopausal status on breast secretor status among healthy Finnish women, who had an overall secretor status frequency of 38%. Petrakis et al. (1987) subsequently observed an age-related increase in the frequency of the dry wax phenotype among White (but not Asian or African) women. The use of exogenous estrogens in postmenopausal women was also associated with an increased frequency of the dry phenotype among women.

Wynder et al. (1985) studied over 1,000 women in New York City and found no association between breast cancer and breast fluid secretor status. However, there was no association between secretor status and parity, age at first pregnancy, or body weight. One group of women with preneoplastic breast abnormalities had a greater proportion of breast fluid secretors. Wynder et al. (1985) also noted, however, that the composition of secretory fluid (which was not actually assessed in their study) is important to the pathogenesis of breast cancer.

## Breast Fluid Composition

Petrakis and coworkers (Petrakis & King, 1981; Petrakis, Maack, Lee, & Lyon, 1980) noted mutagenic activity in nipple aspirates of human breast fluid and identified specific mutagens, including cholesterol-epoxide. Petrakis and King (1981) studied human breast fluid from nearly 1,500 women, aged 20–70 years in San Francisco. Cytologic abnormalities in exfoliated breast epithelial cells were found in women with severe constipation. The authors postulated a mechanism by which mutagenic substances originating in the dietary tract may enter the circulation and reach the breast, where they may be selectively concentrated in breast fluid by the actions of breast apocrine secretory epithelia. The production of fecal mutagens in the colon has been described and the association between breast cancer and bowel function has been confirmed among U.S. women, as reported in the U.S. National Health and Nutrition Examination Survey Epidemiologic Follow-up Study (Micozzi et al 1989).

The production of cytologic abnormalities in breast fluid cells is related to epithelial dysplasia in breast tissue and is regarded as a preneoplastic lesion by Petrakis and King (1981), who observed abnormal cells in nipple aspiration fluid from women with diagnosed atypical proliferative breast disease. Women with atypical proliferative breast disease, particularly in combination with a positive family history for breast cancer, are at a significantly increased risk for the development of breast cancer. Petrakis and King (1981), in a study of over 1,000 White and Asian women in San Francisco, found that the wet–cerumen type was associated with the presence of preneoplastic cytologic atypia in nipple aspiration fluid. It is assumed that the presence of atypical cells in breast fluid is a marker for the presence of epithelial atypical proliferation in the actual breast tissue of women who have the positive secretory status. In turn, women with atypical proliferative breast disease appear to be at significantly increased risk of breast cancer.

The Petrakis model of wet/dry cerumen polymorphism found in different populations may be an indication of predisposition to breast cancer at the population level. However, the final association with breast cancer itself remains to be proven.

# Breast Tissue Microenvironment

In the Petrakis studies, women who were lactating, who were parous, or who had breast-fed had lower levels of cholesterol and potentially carcinogenic cholesterol-epoxide in breast fluid. These low levels persist for 2 years postpartum or postlactation. Because breast fluid levels of potential carcinogens are reduced for relatively long periods after pregnancy or lactation, it has been hypothesized that this biochemical mechanism may help explain the reduction of breast cancer risk associated with parity and breast-feeding.

In addition, low levels of breast fluid estrogens were found following full-term birth and lactation, which may also provide a mechanism to explain why childbearing and breast-feeding may reduce risk. Furthermore, estrogen levels in breast fluid were not significantly related to estrogen levels in blood, which may explain why other studies do not observe relations between blood estrogen levels and breast cancer. Estrogen levels in the breast fluid itself should be far more significant for breast cancer risk, as these are the hormone levels to which breast epithelial tissue is most directly and consistently exposed.

Although Petrakis (1977) originally attempted to account for the association among cerumen type, breast secretory activity, and breast cancer epidemiology on a genetic basis at the population level, the association between breast cancer risk factors and breast secretory activity may also be partially explained on an environmental basis, including the effects of childbearing and breastfeeding.

It should seem obvious that the microenvironment to which normal breast tissue is exposed plays a prominent role in the propensity to develop breast cancer. Factors that promote the growth of breast tissue at the cellular level, such as estrogens and certain nutrients, are associated with the development of breast cancer in women in epidemiologic studies. Those reproductive factors associated with prolonged, unopposed estrogen (Table 9.1) and indeed the breast tissue in nonlactating, nonpregnant women appears to be at significantly greater risk for the development of cancer compared to women who spend much of their adult lives pregnant or lactating. Clearly, breast-feeding is associated with reproductive factors that appear to protect women from breast cancer.

A purely independent effect of breastfeeding has been more difficult to define, although the studies of Petrakis and coworkers point to the importance of hormonal and nutritional microenvironment of breast tissue. The effects of pregnancy and lactation appear to produce a microenvironment that is less carcinogenic for breast tissue and decrease conditions of stasis in the breast.

# Summary

Breast cancer risk, although as yet incompletely defined, appears to be associated with a very complex array of biologic and cultural factors. The dramatic variations in breast cancer risk observed among Japanese and Japanese-American women, for example, indicate the important role of behavioral and environmental influences, including acculturation of diet and lifestyle. Reproductive factors also appear to play an important role, including pregnancy and lactation. However, breast-feeding behavior among women has been incompletely characterized in epidemiologic studies of breast cancer.

Breast-feeding may help lower the risk of breast cancer by two general mechanisms: one associated with whether a woman was breastfed as a baby (early nutritional influences) and the other associated with whether a woman breast-fed her child(-ren). Dietary events relevant to breast cancer risk may have an influence early in the life of the individual. If an individual is not breast-fed (e.g., formula fed), there is the risk of overnutrition in early life.

Formula-fed infants are exposed to higher caloric, fat, and protein intake than those who are breast-fed. They are also not exposed to the immunologic benefits of breast milk, which may lead to an increased incidence of childhood cancer. Numerous human and animal studies are consistent with the hypothesis that overnutrition in infancy is a risk factor for the later development of certain cancers, including breast cancer. Increased childhood nutrition and growth also lead to earlier menarche. Early maturers have a lifelong increase in the risk of developing breast cancer.

In mature women, breast-feeding may affect breast cancer risk by influencing systemic hormone levels and by influencing the microenvironment of the breast tissue. A woman who breast-feeds through the "ancient" or traditional pattern (on demand, through the night, and for a duration of at least 1 year) will experience lactational amenorrhea, usually from 1 to 2 years duration and corresponding high levels of prolactin. Nonpregnant, nonlactating women have higher levels of estrogens, which appear to be associated with increased risk of breast cancer. Prolonged lactation has an effect on the microenvironment of breast tissue and may help minimize exposure of the breast epithelium to carcinogens.

Recent studies indicate that the ancient or traditional pattern of breast-feeding appears to lower the risk of breast cancer. Earlier epidemiologic studies in Western and other populations may not have shown a clear, independent effect of breast-feeding on breast cancer because (1) breastfeeding behavior was incompletely characterized and/or (2) the breastfeeding that does occur in Western populations generally does not follow the ancient or traditional pattern.

Biologically, pregnancy and lactation are linked in both adaptive and physiologic ways. Rapid sociocultural developments have recently resulted in many more years of fertile adult life in women who are not pregnant or lactating compared to past generations. Breast cancer may be one of the biologic consequences.

## REFERENCES AND RESOURCES

Albanes, D. A., Schatzkin, A. G., & Micozzi, M. S. (1987). A survey of time related factors in diet and cancer. *Journal of Chronic Disease, 40*, 395–445.

Armstrong, B., & Doll, R. (1975). Diet and reproductive hormones: A study of vegetarian and nonvegetarian postmenopausal women. *Journal of the National Cancer Institute, 67*(4), 761–767.

Berg, J. W. (1975). Can nutrition explain the pattern of international epidemiology of hormone-dependent cancers? *Cancer Research, 35*, 3345–3350.

Bertwistle, D., & Ashworth, A. (1999). The pathology of familial breast cancer: How do the functions of BRCA1 and BRCA2 relate to breast tumour pathology. *Breast Cancer Research, 1*(1), 41–47.

Brinkley, D., Carpenter, R. G., & Haybittle, J. L. (1971). An anthropometric study of women with cancer. *British Journal of Preventive and Social Medicine, 25*, 65–75.

Buell, P. (1973). Changing incidence of breast cancer in Japanese-American women. *Journal of the National Cancer Institute, 51*, 1479–1483.

Buell, P., & Dunn, J. (1965). Cancer mortality of Japanese Isei and Nisei in California. *Cancer, 18*, 656–664.

Bulbrook, R. D., Swain, M. C., Wang, D. Y., Hayward, J. L., Kumaoka, S., Takatani, O., et al. (1976). Breast cancer in Britain and Japan. *European Journal of Cancer, 12*, 725–735.

Byers, T., Graham, S., Rzepka, T., & Marshall, J. (1985). Lactation and breast cancer: Evidence for a negative association in premenopausal women. *American Journal of Epidemiology, 121*, 664–674.

Carter, C. L., Corle, D. K., Micozzi, M. S., Schatzkin, A., & Taylor, P. R. (1988). A prospective study of the development of breast cancer in 16,692 women with benign breast disease. *American Journal of Epidemiology, 128*(3), 467–477.

Centers for Disease Control Cancer and Steroid Hormone Study (CDC). (1983). Long-term oral contraceptive use and the risk of breast cancer. *Journal of the American Medical Association, 249*(12), 1591–1595.

Chilvers, C. (1993). Breast feeding and risk of breast cancer in young women. United Kingdom National Case-Control Study Group. *British Medical Journal, 307*, 17–20.

Clinton, S. K., Truex, C. R., & Visek, W. J. (1979). Dietary protein, aryl hydrocarbon hydroxlase and chemical carcinogenesis in rats. *Journal of Nutrition, 109*, 55–62.

Cohen, M. N. (1989). *Health and the rise of civilization.* New Haven, CT: Yale University Press.

Craig, J. C., Gruenke, L. D., & Petrakis, N. L. (1982). Measurement of cholesterol epoxide formation and turnover in human breast fluid. In W. P. Duncan & A.B. Susas (Eds.), *Synthesis and applications of isotopically labeled compounds* (pp. 297-298). Amsterdam: Elsevier.

Davis, M. K., Savitz, D. A., & Graubard, B. I. (1988). Infant feeding and childhood cancer. *Lancet, 2*, 365–368.

De Souza, I., Morgan, L., Lewis, U. L., Raggatt, P. R., Salih, H., & Hobbs, J. R. (1974). Growth hormone dependence among human breast cancers. *Lancet, 2*, 182–184.

DeWaard, F. (1975). Breast cancer incidence and nutritional status with particular reference to body weight and height. *Cancer Research, 35*, 3351–3356.

DeWaard, F., & Bancers-van Halewijn, E. A. (1974). A prospective study in general practice on breast cancer risk in postmenopausal women. *International Journal of Cancer, 14*, 153–160.

DeWaard, F., Cornelius, J. P., & Aichi, K. (1977). Breast cancer incidence according to weight and height in two cities of the Netherlands and Japan. *Cancer, 40*, 1269–1277.

Doll, R., Muir, C., & Waterhouse, J. (1970). *Cancer incidence in five continents* (Vol. II). New York: Springer-Verlag.

Drasar, B. S., & Irving, D. (1973). Environmental factors and cancer of the colon and breast. *British Journal of Cancer, 27*, 162–172.

Duncan, A. M., Phipps, W. R., & Kurzer, M. S. (2003). Phyto-estrogens: Best practice and research. *Clinical Endocrinology and Metabolism, 17*, 253–271.

Dunn, J. E. (1977). Breast cancer among American Japanese in the San Francisco Bay Area (National Cancer Institute, Monograph 47, pp. 157–160). Washington, DC: National Cancer Institute.

Dupont, W. D., & Page, D. L. (1985). Risk factors for breast cancer in women with proliferative breast disease. *New England Journal of Medicine, 312*, 146–151.

Eaton, S. B., & Konner, M. (1985). Paleolithic nutrition: A consideration of its nature and current implications. *New England Journal of Medicine, 312*, 283–289.

Eveleth, P. B., & Tanner, J. M. (1976). *Worldwide variation in human growth.* Cambridge, UK: Cambridge University Press.

Ewertz, M., Duff, S. W., Adami, H. O., Kvale, G., Lund, E., Meirik, O., et al. (1990). Age at first birth, parity and risk of breast cancer: A meta-analysis of 8 studies from the Nordic countries. *International Journal of Cancer, 46*, 597–603.

Federation of American Societies for Experimental Biology (FASEB). (1976). *Evaluation of the health aspects of sucrose as a food ingredient.* Unpublished manuscript P-I-III, I-30.

Fishman, J., Fukushima, D., O'Connor, J., Rosenfeld, R. S., Lynch, H. T., Lynch, J. F., Guigis, H., & Maloney, K. (1978). Plasma hormone profiles of young women at risk for familiar breast cancer. *Cancer Research, 38*, 4006–4011.

Gaskill, S. P., McGuire, W. L., Osborne, C. K., & Stern, M. P. (1979). Breast cancer mortality and diet in the United States. *Cancer Research, 39*, 3628–3637.

Goldin, B. R., & Gorbach, S. H. (1984). Alterations of the intestinal macroflora by diet, oral antibiotics, and *Lactobacillus*: Decreased production of free amines from aromatic nitropounds, azo dyes, and glucuronides. *Journal of the National Cancer Institute, 73*, 689–695.

Goldin, B. R., Adlercreutz, H., & Dwyer, J. T. (1981). Effect of diet on excretion of estrogens in pre- and postmenopausal women. *Cancer Research, 41*, 3771–3773.

Goldin, B. R., Adlercreutz, H., Gorbach, S. L., Warram, J. H., Dwyer, J. T., Swenson, L., et al. (1982). Estrogen excretion patterns and plasma levels in vegetarian and omnivorous women. *New England Journal of Medicine, 307*, 1542–1547.

Graham, S., Marshall, J., Mettlin, C., Rzepka, T., Nemoto, T., & Byers, T. (1982). Diet in the epidemiology of breast cancer. *American Journal of Epidemiology, 116*, 68–75.

Gray, G. E., Pike, M. C., & Henderson, B. E. (1979). Breast cancer incidence and mortality rates in different countries in relation to known risk factors and dietary practices. *British Journal of Cancer, 39*, 1–7.

Greulich, W. W. (1957). A comparison of the physical growth and development of American-born and native Japanese children. *American Journal of Physical Anthropology, 15*, 489–515.

Grodin, J. M., Siiteri, P. K., & MacDonald, P. C. (1973). Source of estrogen production in post-menopausal women. *Journal of Clinical Endocrinology and Metabolism, 36*, 207–214.

Gruenke, L. D., Wrensch, M. R., Petrakis, N. L., Miike, R., Ernster, V. L., & Craig, J. C. (1987). Breast fluid cholesterol and cholesterol epoxides: Relationships to breast cancer risk factors and other characteristics. *Cancer Research, 47*, 5483–5487.

Hahn, O., & Koldovsky, O. (1966). *Utilization of nutrients during postnatal development.* Longon: Pergamon.

Haymond, M. W., Karl, I. E., & Pagliara, A. S. (1974). Increased gluconeogic substrates in the small-for-gestational age infant. *New England Journal of Medicine, 291*(7), 322–328.

Hayward, J. L., Greenwood, F. C., & Glober, G. A. (1978). Hormonal status in normal British, Japanese, and Hawaii-Japanese women. *European Journal of Cancer, 14*, 1221–1228.

Hems, G. (1978). Contributions of diet and childbearing to breast cancer rates. *British Journal of Cancer, 37*, 974–982.

Hill, P., Wynder, E. L., Helman, P., Huskisson, J., Sporangisa, E., & Wynder, E. L. (1980). Diet life-styles and menstrual activity. *American Journal of Clinical Nutrition, 33*, 1192–1198.

Hirayama, T. (1978). Epidemiology of breast cancer with special reference to the role of diet. *Preventive Medicine, 7*, 173–195.

Holmes, M. D., & Willett, W. C. (2004). Does diet affect breast cancer risk? *Breast Cancer Research, 6*, 170–178.

Howe, G. R., Hirohata, T., Hislop, T. G., Iscovich, J. M., Yuan, J. M., Katsouyanni, K., et al. (1990). Dietary factors and risk of breast cancer: Combined analysis of 12 case-controlled studies. *Journal of the National Cancer Institute, 82*, 561–569.

Howe, H. L., Wingo, P. A., Thun, M. J., Ries, L. A. G., Rosenberg, H. M., Feigal, E. G., et al. (2001). The Annual Report to the Nation on the Status of Cancer (1973 Through 1998), Featuring Cancers With Recent Increasing Trends. *Journal of the National Cancer Institute, 93*(11), 824–842.

Huang, Z., Hankinson, S. E., Colditz, G. A., Stampfer, M. J., Hunter, D. J., Manson, J. E., et al. (1997). Dual effects of weight and weight gain on breast cancer risk. *Journal of the American Medical Association, 278*, 1407–1411.

Hulka, B. S. (1984). When is the evidence for 'no association' sufficient? *Journal of the American Medical Association, 252*(1), 81–82.

Hunter, D. J., & Willett, W. C. (1993). Diet, body size and breast cancer. *Epidemiology Reviews, 15*, 110–132.

Hutchinson, W. B., Thomas, D. B., Hamlin, W. B., Roth, G. J., Peterson, A. V., & Williams, B. (1980). Risk of breast cancer in women with benign breast disease. *Journal of the National Cancer Institute, 65*, 13–20.

Hilakivi-Clarke, L. (2000). Estrogens, BRCA1, and breast cancer. *Cancer Research, 60*(18), 4993–5001.

Ing, R., Petrakis, N. L., & Ho, J. H. C. (1977). Unilateral breast feeding and breast cancer. *Lancet, 2*, 124–127.

Johnson, R. C., Bowman, K. S., & Schwitters, S. Y. (1984). Ethnic familial and environmental influences in lactose tolerance. *Human Biology, 56*, 307–316.

Juret, P., Couette, J.-E., Burne, D., & Vernhes, J.-C. (1974). Age at first birth: An equivocal factor in human mammary carcinogenesis. *European Journal of Cancer, 10*, 591–594.

Kaufman, D. E., Miller, D. R., Rosenberg, L., Helmrich, S. P., Stolley, P., Schottenfeld, D., et al. (1984). Non-contraceptive estrogen use and risk of breast cancer. *Journal of the American Medical Association, 252*, 63–67.

Kelsey, J. L., & Gammon, M. D. (1991). The epideiology of breast cancer. *CA: Cancer Journal for Clinicians, 41*, 146–165.

Kolonel, L. N., Hankin, J. H., Lee, J. H., Chi, S. Y., Nomura, A., & Hinds, M. W. (1981). Nutrient intakes in relation to cancer incidence in Hawaii. *British Journal of Cancer, 44*, 331–339.

Kondo, S., & Eto, M. (1975). *Physical growth studies on Japanese-American children in comparison with native Japanese.* In Proceedings of Meeting for Review and Seminar of the U.S.-Japan Cooperative Research on Human Adaptabilities (pp. 13–45). Tokyo: University of Tokyo.

Kralj-Cercek, L. (1956). The influence of food, body build, and social origin on the age at menarche. *Human Biology, 28*, 393–406.

Kurihara, M., Aoki, K., & Tominaga, S. (1984). *Cancer mortality statistics in the world.* Nayoga, Japan: University of Nayoga.

Kvale, G. (1992). Reproductive factors in breast cancer epidemiology. *Acta Oncologica, 31*, 187–194.

Kvale, G., & Heuch, I. (1988). Lactation and cancer risk: Is there a relation specific to breast cancer? *Journal of Epidemiology and Community Health, 42*, 30–37.

Kvale, G., & Jacobsen, B. K. (1990). Risk factors for breast cancer. Do epidemiologic findings provide a basis for primary prevention? (Norwegian). *Tidsskrift for den Norske Laegeforening, 110*, 232–235.

Lannin, D. R., Mathews, H. F., Mitchell, J., Swanson, M. S., Swanson, F. H., & Edwards, M. S. (1998). Influence of socioeconomic and cultural factors on racial differences in late-stage presentation of breast cancer. *Journal of the American Medical Association, 279*(22), 1801–1807.

LaPorte, R. E., Adams, L. L., Savage, D. D., Brenes, G., Dearwater, S., & Cook, T. (1984). The spectrum of physical activity, cardiovascular disease and health: An epidemiologic perspective. *American Journal of Epidemiology, 120*, 507–517.

Layde, P. M., Webster, L. A., Boughman, A. L., Wingo, P. A., Rubin, G. L., & Ory, H. W. (1989). The independent associations of parity, age at first full term pregnancy, and duration of breast feeding with the risk of breast cancer. Cancer and Steroid Hormone Study Group. *Journal of Clinical Epidemiology, 42*, 963–973.

London, S. J., Colditz, G. A., Stampfer, M. J., Willett, W. C., Rosner, B. A., Corsano, K., et al. (1990). Lactation and risk of breast cancer in a cohort of U.S. women. *American Journal of Epidemiology, 132*, 17–26.

Lord, R. S., Bongiovanni, B., & Bralley, J. A. (2002). Estrogen metabolism and the diet-cancer connection: rationale for assessing the ratio of urinary hydroxylated metabolites. *Alternative Medicine Review, 7*, 111–129.

Love, R. (1992). Clinical trials on breast cancer. In M. S. Micozzi & T. E. Moon (Eds.), *Macronutrients: Investigating their role in cancer* (pp. 377–406). New York: Marcel Dekker.

Lubin, J. H., Burns, P. E., Blot, W., Ziegler, R. G., Lees, A. W., & Fraumeni, J. F., Jr. (1981). Dietary factors and breast cancer risk. *International Journal of Cancer, 28*, 685–689.

Lynch, H. T., Albano, W. A., Danes, B. S., Layton, M. A., Kimberling, W. J., Lynch, J. F., et al. (1984). Genetic predisposition to breast cancer. *Cancer, 513*, 612–622.

MacMahon, B., Cole, P., Lin, T. M., Lowe, C. R., Mirra, A. P., Ravnihar, B., et al. (1970). Age at first birth and breast cancer risk. *Bulletin of the World Health Organization, 43*, 209–221.

Malcolm, L. A. (1974). Ecological factors relating to child growth and nutritional status. In A. F. Roche & F. Falkner (Eds.), *Nutrition and malnutrition* (pp. 329–353). New York: Plenum.

Matsunaga, E. (1962). The dimorphism in human normal cerumen. *Annals of Human Genetics, 25*, 273–286.

McPherson, K., Neil, A., Vessey, M. P., & Doll, D. (1983). Oral contraceptive and breast cancer. *Lancet, 2*, 1414–1415.

McTiernan, A., & Thomas, D. B. (1986). Evidence for a protective effect of lactation on risk of breast cancer in young women. *American Journal of Epidemiology, 124*, 353–358.

Micozzi, M. S. (1990). Applications of anthropometry to epidemiologic studies of nutrition and cancer. *American Journal of Human Biology, 2*, 727–739.

Micozzi, M. S., Carter, C. L., Albanes, D., Taylor, P. R., & Licitra, L. M. (1989). Bowel function and breast cancer in U.S. women. *American Journal of Public Health, 79*, 73–75.

Micozzi, M. S., & Schatzkin, A. G. (1985). International correlation of anthropometric variables and adolescent growth patterns with breast cancer incidence. *American Journal of Physical Anthropology, 66*, 206–207.

Miller, A. B. (1977). Role of nutrition in the etiology of breast cancer. *Cancer, 39*, 2704–2708.

Miller, A. B., & Bulbrook, R. D. (1980). The epidemiology and etiology of breast cancer. *New England Journal of Medicine, 303*, 1246–1248.

Miller, A. B., Kelly, A., Choi, N. W., Matthews, V., Morgan, R. W., Munan, L., et al. (1978). A study on diet and breast cancer. *American Journal of Epidemiology, 107*, 499–509.

Montoye, H. J., & Taylor, H. L. (1984). Measurement of physical activity in population studies: A review. *Human Biology, 56*, 195–216.

Moolgavkar, S. H., Day, N. E., & Stevens, R. G. (1980). Two-stage model for carcinogenesis: Epidemiology of breast cancer in females. *Journal of the National Cancer Institute, 65*, 559–569.

Muti, P., Bradlow, H. L., Micheli, A., Krogh, V., Freudenheim, J. L., Schunemann, H. J., et al. (2000). Estrogen metabolism and risk of breast cancer: A prospective study of the 2:16 alphahydroxyestrone ratio in premenopausal and postmenopausal women. *Epidemiology, 11*, 635–640.

Newcomb, P. A., Storer, B. A., Longnecker, M. P., Mittendorf, R., Greenberg, E. G., Clapp, R. W., et al. (1994). Lactation and reduced risk of premenopausal breast cancer. *New England Journal of Medicine, 330*, 81–87.

Newman, M. T. (1975). Nutrition and adaptation in man. In A. Damon (Ed.), *Physiological anthropology* (pp. 210–259). London: Oxford University Press.

Nomura, A., Henderson, B. E., & Lee, J. (1978). Breast cancer and diet among the Japanese in Hawaii. *American Journal of Clinical Nutrition, 31*, 2020–2025.

O'Rourke, D. H., & Petersen, G. M. (1983). Biological anthropology and genetic disease research: Introduction. *American Journal of Physical Anthropology, 62*, 1–21.

Paffenbarger, R. S., Kampert, J. B., & Chang, H. (1980). Characteristics that predict the risk of cancer before and after menopause. *American Journal of Epidemiology, 112*, 258–268.

Page, D. L, Vander Zwaag, R., Rogers, L. W., Williams, L. T., Walker, W. E., & Harmann, W. H. (1978). Relation between component parts of fibrocystic disease complex and breast cancer. *Journal of the National Cancer Institute, 61*, 1055–1063.

Petrakis, N. L. (1977). Genetic cerumen type breast secretory activity and breast cancer epidemiology. In J. J. Mulvill, R. W. Miller, & J. F. Fraumeni (Eds.), *Genetics of human cancer* (pp. 297–299). New York: Raven.

Petrakis, N. L., Dupuy, M. E., Lee, R. E., Lyon, M., Maack, C. A., Gruenke, L. D., et al. (1982). Mutagens in nipple aspirates of breast fluids. In B. A. Bridges, B. E. Butterworth, & I. B. Weinstein (Eds.), *Banbury Report 13: Indicators of genotoxic exposure* (pp. 67–82). Cold Spring Harbor, NY: Cold Spring Harbor Laboratory.

Petrakis, N. L., & King, E. B. (1981). Cytological abnormalities in nipple aspirates of breast fluid from women with severe constipation. *Lancet, 2*, 1203–1205.

Petrakis, N. L., Maack, C. A., Lee, R. E., & Lyon, M. (1980). Mutagenic activity in nipple aspirates of human breast fluid. *Cancer Research, 40*, 188–189.

Petrakis, N. L., Mason, L., Lee, R., Sugimoto, B., Pawson, S., & Catchpool, F. (1975). Association of race, age, menopausal status and cerumen type with breast fluid secretion in nonlactating women as determined by nipple aspiration. *Journal of the National Cancer Institute, 54*, 829–833.

Petrakis, N. L., Wrensch, M. R., & Ernster, V. L. (1987). Influence of pregnancy and lactation on serum and breast fluid estrogen levels: Implications for breast cancer risk. *International Journal of Cancer, 40*, 587–591.

Phillips, R. L. (1975). Role of life-style and dietary habits in risk of cancer among Seventh-Day Adventists. *Cancer Research, 35*, 3513–3522.

Pike, M. C., Henderson, B. E., Krailo, M. D., Duke, A., & Roy, S. (1983). Breast cancer in young women and use of oral contraceptives: Possible modifying effect of formulation and age at use. *Lancet, 2*, 926–930.

Prentice, R. (1992). Rationale, feasibility, and design of a low fat diet intervention trial among post-menopausal women. In M. S. Micozzi & T. E. Moon (Eds.), *Macronutrients: Investigating their role in cancer* (pp. 356–376). New York: Marcel Dekker.

Roberts, M. M., Jones, V., Elton, R. A., Fortt, R. W., Williams, S., & Gravelle, I. H. (1984). Risk of breast cancer in women with history of benign disease of the breast. *British Medical Journal, 228*, 275–278.

Roche, A. F. (1984). Anthropometric methods: New and old. What they tell us. *International Journal of Obesity, 8*, 509–523.

Ross, M. H. (1977). Dietary behavior and longevity. *Nutrition Reviews, 35*, 257–265.

Ross, M. H., & Bras, G. (1965). Tumor incidence patterns and nutrition in the rat. *Journal of Nutrition, 87*, 245–250.

Ross, M. H., Bras, G., & Lustbader, E. D. (1983). Diet, body weight and tumor susceptibility. *Twenty-eighth Scientific Report, Institute for Cancer Research* (pp. 18–20). Philadelphia, PA: Fox Chase Cancer Center.

Rothman, K. J., MacMahon, B., Lin, T. M., Lowe, C. R., Mirra, A. P., Ravnihar, B., et al. (1980). Maternal age and birth rank of women with breast cancer. *Journal of the National Cancer Institute, 65*, 719–722.

Royal College of General Practitioners. (1981). Breast cancer and oral contraceptives. *British Medical Journal, 282*, 2089–2093.

Sherman, B., Wallace, R., Bean, J., & Schlabaugh, L. (1981). Relationships of body weight to menarche and menopausal age: Implications for breast cancer risk. *Journal of Clinical Endocrinology and Metabolism, 52*, 488–493.

Simoons, F. J. (1969). Primary adult lactose intolerance and the milking habit: A problem in biological and cultural interrelations. I. Review of the medical literature. *American Journal of Digestive Disease, 14*, 819–836.

Siskind, V., Schofiels, F., Rice, D., & Bain, C. (1989). Breast cancer and breastfeeding: Results from and Australian case-control study. *American Journal of Epidemiology, 130*, 229–236.

Smith-Warner, S. A., Spiegelman, D., & Yuan, S. S. (1998). Alcohol and breast cancer in women: A pooled analysis of cohort studies. *Journal of the American Medical Association, 279*, 535–540.

Sreekumar, O., & Hosono, A. (2000). Immediate effect of *Lactobacillus acidophilus* on the intestinal flora or rats and the in vitro inhibition of *E. coli* in coculture. *Journal of Dairy Science, 83*, 931–939.

Staszewski, J. (1971). Age at menarche and breast cancer. *Journal of the National Cancer Institute, 47*, 935–940.

Stini, W. A. (1978). Early nutrition, growth, disease, and human longevity. *Nutrition and Cancer, 1*, 31–39.

Taitz, L. S. (1971). Overnutrition among artificially fed infants in Sheffield regions. *British Journal of Medicine, 1*, 315–316.

Takahashi, E. (1984). Secular tend in milk consumption and growth in Japan. *Human Biology, 56*, 427–437.

Tanner, J. M. (1968). Earlier maturation in man. *Scientific American, 218*, 21–27.

Tanner, J. M., & Eveleth, P. B. (1975). Variability between populations in growth and development at puberty. In S. R. Berenberg (Ed.), *Puberty: Biologic and psychosocial components* (pp. 256–273). Leiden: H. E. Stenfert Kroese B.V.

Tao, S. C., Yu, M. C., Ross, R. K., & Xiu, R. W. (1988). Risk factors for breast cancer in Chinese women of Beijing. *International Journal of Cancer, 42*, 495–498.

Tashiro, H., Nomura, Y., & Hisamatu, K. (1990). A case-control study of risk factors of breast cancer detected by mass screening (Japanese). *Gan No Rinsho, 36*, 2127–2130.

Thomas, D. B. (1983). Factors that promote the development of human breast cancer. *Environmental Health Perspective, 50*, 209–218.

Trichopoulos, D., Cole, P., Brown, J. B., Goldman, M. B., & MacMahon, B. (1980). Estrogen profiles of primaparous and nulliparous women in Athens, Greece. *Journal of the National Cancer Institute, 55*, 43–46.

Van den Brandt, P. A., Spiegelman, D., Yuan, S. S., Adami, H. O., Beeson, L., Folsom, A. R., et al. (2000). Pooled analysis of prospective cohort studies on height, weight and breast cancer risk. *American Journal of Epidemiology, 152*, 514–527.

Waterhouse, J., Correa, P., Muir, C., & Powell, J. (1976). *Cancer incidence in five continents* (Vol. III). Lyons, France: International Agency for Research on Cancer.

Waterhouse, J., Muir, C., Shanmugaratnam, K., & Powell, J. (1982). *Cancer incidence in five continents* (Vol. IV). Lyons, France: International Agency for Research on Cancer.

Wenten, M., Gilliland, F. D., Baumgartner, K., & Samet, J. M. (2002). Associations of weight, weight change and body mass with breast cancer risk in Hispanic and non-Hispanic white women. *Annals of Epidemiology, 12*, 435–444.

Widdowson, E. M. (1974). Changes in pigs due to undernutrition before birth and for one, two, and three years afterward, and the effects of rehabilitation. In A. F. Roche & F. Falkner (Eds.), *Advances in experimental medicine and biology: Vol. 49. Nutrition and malnutrition: Identification and measurement* (pp. 165–181). New York: Plenum.

Wilson, D. C., & Sutherland, I. (1960). Further observations on the age of menarche. *British Medical Journal, 2*, 864–867.

Wood, J. W., Milner, G. R., Harpending, H. C., & Weiss, K. M. (1992). The osteological paradox: Problems of inferring prehistoric health for skeletal samples. *Current Anthropolgy, 33*, 343–370.

Wynder, E. L., Laht, H., & Laakso, K. (1985). Nipple aspirates of breast fluid and the epidemiology of breast disease. *Cancer, 56*, 1473–1479.

Yuan, J. M., Yu, M. C., Ross, R. K., Gao, Y. T., & Henderson, B. E. (1988). Risk factors for breast cancer in Chinese women in Shanghai. *Cancer Research, 48*, 1949–1953.

Ziegler, R. G. (2004). Phytoestrogens and breast cancer. *American Journal of Clinical Nutrition, 79*, 183–184.

# Prevention of Cancer With Nutrients and Whole Foods

10

Marc S. Micozzi

## Introduction

Most people can fully expect to live well into their seventies; at the same time, cancer has been identified as the second leading cause of mortality in many Western countries. More than 800,000 new cases of cancer occur each year in the United States, and over 20% of the approximately 2 million annual deaths in the United States are because of cancer. The search for the causes of cancer and possible controls remains intense. At the same time, however, the potential role of dietary factors in the etiology and prevention of cancer has gained considerable attention Since Doll and Peto (1981) raised the possibility that a high dietary intake of beta-carotene might decrease the risk of human cancer, considerable interest has been focused on micronutrients and cancer prevention. These investigators provided a wide range of estimates (10%–70%) for the proportion of deaths from cancer that could be reduced by practical dietary means, concluding that dietary modification might eventually result in a 35% reduction in cancer mortality in the United States.

In 1982, the National Research Council Committee on Diet, Nutrition, and Cancer, part of the National Academy of Sciences, first conducted an in-depth review of the literature and concluded that cancers of most major cancer sites are influenced by dietary patterns. However, the data were found to be insufficient to quantitate the contribution of diet to overall cancer risk or to determine the percentage reduction in risk that might be achieved by dietary modification. This chapter examines the general activities and the evidence for anticancer effects of the best studied nutrients, vitamin A, vitamin E, vitamin C, selenium, and fiber, and presents mechanisms for the possibility of an effect of vitamin D, calcium, B vitamins, choline, copper, zinc, and other dietary constituents that may be considered as dietary antioxidants (Borek, 2004).

# Cancer as a Preventable Disease

The idea of cancer as a preventable disease has evolved from studies to identify carcinogens (chemicals in the environment that cause cancer). The concept that cancer can be prevented by selectively altering the intake of specific foods or nutrients in the diet has gained importance. Ideas about the relations between micronutrients (vitamins and minerals) and cancer prevention have come from studies of dietary intake and cancer rates. Science has moved from the study of complex foods and dietary intake to the testing of specific food constituents (e.g., micronutrients) that might prevent cancer.

One approach to the development of micronutrients as cancer preventive agents followed clinical pharmacology for development of cancer chemotherapeutic agents. The drug development and clinical trials program of clinical pharmacology, applied to many areas of medical science, provides one model for scientific inquiry into cancer prevention.

In cancer prevention research, whether testing a product (such as a micronutrient) as a food or a drug, the process of clinical trials remains important to establishing end results. The small effects estimated for most nutritional factors in cancer also impose the requirement for large-scale clinical trials to obtain definitive, statistically significant results. The long duration of most clinical trials and great publicity surrounding them allows for the influence of secular trends on treatment, which may influence results, as the general population changes dietary patterns.

# Prevention of Cancer by Nutrients

Nutritional prevention of cancer may be defined as the prevention of cancer in human populations by dietary agents that inhibit carcinogenesis. This concept is based on the cancer-inhibiting potential of certain chemical compounds in the diet. The important characteristics of dietary agents relevant to human cancer prevention include their mechanisms of action, toxicity, and effectiveness. Dietary agents used in clinical trials for cancer prevention include various micronutrients and their synthetic analogs.

Cancer prevention through nutrition offers considerable opportunities for the improvement of human health. Many chronic diseases may be preventable. Cancer is no longer considered an inevitable part of the aging process. Environmental factors, acting in the presence of genetic factors, are now recognized as important determinants of human cancer. These environmental determinants include dietary habits and lifestyle.

## Levels of Prevention

Cancer prevention may focus on several levels in the effort to reduce cancer incidence and mortality in human populations. For example, reduction in exposure to environmental risk factors may reasonably be expected to reduce cancer incidence. Within the United States, it has been estimated that 80%–90% of cancers may be attributable at least in part to environmental factors and that diet and nutrition may account for approximately 30% of that attributable risk.

Other risks, such as smoking and various occupational exposures to industrial carcinogens, are also recognized. Strategies for recognition of individuals at high risk may result in more effective allocation of health resources and may create special opportunities for cancer prevention. There is increasing evidence that chemical carcinogenesis can be reversed if the chemical insult is removed or neutralized. The slow process of cancer promotion may be reversed or slowed to the point of never reaching tumor.

## Identification of Dietary Factors

Identification of agents in the diet that may inhibit the multistage process of carcinogenesis and prevent the occurrence of cancer has been underway. It may be easier or more appropriate in some situations to prescribe preventive agents than to proscribe unhealthy diets and other practices. For example, cancer prevention may be more readily achieved by prescription of a specific micronutrient than by attempting major modifications of the human diet.

Because many carcinogens are viewed as environmental chemicals that enter the body, metabolic processing of chemical carcinogens is relevant to cancer prevention. A *procarcinogen* is a chemical absorbed into the metabolic system from the environment that is subsequently transformed into a proximate carcinogen. The *proximate* carcinogen is then metabolically converted into the *ultimate* carcinogen, which displays its final activity at the molecular or cellular level. Preventive compounds may act at different steps in the metabolic processing of a carcinogen. Thus, a dietary agent may (1) prevent formation or absorption, (2) modulate metabolism, (3) accelerate excretion or (4) block the action of ultimate carcinogens once they are formed.

Other characteristics of dietary agents include their structure/activity relationships, toxicity, efficacy, dose, and dosage form. A wide range of compounds have been noted to manifest cancer-inhibiting potential. These observations indicate that structurally related compounds share cancer-inhibiting potential and suggest avenues for development of cancer preventive agents. Agents that inhibit later stages in the process of carcinogenesis may be particularly useful for preventing cancer in populations already exposed to carcinogens.

## Low Toxicity

An important characteristic of dietary preventive agents is low toxicity, because the target population includes individuals who are not ill but only at risk of cancer and may also include individuals with only a "normal" risk of exposure to environmental carcinogens. This requirement for low toxicity is in contrast to the typical features of chemotherapeutic agents for cancer therapy (see Chapters 1 and 2).

Potential chemical inhibitors of carcinogenesis occur in the human diet and include micronutrients, other metabolically active constituents, or food additives. Micronutrients are present in low concentrations and mediate critical aspects of human biochemistry and metabolism. Synthetic analogues of micronutrients that have greater efficacy (and less toxicity) than the parent compound may be of particular interest for use as cancer-preventive agents.

# Nutritional Inhibition of Cancer by Selected Nutrients

The relations between dietary practices and human cancer are supported by a variety of sources. Dietary practices may increase or decrease cancer risk depending on intakes of individual nutrients and their interactions. The multitude and complexities of relations among dietary constituents possibly accounts for reported inconsistencies among human studies. Nevertheless, based on laboratory, epidemiological, and clinical data, modification in diet appears to offer a means of reducing cancer risks.

Selected dietary factors have long been recognized as influencing the development of tumors in experimental animals. The intake of various micronutrients has been observed to significantly alter cancer incidence and severity by modifying specific phases of carcinogenesis. Thus, dietary constituents can alter the formation of carcinogens, modify the promotion and progression of cancer cells, modulate the immune system, and lead to variations in rates of tumor growth. The influence of individual micronutrients on the steps of carcinogenesis is discussed later in this chapter.

It has long been known that dietary modifications can alter the course of tumor formation and development. In recent years studies have actively examined specific dietary constituents for their impact on the cancer process. Attention also has been given to the influence of dietary intakes of the macronutrients, including fiber, as factors in cancer development. Continued examination of dietary constituents will likely result in more specific dietary recommendations for the general population and indicate critical times in life when nutritional intervention may be most beneficial. Micronutrients in the diet are not consumed alone but as part of foods and together with other constituents. Results must be reviewed as a reflection of the interactions of specified micronutrients with the other constituents of the diet. Nutritionists have long recognized that the *quantity* of a dietary constituent alone does not determine its relative importance in either disease prevention or treatment.

# Process of Carcinogenesis

The process of carcinogenesis may be separated both mechanistically and temporally. Normally, the first phase of this process is metabolic activation of the carcinogens that react with critical factors within the cell. This process, occurring within a few hours after exposure, can be repaired by many cells, thereby presumably leaving the normal cell unaltered. However, cells unable to remove this damage either die or become precancerous cells. For nutrients to impact this first phase of carcinogenesis, they must modify the biological behavior of the cell prior to, or at the time of exposure to, the carcinogen.

In contrast to the short duration of the first phase, the second phase of promotion is a prolonged process that is considered to last decades in human beings. This phase of carcinogenesis is extremely complex, with a variety of cellular changes occurring. Nutrients can have an influence during the early or late stages of the promotion phase. The final phase of carcinogenesis is progression. This phase results in the conversion of the premalignant cell to a malignant cell of increased virulence. In some circumstances the early changes occurring in these cells appear to be reversed by known dietary constituents, such as ascorbic acid (vitamin C) and vitamin A and retinoids. However, it is unknown whether this response represents complete reversibility to the normal cell. Information is limited on the effects of specific nutrients on the later progression of malignant cells' increasing invasiveness or metastatic properties, which is relevant to cancer treatment (see Chapter 11).

## Exposures in the Course of Life

In the course of living, humans will inevitably be exposed to compounds that are not essential for life or "natural" from the standpoint of evolution. Such agents may be acutely toxic or potentially toxic following metabolic activation or exhibit long-term effects such as cancer development. The ability of a dietary constituent to modify the formation of a potential carcinogenic agent is shown by the fact that vitamin C can reduce the formation of nitrosamines, for example. Most nitrosamines are very strong carcinogenic compounds and induce tumors in various species. Although ascorbic acid may be a significant factor in reducing formation of this carcinogen, other dietary constituents may have the opposite effect. The intake of some phenols, or thiocyanates and iodides, as present in green leafy vegetables, may paradoxically enhance cancer development by stimulation of the formation of carcinogenic compounds.

Thus, dietary constituents may impact the development of cancer by modifying the formation of specific carcinogens, altering the metabolic activation of carcinogens, or influencing the occurrence of anticarcinogens. The ability of selected micronutrients, such as vitamin A and selenium, to modify the metabolic activation of carcinogens is well appreciated. Similarly, a change in the metabolism of some carcinogens by a nonnutrient food additive, such as the common preservative butylated hydroxytoluene (BHT), has the effect of reducing carcinogenicity.

Minor constituents of commonly consumed plant foods, such as flavones, isothiocyanates, phenols, and indoles, also have the ability of altering the metabolic activation of carcinogens. The inverse association between the risk of cancer of the gastrointestinal tract and the consumption of selected vegetables, particularly the cruciferous vegetables, suggests a role of nonnutrient dietary constituents in the risk of human beings to cancer, in addition to the role of the recognized micronutrients in cancer prevention (see Chapter 13).

# Vitamin A and Retinoids

Vitamin A and retinoids have been identified as having a potential role in cancer prevention and treatment (Dragnev et al., 2003). Vitamin A (retinol) functions as a constituent of visual pigments, allows for normal reproductive capacity in both males and females, and allows for normal cellular growth and differentiation. Only retinol and its chemical derivatives can serve all of these functions. Interest in retinol has stemmed from several investigations noting an inverse relationship between vitamin A intake and the risk of developing cancer. Since the early 1940s, a deficiency of this vitamin has been recognized to increase the susceptibility of experimental animals to tumors. Moreover, some carcinogens result in a marked reduction in the liver stores of this vitamin. Thus, marginal vitamin A deficiencies may become evident following exposure to some carcinogens.

## Mechanisms of Action

The ability of vitamin A to modify cellular differentiation has often been cited as the mechanism by which this vitamin modifies the susceptibility of animals to cancer. Cancer cells are inherently characterized by a defect or change in the process of differentiation. The importance of this observation in human cancer is emphasized by the fact that most primary cancers in humans arise in epithelial tissues that depend on vitamin A for normal cellular differentiation.

The term *retinoids* refers to both natural and synthetic analogues of retinol. These compounds possess varying amounts of vitamin A activity depending on their specific structural characteristics. Various retinoid supplements have been shown to be effective inhibitors of chemical carcinogenesis in the skin, breast, esophagus, respiratory tract, pancreas, and urinary bladder of animals. Continuous retinoid administration is required for the continued inhibitory effects of this nutrient. Although the retinoids are generally most effective when administered shortly after the carcinogenic insult, even when treatment is delayed, these compounds are often effective cancer preventive agents. At least one retinoid without vitamin A activity is able to reduce UV-induced skin cancer animals.

The greatest effect of retinoids appears to be involved primarily in the promotional phase of tumor growth. Vitamin A and the retinoids in general may modify preneoplastic and/or neoplastic cells by stimulating cellular differentiation, blocking cellular division, or enhancing the destruction of cancer cells. None of the possible mechanisms would be mutually exclusive.

## Discovery and Observations of Effects

Wolbach and Howe (1925) were the first investigators to discover a relation between vitamin A and neoplasia; that is, dietary deficiencies in rats led to "preneoplastic abnormalities," and restoration of vitamin A to their diet reversed the neoplastic process. Wolbach and Howe's classic report followed the recognition in 1909, and naming in 1920, of the fat-soluble substance essential for normal growth we now call vitamin A. Preformed vitamin A, or the aldehyde and alcohol forms and their esters, is found mainly in animal products, including milk, eggs, meat, and fish and is not synthesized by plants. However, provitamin A, which includes beta-carotene among several other carotenoids, is found in plant sources and cannot be synthesized either by humans or animals. Both forms are also commonly found in over-the-counter pharmaceutical compounds. For the most part, beta-carotene is converted to vitamin A during absorption through the intestinal mucosa, where it and preformed vitamin A are transported in the plasma by lipoproteins. Vitamin A is then stored in the liver in fat cells.

## Toxicity

Many subsequent studies, including that in 1941 by Abels et al. that associated vitamin A deficiency with human cancer, strongly supported the link between vitamin A and neoplastic disease. Recognition that vitamin A deficiency leads to abnormal growth of the skin and to preneoplastic changes spurred an initial rush to treat skin disorders with this new drug; however, early excitement was tempered in light of toxic effects in many patients, especially on the liver. Excessive intake of vitamin A, or hypervitaminosis A, was first reported over 100 years ago, many years before vitamin A had even been positively identified. These reports involved the ingestion of polar bear and seal livers (5–8 mg retinal/g liver) by Eskimos and Arctic explorers. Their acute symptoms included severe headaches, drowsiness, irritability, nausea, and vomiting. Twelve to 24 hours after ingestion, redness and skin loss of the face, trunk, palms, and soles developed. Seven to 10 days later, all symptoms resolved.

Subsequent clinical observations verified these major acute symptoms of hypervitaminosis A, which occur when the intake of vitamin A exceeds the liver's capacity to remove and store it and after ingestion of a dose of at least 350,000 international units (IU) of vitamin A by infants and 1,000,000 IU by adults. Minor acute side effects are more frequent and better described and include dryness of skin and mucous membranes and ocular, gastrointestinal, and musculoskeletal complaints such as tenderness of long bones. Specific major chronic vitamin A toxicities include abnormalities of the following: reproductive function and embryological development, serum lipids, the liver, and the skeletal system. A partial hominid or prehuman (*Homo erectus*) skeleton discovered in Kenya exhibited the earliest pathologically documented changes consistent with chronic hypervitaminosis A. Minor chronic side effects resemble the minor acute toxicities described above but are more subtle.

## Retinoids: Synthetic Analogues of Vitamin A

The severe side effects of vitamin A, primarily liver toxicity, led to the search for vitamin A derivatives with improved therapeutic safety. New drugs began to be synthesized in the mid-1950s and were called *retinoids*—a term encompassing the entire natural (excluding carotenoids) and synthetic compounds having some or all of the biological activities of vitamin A.

Laboratory data have clearly demonstrated the potent cell differentiation-inducing and antiproliferative effects of many of the newer synthetic retinoids (Dragnev, 2003). Retinoids prevent cancer in the skin, breast, bladder, lung, and other sites in experimental animals.

## Vitamin A and Retinoids in Human Cancer

Vitamin A is critical to skin and epithelial cell growth and differentiation. There has been great interest in epidemiological studies of vitamin A and cancer, since an estimated 35% of U.S. cancers are because of dietary factors and over 90% of all human cancers are of epithelial origin. Evidence from several epidemiological studies suggests relations among dietary intake, serum levels of vitamin A, and cancer risk. However, dietary studies do not clearly distinguish between the relative protective effects of vitamin A and those of carotenoids (which the body converts in part to vitamin A). The next section focuses on epidemiological studies of lung cancer, as this is the best studied cancer and serves as a prototype for the limited studies of other malignancies.

## Lung

There are six major types of epidemiological studies in this field: (1) dietary studies relating variations in diet to cancer rates among different populations, (2) dietary studies of patients with diagnosed cancers that asked about consumption of foods "rich in vitamin A," (3) prospective or cohort dietary studies, (4) dietary studies with supplement pills with a known vitamin A content, (5) correlation between serum vitamin A levels and disease in patients with established diagnoses of cancer, and (6) correlation between serum vitamin A levels taken from apparently healthy individuals and the later development of cancer.

Different population studies have yielded conflicting results. For example, studies from Japan showed an inverse correlation between vitamin A intake and certain cancers; however, large studies from Hawaii and China failed to confirm this finding. Case-control dietary studies from England, Buffalo (New York), New Jersey, New Mexico, and Hawaii indicated an inverse correlation between vitamin A and lung cancer, especially in populations with marginal intake of vitamin A. The relative importance of carotenoids versus vitamin A is especially difficult to sort out with this retrospective study design. In 1975, Bjelke reported the first prospective study showing an inverse relationship between vitamin A intake and lung cancer. Over the succeeding years, several other follow-up studies were reported, including those conducted in Chicago (Western Electric), Boston, Norway, and Japan. Several of these studies suggest a relatively greater protective effect with vegetables (carotenoids) than with preformed vitamin A, although this result is still questioned. Dietary vitamin A supplementation (pills) may modestly increase serum vitamin A levels, but it remains questionable whether this effect provides protection against lung cancer, especially when the level varies only within the physiologic range.

Other studies have attempted to correlate vitamin A levels of serum (stored samples) with the development of lung cancer many years later. The first two studies were conducted in England and in Evans County, Georgia, and indicated a strong inverse relation between serum vitamin A and the development of lung cancer. However, several subsequent negative studies, including another study from Evans County, showed only an insignificant trend correlating low serum vitamin A with lung cancer development. Also negative was a study in Washington County, Maryland, in which low levels of beta-carotene (but not preformed vitamin A) correlated with the development of cancer of the lung. These conflicting results caused some confusion. The differences may reflect different cancer subtypes, small patient numbers, other covarying micronutrients (e.g., selenium and zinc), or factors such as sex, age, and smoking.

Beginning with Abels' classic report in 1941, several other studies have observed low plasma retinol levels in patients with established diagnoses of lung cancer. These studies are difficult to interpret because the effect of the malignancy on a patient's general nutritional status and the metabolism of vitamin A is unknown.

Studies linking nutritional intake with risk of cancer suffer the difficulty of obtaining information from personal diet history and then trying to translate food intake into nutrients from the existing food tables, which may be quite faulty. Carcinogenic agents (e.g., smoking and dietary initiators and promoters such as saturated fats) and anticancer factors (e.g., interactive micronutrients such as selenium) are also difficult to specifically quantify in dietary studies. Some of the epidemiological associations are supported by laboratory findings and current understanding of vitamin A metabolism while others have no laboratory correlations.

Because the epidemiological and laboratory work alone cannot firmly establish this link, carefully controlled, clinical trials have been required to establish a direct vitamin A intake/risk relationship. These trials, however, are extremely expensive and require substantial evidence from laboratory scientists and epidemiologists before they can be started. If the association becomes proven, it will have a significant impact on the public's health and on public health policy. It may become desirable to assay for serum vitamin A levels and serum retinol-binding protein (which corresponds strongly with serum vitamin A) as part of general health exams to identify people with higher risks of developing cancer. Establishing a positive association between vitamin A and cancer risk would also promote developing safer methods for increasing serum vitamin A.

## Interactions With Other Micronutrients

At least in part, the possible anticancer effects of vitamin A depend on interactions with other micronutrients, which also help to confound the interpretation of epidemiological studies. The principal micronutrients shown to interact with vitamin A are selenium, zinc, vitamins E and C, and iron. Selenium is an effective cancer-preventive agent in its own right, and its mechanism of action may be similar to that of vitamin A.

Several studies have indicated interactions between zinc and vitamin A at many levels of cellular activity. Some human enzyme systems requiring zinc are directly and indirectly critical to vitamin A metabolism. Zinc reportedly influences the enzyme that catalyzes the conversion of retinaldehyde to retinoic acid. Indirectly, zinc may affect vitamin A through zinc-dependent enzymes, which may be involved in the synthesis of vitamin A carriers and cellular-binding proteins.

Research suggests potentially important interactions between both vitamins E and C and vitamin A. Some investigators believe that vitamin E has only a nonspecific, antioxidant role in its relationship with vitamin A. Vitamin E stabilizes cell membranes, and vitamin E deficiency shortens the survival time of red blood cells and accelerates the depletion rate of liver stores of vitamin A. Vitamin E provides vitamin A and carotenoids with protection from oxidation in mixed diets. This protection results in higher levels of liver vitamin A and, under certain circumstances, higher circulating vitamin A levels. Studies of vitamin E-deficient rats fed vitamin A indicate that vitamin E protects vitamin A at a cellular level as well. Vitamin E may also reduce vitamin A toxicity. Vitamin A deficiency and excess appear to influence the liver's synthesis of vitamin C (ascorbic acid), and vitamin C apparently acts as an antioxidant for vitamin A. Some reports claim to demonstrate a direct association between vitamin A deficiency and vitamin C synthesis.

High levels of iron in the intestine may contribute to destruction of vitamin A-active compounds. However, no data indicate that intake of high levels of inorganic iron causes vitamin A deficiency. Studies of human volunteers have revealed that vitamin A deficiency produces the gradual onset of anemia that responds to vitamin A but not to medicinal iron supplementation. Nutrition surveys commonly reveal an association between anemia and inadequate dietary vitamin A.

Epidemiological studies of children in developing countries showed a parallel increase in hemoglobin and serum iron with increasing blood levels of vitamin A. Experimental studies of the interaction between iron and vitamin A show that iron absorption is not altered by vitamin A deficiency and that vitamin A appears to help mobilize stored iron and incorporate it into red blood cells.

## Dose and Requirements

The recommended daily allowance (RDA) for vitamin A is set well above the level required for most people who ingest substantial amounts of animal protein to compensate amply for adverse nutrient interactions that could influence levels of vitamin A. One can assume that micronutrient interactions with vitamin A–active compounds are similar in effect to interactions with the synthetic analogues or retinoids. Differences in clinical responses to retinoid therapy, varying levels of interactive micronutrients in patients with the same disease, and standard medical screening of patients in the future may include serum analyses of micronutrients that affect vitamin A in the body.

## Therapeutic Anticancer Activity

In addition to the recognized cancer preventive effects, these agents have also shown antitumor activity in several clinical studies (Chapter 11). The growing clinical experience with retinoid therapy in established cancers includes significant results in skin cancers and acute leukemia. Several other cancers, including head and neck cancer, eccrine poroma, melanoma, and several other leukemias, have also been studied for responses to retinoids.

Topical and systemic retinoids have been used to treat basal cell skin cancer. A total of 49 patients were treated in several different studies of topical retinoic acid, which produced 16 complete (33%) and 32 partial responses. Early observations that a therapeutic effect occurred after 6 to 8 weeks of treatment and that a significant number of patients recurred at follow-up 10 months later were characteristic of all these topical studies. Three other studies totaling 55 patients employed oral retinoids, either isotretinoin or another synthetic derivative. Data from these studies were also promising, with a response rate over 50%, although both complete and partial responses required maintenance therapy to prevent recurrences.

While the number of studies on retinoid treatment for squamous cell skin cancer in humans has been limited, results in animals have been promising and studies involving patients with cancers of the skin have netted promising results. The retinoids were also well tolerated by these patients. These results are encouraging because no standard effective systemic therapy for advanced or metastatic squamous cell cancer of the skin currently exists.

Primarily involving the skin for most of its natural history, mycosis fungoides is an uncommon disorder. Single-agent retinoid treatment of this disease on nearly 100 patients has produced impressive results with an overall response rate of 62%. Responses in these studies generally require maintenance retinoid treatment to avoid relapse.

Acute promyelocytic leukemia is the most promising leukemic disorder to undergo clinical study with retinoids. In general, data encourage the use of retinoids in treating leukemia.

# Beta-Carotene and Carotenoids

## Epidemiological Studies

Early epidemiological studies relating total dietary vitamin A intake to cancer (e.g., Bjelke, 1975) could not distinguish intake of specific carotenoids from intake of total carotenoids or vitamin A. Natural preformed vitamin A is found only in animals, whereas plants contain provitamin A (alpha- and beta-carotene) and other carotenoids with lower or absent vitamin A activity. All of these studies used crude estimates of carotenoids and vitamin A (Shekelle et al., 1981), which did not permit differentiation of beta-carotene. Most early dietary studies utilized dietary intake indices based predominantly on plant foods (Peto, Doll, Buckley, & Sporn, 1981), and thus the evidence relates primarily to the effects of total carotenoids rather than total vitamin A or beta-carotene specifically. In a prospective study where a dietary distinction was drawn between plant (carotenoid) and animal vitamin A food sources of vitamin A (Shekelle et al., 1981), plant-source foods, but not animal-source foods, were found protective against cancer.

Accordingly, early dietary intake studies did not generally have high specificity for individual carotenoid-containing foods. However, the broad categories of "fruits, and green and yellow vegetables" are notable for the preponderance of food items that are low or absent in beta-carotene and relatively high in other carotenoids.

Increased risks of cancer have been seen with higher dietary intake of preformed vitamin A but such observations are confounded by the association of fat and protein intake (Armstrong & Doll, 1975) with animal products high in vitamin A. In studies where individual carotenoid sources are considered separately, there is often no effect of beta-carotene specifically. It is likely that constituents of green and yellow vegetables other than beta-carotene may actually reduce cancer incidence. Nutrient analyses of carotenoid-containing foods substantiated that beta-carotene is not an abundant constitute of foods found protective against cancer in epidemiological studies (Micozzi, Beecher, Taylor, & Khachik, 1990; see also Whole Foods). Nonetheless the National Cancer Institute has proceeded with complex and costly studies to evaluate the effects of beta-carotene and other constituents on the occurrence of cancer. These misguided experiments and experiences have motivated considerable reflection on the part of cancer researchers (Duffield-Lillico & Begg, 2004).

## Clinical Trials

Early trials using retinoids included a trial in head and neck cancer patients where 13-*cis* retinoic acid was given to patients and they were observed for recurrence or secondary cancers. The frequency of secondary cancers was observed to be significantly lower in the treatment arm (4% vs. 24%) when compared to the nontreatment arm. A subsequent trial was published that involved 307 patients with resected lung cancer randomized to receive either vitamin A or supportive care. The authors observed again a lower incidence of secondary cancers (12% vs. 21%).

However, two large randomized chemoprevention trials were published in the 1990s that underscore the necessity of large randomized confirmatory trials. The Alpha Tocopherol Beta Carotene (ATBC) trial examined the efficacy of beta-carotene and alpha-tocopherol supplementation in male smokers in Finland. Not only did the treatment fail to show any protective effects, but beta-carotene was associated with a significant increase in lung cancer incidence and mortality. This observation was confirmed in the Beta Carotene and Retinol Efficacy (CARET) trial, which examined patients who were smokers and ex-smokers and those exposed to asbestos. The trial concluded that those supplementing with beta-carotene were at a 28% higher risk of developing lung cancer and at a 17% higher mortality rate than those not supplementing. In both the animal and human models, it has been demonstrated that cigarette smoking and beta-carotene yield unstable oxidants and probably contribute to risk of bronchogenic carcinoma.

Since these very publicized studies, a European group and the NCI have confirmed ATBC and CARET. EuroScan examined the effects of retinyl palmitate and *N*-acetylcysteine (NAC) in patients with lung as well as head and neck cancer. No reduction in secondary cancers or recurrences were noted. The NCI Intergroup trial with 13-*cis* retinoic acid in patients with early-stage nonsmall cell lung cancer also failed to show improvement in secondary cancers or recurrence rates in the interventional arm. However, subgroup analyses suggested that retinoic acid may have been harmful in smokers and perhaps beneficial for those who had never smoked.

Omenn (1998) chronicles the rise and demise of the beta-carotene hypothesis. One conclusion of findings such as these points to the importance of the complex mix of other constituents such as polyphenols in whole foods for the prevention of cancer (Hercberg, 2005), as observed with the green leafy vegetables and with soy, for example.

# Vitamin C (Ascorbic Acid)

Vitamin C is an essential nutrient for humans and has been proposed as protective against cancer since the late 1940s. In 1936, it was proposed that vitamin C influences neoplastic white blood cells and vitamin C was used in the successful treatment of a patient with leukemia. Since this early observation, vitamin C has been implicated in human cancer prevention largely on the basis of several studies showing that consumption of foods containing high concentrations of this vitamin is associated with a reduction in cancer incidence, especially cancer of the stomach and esophagus.

## Mechanisms of Action

Evidence exists to support several mechanisms by which ascorbic acid may act in cancer prevention. Such mechanisms include blocking the formation of a carcinogen or tumor promoter, converting it to a less harmful metabolite, or enhancing host resistance to tumor progression and dissemination.

Experimental data from animals and cell culture systems suggest several mechanisms by which vitamin C might interfere with the cancer process. An important mechanism by which vitamin C may interfere with cancer development is by inhibiting nitrosamine formation. Nitrosamines and their potential hazards have been recognized for many years. Vitamin C treatment reduced *N*-nitroso compound formation in a selected group of human subjects at risk for gastric cancer. Supplementation of the diet with ascorbic acid and vitamin E was also found to reduce carcinogenic compounds excreted in human feces.

The ability of vitamin C to modify cancer cells has been documented through studies examining synergism with various drugs and interference with tumor cell metabolism. Although metabolic effects may account for the inhibition of some tumor cells, the effectiveness of vitamin C is likely dependent on cellular activities. Under some conditions it is possible to cause a reversal of chemically transformed cells to normal appearing cells by adding ascorbic acid. The exact mechanism by which vitamin C leads to this inhibition and reversion is unknown. Vitamin C also enhances immune function, thereby reducing the risk of certain types of cancer.

Several studies have described the antioxidant and general immunostimulant properties of vitamin C. Specifically, vitamin C is considered one of the most effective and least toxic antioxidants for humans and is thought to enhance the function of lymphocytes. In other experiments, vitamin C has demonstrated chemopreventive effects (preventing the recurrence of transplanted tumor cells), as well as therapeutic effects (inhibiting tumor growth, producing tumor regression of established tumors, or increasing survival of animals with implanted tumors). Results of some studies suggest that ascorbic acid may have a direct cell-killing effect on some types of tumor cells and that it may enhance the cell-killing effect of some drug treatments for cancer. The concentration of vitamin C required to damage tumor cells seems to be much lower than that which will damage normal cells. However, it is not clear if the concentrations necessary to cause these effects on cancer cells can be achieved by oral or even intravenous administration of vitamin C supplements. One study suggested that intravenous administration of vitamin C may be more effective than oral administration, but further clinical trials are needed to confirm this finding.

## Discovery and Observations of Effects

Ascorbic acid, long known for its role in the prevention of scurvy, is becoming increasingly recognized as an important biochemical factor in many physiologic and biochemical systems. It is used in the synthesis of collagen, the most abundant protein in the body; in the synthesis of hormones and neurotransmitters, including norepinephrine, epinephrine, and serotonin; and in hydrogen-ion transfer and regulation of the proper oxidation state of biologically important metal ions such as iron and copper. An antioxidant and free-radical scavenger, it is an effective detoxifier of various poisons and carcinogens and is thought to protect other important antioxidants such as vitamin E, vitamin A, butylated hydroxyanisole (BHA), and glutathione.

Ascorbic acid is a six-carbon molecule only a few biosynthetic steps removed from glucose (or galactose). It is synthesized by amphibians, reptiles, some birds, and most mammals. Among mammals, vitamin C does not appear to be synthesized by guinea pigs, fruit bats, and most primates, including humans.

In mammals, the vitamin is synthesized in the liver. Although microsomal enzymes appear to be responsible for most of the activity, some evidence suggests that mitochondria may be responsible for as much as 25% of the activity in rats. Because mitochondria are self-replicative, contain their own DNA (distinct from that in the nucleus), and are transmitted by maternal inheritance only, their participation in vitamin C biosynthesis deserves further exploration.

In animals that fail to synthesize the vitamin, the deficiency is in one or all of three of the important metabolic enzymes. It has been suggested that the deficiency is a result of a mutation involving a gene deletion. Several lines of evidence, however, suggest that this may not be the case. First, the same gene deletion would have had to occur several times, because the biosynthetic ability is lacking in several branches of the evolutionary tree, in some but not all bats, birds, and primates. Although multiple occurrences of the same mutation are not impossible, it is reasonable to examine alternative mechanisms.

An alternative to the gene-deletion hypothesis raises the possibility of individual variability in the degree to which various suppressor or competitor proteins may be expressed. Such variability in expression is well established for other genes. For example, carriers of the sickle cell gene vary considerably in the degree to which they are affected by oxygen deprivation. Reports find vitamin C-linked enzyme activity in the liver of some guinea pigs and indicate that in a large group of guinea pigs it is possible to find some that do not become vitamin C deficient.

In a group of guinea pigs bred in a region from which some guinea pigs are resistant to scurvy, 10 of 12 animals showed no ascorbic acid-producing enzymes in their liver. On an ascorbic acid-free diet, their serum levels fell to 0.05 mg/dl. An 11th animal also had no enzyme activity, but the serum level fell only to 0.05 mg/dl, presumably reflecting a marked difference in catabolism. The 12th animal had a normal level liver enzyme production and had serum levels of 0.99 mg/dl. These data demonstrate the presence and physiologically adequate level of biosynthetic activity in some individuals of this species. Thus, although it is usually stated that humans and guinea pigs completely lack the ability to synthesize ascorbic acid, there are data indicating the possibility of varying levels of synthesis.

Ascorbic acid is actively transported to numerous tissues. The highest levels are found in the adrenal and pituitary glands, where concentrations are 50–100 times the plasma levels in humans. Very high uptake and concentrations, 30–50 times the plasma levels, are also found in the central nervous system, spleen, testes, salivary glands, eye lens, bone marrow, and leukocytes; a distinct role of ascorbic acid in these tissue seems to be implied.

## Vitamin C and Human Cancer

Most human studies of diet and cancer have not examined the role of vitamin C. Many have used food lists designed to assess only macronutrients such as fats. Others have used lists that included some vegetables but that were not designed to assess vitamin C adequately. Such studies shed little or no light on the role of vitamin C and cancer. The studies reported later in the chapter have explicitly reported on a vitamin C index or on the apparent role of fruits or vegetables that are important sources of vitamin C.

### Lung

A 1-million-person prospective study initiated by the American Cancer Society was analyzed for the role of fruit consumption in subsequent lung cancer among White male cigarette smokers aged 40–75 years. In each of six age groups a protective effect was seen for frequent fruit consumption, with a consistent dose response. Over all age groups, the mortality rate was 1.75 times higher for those who ate fruit only zero to two times per week compared with those who ate it five to seven times per week.

Several studies have examined diet in relation to lung cancer but have not reported specifically on the role of vitamin C, in some cases clearly because the dietary interview was not intended to assess vitamin C. One found a reduced risk associated with high consumption of three leafy green vegetables, typically good sources of vitamin C as well as provitamin A and folate.

Because of limitations in assessment methods or analysis, the available data provide ambiguous evidence regarding an effect of vitamin C in the prevention of lung cancer. In summary, studies offer some suggestion of a protective effect. Additional studies are needed that are large enough to ensure adequate numbers of lung cancer outcomes and with dietary methods capable of assessing vitamin C as well as other nutrients such as carotenoids, folate, and vitamin E.

## Larynx

A report examining the role of diet in cancer of the larynx showed highly significant effects for both vitamin A and vitamin C. After control for the effects of cigarettes and alcohol, a low intake of vitamin C was associated with a relative risk of 2.5, with a clear dose/response relationship.

## Oral

Marshal et al. (1982) examined 427 White male oral cancer patients and 558 controls with nonneoplastic diseases of other sites. After control for smoking, alcohol, and age, vitamin C was associated with a significant risk trend, with an odds ratio of 1.7 for lowest to highest intake. A somewhat stronger association was observed for the vitamin A index. The authors note, however, that "the difference in the estimated effects of vitamin A and vitamin C could also be the result of differential measurement error: the scale measuring vitamin A in the diet may be more accurate than the vitamin C scale. If the effects of these substances were equal, with vitamin A measured more accurately than vitamin C, it would be estimated that the effect of vitamin A is stronger than that of vitamin C." The instrument used in the collection of these data during 1958–1965 certainly resulted in considerable misclassification with respect to vitamin C intake, with consequent reduction in power to detect an effect.

A highly significant protective effect was found for frequent (once a day or more) consumption of fresh fruit. Green leafy vegetables and other vegetables also had an effect in the protective direction. Analyses at the National Cancer Institute of a case-control study of dietary factors in oral cancer showed a strongly protective effect for both fruit and supplemental vitamin C intake.

## Esophagus

For esophageal cancer, the data are reasonably persuasive that vitamin C, or some factor in vitamin C-containing foods, plays a protective role in this disease.

## Stomach

Investigators have found a significant protective role for vitamin C in stomach cancer. In south Louisiana, a high-risk area for gastric cancer, dietary factors were categorized into quartiles based on the control distribution. Even after adjusting for several risk factors, a significant trend for vitamin C intake was observed. For carotenoids, a nonsignificant risk reduction to 0.68 was observed. The protective effect of carotenoids disappeared when vitamin C was controlled, but the strong protective effect from vitamin C persisted after controlling for carotenoid intake.

In Norway, the vitamin C index was the dietary variable that discriminated most strongly in stomach cancer cases. The same significantly protective result was obtained when analysis was restricted to those subjects for whom the food consumption estimates given by spouses for subjects' intake was concordant with the subjects' estimates themselves (a subset with presumably more accurate diet responses). In the latter subset the relative odds for a high intake (approximately upper quartile) of the vitamin A index was 0.87 and for a vitamin C index, 0.64 (more protective).

## Colon and Rectum

A protective effect of ascorbic acid in colorectal cancer could exist by its prevention of fecal nitrosamines or against other fecal mutagens. In addition, a mechanism has been proposed whereby vitamin C inhibits DNA synthesis and proliferation of preneoplastic cells. Administration of ascorbate has been shown to produce a 30%–40% increase in protective enzymes.

Studies of a cancer precursor lesion, rectal polyps among familial polyposis patients, support the possibility of a protective effect of vitamin C in polyp formation and thus possibly in colorectal cancer. With 400 mg of vitamins C and E administered to patients following polypectomy, after 2 years, the recurrence data rate was reduced approximately 20%.

Studies of the fecal mutagen fecapentaene provide evidence of a different mechanism for a protective effect of ascorbic acid. A study of diet and fecapentaene levels conducted at the National Cancer Institute found a strong negative association between fecapentaene levels and both usual dietary vitamin C intake and supplemental vitamin C. Strong negative associations with citrus fruit and with vitamin E were also observed. Consumption of citrus fruit and supplemented vitamin C were two of only four factors significantly correlated with fecal mutagen levels in both study groups. The other two factors were supplemental vitamin E, negatively correlated, and consumption of butter/margarine, positively correlated. Thus, if fecal mutagens play a role in colon cancer, there is evidence that ascorbic acid may function, either independently or synergistically with vitamin E, in preventing or detoxifying the carcinogen.

In Australia, for colon cancer, no consistent results were seen for vitamin C (nor for beta-carotene or vitamin A). A high fiber intake was associated with a significantly *elevated* risk in female colon cancer, which on close inspection was found to be associated solely with cereal fiber; vegetable fiber was not associated with excess risk.

For rectal cancer, however, vitamin C was associated with a reduced risk in both sexes, especially women. Neither carotene nor vitamin A was protective against rectal cancer; cereal fiber, but not vegetable fiber, was associated with a high and significant excess risk.

Several studies have examined the relations between diet and colon cancer by constructing fiber indices, but without estimating the vitamin C content of foods considered, reporting reduced risks with various vegetable foods. Two of four foods consumed significantly *more* by cancer cases (thus suggesting an *elevated* risk) were cereals. In patients with cancer of the stomach, colon, rectum, and other gastrointestinal (GI) sites, a significant trend was noted for carrots and pumpkin, rich sources of carotene but not of vitamin C. In contrast, oranges, tomatoes, and green peppers had the most highly significant trends, and these foods are rich sources of vitamin C but rather poor sources of beta–carotene. (Tomatoes, for example, contain primarily lycopene, not beta-carotene.) These results do suggest that vitamin C (or something else in vegetables and fruits) could be as important, or more important, than dietary fiber.

Thus, it appears possible that what some have interpreted to be a protective effect of fiber may be instead an effect of something else in fruits and vegetables. Although international correlation data are often interpreted as identifying dietary fiber with lower cancer rates, other legitimate candidates include vitamin C, carotenoids, folate, vitamin E, or other factors and their interactions. The evidence for a protective role for vitamin C is suggestive.

## Pancreas

In a study of pancreatic cancer, significant elevations in risk were found for frequent use of fatty foods, margarine, and fried or grilled meat, although the latter were based on very small numbers of exposed persons. A statistically significant protective effect was observed for frequent consumption of carrots and of citrus fruits. Citrus fruits are important sources of vitamin C and unimportant as sources of carotenoids. Inclusion of both foods in a statistical model did not apparently weaken the association of either one. Observations are consistent with the hypothesis of a protective role of vitamin C in pancreatic cancer.

## Cervix

Cervical cancer patients were evaluated using the same dietary questionnaire described above under the study of lung cancer. No relationship was found for vitamin C. However, ascorbic acid was examined in relation to a precancerous condition, cervical dysplasia, and found to support a protective effect. Examination of precursor conditions is useful because it makes less tenable the interpretation that the serum levels are a consequence of the disease. Statistical analysis, controlling for other confounding variables known to be important epidemiological factors in cervical cancer, such as early onset of sexual activity, multiple partners, and multiple pregnancy, established vitamin C as an independent risk factor in all degrees of cervical dysplasia and cancer. This relationship held in both lower and higher socioeconomic groups.

## Interactions With Other Micronutrients

The biological functions of vitamin C are significantly more diverse and more complex than the generally recognized one of preventing the formation of nitrosamines. It is required in the synthesis of an array of major biomolecules, including collagen, nore-pinephrine, and carnitine. In its role as a reducing agent and free-radical quencher, it can prevent the formation of carcinogens and reduce the toxic or carcinogenic effects of numerous chemical and radiologic agents. It plays an important role in many enzyme-mediated reactions that require metal ions to be in the reduced state for full activity. And it may enhance host immune resistance in a variety of ways.

For cancers of the esophagus, oral cavity, and uterine cervix the evidence appears quite strong. For cancers of the stomach and rectum, the evidence is mixed, but some studies suggest a strong protective effect. For cancer of the larynx, results indicated a significant protective effect. Bladder and pancreatic cancer studies also show suggestive results. For lung cancer the current evidence is weak for vitamin C. For prostate cancer there is scant evidence for a protective effect of vitamin C.

With few exceptions, it is highly unlikely that nutrients act singly and without regard to the level and action of other nutrients. For example, ascorbic acid provides electron and hydrogen atom transfer in the reconstitution of active forms of vitamin E, vitamin A, and glutathione. Moreover, numerous free-radical-generating, or oxidizing, reactions in the body may be preferentially scavenged by different agents; because many of these reactions are linked in cascades of interrelated processes, any single agent may be less effective alone than in combination with complementary agents.

## Dose and Requirements

Diets for nonhuman primates and guinea pigs, species that typically do not synthesize ascorbic acid, are formulated at concentrations providing 16–35 mg/kg body wt, equivalent to approximately 1,000–2,000 mg/day for a 60-kg man For humans, estimates of requirements depend on the criteria used to define adequacy. As little as 10 mg/day can alleviate the clinical symptoms of scurvy but allow no reserves. Approximately 60 mg/day will raise serum vitamin C in healthy adults to levels that are adequate to protect against clinical signs of scurvy in the adult male for at lease one month. Little is known regarding requirements in the adult female, but there is some evidence of physiological differences in retention or requirements between the two sexes.

Various physiologic and environmental factors increase the requirement for vitamin C. Smokers have lower blood levels than nonsmokers, and ascorbic acid metabolism in smokers is markedly increased. Smokers would need about twice as much vitamin C as nonsmokers to maintain comparable levels. Use of oral contraceptives is found by most but not all studies to lower plasma levels. Aspirin consumption lowers blood ascorbate levels by increasing its urinary excretion. More important, aspirin dramatically inhibits vitamin C absorption by leukocytes, lowering leukocyte levels to barely above scorbutic levels and raising the possibility of impaired leukocyte function. During pregnancy the placenta transmits ascorbic acid to the fetus against a concentration gradient, resulting in fetal levels 50% higher than maternal at term. This apparent fetal need is associated with lower maternal levels during pregnancy. The elderly are frequently found to have lower serum levels, which can be raised by supplementation. Persons subjected to stress such as heat, cold, surgery, or other trauma require higher intake to maintain normal serum levels than do healthy unstressed volunteers. For example, South African mine workers were found to require 200–250 mg/day to achieve serum levels that, in healthy young volunteers, are normally achieved by 60–75 mg/day.

The RDA set by the Food and Nutrition Board is 60 mg/day, a level that will protect against overt signs of scurvy in the adult male for a period of 30–45 days as observed in studies among healthy young adult male volunteers.

## Physiologic Levels and Effects

The level constituting a "normal" serum concentration varies with different reports: Serum levels below approximately 0.2 mg/dl are very poor and may be associated with clinical symptoms of scurvy. Levels that might be relevant to cancer risk are not established.

Active transport of vitamin C against a concentration gradient occurs in many tissues. Thus, it would appear that blood is primarily a transport vehicle, and it would be more relevant to examine actual tissue levels whenever possible. Leukocytes represent an accessible and relevant tissue, where concentrations are much higher than in serum. The technique is not simple, and values vary.

Ascorbic acid may be administered orally or by intravenous injection. Oral administration should be in divided doses. The more divided doses, the higher the proportion of a given daily amount that will be absorbed. Timed-release tablets would seem to be appealing; however, timed-release tablets have been observed to pass through the gut completely unabsorbed. Regardless of the administration, blood (and leukocyte) levels should confirm that administered doses are in fact being absorbed.

Ascorbic acid is remarkably nontoxic at levels many times the RDA. In studies on guinea pigs, the animals tolerate 500–1,000 times the therapeutic dose of ascorbic acid daily without ill effects. Studies in humans on prolonged high dosage have also found no toxic effects.

The most commonly suggested adverse effects of high doses of ascorbic acid are gastrointestinal disturbances, particularly loose bowels, but also flatulence and nausea and vomiting. In a clinical trial in advanced cancer patients receiving 10 g/day there were no significant differences in nausea and vomiting. In a subsequent study patients tolerated the 10 g/day very well. Two patients reduced the dose and one withdrew from the study because of unacceptable gastrointestinal symptoms.

It seems clear that some individuals do experience gastrointestinal symptoms at high doses, although it is equally clear that many do not. This may simply be the case because of biologic variability in metabolism; however, the above data also raise the possibility that cancer patients, or others with severe biological stress, may be more tolerant than are healthy volunteers of high doses. Indeed, it has been suggested that bowel tolerance may be a fairly reliable indicator of requirement for vitamin C.

Presence of high vitamin C may produce false negatives in gastrointestinal occult blood tests, and persons should stop taking vitamin C 48–72 hr before such a test. When added to blood samples at 2 to 40 times the concentration attainable in blood, there is interference with tests for liver function, bilirubin, uric acid, and glucose. At physiologic levels, however, interference is negligible.

One report suggests that ascorbic acid may shorten prothrombin time in individuals receiving warfarin anticoagulants. It would seem prudent to avoid high doses under such conditions.

Vitamin C substantially increases iron absorption. Thus, high levels of vitamin C could produce iron overload in individuals with inborn errors of iron metabolism or hemochromatosis or in persons for whom iron overload is a problem for other reasons, such as those who must receive regular blood transfusions.

## Formation of Calcium Oxalate Kidney Stones

Formation of calcium oxalate kidney stones has been hypothesized as a possible adverse effect of high doses of vitamin C, because one of the catabolic pathways results in the production of oxalic acid. Studies of urinary oxalate excretion after administration of vitamin C have been variable. One found increased urinary oxalate after 1–9 g/day but no evidence of a dose response; another found large elevations in 3 of 67 volunteers; and others found no statistically significant increase after 3–4 g/day for up to 6 months. However, it is unclear that oxalate excretion is a useful indicator for risk of kidney stones. When 50 normal subjects and 75 patients with kidney stones were tested, their urinary oxalate was virtually identical.

Actual evidence of stone formation associated with use of ascorbic acid is minimal. Only three case reports were found of individuals who presented with kidney stones and who also had consumed ascorbic acid. Of several clinical trials in which large doses of ascorbic acid (up to 10 g/day) were administered to cancer patients for periods of up to 2 years, there were no reports of kidney stones. Several researchers who have regularly prescribed large daily doses have reported no instances of kidney stones. Given the absence of reports of kidney stones in the several large-scale clinical studies that have administered vitamin C, this is very unlikely to be a notable problem.

A few case reports exist of persons who developed clinical symptoms when they suddenly discontinued high doses of ascorbic acid. Studies in guinea pigs both support and refute the induction of a deficiency state after suddenly discontinuing high doses. It is commonly recommended that users taper off rather than stop the dosage suddenly. A few case reports also exist regarding rebound scurvy in newborn infants whose mothers had taken high levels of vitamin C during their pregnancy. Prudence would suggest moderating dosage during pregnancy and alerting the pediatrician to the possible effect.

## Therapeutic Antitumor Effects

In the Vale of Leven studies, 10 g of ascorbic acid per day was administered to patients with advanced cancer. Three of 50 patients, described as terminal but not moribund, suffered rapid deterioration and death within days after initiation of ascorbic acid therapy. All had massive tumor burden, extensive metastatic disease, and aggressive, rapidly dividing tumors. The authors concluded that death was caused by tumor hemorrhage and the toxic effects of massive tumor necrosis. These observations suggest caution in the use of high-dose ascorbic acid in patients with massive aggressive metastatic cancer (see Chapter 11).

# Vitamin D and Calcium

Recently, vitamin D and its analogues have been shown to inhibit the proliferation of some neoplastic cells (Albert et al., 2004). Suppression of growth of these malignant cells point to involvement of vitamin D in cell proliferation and differentiation and suggest that analogues of the vitamin D hormone may be of interest as possible cancer preventive agents. The mechanism of action of vitamin D hormone remains largely unknown.

The function of vitamin D in cellular differentiation may relate to its action on intracellular calcium metabolism. Several studies provide indirect evidence of a possible involvement of calcium in cancer based on the effects of this mineral on the activity of carcinogens and on the ability of carcinogens and tumor proliferation to induce disturbances in calcium homeostasis. Whatever the mechanism, calcium seems to have an active role in cancer.

## Vitamin D

Basic research investigations of the anticancer properties of vitamin D have appeared in light of the suspected regulatory effects on calcium. Another facet of the function of vitamin D must be considered: its potential function alone as a steroid hormone. Receptors for vitamin D have been found in the small intestine, kidney, pituitary, parathyroid, and bone, all considered target organs. Through a series of metabolic steps in liver and kidney, vitamin $D_3$ is transformed into the active metabolite 1,25-dihydroxyvitamin $D_3$, which functions in calcium and phosphorus homeostasis. The suggested functions in cellular growth and differentiation distinguish the action of the active vitamin D metabolite.

Anticancer effects have been reported for vitamin D in leukemic cells and in cancer cells derived from sarcoma and melanoma. A high degree of receptivity for vitamin D was shown in human colon tumors. Vitamin D has a marked effect on cellular membrane composition and the fluidity of membranes. Vitamin D-deficient rats undergo changes in the fatty acid composition of cellular membranes, incorporating more saturated fatty acids. Whether vitamin D has pronounced effects on the colonic epithelium remains to be confirmed. Topical application of 1,25-dihydroxyvitamin $D_3$ inhibited proliferation in skin cells. Whether the parental form of the vitamin $D_3$ shows the same antiproliferative effects has yet to be resolved. Analysis of the diets and the intensity of sunlight (and thus vitamin D levels) at various latitudes in the United States showed increased vitamin D levels to be a protective factor for cancer.

The argument for supplementation of the diet with additional amounts of calcium or vitamin D has been largely derived for the suggested prevention of osteoporosis, an escalating disease in the United States. Evidence from clinical studies of the effects of calcium in the potential prevention of cancer suggest that the RDA for calcium should be increased from 800 mg/day to 1,500 mg/day. It is premature to recommend supplementation to the public until confirmation of the benefit of added calcium has been shown more convincingly. At least one study has indicated an anticancer effect for calcium. Further testing of calcium could include this element in trials featuring reduction of human cell proliferation or precancerous lesions. Human studies of the cancer prevention effects of vitamin D have yet to be proven, and nutritional supplementation may be considered as a prospect of the future.

## Calcium

Calcium figures prominently in many cell functions and is important in survival of the cell through the regulatory nature of this elemental mineral on cellular proliferation and synthesis of DNA. Imbalances in calcium concentration have been correlated to aberrant cellular behavior. From the perspective of calcium/cell interactions, there are a least two mechanisms by which calcium could prevent tumor promotion. The first concerns the active role of dietary lipids and their chemical affinity for calcium. The second concerns the physiological and molecular aspects of cellular proliferation.

The digestion of fat yields aggregates of fatty acids, glycerides, and cholesterol intermixed with bile acids that function to solubilize these compounds. In the upper jejunum glycerols interact with pancreatic lipases to yield free and bound fatty and bile acids. Bound lipids are largely in the form of calcium soaps that are reported to be biologically inert. Unbound fatty and bile acids have a high affinity for calcium. Addition of calcium to the diet does not change serum triglyceride levels, but incorporation of high levels of calcium in the diet significantly increases fecal excretion of saturated fatty acids. Thus, with entry of dietary fat into the colon a significant loss of calcium could occur.

Loss of calcium from colonic epithelial cells could have a number of effects contributing to initiation of the tumor process. In skin, the level of ionized calcium is suspected to regulate the balance of growth of skin cells and induce differentiation.

That calcium could offset abnormal cellular proliferation has been tested clinically. Investigations found that supplementation by 1,250 mg of calcium/day significantly reduced cell proliferation in patients at high risk for large bowel cancer. Epidemiological studies support the hypothesis that a higher calcium intake may reduce risk for colon cancer. One large study showed that people who took calcium supplements of 1200 mg/day showed a decreased risk of colorectal polyps (Baron et al., 1999).

Addition of calcium to the diet is not simple; calcium is bound by many dietary factors, including phosphate, fiber, phytate, and oxalates. Phytate, found in fibrous foods, stimulates colonic proliferation. Phytate binds with strong affinity to calcium and may lead to dietary insufficiency of this element in humans. The interplay between calcium and dietary lipids is complex. Understanding of the molecular processes of tumor promotion points to importance of calcium as a regulatory element. Also critical are agents that facilitate calcium transport, such as vitamin D. In terms of cancer prevention, there is speculation that vitamin D and its metabolites may be prominent in inhibiting tumor.

# Vitamin E (Alpha-Tocopherol)

Vitamin E (alpha-tocopherol) is a major free radical trap (antioxidant) in lipid cell membranes. Few studies have adequately evaluated the role of the lipid phase antioxidants in cancer. However, their potential role is supported by the hypothesis that cellular damage produced by oxidants contributes to the promotional of cancer and that antioxidants such as alpha-tocopherol can, at times, protect against this damage. Consumption of a diet devoid of vitamin E for extended periods has been shown to influence carcinogen activation. Also, alpha-tocopherol has been shown to inhibit the formation of carcinogenic nitrosamines. Administration of vitamin E and ascorbic acid to volunteers on Western diets causes dramatic reduction in fecal carcinogens. The anticarcinogenic effects of vitamin E have largely been observed with high and nonphysiological concentrations of this vitamin. Vitamin E may also potentiate the inhibitory effects of selenium on the promotion cancer.

The toxicity of vitamin E in adults is low. Clinical trials in humans have demonstrated that large doses (e.g., 200–800 mg/day) of vitamin E do not have serious side effects for most adults with the possible exception of individuals taking oral anticoagulants and those with other clotting disorders. These patients should ensure that they obtain medical advice before taking vitamin E supplements. Long-term use of high doses (greater than 300 IU daily of vitamin E) may cause transient nausea, diarrhea, and blurred vision. High-dose treatment of infants may be associated with more serious side effects.

## Discovery and Observations of Effects

In 1922, Evans and Bishop started a series of investigations on the influence of nutrition on reproduction in the laboratory rat that eventually led to the establishment of vitamin E as an essential micronutrient for animals and humans. Following the decades of exploration since these original studies, it is now well established that vitamin E deficiency can result in abnormalities of the vascular, nervous, and reproductive systems and tissues such as liver. In some species, vitamin E alone is not effective to correct the deficiency symptoms if the diet is also low in selenium. In adult humans, chronic ingestion of a low vitamin E diet leads to a decrease in red blood cell survival. Anemia has been observed in premature infants with low plasma vitamin E levels. Cystic fibrosis patients have low plasma vitamin E levels, decreased red blood cell survival times, and muscle, heart, and testicular degeneration.

## Deficiency

Frank vitamin E deficiency secondary to fat malabsorption has been well documented in humans and is correlated with specific neurological and neuromuscular symptoms. The condition can be corrected by vitamin E treatment if started promptly. Many studies have appeared in the literature about its relationship to human cancer. The potential role of vitamin E is not just related to deficiency states but, rather, an optimal nutritional intake that is likely to reduce the risk of cancer.

## Cancer Prevention

Positive results have been observed for vitamin E (alpha-tocopherol) inhibition of tumor formation in all classes of animal studies. There is experimental evidence to support the role of alpha-tocopherol inhibiting (1) the formation of carcinogens, (2) the initiation of carcinogenic-related events, and (3) the expression of tumors. The results, however, have not been consistent. Ranges of effectiveness, vary widely. One possible explanation is that alpha-tocopherol is simply not effective against certain specific chemical carcinogens. This might prove to be true as more environmental cancer-causing agents are identified and/or evaluated in animals. Alpha-tocopherol has been found to inhibit tumor formation to a lesser or greater degree in the same model.

Composition of the diet, particularly unsaturated fat, has been another factor that influences the effectiveness of alpha-tocopherol as an antitumor agent. It has been fairly well established that the intake of dietary fat, especially polyunsaturated fat, must be accompanied by an elevated level of antioxidant to prevent tissue damage. However, when the combination of stress factors (e.g., carcinogenic agent plus unsaturated fat) becomes too high, inhibitory effects of alpha-tocopherol are overridden. The relevance of this finding to the human experience relates directly to an understanding of how well animal experiments approximate human exposure to carcinogens and promoters as well as composition of the diet.

An equally important finding is data suggesting that alpha-tocopherol and selenium act together to inhibit tumor formation. This is not surprising in light of the known need for and complimentary roles these two micronutrients play as cellular antioxidants. The question arises: Are these the only micronutrients that can act in symphony to optimize the body's antioxidant defense system against cancer?

In summary, animal studies indicate that alpha-tocopherol does exhibit anticancer properties. Its role in cancer prevention is probably not a solitary one but likely related to its synergy with other key molecules that contribute to the body's antioxidant defense system.

## Epidemiological Studies

There is epidemiological evidence to support the role of vitamin E in preventing human cancer. Vitamin E is present in a wide variety of foods of both plant and animal origin, and although this makes it difficult to identify large population groups with vastly different intakes, recent findings are suggestive of relatively low vitamin E status being associated with increased risk for certain types of cancer.

Animal studies suggest that it can prevent some chemically induced cancers and it may reduce the size of tumors. One study, in humans, suggested a beneficial effect associated with the use of vitamin E in patients with superficial premalignant lesions in the mouth. In a laboratory study using breast cancer cells, vitamin E inhibited their growth. Results of animal studies examining the effect of vitamin E on mammary cancers have been contradictory. However, it has been reported that a supplement of 800 mg/day of alpha-tocopherol, taken during radiation therapy for breast cancer, reduced side effects and improved general well-being. In one study of patients with benign breast disease, vitamin E supplements were not beneficial.

An epidemiological study on the incidence of esophageal cancer in Calvados, France, showed alcohol and tobacco were the major risk factors. A systematic analysis of nutrients, corrected for alcohol and tobacco consumption, revealed a clear protective effect for nicotinic acid, vitamin C, and vitamin E, with sizably reduced risks in high consumers. The Melbourne Colorectal Cancer (CRC) Study, which is a case-control study and part of a large-scale investigation of CRC incidence, etiology, and survival, found that the use of vitamin supplements, which included vitamin E, was a protective factor.

Most studies in the literature have attempted to relate serum vitamin E levels to be the subsequent development of cancer. Some of the studies have found that low serum vitamin E correlates with an elevated risk of cancer.

## Breast

A prospective epidemiological study of breast cancer had been conducted with blood from 5,000 women in the Channel Islands, England, stored deep-frozen for up to 14 years. During this time, 39 subjects developed breast cancer. The original serum level of vitamin E and beta-carotene was compared with the serum levels in two matched controls (i.e., subjects who did not develop cancer). Consistently in all age groups, significantly lower serum concentrations of vitamin E were found in cancer cases than in controls. Those subjects who had the lowest serum levels (less than 3.3 mg/L) had an incidence of breast cancer five times higher than those with the higher serum levels of vitamin E (greater than 5 mg/L). The results thus show that a relatively high serum level of vitamin E is protective with respect to breast cancer. The long interval between the time when blood samples were collected and when breast cancer was diagnosed (an average of 5 years) makes it unlikely that cancer caused the decrease in serum vitamin E levels.

## Lung

In 99 cases of lung cancer from the Washington County, Maryland, cancer registry of approximately 26,000 participants, serum levels of beta-carotene and alpha-tocopherol were both significantly higher in the controls than in the cases. These data support the association between low levels of serum vitamin E and the risk for lung cancer. Small to moderate reductions in the risk for cancer attributable to the micronutrients seem plausible.

## Stomach

As part of an ongoing cohort study of stomach cancer in Colombia, blood levels of vitamin C, vitamin E, vitamin A, prealbumin, and carotenoids were measured and correlated with findings of stomach biopsies. The data show that circulating carotene levels in both sexes and vitamin E in males were significantly lower in subjects with precancerous stomach cells than in subjects with normal stomachs.

## All Cancer Sites

There was no association between serum vitamin E levels and subsequent development of lung, colon, rectum, stomach, or bladder cancer in men of Japanese ancestry living in Hawaii. The British United Provident Association study of adult male cancer involved about 22,000 men aged 35–64. An inverse relation between vitamin E status and cancer incidence was found. However, it was suggested that this association was a consequence of early cancer rather than low plasma vitamin E levels. In the prospective Basel study on cardiovascular and peripheral arterial disease, cancers of the lung, stomach, large bowel, and all other sites were treated separately. The absolute plasma level of vitamin E was significantly lower at baseline in subjects who later died from combined gastrointestinal cancers (stomach and colorectal). Serum vitamin E levels in subjects in the Hypertension Detection and Follow-up Program who later developed cancer were lower than those of controls matched for age, sex, race, and time of blood collection. Serum vitamin E levels were lower in subjects who later had cancer as compared with controls.

The observation that vitamin E is inversely related to lung cancer prompted an analysis of 10,532 subjects in the Netherlands. Risk analysis according to quintile showed a strong negative trend for vitamin E, suggesting an increased risk of all cancers associated with lower serum levels of vitamin E. The Eastern Finland Heart Survey data suggested that dietary selenium deficiency is associated with an increased risk of fatal cancer, that low vitamin E intake may enhance this effect, and that decreased vitamin A or provitamin A intake contributes to the risk of lung cancer among smoking men with a low selenium intake.

Data from several prospective studies support an association of lower plasma alpha-tocopherol levels with an increased risk of cancer, particularly lung, breast, and gastrointestinal. In a controlled clinical trial, vitamin E has recently been found to decrease the incidence and mortality of prostate cancer (Heinonen et al., 1998). Although the data are encouraging, they are not conclusive.

## Dose and Requirements

The "vitamin E" of commerce is a loose term that includes several different tocopherol molecules. All of these molecules have three active centers which appear to have some effect on the biological activity. The biological activity is based on animal bioassays, and, consequently, the activity of the various forms is given in units of activity and not milligrams.

## Formulations

Most commercially available forms of vitamin E are the esters, particularly the acetate. These esters are not naturally occurring but were developed as a means to stabilize the tocopherol molecule for use in foods and pharmaceuticals that prevent problems with processing and long-term stability. It is important to recognize that these esters of vitamin E are not active per se as antioxidants or free radical scavengers. This is a significant distinction because applications involving inhibition of lipid peroxidation, carcinogen formation, and so on, require the free tocopherol molecule. This is also true of studies seeking to evaluate the activity of alpha-tocopherol in the upper portion of the GI tract (e.g., stomach and duodenum) because little or no activation of these esters can be expected to occur in these regions.

All of these forms of the vitamin E molecule are either oils or, at best, low-melting solids. Their use in solid dosage forms requires that these physical properties be altered to yield forms that can withstand the rigors of a tablet press and not affect the desired physical properties of the tablet. Similarly, hard shell gelatin capsule formulations generally also require a solid material. Successfully marketed forms of vitamin E accomplish this goal by employing microencapsulation techniques using a number of substrates as a matrix (e.g., gelatin, starch, and gums). This approach not only addresses the physical requirements but also produces vitamin E forms with enhanced absorption. The latter is the result of emulsifying and subdividing the pure material into a range of particle sizes that aid the absorption process in the lower GI tract. The same approach has been used to develop oily forms of vitamin E for use in applications such as soft elastic gelatin capsules. The proper use of emulsifying agents and carefully selected triglycerides facilitate dispersion of these oily forms in the GI tract, providing optimum absorption.

As the relationship of vitamin E to cancer in humans becomes clearer, a more definitive picture should develop on target plasma levels. Dosage forms and regimens to achieve these targets should be met with currently available commercial forms of vitamin E and formulation technology.

## Dietary Sources

Vitamin E occurs widely in nature in foods of animal and plant origin as well as vegetable oils. Although estimates of dietary intake are theoretically possible to calculate from food tables, in practice, a poor correlation is often found because of the many influences (e.g., seasonal, age, and processing) on the actual content of many foods. A typical "well-balanced" U.S. diet is expected to provide about 15 IU of vitamin E daily, and the RDA for vitamin E has been based on this premise. In a normal adult American not taking any supplements, serum plasma levels of vitamin E are generally in the range of 0.8–1.0 mg/dl. This is adequate to prevent deficiency, and plasma levels below 0.5 mg/dl will lead to deficiency. The definition of adequacy with respect to preventing deficiency states does not necessarily apply to optimal plasma levels to reduce risk for cancer. Some preliminary data suggests that for lowering the risk for intestinal cancer, for instance, plasma vitamin E levels would have to be greater than 1.29 mg/dl. This requirement would translate to a daily intake of 60–100 IU.

Polyunsaturated fatty acids (PUFA) are macronutrients that have an impact on vitamin E status, and there is a direct relationship between the PUFA content of diet and vitamin E needs. Approximate requirements for vitamin E in terms of PUFA intake have been calculated and the source of dietary fat has an effect on vitamin E needs.

# B Vitamins and Choline

Because the B vitamins are essential components of any adequate diet and are necessary for the continued maintenance of cellular integrity and metabolic function, severe deficiencies generally reduce the growth rate of tumor cells and interfere with the normal functioning of the organism. A few studies are available to adequately evaluate the impact of B vitamin intake on the process of cancer (Matsubara et al., 2003). The effects of B vitamins on carcinogenesis cannot be easily ascribed to specific effects on initiation and promotion. Thus, the B vitamins in general may function by modulating cellular processes, including growth and immunosurveillance. However, at least two B vitamins appear to significantly modify cancer. A significant amount of data suggest that a deficiency of either vitamin $B_{12}$ or folic acid enhances the activity of various chemical carcinogens in various organs, suggesting a carcinogenic effect of inadequate intake of these vitamins. A deficiency of either may have similar results as choline deficiency. Failure of the immune system to defend the host may also account for the increased tumor development observed in cases of deficiencies of these vitamins. Wu and coworkers (1999) reported an association of low levels of vitamin $B_{12}$ with breast cancer in postmenopausal women and have suggested an association. Another recent study has shown a protective effect of dietary folate against the development of colon cancer (Giovannucci et al., 1998).

Choline deficiency produces various pathologic lesions in virtually every organ of the body. A vast body of literature describes the consequences of dietary choline deficiency on tissue growth and development. A deficiency of choline enhances the potency of several carcinogens. Cellular alterations, either individually or in combination, may play a critical role in the ability of this nutrient to modify cancer.

# Copper and Zinc

Copper is an essential nutrient implicated as a positive factor in cancer susceptibility. Although some studies concerning exposure to copper have suggested a direct relationship with cancer risk, little evidence is available relating dietary intakes to cancer development. Experimental studies in animals indicate that large dosages of copper protect against chemically induced tumors.

Zinc, an essential constituent of numerous enzymes, functions in cell replication and tissue repair. The data on effects of excess zinc on chemically induced tumors have been mixed, some showing increased and others decreased tumor development. Zinc deficiency is also known to modify the growth of cancer. Whether these effects on the growth of established tumors are a result of alterations in the immune system or on cell proliferation is not completely resolved.

# Selenium

The inhibitory effect of selenium on experimentally induced tumors is well documented. Dietary supplementation has been shown to be effective in inhibiting the formation of chemically induced tumors in the gastrointestinal tract, liver, breast, skin, and pancreas. Generally, selenium (as sodium selenite) is effective in inhibiting chemically and virally induced tumors. Selenomethionine or other organic selenium compounds present in foods have not been as extensively examined but appear to be less effective than selenite supplementation. The ability of this trace element to exhibit such dramatic effects across such a variety of experimental conditions suggests a generalized mechanism rather than a tissue or cell specific reaction. The protection offered by selenium is generally observed at concentrations greater than those known to meet the requirements for normal growth and metabolic activity. As observed with vitamin A, continuous intake of selenium is necessary for maximum inhibition of cancer.

## Mechanisms of Action

The mechanism of selenium inhibition of cancer appears complex and is poorly understood. Studies have shown that selenium inhibits the initiation phase. At least part of the protection appears to relate to the inhibition of an enzyme(s) responsible for the formation of carcinogens. Other studies have clearly shown effects of this trace element when given after carcinogen exposure. Such results suggest that selenium owes at least part of its effects to a decrease in the proliferation of cancer cells. The active form of selenium within these cells leading to cancer inhibition is unknown.

## Discovery and Observations of Effects

Questions were first raised concerning the possibility of a relationship between selenium (Se) and carcinogenesis in the 1940's with apparently discrepant reports. One report suggested that relatively high dietary levels of Se (i.e., several parts per million) could produce benign liver cell tumors or low-grade cancer in rats that first developed liver cirrhosis. A later report, however, indicated that high levels of Se protected against carcinogen-induced liver tumors in rats. Thus, for a decade before the discoveries that low levels of Se are important in the nutrition of experimental animals, it was unclear whether the element could be carcinogenic or anticarcinogenic.

In the latter part of the 1950s, independent studies showed that Se prevents tissue degeneration in the vitamin E-deficient rat and in the vitamin E-deficient chick, thus demonstrating for this element a nutritional role related to that of vitamin E. It was not until 1970 that Se was found to have a nutritional activity beyond that of vitamin E, that is, that it prevents the degeneration of pancreas in the vitamin E-fed chick; this discovery established Se as an essential nutrient. By the 1970s, Se was recognized as having nutritional activity, much but not all of which related to vitamin E in a variety of species. This recognition and consideration of the use of Se compounds as nutritional supplements to formulated animal feed again put focus on the possibility of a relationship of Se and cancer.

At about the same time, in the late 1960s it was reported that cancer mortality rates in the United States were inversely associated with the geographic distribution of Se, as indicated by the Se contents of forage crops. When it was shown that the levels of Se in selected urban blood bank samples demonstrated geographic variations similar to those of forage crop Se, calculations determined the cancer mortality rate to be correlated negatively with blood Se level in the same communities. Thus, in addition to its known nutritional role, Se was seen to function in some way to reduce cancer risk. A biochemical basis for the nutritional action of Se, is provided in that it is an essential constituent of the hydroperoxide-metabolizing enzyme glutathione peroxidase.

While a substantial body of research has yielded insight into the function of Se both in normal health and in cancer, much remains to be elucidated concerning the role of nutritional Se status and cancer risk.

## Selenium and Human Cancer

The Se status of a population tends to be determined in large part by the geochemical environment of the primary areas of food production, which, in many countries, remains local to the population. That is, human populations tend to show indices of Se status (e.g., blood or hair Se contents) that correspond to the Se contents of locally produced plant crops. Therefore, the results of geographical studies of the relations of Se status and cancer incidence in human populations have been of interest. Several such studies have been conducted; each has indicated an inverse association of Se status and cancer mortality. In over 27 developed countries, the overall cancer mortality rate as well as age-corrected mortality rates because of leukemia and cancers of the colon, rectum, breast, ovary, and lung correlated inversely with estimates of the average per capita intakes of Se in those countries. Age-adjusted mortality rates within the United States for cancers of the breast, colon, rectum, and lung were inversely related to whole blood Se concentrations as estimated on the basis of average values obtained from blood bank samples. Similar results were reported from mainland China; in a study conducted in 24 locations in a total of eight provinces in that country, there was a significantly negative correlation between age-adjusted total cancer mortality rate and whole blood Se concentration. Further, in a county with a particularly high incidence of hepatoma (Qidong County, Jiangsu Province), the geographic distribution of liver cancer incidence was inversely related to either blood Se level or to the Se contents of locally available food grains.

A number of studies have been conducted to examine the hypothesis that Se status is related to cancer risk in human populations. Most of these have been cross-sectional in nature; their value is in challenging the plausibility of the hypothesis and not in testing the hypothesis itself. The results of theses studies would appear to support the hypothesis that low Se status can increase cancer risk; they indicate that cancer patients are generally of lower Se status, as indicated by tissue Se levels, than healthy controls. However, the careful evaluation of these types of results necessitates determining whether the controls were actually drawn from the same population as the cancer cases and whether the indices of Se status may have been affected by the cancer. For example, because many cancer patients, particularly those with late-stage and debilitating conditions, are likely to have patterns of food intake that are different from those of healthy people, case-control studies that assess the Se status of prevalent cases may easily yield associations that do not discriminate between effects resulting from cancer and those causing it. The difficulty in making this distinction for the majority of these published studies limits their usefulness in determining whether Se status can affect cancer risk. Studies that have measured selenium levels and then followed people over time for the development of cancer have shown mixed results (Knekt et al., 1991; Koo, 1997). Three studies observed the effects on supplementation with selenium on the subsequent development of cancer (Blot et al., 1993; Clark et al., 1996; Yu et al., 1990). Although these reports are encouraging, questions remain about dose, who it may protect from cancer (smokers vs. nonsmokers or people with low levels of selenium vs. those with normal levels), and the length of time needed to attain the protective effect (Cirigliano & Szapary, 1999).

## Interactions With Other Micronutrients

A variety of studies show the interactive nature of selenium with other dietary constituents. Two of the most promising candidates for cancer prevention, vitamin A and selenium, have been shown to act additively in the inhibition of breast cancer. Likewise, vitamin E apparently provides a more favorable environment against oxidative stress, thereby potentiating the action of selenium. Other nutrients may have the opposite influence on the beneficial action of selenium. Vitamin C appears to be one such nutrient, because it has been reported to nullify the preventive action of selenite.

## Therapeutic Antitumor Effects

Despite early claims of the value of Se in cancer chemotherapy most animal tumor model studies have evaluated Se as a cancer-preventative agent. Those that have tested the chemotherapeutic efficacy of Se have yielded mixed results. Several studies with transplanted tumors have shown high levels of Se to retard tumor growth, whereas others have failed to demonstrate significant effects of Se. Therefore, although the potential for Se to be useful in cancer chemotherapy would appear clear, many questions remain concerning the types of tumors that may be affected, the compounds of Se that may be effective, and the dose regimens that may be appropriate.

The case for considering Se compounds as possible cancer-preventative agents is strong by virtue of the results of quite a number of studies both with animal tumor models and of basic metabolism. These issues involves questions of Se toxicity that cannot be resolved readily on the basis of present information concerning the toxicity of Se for humans. It will be necessary to have intervention trials of food forms of Se (e.g., selenoaminoacids, high-Se wheat, Se-enriched yeasts) roughly comparable to those within the normal dietary experience of human populations and at levels similar to the Se intakes of healthy populations residing in regions of the world naturally high in the element (e.g., parts of Venezuela, Colombia, and the People's Republic of China).

Determining whether selenium has a role in human carcinogenesis necessitates more extensive studies of the metabolism and toxicology of various chemical forms of the element selenium.

---

### Experiments of Humans and Nature:

Selenium in the Peoples Republic of China

Whereas some areas of China are high in selenium, in the heartland of China lies an inland region drained by the Yangtze River where the soil is very low in selenium—so low that clinical selenium deficiency has a name: "ke-shan" disease. Over the past century new land has been deposited in the Yangtze River Delta from soils washed down from the upland region. This new soil is likewise low in selenium, in marked contrast to the surrounding regions of Jiangsu Province where _terra firma_ has normal or high selenium levels.

The new lands in the Yangtze Delta such as Chong Ming Island (the "isle of wisdom") were forcibly resettled with "intellectuals" from nearby Shanghai during the Cultural Revolution of the 1960s. Although their rates of cancer risk factors, such as hepatitis, are comparable to those found on the mainland, their rates of liver cancer are much higher. In the 1980s my mentor, Nobel laureate Barry Blumberg, developed a hypothesis that lack of selenium was responsible for higher rates of liver cancer, and that providing normal selenium intake would reduce the occurrence of cancer. The National Cancer Institute supported our study led my late colleague, Larry Clark, to conduct dietary selenium supplementation in an attempt to reduce liver cancer rates in Jiangsu Province, where an experiment of nature placed two areas of such different selenium levels in close proximity and where an experiment of humans (Mao's Cultural Revolution) had placed a new population.

The negotiations with the Chinese government and pilot studies in Jiangsu in 1987 were successful. However, the events at Tiananmen Square in June 1989 precluded the study from being completed as U.S. participation was withdrawn from China as a result. This occurrence provided a dramatic example of the influence of politics at many levels in cancer research.

# Dietary Fiber

Dietary fiber is an important component of daily diet. It influences metabolic functions and physiologic process in a variety of human diseases.

## Discovery and Observations of Effects

Most research in dietary fiber, including its chemistry, analysis, metabolic functions, and health effects, has been made since the early 1990s. However, the idea of physiological benefits from dietary fiber is not new. Hippocrates spoke of the benefits of wheat with bran over refined flour, and medical scientists in the 19th and 20th centuries noted the laxative properties of fiber. Current interest in the role of dietary fiber in the etiology of diseases common in Westernized countries are because of the observation of Burkitt that diseases such as colon cancer, diverticular disease, gallstones, and ischemic heart disease are rare in most African populations. He had hypothesized a link between a diet high in fiber and low risk for these diseases (Chapter 8).

## Definitions of Dietary Fiber

Prior to the 1970s the term *fiber* or *roughage* was used to describe the components of food not digested by humans. However, little research was done to assess the constitution of these substances, because fiber was considered to have limited physiological effects. Scientists understood that fiber is not one substance, but a heterogeneous mixture of complex polysaccharides and nonpolysaccharide polymers. Trowell offered a definition of the term *dietary fiber*, calling it the components of the plant cell wall that resist digestion by secretions of the human alimentary tract.

This biological definition grouped together a number of substances, including proteins, lipids, and inorganic substances, that are resistant to digestion but that are not usually considered to be dietary fiber components. A Canadian government report proposed the following definition: "the endogenous components of plant material in the diet which are resistant to digestion by enzymes produced by man. They are predominantly nonstarch polysaccharides and lignin and may include associated substances." This definition attempted to be broad enough to encompass the biological definition and at the same time specific enough to be meaningful to international and health communities. This definition was subsequently used by Federation of American Societies for Experimental Biology Report on Dietary Fiber and Health. Although this definition is widely shared by the scientific community, there is still controversy. The problem with defining dietary fiber stems from its heterogeneous nature from both a physiologic and analytic perspective.

## Types of Fiber

Most dietary fibers are polysaccharides and can be classified as pectin, hemicellulose, or cellulose. The other major fiber class is lignin, which is a nonpolysaccharide. The structural fibers in cellulose, lignin, and some hemicelluloses tend to be nonfermentable by colonic bacteria and less soluble in water, whereas the natural gel-forming fibers, including pectins, gums, mucilages, and the remaining hemicelluloses, are more fermentable and water soluble.

Cellulose, a simple linear polymer of glucose, is one of the most abundant molecules in nature and is the principal plant cell wall structural material. The term *hemicelluloses* was originally applied to polysaccharides that were structurally related and associated with cellulose. The structure of hemicelluloses is quite diverse, with over 250 different known hemicelluloses. These plant polysaccharides consist mostly of branched polymers of pentose and hexose sugars such as mannose, glucose, galactose, xylose, and arabinose. Pectins are a mixture of colloidal polysaccharides present in the cell wall matrix that bind adjacent cell walls. Other polysaccharides include gums, which are found as exudates at the sites of injury to plants and consist primarily of galactose, glucose, and galacturonic acid; mucilages, which are a mixed group of complex polysaccharides that are not generally part of the cell wall; and algal polysaccharides, which are derived from algae and seaweed and are used as food ingredients. Lignin can be described as three-dimensional networks of phenylpropane units. The precursors of these consist of aromatic alcohols, cinnamyl, coniferyl, *p*-coumaryl, and sinapyl alcohols, which are formed into lignin by a complex polymerization process.

## Foods and Fiber

Foods differ in both the amount and types of dietary fiber they contain. Cereals, except for oats and barley, contain only insoluble fibers and are especially rich in hemicelluloses. Vegetables and fruits tend to be higher in cellulose than most cereals and contain a range of soluble to insoluble fibers. Legumes are a rich source of both total dietary fiber and the highly water-soluble gums. Seaweeds and oats are also rich sources of gums. Pectins are found mostly in fruits, especially apples and citrus fruits. Lignin is highest in fruits with edible seeds or in mature vegetables such as carrots and other root vegetables.

Until recently, food composition tables presented data for crude fiber. The method for measuring crude fiber was developed as early as 1800 to analyze animal feed. Crude fiber data is of no practical value because it underestimates dietary fiber content. The next generation of fiber analysis methods utilized detergents to remove the nonfiber components from animal feeds. This procedure could be used only for foods containing insoluble fibers, such as wheat products.

## Measurement of Fiber

Measurement of fiber has always been approached by quantifying the residue left after all other macronutrients such as starches, proteins, and fats are removed from the food.

One difficulty is the complete removal of starch. During food processing, some starch becomes resistant to both enzymatic and chemical removal. This occurs in a variety of foods, including corn flakes and potato chips. Whether this resistant starch behaves like dietary fiber in the intestine and therefore should be included in the fiber measurement is controversial.

Another recent problem is the classification of dietary fiber as either soluble or insoluble, with different procedures yielding quite different results. For most foods, there is no clear distinction between soluble and insoluble dietary fiber fractions, and the ratio of these components is strictly dependent on the pretreatment or the analytical method itself. Grouping dietary fiber according to solubility must be considered a rather arbitrary classification, and data on soluble and insoluble fiber should be used cautiously.

## Dietary Consumption

Data on dietary fiber intake in the U.S. population is limited as there remain limitations regarding data on the dietary fiber content of foods. Crude fiber values provide a poor estimate of dietary fiber intake. Data suggest a 30% decrease in crude fiber consumption in the United States from 1901 to 1975. The largest decrease has been in cereal fiber, followed by legumes and potatoes. For other vegetables there has been relatively little change. There has also been a considerable decrease in crude fiber consumption from fruits. The only increase is seen for nut consumption, also a high source of fiber. Although crude fiber is only a rough estimate, fiber relative to changes across food groups is instructive.

The first estimate of dietary fiber intake in the U.S. population from a cross-sectional national survey found a mean intake of 11.1 g/day of dietary fiber. This estimate was derived by examining 24-hr recall data from 11,658 adult respondents in the second National Health and Nutrition Examination Survey (NHANES II, 1976–1980).

Other studies have confirmed low levels of dietary fiber intake in the United States.

The major source of dietary fiber in the United States and in many Western countries is from vegetables. This is important to remember when interpreting epidemiological association between dietary fiber and cancer. Vegetables (including potatoes and salads) represent 28% of dietary fiber intake. If one adds to this the 14% from beans and legumes, a total of 42% of dietary fiber comes from vegetables. This compares to 17% from fruits and only 24% from cereals and grains (19% bread and 5% breakfast cereals). Thus, 59% of dietary fiber comes from fruits and vegetables, and only 24% from cereals. Legumes, despite their relatively infrequent consumption (approximately 10% of the population on any day), are the fourth most important contributor of dietary fiber by virtue of their high fiber content.

## Fiber and Cancer

### Colon

Dietary fiber offers numerous plausible mechanisms by which it could prevent the development of cancer, especially colon cancer. Probably the most widely accepted hypothesis for the development of colon cancer is that fecal bile acids cause small adenomas (with a low malignant potential) to grow to a large size (with a correspondingly high malignant potential) and to become precancerous. Colonic bile acid concentration is thought to increase with a high fat diet. Colonic bacteria may convert these bile acids to secondary bile acids. These secondary bile acids have been shown in laboratory models to promote tumors. In addition, the amount of fat in the diet directly affects the amount of free fatty acids in the bowel, and these free fatty acids have been shown to damage bowel. Fiber is postulated to reduce the adverse affects of fat and bile acids. However, the results of the Polyp Prevention Trial did not show that a diet high in fiber, fruit, and vegetables and low in fat prevented recurrence of colorectal polyps (Schatzkin et al., 2000). A recent controlled clinical trial failed to show that fiber supplementation protected against colorectal tumors (Alberts et al., 2000). As discussed in Chapter 8, fiber may have variable effects on the development of cancer.

## Breast

Recent evidence suggests that certain types of fibers may modify the biological action of hormones and thus may reduce the risk of hormone-related cancers, especially breast cancer. The lower plasma prolactin and estrogen levels and higher fecal estrogen levels found in women consuming high-fiber diets are generally associated with a lower breast cancer risk. These hormone changes could occur through fiber-mediated changes in the intestinal bacteria. An additional mechanism by which dietary fiber may exert it influences is the direct binding of the unconjugated estrogens to fibers.

## Ovary

Several case-control studies have examined the effect of fiber or fruit and vegetable intake on epithelial ovarian cancer risk. Byers and colleagues observed an increase in risk for women aged 30–49 with low vitamin A intake from fruits and vegetables. La Vecchia and colleagues also observed significantly lower risk with high intake of green vegetables and whole grain bread or pasta. No association was observed for fruit, and an association with beta-carotene disappeared after adjustment. It should be noted that none of these studies adjusted for energy intake. However, energy intake, fat, and protein were not associated with risk in one study, fat and protein intake were unrelated to risk in another study, and all studies adjusted for body mass index.

## Endometrium

An inverse association between endometrial cancer risk and high intake of both beta-carotene and whole grain bread or pasta has been reported. However, there were limitations to the study. Energy intake was not determined, and only a limited number of dietary items were included in the questionnaire. Adjustment was not carried out for more than one dietary factor simultaneously. An association with fat was limited to consumption of butter, margarine, and oil; no association with other fat sources was observed.

## Prostate

A metabolic epidemiology study among Seventh-Day Adventist men revealed significant associations between fiber intake and fecal concentration of sex hormones. Three groups of men were compared: nonvegetarians (NV), lacto-ovo-vegetarians (LOV), and vegans (V). Fecal concentration of estrone and estrone plus estradiol were significantly higher among V compared to LOV and NV. Furthermore, fecal estradiol and testosterone were each higher in V by more than 20%, but the difference was not statistically significant. Among plasma hormones, only prolactin was significantly lower among V than either LOV or NV, and serum prolactin was positively correlated with saturated fat intake. Regression analyses revealed significant correlations between both dietary and crude fiber intake and fecal estrone, estradiol, and testosterone levels among all three groups combined. Fecal weight and fecal concentration of fiber components were all significantly higher among V than LOV or NV, and in vitro assays determined that the percentage of bound steroid hormones increased with the dietary concentration of lignin. However, it is unclear from the reports whether adjustment was made for body mass index, which was significantly lower in both V and LOV compared to NY, or energy intake, which was significantly higher in V compared to either group.

One other epidemiological study has assessed prostate cancer risk associated with dietary fiber; no effect was observed. A number of case-control studies have examined associations with intake of vegetables, vitamin A, or beta-carotene. Results have been inconsistent, with several finding excess risk, whereas others have found protective effects, and one cohort study has observed both protective and adverse effects according to age. None of these studies had adequate adjustment for energy intake, and several of the observed effects were age dependent. Thus although an effect of fiber or high fruit and vegetable intake on prostate cancer risk is biologically plausible through an influence on circulating hormone levels, available epidemiological data are inadequate to determine whether risk modification actually occurs.

### Other Sites

Although high intake of "starchy" foods has been associated with increased stomach cancer risk, these foods include pastry and other digestible carbohydrates in addition to the nondigestible carbohydrates. Pancreatic cancer risk has been shown to be inversely correlated with fruit and vegetable intake. Simultaneous inclusion of total fiber, fruit, and vegetable intake in a statistical model resulted in a significant protective effect only for fiber, suggesting that fiber was not just an indicator of fruit and vegetable intake. These data suggest that pancreatic cancer risk may also be modified by a diet higher in fruits, vegetables, and grains.

## Mechanisms of Action

The mechanism(s) by which fiber might be protective for cancers of the esophagus, oral cavity and pharynx, stomach, and rectum is not known. Since the early 1980s research has demonstrated that fiber is not merely an inert component of the diet, but one that elicits a variety of physiologic effects. In some studies it is not known whether protection is because of fiber or other components present in the fiber-rich foods such as carotenoids, vitamin C, micronutrients, or other plant substances such as indoles, flavonoids, lignans, and phytates. In addition, because high-fat diets are also usually low in fiber, an indirect role for dietary fiber can be accordingly constructed for all cancers positively associated with high-fat diets.

Diets high in fiber or fruits and vegetables have been associated with reduced risk for a number of cancers. These associations have been less well studied than those for colorectal cancer or breast cancer. Furthermore, the etiology of most of these other cancer sites is, for the most part, unknown. Nevertheless, the effects of fiber on circulating sex hormone levels suggest that risk for cancers with a probable endocrine component may be modifiable by a diet high in vegetables, grains, or fruit. Etiological mechanisms for a fiber effect on nonendocrine cancers are less readily apparent.

A very large body of evidence from diverse populations suggests that diets high in vegetables, grains, and fruits may modify risk from several cancers. The strongest evidence to date is for a protective effect on colorectal cancer, although the data for breast cancer is also consistent. Evidence for other sites is based on limited investigation. The current data do not allow discrimination between effects of dietary fiber and the nonfiber components of fiber-rich diets. Determination of the specific nutrients or dietary components conferring protection may not be possible with retrospective data.

## Dose and Requirements

The dietary fiber recommendations of a number of organizations in North America since 1977 have been for generally good health, disease prevention, and cancer prevention. A step forward was taken by the Canadian Government Expert Advisory Committee on Dietary Fiber when they quantitated the fiber recommendation (double the current intake of dietary fiber). The NCI recommendation has been to consume 20–35 g dietary fiber/day from a variety of food sources, including fruits, vegetables, and cereal products. This level of intake is roughly twice our current dietary fiber intake level of 10–15 g/day. Because the evidence for a protective effect of fiber is generally from an association of dietary patterns in which fiber occurs as a complex mixture with other foods, the extrapolation to the possible beneficial effects from fiber supplements cannot be made at this time. Totally independent effects of individual dietary components, especially for macronutrients such as dietary fiber, are difficult to establish. Recommendations for increasing dietary fiber for cancer prevention should be made in the context of the total diet.

Despite the uncertainties associated with the observations about dietary fiber, the possible public health implications of this research are significant. Increasing intake of grains, fruits, and vegetables, whereas concomitantly decreasing fat intake, has the potential to reduce risk from two of the major causes of cancer (colon and breast) mortality and possibly from a number of other cancers as well. Risk for cancers of the head and neck also appears to reduce by dietary fruit and vegetable intake. Furthermore, such a diet has cardiovascular benefits and no apparent adverse effects. Thus, even in the absence of detailed knowledge of the specific causative mechanisms, it is likely that meaningful risk reduction can be achieved by dietary modification.

# Other Dietary Constituents

Considerable evidence indicates that oxidation, or the liberation or generation of activated oxygen species (e.g., hydrogen peroxide, superoxide anions, are hydroxyl radicals) with the cell is highly damaging and may directly or indirectly contribute to cancer. Food additives, such as synthetic antioxidants, including BHA and BHT, as well as dietary constituents such as certain carotenoids, ascorbic acid, or alpha-tocopherol, may reduce cancer. Although the evidence for the role of antioxidants in the prevention of cancer show inconsistencies, there is a strong rationale for their potential protective effect. Various studies have suggested that antioxidants such as BHT and BHA possibly inhibit cancer by alteration in metabolic activation and not by their antioxidant properties. Some carotenoids could likewise owe any anticarcinogenic effects to properties other than their properties as antioxidants. The role of beta-carotene specifically in cancer prevention, as above, has been seriously questioned.

Nutrient intake is not the sole determinant of the observed patterns of human cancer. Adjustment of dietary practices to conform to recommended dietary goals may not be possible for all segments of the population. Sophisticated techniques and procedures are needed to adequately assess clinically the potential merit of nutritional intervention in each individual in relationship to cancer prevention. However, it is clear that a variety of essential nutrients may modify the cancer process at specific sites.

# Whole Foods

The purpose of this section is to (1) present the whole foods widely found to be protective against various cancers in human epidemiological studies, (2) present findings on the effects of food preparation on these foods as actually consumed by humans, and (3) evaluate the possibilities of various chemical constituents of foods being responsible for observed reduction in human cancer rates.

As presented in the previous sections, investigations focusing on individual nutrients as potential cancer-preventive agents have been stimulated by laboratory findings on the possible cancer-modifying activity of these natural substances. However, *people eat foods, not nutrients*. Although scientific investigation isolates individual nutrients, the experience of people consuming diets points consistently to the importance of the consumption of certain foods in reducing risks of cancer.

For a considerable period of time, studies on diet and cancer investigated relations between the consumption of certain foods or classes of foods (e.g., green vegetables) with the risk of various cancers in humans. Analyzing foods found to be protective against cancer rather than presumed dietary intake of a specific component is important. People consume (and epidemiological studies inquire about) foods, culturally processed in various ways, as opposed to nutrients. The cultural processing of foods includes agriculture (domestication, cultivation, harvesting, and storage), cuisine (preparation, seasoning, cooking, and eating), and various intermediate processes. These cultural processes may introduce variability into nutrient composition and nutrient bioavailability of foods, in addition to the variability introduced by environmental factors (e.g., climate, soil, rainfall, and seasonality).

## Foods Protective Against Cancer

Early studies of diet and cancer took a broad approach to dietary assessment. During 1929–1932, the British Empire Cancer Campaign conducted a case-control study of diet and all-sites cancer on nearly 500 cancer patients in Wales and found beetroot, bread (whole meal), cabbage, carrots, cauliflower, milk (unboiled), onions, turnips, and watercress to be protective against cancer. No associations were found for 25 other food items. This suggested that milk and green vegetables might contain a cancer-protective factor. These observations provide a useful framework for considering subsequent studies on foods and cancer:

Little work has been done to investigate the possible influences of dietary habits on the incidence of cancer. Such studies are difficult because it is to be expected that carcinogenic action of a particular kind of food would become manifest only after a long period of years, and histories have to be retrospective and must be compared with those of control groups of people without cancer. In such enquires, error can arise from poor memory and careless answers, changes in habits that may be connected with onset of a precancerous condition, different ways the interviewer may phrase the question, and different ways the patient and informant may interpret the question.

### Green and Yellow Vegetables

Stocks (1957) repeated the British Empire Cancer Campaign study 15 years later in over 1,750 cancer cases, ages 45–74, in North Wales and Liverpool. There were inverse associations between daily consumption of green vegetables and lung, gastric, intestinal, and other cancers. Eating green vegetables less often than once a day had a significant risk for gastrointestinal cancer. However, these associations were found only in areas where average green vegetable intake was highest.

In 1961, it was suggested that increased dietary intake of green and yellow vegetables was protective against cancer of the esophagus. Subsequently, a heterogeneous dietary intake index, including a spectrum of red, orange, yellow, and green vegetables was used in studies of gastric cancer. Among these vegetables, consumption of raw carrots, coleslaw, red cabbage, lettuce, and tomatoes were found to be protective against cancer.

While fruits and vegetables were found protective against oral and pharyngeal cancer fresh fruits and green leafy vegetables were also examined individually and found to have protective effects. In a case-control study of prostate cancer using both hospital-based and community-based controls a series of green and yellow vegetables were found protective. Carrots and beans were also protective against cancer.

# Epidemiological Studies

## Chinese Populations

MacLennan et al. (1977) investigated dietary risk factors for lung cancer in Singapore Chinese women. This Chinese population comes primarily from southeast China and is composed of a variety of cultural groups speaking different Chinese dialects, including Cantonese, Hokkein, and Teachew. Traditional dietary practices in these groups were derived. Dietary questionnaires asked frequency of consumption of common dark green leafy vegetables. Low consumption of vegetable constituents of the diet was associated with increased lung cancer risk in women. A dietary intake index was constructed using combinations of six common leafy vegetables, eggplant, and beans. Of these eight, an

---

## Yunan China Tin Mines and Lung Cancer

In Yunan Province in southeastern China, the area is rich in tin as is true of neighboring Indo–China and the Malay Peninsula. Foreign interests in this mineral asset have prompted interest from the British in Malaya to the French and United States in Vietnam. Traditional mines in Yunan Province extracted tin for many years without benefit of occupational protection. Tin is naturally contaminated with arsenic, a carcinogenic poison. Early studies in Central Europe first pointed out the association between tin mining and lung cancer. Further, tobacco was historically introduced by Moslem influences into the region and Yunan tin miners have also taken up the use of the water pipe for smoking.

After the Communist Revolution in 1949, the Chinese Labor Protection Institute eventually cleaned up the mines, providing miners with respiratory protection, paying better wages, and discouraging the traditional use of tobacco in water pipes. However, instead of decreasing, lung cancer rates were found to increase. This result turned out to be a "wealth effect," whereby newly prosperous miners, deprived of cultural traditions, had extra income to spend on manufactured cigarettes (a state monopoly in the Peoples Republic of China).

Thus, the wealth effect placed prosperity as a root cause of increasing cancer. Industrialization, urbanization, and economic prosperity may lead to higher rates of certain cancers. States such as New Jersey witnessed increases in cancer in the post WWII period for similar reasons.

---

index giving equal weight to four items, mustard greens (*chaisim*), kale (*tua-chai*), eggplant (*brin-jal*) and long beans was as predictive of cancer as any other index using all eight foods.

## Japanese Populations

Studies of diet and gastric cancer in Japan and Japanese Hawaiians found increased fruit and vegetable intake to be protective. Low cancer risk was suggested for several Western-style vegetables, many of which were eaten raw. The associations for uncooked vegetables appeared to be independent of those found for pickled vegetables and persisted after controlling other aspects of vegetable consumption. Nine food items were analyzed in detail, and tomatoes and corn exhibited inverse dose/response relationships with gastric cancer, whereas lettuce and green onions were marginally protective. Construction of various "vegetable consumption profiles" using these food items did not alter the low risks noted for individual vegetables.

## Israel

Studies in Israel found increased intake of fruits and vegetables to be protective against stomach and colon cancer, especially squash and eggplant for the former. The role of dietary fiber was also considered in these studies.

## United States

A study of Seventh-Day Adventists (Phillips, 1975) found consumption of milk and green leafy vegetables to be protective against overall cancer rates, including colon cancer. Bjelke (1975) found consumption of carrots, eggs, and milk to be protective against lung cancer. Distinguishing smokers and nonsmokers also found carrots and milk to be protective against lung cancer. The protective effects were greater in smokers than in nonsmokers. The consumption of carrots had a lesser effect than did the total dietary intake index and was probably associated with consumption of other green and yellow vegetables (Graham et al., 1972). The same group of investigators found carrots, cruciferous vegetables, and milk to be protective against bladder cancer. Green and yellow vegetables were also found protective against laryngeal cancer as were fruits and vegetables against esophageal cancer (Mettlin et al., 1981).

---

**Complexities of Multicausal Cancer Studies:**

"Does New Jersey Cause Cancer?"

Following WWII, there were dramatic increases in cancer rates among the citizens of New Jersey, as industrialization brought economic growth. The question was asked in public policy debate: "Does New Jersey Cause Cancer?" At first, it was thought that pollution from new highways and growing industrial plants might primarily be responsible. However, richer diets, excess weight, sedentism, and increased consumption of luxuries such as tobacco and alcohol (the "good life" of the 1950s) were ultimately recognized as the contributing factors to increasing cancer.

---

## Older Americans

A study of cancer in older Americans attempted to differentiate individual food items with respect to cancer risk (Colditz et al., 1985). A strong protective effect was found for strawberries and tomatoes, and a moderate protective effect was found for dried fruits (apricots, raisins, and prunes) and broccoli. No protective effect was found for carrots or squash or for salads. Although frequent strawberry consumption is probably a proxy for high SES, strawberries contain no carotenoids, and dried fruits represent a natural form of concentrated whole food dietary "supplement."

Investigators at the NCI found that inverse associations with lung cancer risk were more pronounced for intake of vegetables, dark green vegetables, and dark yellow-orange vegetables than for vitamin A intake. Micozzi et al. (1990) suggested the explanation for these observations: the protective agent in vegetables is not beta-carotene but rather other carotenoids, vitamin C, indoles, plant phenols, and/or trace minerals, such as selenium. At least 14 additional diet and cancer studies cited in this chapter are consistent with this overall pattern of foods associated with decreased risk of cancer.

### Soy

In addition to the green leafy vegetables and carotenoid-containing foods, attention has focused on soy in the prevention of cancer. Women have been encouraged to eat a diet rich in phytoestrogens that includes soy products to counter some of the effects of menopause. Soy may be taken as a whole food or as isolated isoflavone constituents. A review by the National Institutes of Health in 1999 found that whole soy foods seemed to provide greater health benefits than isolated isoflavones. Soy food consumption, in such foods as tofu, soy milk, and tempeh, is generally associated with a reduced risk of breast cancer. However, laboratory studies have shown variable effects of isolated isoflavones on cancer cells.

Soy protein has also been observed to inhibit the growth of prostate cancer cells (Fair et al., 1997). In one report, men who drank several glasses of soy milk daily lowered their risk of prostate cancer by 70% (Jacobsen et al., 1998).

### Fish and Omega-3 Fatty Acids

Although interest in dietary fat and cancer has generally focused on its role as a possible cause of cancer (Chapter 8), omega-3 essential fatty acids may offer protection against the development of cancer. Omega-3 fatty acids demonstrate a wide range of health benefits. They are found in the diet in cold water fish, such as salmon, sardines, and cod liver, and in certain nuts, seeds, and cooking oils. In the latter category are walnuts, flax oil and seeds, hemp seeds, and canola oil. The typical American diet is deficient in omega-3 as the best dietary sources do not feature prominently in the modern Western diet. Some benefits of the Mediterranean diet and the traditional Japanese diet may derive from foods that are high in this constituent.

Studies have linked omega-3 from fish and other foods with a reduced risk of various types of cancer, including breast, prostate, and colon. Omega-3 fatty acids demonstrate inhibitory effects against cell division in some human cancer cell lines and inhibit growth of cultured metastatic malignant melanoma cells. Omega-3 fatty acids also decreased endothelial adhesion of human colorectal cancer cells (Kontogiannea et al., 2000).

In 2001 *The Lancet* reported that in a prospective study of over 6,000 Swedish men, those who ate no fish had a two- to threefold increased frequency of prostate cancer than in those who ate moderate to high amounts. In undernourished patients with breast, lung, liver, gastrointestinal, and pancreatic cancers, omega-3 with vitamin E showed immunomodulating effects and prolonged survival (Gogos et al., 1998).

Laboratory studies have shown that flax oil (as a source of omega-3) may increase the growth of human prostate cancer cells, but these findings have not been confirmed clinically. By contrast, flax seeds appear to be safe.

## Effects of Food Processing, Cooking, and Digestion

Some epidemiological studies have emphasized that the consumption of raw versus cooked vegetables was associated with decreased risk of cancer although raw and cooked vegetable consumption may be correlated. Many studies have not distinguished between raw versus cooked vegetable consumption or have only indicated which vegetables are normally eaten raw or normally eaten cooked. Therefore, the effects of cooking on nutrient content and profile in foods must also be considered.

Many food constituents are sensitive to traces of acids and are rapidly subjected to rearrangement, isomerization, and rearrangement in a low-pH environment as in the stomach. Even if vegetables are ingested in raw form, many of the changes associated with cooking may be expected to occur because of the presence of acids in the stomach.

# Summary

This chapter has provided a review of nutrients and of foods in relation to cancer prevention, from alpha-tocopherol to omega-3 fatty acids. The cancer-modifying effects of foods identified in studies of diet and cancer cannot be explained primarily by the assumption that these foods are high in any one nutrient versus being abundant sources of many nutrients and other biologically active constituents. The preponderance of foods found protective against cancer, including the cruciferous vegetables, are high in a number of biologically active compounds, such as vitamin C, which have cancer-modifying effects. Soy and food sources of omega-3 fatty acids also have been shown to reduce the risk of cancer. The nutrient composition of whole foods found protective against cancer requires primary consideration regarding the potential cancer-modifying effects of the human diet.

## REFERENCES AND RESOURCES

Albert, D. M., Kumar, A., Strugnell, S. A., Darjatmoko, S. R., Lokken, J. M., Lindstrom, M. J., et al. (2004). Effectiveness of vitamin D analogues in treating large tumors during prolonged use in murine retinoblastoma models. *Archives of Ophthalmology, 122,* 1357–1362.

Alberts, D. S., Martinez, M. E., Roe, D. J., Guillen-Rodriguez, J. M., Marshall, J. R., van Leeuwen, J. B., et al. (2000). Lack of effect of high fiber cereal supplement on the recurrence of colorectal adenomas. *New England Journal of Medicine, 342,* 1156–1162.

Alekel, D. L., Germain, A. S., Peterson, C. T., Hanson, K. B., Stewart, J. W., & Toda, T., (2000). Isoflavone-rich soy protein isolate attenuates bone loss in the lumbar spine of perimenopausal women. *American Journal of Clinical Nutrition, 72,* 844–852.

Armstrong, B., & Doll, R. (1975). Environmental factors and cancer incidence and mortality in different countries, with special reference to dietary practices. *International Journal of Cancer, 15,* 617–631.

Baron, J. A., Beach, M., Mandel, J. S., van Stolk, R. U., Haile, R. W., Sandler, R. S., et al. (1999). Calcium supplements for the prevention of colorectal adenomas. *New England Journal of Medicine, 340,* 101–107.

Basu, T. K., Chan, U., & Fields, A. (1984). Vitamin A (retinol) and epithelial cancer in man. In K. Prasad (Ed.), *Vitamins, nutrition, and cancer* (pp. 35–45). Basel: Karger.

Bendich, A., Gabriel, E., & Machlin, L. J. (1986). Dietary vitamin E requirement for optimum immune response in the rat. *Journal of Nutrition, 116,* 675.

Bjelke, E. (1975). Dietary vitamin A and human lung cancer. *International Journal of Cancer, 15,* 561.

Blot, W. J., Li, J. Y., Taylor, P. R., Guo, W., Dawsey, S., Wang, G. Q., et al. (1993). Nutrition intervention trials in Linxian, China. *Journal of the National Cancer Institute, 85,* 1483–1492.

Borek, C. (2004). Dietary antioxidants and human cancer. *Integrative Cancer Therapies, 3,* 333–341.

Boutwell, R. K. (1974). The function and mechanism of promoters of carcinogenesis. *Critical Reviews in Toxicology, 2,* 419.

Bright-See, E. (1984). Role of vitamins C and E in the etiology of human cancer. In K. N. Prasad (Ed.), *Vitamins, nutrition, and cancer* (pp. 68–75). Karger: Basel.

Buell, P. (1973). Changing incidence of breast cancer in Japanese-American women. *Journal of the National Cancer Institute, 51,* 1479–1483.

Buell, P., & Dunn, J. E. (1986). Cancer mortality of Japanese Isei and Nisei of California. *Cancer, 18,* 656–664.

Cameron, E., Pauling, E., & Leibovitz, B. (1979). Ascorbic acid and cancer: A review. *Cancer Research, 39,* 663.

Carter, C. L., & Micozzi, M. S. (1986). The genetics of human breast cancer. *Yearbook of Physical Anthropology, 29,* 161–180.

Chow, C. K., & Gairola, G. C. (1984). Influences of dietary vitamin E and selenium on metabolic activation of chemicals to mutagens. *Journal of Agricultural and Food Chemistry, 32,* 443.

Cirigliano, M. D., & Szapary, P. O. (1999). Selenium supplementation for cancer prevention. *Alternative Medicine Alert, January*, 3–7.

Clark, L. C. (1985). The epidemiology of selenium and cancer. *Federation Proceedings, 44*, 2584.

Clark, L. C., et al. (1996). Effects of selenium supplementation for cancer prevention in patients with carcinoma of the skin. *Journal of the American Medical Association, 276*, 1957–1963.

Cochrane, W. (1965). Overnutrition in prenatal and neonatal life: A problem? *Canadian Medical Association Journal, 93*, 893.

Colditz, G. A., Branch, L. G., Lipnick, R. J., Willett, W. C., Rosner, B., Posner, B. M., & Hennekens, C. H. (1985). Increased green and yellow vegetable intake and lowered cancer death in an elderly population. *American Journal of Clinical Nutrition, 4*, 32–36.

Committee on Diet, Nutrition and Cancer, Assembly of Life Sciences, National Research Council. (1982). *Diet, Nutrition, and Cancer*. Washington, DC: National Academy Press.

Cook-Mozaffari, P. J., Azordegan, F., Day, N. E., et al. (1979). Oseophageal cancer studies in the Caspian littoral of Iran: Results of a case-control study. *British Journal of Cancer, 39*, 293.

Creagan, E. T., Moertel, C. G., & O'Falloon, J. R. (1979). Failure of high-dose vitamin C (ascorbic acid) therapy to benefit patients with advanced cancer. *New England Journal of Medicine, 301*, 687.

DeCosse, J. J., Adams, M. B., & Kuzma, J. F. (1975). Effect of ascorbic acid on rectal polyps of patients with familial polyposis. *Surgery, 78*, 608.

Doll, R., & Peto, R. (1981). The cause of cancer. *Journal of the National Cancer Institute, 66*, 1191–1308.

Dragnev, K. H. (2003). Retinoid targets in cancer therapy and chemoprevention. *Cancer Biology and Therapy, 2*(4 Suppl. 1), S150–S156.

Duffield-Lillico, A. J., & Begg, C. B. (2004). Reflections on the landmark studies of beta-carotene supplementation. *Journal of the National Cancer Institute, 96*, 1729– 1731.

Dunn, J. E. (1977). Breast cancer among American Japanese in the San Francisco Bay area. In *Epidemiology and Cancer Registries in the Pacific Basin*. [DHEW Pub. No. (NIH) 77-1223, NCI Monograph, No. 47, pp. 157–160]. Washington, DC: U.S. Government Printing Office.

Evans, H. E. (1962). The pioneer history of vitamin E. *Vitamins and Hormones, 20*, 379.

Fair, W. R., et al. (1997). Cancer of the prostate: A nutritional disease? *Urology, 50*, 843.

Fairfield, K. M., & Fletcher, R. H. (2002). Vitamins for chronic disease prevention in adults: Scientific review. *Journal of the American Medical Association, 287*, 3116– 3126.

Fletcher, R. H., & Fairfield, K. M. (2002). Vitamins for chronic disease prevention in adults: Clinical applications. *Journal of the American Medical Association, 287*, 3127–3129.

Giovanucci, E., et al. (1998). Multivitamin use, folate and colon cancer in women in the Nurses Health Study. *Annals of Internal Medicine, 129*, 517–524.

Gogos, C. A., et al. (1998). Dietary omega-3 polyunsaturated fatty acids plus vitamin E restore immunodeficiency and prolong survival for severely ill patients with generalized malignancy. American Cancer Society.

Gori, G. B. (1979). Dietary and nutritional implications in the multifactorial etiology of certain prevalent human cancers. *Cancer, 43*, 2151.

Haenszel, W., & Kurihara, M. (1968). Studies of Japanese Migrants. I. Mortality from cancer and other disease among Japanese in the United States. *Journal of the National Cancer Institute, 40*, 43.

Hercberg, S. (2005). The history of beta-carotene and cancers: From observational to intervention studies. What lessons can be drawn for future research on polyphenols? *American Journal of Clinical Nutrition, 81*, 218S–222S.

Heinonen, A., et al. (1998). Prostate cancer and supplementation with alpha-tocopherol and beta-carotene: Incidence and mortality in a controlled trial. *Journal of the National Cancer Institute, 90*, 440–446.

Hirayama, T. (1978). Epidemiology of breast cancer with special reference to the role of diet. *Preventive Medicine, 7*, 173–195.

Hoffer, A. (1971). Ascorbic acid and toxicity. *New England Journal of Medicine, 285*, 635.

Horvath, P. M., & Ip, C. (1983). Synergistic effect of vitamin E and selenium in the chemoprevention of mammary carcinogeenasis in rats. *Cancer Research, 43*, 5335.

Institute of Medicine. (2001). *Dietary reference intakes*. Washington, DC: National Academy Press.

Ip, C. (1982). Dietary vitamin E intake and mammary carcinogenesis in rats. *Carcinogenesis, 3*(12), 1453.

Ip, C., & Horvath, P. (1983). Synergistic effect of vitamin E and selenium in the chemoprevention of mammary carcinogeenasis in rats. *Proceedings of the American Association of Cancer Research, 24*, 382.

Ip, C., & Ip, M. (1981). Chemoprevention of mammary tumorigenesis by a combined regimen of selenium and vitamin A. *Carcinogenesis, 2*, 915.

Jacobsen, B. K., et al. (1998). Does high soy milk intake reduce prostate cancer incidence? The Adventist Health Study (United States). *Cancer Causes and Control, 9*, 553–557.

Knekt, P., et al. (1991). Dietary antioxidants and risk of lung cancer. *American Journal of Epidemiology, 134*, 471–479.

Kontogiannea, M., et al. (2000). Omega-3 fatty acids decrease endothelial adhesion of human colorectal carcinoma cells. *Journal of Surgical Research, 92*, 201–205.

Koo, L. C. (1997). Diet and lung cancer 20+ years later. *International Journal of Cancer, 10*, 22–29.

Lipkin, M., & Newmark, H. L. (1985). Effect of added dietary calcium on colonic epithelial-cell proliferation in subjects at high risk for familial colon cancer. *New England Journal of Medicine, 313*, 1381.

Lipkin, M., Sherlock, P., & Bell, B. (1963). Cell proliferation kinetics in the gastrointestinal tract. *Gastroenterology, 45*, 721.

Marmot, M. G., & Syme, S. L. (1976). Acculturation and coronary heart disease in Japanese Americans. *American Journal of Epidemiology, 104*, 171–200.

MacLennan, R., DaCosta, J., Day, N. E., et al. (1977). Risk factors for lung cancer in Singapore Chinese, a population with high female incidence rates. *International Journal of Cancer, 20*, 854.

Matsubara, K., et al. (2003). Vitamin B6-mediated suppression of colon tumorigenesis, cell proliferation and angiogenesis: Review. *Journal of Nutritional Biochemistry, 14*, 246–250.

Menkes, M. S., Comstock, G. W., Vuilleunmier, J. P., Helsing, K. J., Rider, A. A., & Brookmeyer, R. (1986). Serum beta-carotene, vitamin A and E, selenium, and the risk of lung cancer. *New England Journal of Medicine, 315*, 1250.

Menzel, D. B. (1970). Toxicity of ozone, oxygen and radiation. *Annual Review of Pharmacology, 10*, 379.

Micozzi, M. S. (1987). Cross-cultural correlations of childhood growth and adult breast cancer. *American Journal of Physical Anthropology, 73*, 525–537.

Micozzi, M. S., Beecher, G. R., Taylor, P. R., & Khachik, F. (1990). Carotenoid analysis of foods associated with a lower risk of cancer. *Journal of the National Cancer Institute, 82*, 292–285.

Milner, J. A. (1986). Inhibition of chemical carcinogenesis and tumorigenesis by selenium. In L. A. Poirier, P. M. Newberne, & M. W. Pariza (Eds.), *Essential nutrients in carcinogenesis* (p 449). New York: Plenum.

Moon, R. C., & Itri, L. M. (1984). Retinoids and cancer. In M.B. Sporn, A. B. Roberts, & D. S. Goodman (Eds.), *The Retinoids* (Vol. 2, p. 327). New York: Academic Press.

Mori, S. (1922). The changes in the paraocular glands which follow the administration of diets low in fat-soluble A with notes of the effects of the dame diets on the salivary glands and the mucosa of the larynx and trachea. *Johns Hopkins Hospital Bulletin, 33*, 357.

National Center for Health Statistics, R. Fullwood C. L. Johnson J. D. Bryner, et al. (1982). Hematological and nutritional biochemistry reference data for persons 6 months–74 years of age: United States, 1976–80. Vital and Health Statistic. Series 11-No. 232. DHHS Pub. No. (PHS) 83-1682. Public Health Service. Washington, DC: U.S. Government Printing Office.

Newmark, H. L., Wargovich, M. J., & Bruce, W. R. (1984). Colon cancer and dietary fat phosphate, and calcium: A hypothesis. *Journal of the National Cancer Institute, 72*, 1321.

Nomura, A. M. Y., Stemmerman, G. N., Heilbrun, L. K., Salkeld, R. M., & Vuillemier, J. P. (1985). Serum vitamin levels and the risk of cancer of specific sites in men of Japanese ancestry in Hawaii. *Cancer Research, 45*, 2369.

Omenn, G. S. (1998). Chemoprevention of lung cancer: The rise and demise of beta-carotene. *Annual Review of Public Health, 19*, 73–99.

Peleg, I., Morris, S., & Hames, C. G. (1985). Is selenium a risk factor for cancer? *Medical Oncology and Tumor Pharmacotherapy, 2*, 137.

Peto, R., Doll, R., Buckley, J. D., & Sporn, M. B. (1981). Can dietary beta-carotene materially reduce human cancer rates? *Nature, 290*, 201–208.

Phillips, R. L. (1975). Role of lifestyle and dietary habits in risk of cancer among Seventh Day Adventists. *Cancer Research, 35*, 3513–3522.

Potter, J. D., & McMichael, A. J. (1986). Diet and cancer of the colon and rectum: A case-control study. *Journal of the National Cancer Institute, 76*, 557.

Rittenbaugh, C. K., & Meyskens, F. L., Jr. (1986). Analysis of dietary associations of vitamin A with cancer. In J. Bland (Ed.), 1986: *A year in nutritional medicine* (pp. 264–291). New Canaan, CT: Keats.

Rivers, J. M. (1975). Oral contraceptives and ascorbic acid. *American Journal of Clinical Nutrition, 28*, 50.

Rivers, J. M., & Devine, M. M. (1975). Relationships of ascorbic acid to pregnancy and oral contraceptive steroids. *Annals of the New York Academy of Sciences, 258*, 465.

Rosenthal, G. (1971). Interaction of ascorbic acid and warfarin. *Journal of the American Medical Association, 215*, 1671.

Rywlin, A. M. (1984). Terminology of premalignant lesions in light of the multistep theory of carcinogeenesis. *Human Pathology, 15*, 806–807.

Sahud, M. A., & Cohen, R. J. (1971). Effect of aspirin ingestion on ascorbic acid levels in rheumatoid arthritis. *Lancet, 1*, 937.

Schatzkin, A., et al. (2000). Lack of effect of low-fat, high fiber on the recurrence of colorectal adenomas. *New England Journal of Medicine, 342*, 1149–1155.

Schrauzer, G. N., Molenaar, T., Mead, S., Kuehn, K., Uamamoto, H., & Araki, E. (1985). Selenium in the blood of Japanese and American women with and without breast cancer and fibrocystic disease. *Japanese Journal of Cancer Research, 76*, 374.

Schrauzer, G. N. (1979). Vitamin C: Conservative human requirements and aspects of overdosage. *International Review of Biochemistry, Biochemistry of Nutrition, 27*, 167.

Schrauzer, G. N., & Rhead, W. J. (1973). Ascorbic acid abuse: Effects of long-term ingestion of excessive amounts on blood levels and urinary excretion. *International Journal for Vitamin and Nutrition Research, 43*, 201.

Shamberger, R. J. (1970). Relationship of selenium to cancer. I. Inhibitory effect of selenium on carcinogenesis. *Journal of the National Cancer Institute, 44*, 931.

Shamberger, R. J., & Rudolph, G. (1966). Protection against carcinogenesis by antioxidants. *Experientia, 22*, 116.

Shekelle, R. B., Lepper, M., Liu, S., et al. (1981). Dietary vitamin A and risk of cancer in the Western Electric Study. *Lancet, 2*, 1185–1190.

Sporn, M. B., & Roberts, A. B. (183). Role of retinoids in differentiation and carcinogeenesis. *Cancer Research, 43*, 3034.

Wargovich, M. J., Eng, V. W. S., Newmark, H. L., & Bruce, W. R. (1983). Calcium ameliorates the toxic effects of deoxycholic acid on colonic epithelium. *Carcinogenesis, 4*(9),1205.

Wargovich, M. J., Eng, V. W. S., & Newmark, H. L. (1984). Calcium inhibits the damaging and compensatory proliferative effects of fatty acids on mouse colon epithelium. *Cancer Letters, 23*, 253.

Wattenberg, L. W. (1972). Inhibition of carcinogenic and toxic effects of polycyclic hydrocarbons by phenolic antioxidants and ethoxyquin. *Journal of the National Cancer Institute, 48*, 1425.

Wattenberg, L. W. (1978). Inhibitors of chemical carcinogeenesis. *Journal of the National Cancer Institute, 60*, 11.

Wattenberg, L. W. (1983). Inhibition of neoplasia by minor dietary constituents. *Cancer Research, 43*, 2448S.

Wattenberg, L. W. (1978). Inhibitors of chemical carcinogenesis. *Advances in Cancer Research, 26*, 197-226.

Weisburger, J. H., & Horn, C. (1982). Nutrition and cancer: Mechanisms of genotoxic and epigenetic carcinogens in nutritional and carcinogenesis. *Bulletin of the New York Academy of Sciences, 58*, 296.

Weisburger, J. H., Marquardt, H., Mower, H. F., et al. (1980). Inhibition of carcinogenesis: Vitamin C and the prevention of gastric cancer. *Preventive Medicine, 9*, 352.

Weisburger, J. H., & Ranieri, R. (1975). Dietary factors and the etiology of gastric cancer. *Cancer Research, 35*, 3469.

Willett, W., Polk, B. F., Hames, C., et al. (1983). Prediagnostic serum selenium and the risk of cancer. *Lancet, 2*, 130–134.

Willet, W. C., Polk, B. F., Underwood, B. A., & Hames, C. G. (1984). Hypertension detection and follow-up program study of serum retinol, retinol-binding protein, total carotenoids, and cancer risk: A summary. *Journal of the National Cancer Institute, 73*, 1459.

Wolbach, S. B., & Howe, P. R. (1925). Tissue changes following deprivation of fat soluble A vitamin. *Journal of Experimental Medicine, 42*, 753.

Wu, K., Helzlsouer, K. J., Comstock, G. W., et al. (1999). A prospective study on folate, B-12 and pyridoxal-phosphate (B6) and breast cancer. *Cancer Epidemiology Biomarkers & Prevention, 8*, 209–217.

Yu, S. Y., et al. (1990). Intervention trial with selenium for the prevention of lung cancer in miners in Yunnan. *Biological Trace Element Research, 24*, 105–108.

Marc S. Micozzi

## Introduction

Attempts to treat or ameliorate cancer in patients with active disease have focused on the use of high doses of established nutrients with proven anticancer and/or antioxidant properties, such as vitamins A, C, and E (Block, 2004; Ladas et al., 2003; Norman et al., 2003). Other approaches have utilized certain foods to the exclusion of others, for example, macrobiotic, Gerson, and Livingstone–Wheeler diets, or focused on substitution of digestive enzymes, for example, Kelley–Gonzalez diet (Chapter 12). Although these special diets continue to be used by cancer patients, it remains open as to whether diet in adults may alter the risk of developing cancer in the first place or influence the progress of existing cancers.

Moreover, whether certain nutritional or diet therapies, adopted once cancer has developed, can influence care, survival, and/or quality of life remains controversial. Reviewing the available information on cancer diets provides guidance regarding reasonable recommendations to cancer patients and suggests current directions for investigation. The large amount of basic science and clinical research on micronutrients, carcinogenesis, and cancer prevention in the previous chapter can be compared to clinical experience with the use of vitamins A, C, and E supplementation in cancer patients.

## Vitamins A, C, and E Supplements

In human nutrition, vitamins are essential for normal development and good health. Most cannot be made by the body and must be obtained from foods or supplements.

If supplements are used, they should be taken with meals to ensure absorption, and fat soluble vitamins (including vitamin A, beta-carotene, and vitamin E) should be taken with at least a little dietary fat.

Some vitamin supplements are manufactured from natural or synthetic sources. For example, vitamin E may be isolated from soybean oil or made from petroleum derivatives. However, despite the appeal of "natural" vitamins, research has not found important differences in their effects.

Guidelines are set for recommended daily allowances (RDAs) of vitamins and minerals. Many people eating a balanced diet, choosing foods from each of the four basic food groups and emphasizing fresh fruits and vegetables, may meet the RDA for vitamins. However, individuals who are not eating well as a result of ill health require supplements. Advice on the specific supplement(s) necessary should be obtained from the health care practitioner.

Many people use vitamin supplements either of their own volition or on the advice of their health care practitioner. It is not surprising that many individuals dealing with cancer take vitamin supplements to enhance well-being, particularly when these agents are available at a reasonable price from any pharmacy or health food store. Some vitamins, specifically vitamin A, beta-carotene (a precursor of vitamin A), vitamin C, and vitamin E, are believed to affect the cancer process, perhaps by strengthening the immune system or as a result of their antioxidant properties. Cancer patients may therefore receive advice from friends and some health care professionals to supplement their diets with these vitamins. Proponents of vitamin therapy often recommend daily doses of vitamins that greatly exceed the RDA (megavitamin therapy) and vastly exceed physiologic levels (see Chapter 10).

# Vitamin A (Including Beta-Carotene and Retinoids)

Vitamin A is one of a group of substances with similar structure and activity called retinoids. Vitamin A is necessary for normal growth, bone development, vision, reproduction, and the maintenance of the integrity of the skin and mucous membranes. Clinical deficiency of vitamin A leads to night blindness, abnormalities of the skin, and decreased resistance to infection, but is rare in developed countries.

## Toxicity

Serious vitamin A toxicity (adverse effects) as a result of taking supplementary vitamin A is relatively rare but may result in headache, irritability, drowsiness, dizziness, itchiness, scaling of the skin, and peeling of the skin around the mouth. High dosages may cause temporary or permanent liver damage. Individuals with kidney disorders and pregnant women should be especially careful when taking vitamin A supplements and should seek medical advice. Recognition of the toxicity of vitamin A seriously limits its clinical value and has led to a major effort to identify other less toxic retinoids that have beneficial effects. This has led to the development and testing of more than 1,500 compounds. Some of these are being evaluated for their anticancer activity (see Chapter 10).

# Beta-Carotene

Several retinoids are provitamins (substances known to be transformed into vitamins in the body) for vitamin A. Of these, beta-carotene, which occurs naturally in many foods, has the greatest provitamin activity and is used generally by individuals seeking to increase their intake of vitamin A. It has many advantages over vitamin A: not only is it much less toxic in its own right, but also the body physiologically limits the amount of beta-carotene that is transformed into vitamin A to levels that are nontoxic. In addition, beta-carotene is beneficial in other ways that are independent of its transformation to vitamin A (see below). Daily supplements of beta-carotene taken by individuals who are deficient in vitamin A have been shown to increase its serum level. However, in individuals not deficient in vitamin A, beta-carotene supplements do not physiologically increase the serum levels of vitamin A.

Epidemiological studies have shown the risks of some cancers are higher in individuals with low dietary intakes of foods rich in vitamin A and beta-carotene, as well as in individuals with low serum levels of vitamin A and beta-carotene. In some studies, higher serum levels were found in cancer patients who subsequently responded well to chemotherapy. However, the consumption of nutritional supplements of vitamin A and beta-carotene in amounts sufficient to increase serum levels has not been proven to have an important treatment effect on the cancer process.

The toxicity of beta-carotene is low even at relatively high doses although some individuals may develop temporary hypercarotenemia (yellowing of the skin), especially of the palms of the hands and the soles of the feet. (Micozzi et al, 1988) Of more concern is recent evidence that suggests that beta-carotene supplements may actually increase the risk of lung cancer and lung cancer recurrence among smokers (see Chapter 10).

# Retinoids

The relationship between the serum levels of other retinoids and cancer risk is not clearly understood. However, research has shown that different retinoids have different effects on different types of tumors and that the effects also vary depending on the animal species being studied (Dragnev et al., 2004). Clearly, this variation makes it difficult to select the particular retinoid supplement most likely to be of use to an individual with cancer.

A large number of cellular, animal, and human studies have shown several naturally occurring and synthetic vitamin A derivatives (retinoids) to inhibit tumor development. However, in human cell lines and in patients studies their effectiveness seems to be greatest in cancers of the airway, upper bowel, certain rare forms of leukemia, some skin cancers, cancer of the bladder, and cancer of the cervix.

## Effects on Cellular Differentiation

The anticancer effects of the retinoids are thought to be because of their ability to slow the rate at which cancer cells grow and multiply and to promote cell differentiation. However, as noted above the various retinoids differ in their capacity to cause these anticancer effects.

### Effects on Oncogenes

More specifically, retinoids are thought to change the structure and function of oncogenes associated with the development of cancer thereby delaying the promotion and/or spread of cancer. At a cellular level, they are thought to connect to receptors on cell nuclei. The discovery of these "nuclear retinoid receptors" has contributed greatly to understanding the possible anticancer effects of retinoids.

### Effects on Immune Response

Some animal studies have demonstrated the ability of vitamin A and other retinoids to enhance the immune response increasing the number of immune cells and making them more active, to retard tumor growth, and/or to decrease the size of already established tumors. The immunoenhancing and anticarcinogenic activity of beta-carotene does not require that it be converted to vitamin A and is therefore distinct from its function as a provitamin. In addition, in certain types of cancers the concurrent use of retinoid supplements has enhanced the effectiveness of some cancer treatments. For example, the ability of some retinoids to induce cell differentiation in one form of leukemia has been confirmed in both animal and human studies and it has been shown that these effects are greater and last longer if the retinoids are given in combination with other agents such as interferon or drugs used in chemotherapy. A number of clinical studies designed to investigate the role of retinoids in cancer treatment are underway.

### Effects on Breast Cancer

With respect to breast cancer, some preclinical studies have suggested that retinoids can inhibit cell proliferation and regulate gene expression in breast cancer cells (Lesperance et al., 2002). A specific retinoid, fenretinide, shows activity in both the prevention and treatment of breast cancer. Animal studies using experimental rats have shown that fenretinide can inhibit mammary gland formation in developing animals, can suppress carcinogen-induced mammary cancer, and can lead to regression of invasive mammary cancer. Fenretinide has also demonstrated activity against human breast cancer cell lines in laboratory studies. More clinical studies are needed (see Chapter 9).

# Vitamin C

Vitamin C (ascorbic acid) is a water soluble vitamin found in many fruits and vegetables. Many preparations of vitamin C are available. These preparations may contain different forms of vitamin C that may have different effects and potencies. It has an important role in the formation of collagen (a key component of skin, bone, and cartilage), as well as in the manufacture of various other chemicals required by the body for health function. It is also necessary for wounds to heal effectively, and it influences many immunological and biochemical reactions in the body (see Chapter 10).

In addition to these functions, vitamin C has well-established antioxidant properties. More recently, studies have suggested that vitamin C may have other functions, including an effect on the structure of cell membranes and on the promotion of cell differentiation.

## Vitamin C Deficiency

Vitamin C deficiency, which results in scurvy (a condition marked by anemia, spongy gums, and bleeding into the skin and mucous membranes) is rare in individuals eating a normal diet. However, evidence exists that the body's requirement for ascorbic acid may increase during periods of physical or chemical stress and in the elderly. Most health care professionals recommend the consumption of fresh fruits and vegetables to maintain appropriate levels of vitamin C. If supplements are recommended, doses consistent with the RDA are generally advised. Proponents of high-dose vitamin C for the treatment of cancer (and some other scientists) consider that the daily intake of vitamin C should be much higher than the current recommended dosage of 60 mg/day (designed to protect against clinical vitamin C deficiency). However, more research is needed to determine the appropriate dosages for vitamin C supplements.

## Antioxidant Properties

There is epidemiological evidence that populations who consume diets high in vitamin C have a lowered risk for some cancers. This effect may be because of the antioxidant function of vitamin C and its ability to block the formation of $N$-nitrosamines (cancer-causing substances formed in the stomach from certain foods). The strongest epidemiological finding has been the association between high intakes of foods rich in vitamin C and a reduced risk of stomach cancer. There is a weaker link to a decreased risk of cervical cancer in smokers. The protective effect of vitamin C with respect to other cancers, including lung cancer and breast cancer, remains controversial.

## Side Effects

Ascorbic acid is generally tolerated well, but at high doses it may cause stomach irritation, heart-burn, nausea, vomiting, drowsiness, and headaches. High doses of vitamin C may also acidify the urine and alter the results of urine tests. It is unlikely to increase the risk of kidney or bladder stones in susceptible individuals. Although some oncologists are concerned that high-dose vitamin C may alter the absorption and excretion of some drugs used in the treatment of cancer, there are no clinical studies documenting this effect. Vitamin C may interfere with the absorption or activity of a number of other agents, including anticoagulants, vitamin $B_{12}$, and vitamin E. High doses of vitamin C during pregnancy may be associated with subsequent vitamin C deficiency in newborns, perhaps by inducing vitamin C metabolism in the fetus. In adults, there is significant anecdotal evidence that vitamin C is safe at dosages of 1 g/day and very minimal toxicity has been reported even at much higher dosages. However, there are few controlled studies of the toxicity of vitamin C (see Chapter 10).

## Vitamin C for Cancer Patients

A recommendation that vitamin C supplements be used by cancer patients is based on its reported activity as (1) an antioxidant; (2) an immunoenhancing agent; (3) neutralizing agent for certain cancer-causing chemicals (such as $N$-nitrosamines); (4) an agent having a direct antitumor effect on cancer cells; (5) an agent that might counteract the toxicity of some conventional cancer treatments; and (6) an agent that can strengthen the structural integrity of tissues, thus increasing resistance of these tissues to invasive cancer cells; and (7) an agent that can kill cancer cells directly is sufficient dose (Chen et al., 2005). These reported effects are supported by some research. However, many of the findings cannot be considered conclusive and this list of reported effects is useful as a framework for investigation.

Several studies have described the antioxidant and general immunostimulant properties of vitamin C. Specifically, vitamin C is considered one of the most effective and least toxic antioxidants for humans and is thought to enhance the function of lymphocytes. In other experiments, vitamin C has demonstrated chemopreventive effects (preventing the recurrence of transplanted tumor cells), as well as therapeutic effects (inhibiting tumor growth and producing tumor regression of established tumors or increasing survival of animals with implanted tumors). Results of some studies suggest that ascorbic acid may have a direct cell-killing effect on some types of tumor cells and that it may enhance the cell-killing effect of some drug treatments for cancer. The concentration of vitamin C required to damage tumor cells seems to be much lower than that which will damage normal cells. However, it is not clear if the concentrations necessary to cause these effects on cancer cells can be achieved by oral or even intravenous administration of vitamin C supplements. One study suggested that intravenous administration of vitamin C may be more effective than oral administration, but further clinical trials are needed to confirm this finding.

## Vitamin C and Cancer Survival

Some preliminary clinical data suggest that vitamin C may be useful in improving the survival of cancer patients, but the designs of these studies and the results are limited. The studies suggesting that there is no significant effect as a result of vitamin C supplementation are better designed but their results are still not definitive because only relatively small groups of patients, usually with advanced cancer, were studied.

## High-Dose Vitamin C

Major proponents of cancer treatments that include high-dose vitamin C supplements were the late Nobel laureate Dr. Linus Pauling and Dr. Ewan Cameron. They provided a number of anecdotal reports, case studies, and pilot studies involving large numbers of advanced cancer patients to whom they administered high-doses of vitamin C. They reported that vitamin C appeared to improve overall well-being and quality of life, as well as resulting in a significant increase in the survival of patients with various types of advanced cancer. However, the research designs and statistical techniques used in these studies have been superseded and are no longer regarded as sufficiently rigorous to guide clinical treatment.

High-dose vitamin C levels can be achieved through intravenous as well as oral administration (Padayatty et al., 2004). Vitamin C may also have an adjunctive role in cancer chemotherapy (Drisko et al., 2003; Kurbacher et al., 2004).

In one animal study, vitamin C (administered in high dosages) was found to reduce the toxicity of adriamycin (a chemotherapeutic drug used in the treatment of breast cancer) on heart muscle. If this effect is confirmed at lower dosages and in human studies, vitamin

C could be of considerable clinical value because the use of adriamycin is often limited by its toxic effect on the heart.

# Vitamin E

Vitamin E is a fat-soluble vitamin existing in a variety of forms in many foods. The most common form of vitamin E in a Western diet is alpha-tocopherol. Only 20%–60% of the vitamin from dietary sources is absorbed and, as the dosage of vitamin E increases (as in megadose therapy), the fraction of vitamin E absorbed decreases. Nonetheless, vitamin E deficiency is rare in adults.

Vitamin E is considered to have antioxidant properties and vitamin E supplements have been tested in a number of conditions, including malabsorption disorder, hematologic disorders, cardiovascular disease, precancerous conditions in the oral cavities, and cancer itself.

Descriptive studies have shown that low serum levels of vitamin E are associated with a slightly increased risk of cancer in some populations but data describing the relations between serum levels of vitamin E and the risk of cancer are limited and inconsistent. Daily supplements of alpha-tocopherol have been shown to increase the serum level, but the effect of this increase on the risk of cancer is unknown.

## Toxicity

The toxicity of vitamin E in adults is low. Clinical trials in humans have demonstrated that large doses (e.g., 200–800 mg/day) of vitamin E do not have serious side effects for most adults with the possible exception of individuals taking oral anticoagulants and those with other clotting disorders. These patients should ensure that they obtain medical advice before taking vitamin E supplements. Long-term use of high doses (greater than 300 IU daily of vitamin E) may cause transient nausea, diarrhea, and blurred vision. High-dose treatment of infants may be associated with more serious side effects. Vitamin E's mechanism of action (the precise way in which it has its effects on the body), pharmacokinetics (the way in which it is absorbed, used and excreted), and effects require more study and clarification.

## Vitamin E in Cancer Treatment

Although research addressing the role of vitamin E in the prevention of cancer has been conducted (see Chapter 10), relatively little is known about its effects in cancer treatment. Some studies have shown that alpha-tocopherol can neutralize the effects of certain cancer-causing compounds (such as $N$-nitrosamines) and that it may stimulate the release of antitumor factors from the immune system. Animal studies suggest that it can prevent some chemically induced cancers and it may reduce the size of tumors. One study in humans suggested a beneficial effect associated with the use of vitamin E in patients with superficial premalignant lesions in the mouth.

In a laboratory study using breast cancer cells, vitamin E inhibited their growth. Results of animal studies examining the effect of vitamin E on mammary cancers have been contradictory. However, it has been reported that a supplement of 800 mg/day of alpha-tocopherol, taken during radiation therapy for breast cancer, reduced side effects and improved general well-being. In one study of patients with benign breast disease, vitamin E supplements were not beneficial.

# Summary: Use and Combination of Vitamins

Vitamin supplements may be seen by some as alternative therapies, although there is a great deal of research activity related to vitamin supplements being carried out by the conventional research community. As a result of these efforts, some therapies may be integrated into standard (conventional medical) treatment and others may remain unconventional.

With respect to vitamins, there is some laboratory evidence, and some clinical evidence, that they have potential as anticancer therapies. Although this limited evidence is the basis for recommending the use of vitamin A, C, and E supplements to some cancer patients, it falls short of the solid scientific evidence that should be available before an agent is provided to the general public other than those individuals participating in research trails.

The advantages of vitamin supplements are that they are readily available and can usually be self-provided. Consultation with the oncologist should ensure that undesirable interactions are avoided to the greatest extent possible.

There are a few preliminary clinical studies using combinations of vitamin supplements that have reported improvements in quality of life and survival. These studies suggest that combinations of vitamin supplements confer a greater benefit than might be expected from the use of each agent used separately. Further research to confirm these findings and to identify the particular combinations that are most effective is needed. Factorial design is an appropriate methodology for combination trials.

The complexity of the research required in this area should not be underestimated. In studies of the protective or therapeutic effects of vitamin supplements it is often difficult to determine if any observed improvements are because of supplements, diet, or other factors. In addition, many protocols for the use of supplements combine several agents, thus making it difficult to establish cause and effect or to attribute an observed improvement to any particular agent.

There is a need for additional laboratory research to improve understanding of the functions of these vitamins and to establish their potential role in the treatment of cancer. There is also a need for well-designed clinical studies to examine the transferability of positive laboratory finds to cancer patients. The value of vitamin A, C, and E supplements, alone or in combination, in the prevention and treatment of cancer will be further established as additional scientific studies are conducted to determine the effectiveness of these agents as well as their appropriate clinical indications and dosages.

## REFERENCES AND RESOURCES

Alpha Tocopherol, Beta Carotene Cancer Prevention Study Group. (1994). The effect of vitamin E and beta carotene on the incidence of lung cancer and other cancers in male smokers. *New England Journal of Medicine, 330*(15), 1029–1035.

American Cancer Society. (1993). Questionable methods of cancer management: 'nutritional' therapies. *CA: A Cancer Journal for Clinicians, 43*(5), 28–33.

Baer, R., Cassidy, C., Cheung, L., Harvey, H., Hildenbrand, G., Hoffer, L. J., et al. (1994). Diet and nutrition in the prevention and treatment of chronic disease. In: *Alternative medicine: Expanding medical horizons: A report to the National Institutes of Health on alternative medical systems and practices in the United States* (NIH Publication No. 94-066) (pp. 207–270). Washington, DC: U.S. Government Printing Office.

Barinaga, M. (1991). Vitamin C gets a little respect. *Science, 254*, 374–376.

Bates, C. J. (1995). Vitamin A. *Lancet, 345*, 31–35.

Bendich, A. (1991). Beta-carotene and the immune response. *Proceedings of the Nutrition Society, 50*, 263–274.

Bendich, A., & Langseth, L. (1995). The health effects of vitamin C supplementation: A review. *Journal of the American College of Nutrition, 14*(2), 124–136.

Bieri, J. G., Corash, L., & Hubbard, V. S. (1983). Medical uses of vitamin E. *New England Journal of Medicine, 308*(18), 1063–1071.

Block, K. I. (2004). Antioxidants and cancer therapy: Furthering the debate. *Integrative Cancer Therapies, 3*, 342–348.

Boik, J. (1996). Dietary micronutrients and their effects on cancer. In *Cancer and natural medicine: A textbook of basic science and clinical research* (pp. 142–147). Princeton, MN: Oregon Medical Press.

Bollage, W., & Holdener, E. E. (1992). Retinoids in cancer prevention and therapy. *Annals of Oncology, 3*, 513–526.

Bourne, G. H. (1948–1949). Vitamin C and immunity. *British Journal of Nutrition, 2*, 341–347.

Cameron, E., & Campbell, A. (1974). The orthomolecular treatment of cancer. II. Clincal trial of high-dose ascorbic acid supplements in advanced human cancer. *Chemico-Biological Interactions, 9*, 285–315.

Cameron, E., & Pauling, L. (1978). Supplemental ascorbate in the supportive treatment of cancer: Reevaluation of prolongation of survival times in terminal human cancer. *Proceedings of the National Academy of Sciences of the USA, 75*(9), 4538–4542.

Cameron, E., & Pauling, L. (1979). Ascorbic acid as a therapeutic agent in cancer. *Journal of International Academy of Preventive Medicine, V*(1), 8–29.

Cameron, E., Pauling, L., & Leibovitz, B. (1979). Ascorbic acid and cancer: A review. *Cancer Research, 39*, 663–681.

Canadian Cancer Society. (1996). *CCS position on antioxidant vitamins and cancer.* Toronto: Author.

Chen, Q., et al. (2005). Pharmacologic ascorbic acid concentrations selectively kill cancer cells: Action as a pro-drug to deliver hydrogen peroxide to tissues. *Proceedings of the National Academy of Sciences of the USA, 102*, 13604–13609.

Creagan, E. T., Moetel, C. G., O'Fallon, J. R., Schutt, A. J., O'Connell, M. J., Rubin, J., et al. (1979). Failure of high-dose vitamin C (ascorbic acid) therapy to benefit patients with advanced cancer: a controlled trial. *New England Journal of Medicine, 301*(13), 687–690.

Diplock, A. T. (1995). Safety of antioxidant vitamins and Beta-carotene. *American Journal of Clinical Nutrition, 62*(Suppl.), 1510S–1516S.

Dragnev, K. H., et al. (2004). Retinoid targets in cancer therapy and chemoprevention. *Cancer Biology & Therapy, 2*(4 Suppl. 1), S150–S156.

Drisko, J. A., et al. (2003). The use of antioxidant therapies during chemotherapy. *Gynecological Oncology, 88*, 434–439.

Frey, J. R., Peck, R., & Bollag, W. (1991). Antiproliferative activity of retinoids, interferon alpha and their combination in five human transformed cell lines. *Cancer Letters, 57*, 223–227.

Fugh-Berman, A. (1996). Dietary supplements and nutrition. In *Alternative medicine: What works* (pp. 61–93). Tucson, AZ: Odonian Press.

Gershoff, S. N. (1993). Vitamin C (ascorbic acid): New roles, new requirements? *Nutrition Reviews, 51*(11), 313–326.

Hoffer, A., & Pauling, L. (1990). Hardin Jones biostatistical analysis of mortality data for cohorts of cancer patients with a large fraction surviving at the termination of the study and a comparison of survival times of cancer patients receiving large regular oral doses of vitamin C and other nutrients with similar patients not receiving those doses. *Journal of Orthomolecular Medicine, 5*(3), 143–154.

Hoffer, A., & Pauling, L. (1993). Hardin Jones biostatistical analysis of mortality data for a second set of cohorts of cancer patients with a large fraction surviving at the termination of the study and a comparison of survival times of cancer patients receiving large regular oral doses of vitamin C and other nutrients with similar patients not receiving these doses. *Journal of Orthomolecular Medicine*, *8*(3), 157–167.

Ingram, D. (1994). Diet and subsequent survival in women with breast cancer. *British Journal of Cancer*, *69*(3), 592–696.

Jackson, J. A., Riordan, H. D., Hunningkake, R. E., & Riordan, N. (1995). High dose intravenous vitamin C and long term survival of a patient with cancer of the head of the pancreas. *Journal of Orthomolecular Medicine*, *10*(2), 87–88.

Jaffey, M. (1982). Vitamin C and cancer: Examination on the Vale of Leven trial results using broad inductive reasoning. *Medical Hypotheses*, *8*, 49–84.

Knekt, P. (1991). Role of vitamin E in the prophylaxis of cancer. *Annals of Medicine*, *23*, 3–12.

Kurbacher, C. M., et al. (1996). Ascorbic acid improves the antineoplastic activity of doxorubicin, cisplatin and paclitaxel in human breast carcinoma cells *in vitro*. Cancer Letter, *103*, 183–189.

Ladas, E. J., et al. (2004). Antioxidants and cancer therapy: A systematic review. *Journal of Clinical Oncology*, *22*, 517–528.

Lamm, D. L., Riggs, D. R., Schriver, J. S., vanGilder, P. F., Rach, J. F., & DeHaven, J. I. (1994). Megadose vitamins and bladder cancer: A double-blind clinical trial. *Journal of Urology*, *151*(1), 21–26.

Lerner, M. (1994). Can vitamins and minerals help: The scientific view: Micronutrients. In *Choices in healing: Integrating the best of conventional and complementary approaches to cancer* (pp. 219–250). Cambridge, MA: MIT Press.

Lesperance, M. L., et al. (2002). Megadose vitamins and minerals in the treatment of non-metastatic breast cancer: A historical cohort study. *Breast Cancer Research and Treatment*, *76*, 137–143.

Lupulescu, A. (1993). The role of vitamins A, beta-carotene, E and C in cancer cell biology. *International Journal for Vitamin and Nutrition Research*, *63*, 3–14.

Meydani, M. (1995). Vitamin E. *Lancet*, *345*, 170–175.

Meyer, E. C., Sommers, D. K., Reitz, C. J., Mentis, H. (1990). Vitamin E and benign breast disease. *Surgery*, *107*, 549–551.

Micozzi, M. S., Brown, E. D., Taylor, P. R., & Wolfe, E. (1988). Carotenodermia in men with elevated carotenoid intake from foods and beta-carotene supplements. *American Journal of Clinical Nutrition* *48*, 1061–1064.

Moertel, C. G., Fleming, T. R., Creagan, E. T., Rubin, J., O'Connell, M. J., & Ames, M. M. (1985). High-dose vitamin C versus placebo in the treatment of patients with advanced cancer who have had no prior chemotherapy: A randomized double-blind comparison. *New England Journal of Medicine*, *312*(3), 137–141.

Morishige, F., & Murata, A. (1978). Prolongation of survival times in terminal human cancer by administration of supplemental ascorbate. *Journal of International Academy of Preventive Medicine*, *V*(1), 47–52.

Moss, R. W. (1992). Vitamins. In *Cancer therapy: The independent consumer's guide to non-toxic treatment and prevention* (2nd ed., pp. 27–86). New York: Equinox.

Norman, H. A., et al. (2003). The role of dietary supplements during cancer therapy. *Journal of Nutrition*, *133*, 3794S–3799S.

Omenn, G. S., Goodman, E. G., Thornquist, M. D., Balmes, J., Cullen, M. R., Glass, A., et al. (1996). Effects of a combination of beta carotene and vitamin A on lung cancer and cardiovascular disease. *New England Journal of Medicine*, *334*(18), 1150–1155.

Ontario Breast Cancer Information Exchange Project. (1994). Vitamins. In *A guide to unconventional cancer therapies* (pp. 117–136). Toronto: Author.

Padayatty, S. J., et al. (2004). Vitamin C pharmacokinetics: Implications for oral and intravenous use. *Annals of Internal Medicine*, *140*, 533–537.

Pastorino, U., Infante, M., Maioli, M., Chiesa, G., Buyse, M., Firket, P., et al. (1993). Adjuvant treatment of stage I lung cancer with high-dose vitamin A. *Journal of Clinical Oncology*, *11*(7), 1216–1222.

Prasad, K. N. (1980). Modulation of the effects of tumor therapeutic agents by vitamin C. *Life Sciences*, *27*(4), 275–280.

Riordan, N., Jackson, J. A., & Riordan, H. D. (1996). Intravenous vitamin C in a terminal cancer patients. *Journal of Orthomolecular Medicine*, *11*(2), 80–82.

Roberts, H. J. (1981). Perspective on vitamin E as therapy. *Journal of the American Medical Association*, *246*(2), 129–131.

Schmidt, K. (1991). Antioxidant vitamins and Beta-carotene: Effects on immunocompetence. *American Journal of Clinical Nutrition*, *53*(Suppl.), 383S–385S.

Shimpo, K., Nagatsu, T., Yamada, K., Sato, T., Niimi, H., Shamoto, M., et al. (1991). Ascorbic acid and adriamycin toxicity. *American Journal of Clinical Nutrition*, *54*(Suppl.), 1298S–1301S.

Smith, M. A., Parkinson, D. R., Cheson, B. D., & Friedman, M. A. (1992). Retinoids in cancer therapy. *Journal of Clinical Oncology*, *10*(5), 839–864.

Stahelin, H. B. (1993). Critical reappraisal of vitamins and trace minerals in nutritional support of cancer patients. *Supportive Care in Cancer*, *1*(6), 295–297.

Tallman, M. S., & Wiernik, P. H. (1992). Retinoids in cancer treatment. *Journal of Clinical Pharmacology*, *32*, 868–888.

Tengerdy, R. P. (1990). The role of vitamin E in immune response and disease resistance. *Annals of New York Academy of Sciences*, *587*, 24–33.

United States Office of Technology Assessment. (1990). Pharmacologic and biologic treatments. In *Unconventional cancer treatments* (pp. 90–126). Washington, DC: U.S. Government Printing Office.

Wittes, R. E. (1985). Vitamin C and cancer. *New England Journal of Medicine*, *312*(3), 178–179.

Willett, W. C., Stampfer, M. J., Underwood, B. A., Taylor, J. O., & Hennekens, C. H. (1983). Vitamins A, E, and carotene: Effects of supplementation on their plasma levels. *American Journal of Clinical Nutrition*, *38*, 559–566.

I n addition to the supplementation of individual nutrients and dietary constituents, complete dietary regimens have been developed to help support care of the cancer patient. Although many people with cancer have adopted various cancer diets over many years, evidence on their benefits has been limited. The best documented accounts are presented in detail, and reference is made to some additional cancer diets that are less well documented.

Marc S. Micozzi

## Macrobiotic Diet

Macrobiotics is arguably the most widely used alternative nutritional approach to cancer in the United States. Known for its primarily vegetarian, high complex carbohydrate, low-fat diet, macrobiotics also offers a spiritual philosophy embraced to varying degrees by many thousands of practitioners around the world. Michio Kushi is an influential macrobiotic teacher who has made significant claims for success with cancer. Kushi is a wide-ranging philosopher of human health, history, and evolution, reminiscent of Rudolf Steiner, founder of anthroposophy (see Iscador, Chapter 13).

### History

In its current manifestation, macrobiotics originated in the late 19th and early 20th centuries with an educator named Yukikazu Sakurazawa and a physician named Sagen Ishisuka. They reportedly cured themselves of serious illnesses by changing from the modern refined diet then transforming Japan to a simple diet of brown rice, miso soup, sea vegetables, and other traditional Japanese foods. After restoring their health, they went on to integrate traditional Oriental medicine and philosophy with Vedanta (a Hindu spiritual tradition), original Judeo-Christian teachings, and holistic perspectives in modern science and medicine. Some have asserted that Sakurazawa and Ishisuka never intended a spiritual basis and that later proponents of macrobiotics, particularly Michio Kushi, were responsible for the introduction of this element. When Sakurazawa came to Paris in the 1920s, he adopted George Ohsawa as his pen name and called his teachings macrobiotics. The word *macrobiotics* originally came from the Greek *macro*, meaning "great" or "large" and *bios*, meaning "life."

Before leaving Japan, Kushi studied briefly with George Ohsawa. It was Ohsawa's belief that food was the key to health. By returning to a traditional diet of whole, natural foods, he believed that humanity could regain its physical and mental balance. Although living in New York, Kushi experienced positive changes in his own health and consciousness after changing his own diet. Over the next 10 years, with the support of his wife, Aveline, he began to study traditional and modern approaches to diet and health and to teach macrobiotics.

In the 1960s, Kushi moved to Boston and founded Erewhon (one of the early natural foods distributors) to make available the foods necessary for a macrobiotic life-style. In 1971, his followers founded *East West Journal*, and the following year the East West Foundation was started to support macrobiotic education and research. In 1978, Michio and Aveline Kushi founded the Kushi Institute, with affiliate organizations throughout Europe. Aveline died in 2001 of cancer at a relatively young age.

Twenty-five years ago, Kushi decided to present macrobiotics with a major emphasis on its role in the prevention and alleviation of cancer. His son, Lawrence Kushi, PhD, a respected nutrition researcher, has commented that macrobiotics was generally seen in its role as a philosophy of life. Later it became widely known as a cancer diet. Michio Kushi also moved in that direction. Some would question whether that was the right decision, or whether cancer was necessarily the right disease, because a macrobiotic diet has not been scientifically demonstrated to be effective against cancer.

Macrobiotics and similar vegetarian diets are arguably preventive for those cancers most closely associated with a high-fat Western diet, although this relationship is not clear (see Chapter 8). These diets may some day prove to be effective for patients with some types of cancer, in inhibition or reversal of tumor progression, as well as extension of disease-free interval and overall survival after surgical or medical treatment. However, well-designed scientific research to determine whether, and in what ways, macrobiotics is helpful with cancer has not been done.

Kushi cites a number of intriguing findings from history and contemporary science. There is some evidence to support his view that a grain-based diet can relieve cancer and permit the patient to survive over time, that artificial infant feeding is associated with an increased incidence of breast cancer among mothers (see Chapter 9), that caloric restriction results in a lower incidence of breast cancer in animals, and that a vegetarian diet prevents breast cancer (see Chapter 8).

## Dietary Recommendations

Kushi recommended the following diet for breast cancer, with relatively small modifications of his basic cancer prevention diet:

- 50%–60% of daily consumption, by volume, should be whole-cereal grains. The most preferred are pressure-cooked small-grain brown rice, and frequently, millet or barley.
- 5%–10% soup, consisting of two bowls per day of miso soup or tamari soy sauce broth cooked with kombu, wakame, or other sea vegetables and various land vegetables such as onions and carrots.
- 20%–30% vegetables, cooked in a variety of forms.
- 5% small beans, such as azuki or lentils, may be used daily, cooked together with sea vegetables such as kombu or with onions and carrots.
- 5% or less sea vegetable dishes.
- Condiments (sesame salt, kelp, or wakame powder).

Finely chopped scallions are mixed and heated with an equal volume of miso and a small portion of grated ginger.

Kushi's dietary recommendations may provide a healthy and nutritionally balanced diet, but are based on a complex macrobiotic dietary theory that does not have foundation in medical science. The specific foods included and excluded by macrobiotics for cancer differ from those recommended by other systems of diet coming from traditional medicine (see Part 4). Macrobiotics has a dietary theory that is unproven from a mainstream perspective, and in many respects, contradicts other traditional dietary regimens, such as naturopathic (see Chapter 14) or Ayurvedic (see Chapter 16) dietary programs. Ayurvedic medicine from India, for example, gives dietary recommendations for cancer that differ from, and often contradict, macrobiotic recommendations (see Chapter 16). Systems of traditional medicine differ in detail but generally recommend fresh whole foods. Kushi's recommendation of sea vegetables is supported by suggestive scientific evidence.

## Kushi's Cancer Diet

Kushi does not call his approach a cure for cancer. Although he gives examples of patients who reportedly recovered from metastatic or otherwise life-threatening cancers using macrobiotics, the cases often include explicit evidence that misdiagnosis might have been involved or that the case was not entirely hopeless from a mainstream perspective. By avoiding the representation of macrobiotics as a cancer cure, Kushi has avoided serious conflict with mainstream medicine.

Other groups of practitioners who have avoided serious conflict with mainstream medicine are practitioners of traditional Chinese medicine. They have often been even more cautious than Kushi. They make no special claims about cancer; many practitioners even refuse to treat cancer; and those who do treat it emphasize the purely adjunctive nature of their treatment. As a result, tens of thousands of American cancer patients avail themselves of the supportive treatment of traditional Chinese medicine (see Chapter 15). Careful use of treatments outside the medical mainstream is one of the attributes of Asian culture, accustomed to taking the long view and to achieving goals by indirect means when direct confrontation would be counterproductive.

## Case Histories

Case histories, physician reports, and scientific studies that relate to the use of macrobiotics in cancer are limited. They are suggestive that macrobiotics may have some positive impact for some people with cancer.

One of the most credible independent accounts for a macrobiotic approach to cancer was provided by Anthony Sattilaro, MD, whose book, *Recalled by Life* (1982), describes his recovery from metastatic prostatic cancer. He underwent conventional therapy, but his physician told him that he had at best only a few years to live. Then he turned to macrobiotics, experienced a spiritual awakening, and subsequently recovered. The story of his recovery did for macrobiotics what the story of *New York Times* columnist James Reston's experience in China did for acupuncture. It brought an alternative therapy to public attention through a single personal account. Both authors had credibility. Reston was a respected reporter and columnist. Sattilaro was chief medical executive of Methodist Hospital in Philadelphia, having previously served as chairman of the anesthesiology department. After his initial recovery using macrobiotics, Sattilaro distanced himself from the macrobiotic movement, especially from its more spiritual components and its belief system. But his belief in the importance of his own spiritual awakening and the whole foods vegetarian diet persisted. Some mainstream critics questioned whether Sattilaro's cancer was as life threatening as he portrayed it. Sattilaro died of a recurrence of his cancer in 1989.

## Clinical Studies

Although the scientific literature contains no published studies on macrobiotics and cancer treatment, there are three unpublished studies, each of them flawed. Vivien Newbold, MD, documented the results of cancer patients who (1) used macrobiotics with or without chemotherapy; (2) used macrobiotics for pancreatic or brain cancers; (3) used macrobiotics for other serious illnesses; and (4) had documented cases of medically advanced, incurable cancer, followed macrobiotics, and recovered completely. She ultimately found six cases of complete remission from advanced malignant disease using both conventional therapies and macrobiotic diet. Newbold had the cases reviewed independently, and the diagnoses confirmed by pathologists and radiologists, and offered copies of clinical records to other researchers for confirmation.

### Pancreatic Cancer

Saxe and colleagues conducted two retrospective studies on the effects of the macrobiotic diet. The first study examined primary cancers of the pancreas to determine if patients following a macrobiotic diet survived longer than pancreatic cancer patients from the National Cancer Institute's SEER (Surveillance Epidemiology and End Results) cancer registry data from the same period. Pancreatic cancer was chosen because it has very poor prognosis, is rapidly fatal (therefore a relatively short period of follow-up is required to see evidence of life extension), and is a cancer for which macrobiotics claims positive results.

The 1-year survival rate was over 50% for the macrobiotic group compared with only 10% for the SEER subjects. Carter and Saxe observed that macrobiotic patients lived significantly longer than the nonmacrobiotic population but that this difference may have resulted from selection or other biases. They concluded that these results did not prove that dietary modification was the reason for the longer survival. However, they noted that these findings, taken together with several medically documented reports of remission in macrobiotic pancreatic cancer patients, was suggestive of a possible dietary effect.

### Prostate Cancer

In a second study, Carter and colleagues examined 11 cases of prostate cancer, all of whom were receiving conventional treatment and following a macrobiotic diet. The median survival of the macrobiotic group was 81 months compared to 45 months for the nonmacrobiotic population. In describing the study, the Congressional Office of Technology Assessment report *Unconventional Cancer Treatments* concluded that the same methodologic difficulties that were present in the first study also made it impossible to interpret the results of the second.

### Gastric Cancer

In 1981, Takeshi Hirayama of the National Cancer Research Institute in Japan reported that daily intake of soybean (miso) soup correlated with dramatically reduced gastric cancer rates in a large-scale prospective study of over 260,000 Japanese men and women. The standardized mortality rates for men who drank miso soup daily was 172 per 100,000 compared to a rate of 256 for men who never drank miso soup, with intermediate values for men who drank miso soup occasionally or rarely. The rates for women were 78 for daily miso soup drinkers and 114 for women who never drank miso soup. Hirayama noted that the results could result from beneficial compounds such as protease inhibitors or other nutritious factors in the soybean paste or that it could reflect other beneficial foods that frequently accompany soybean soup consumption, such as intake of green and yellow vegetables (see Chapter 10).

### Seaweed Studies

Two studies on seaweeds used in macrobiotics are of interest. Teas and colleagues (1984) looked at the possibility that brown seaweed (kelp), which is widely consumed by Japanese women, could be prophylactic for carcinogen-induced mammary tumors in rats.

Experimental rats fed kelp took almost twice as long to develop tumors as the control rats and had a 13% reduction in the number of cancers that developed. A second seaweed study looked at the role of polysaccharides from brown seaweed (kelp) in inhibiting the intestinal absorption of radioactive strontium.

## Macrobiotic Diet as Cure?

The macrobiotic program is clearly not a cure for cancer. If it were, the researchers who gathered cases for analysis would have found more examples. However, there are a considerable number of well-documented, unexpected recoveries, including recoveries from metastatic cancers. The available data suggest that the kind of person who chooses the rigors of the macrobiotic program may be likely, for psychologic reasons, to have a somewhat more optimistic outlook regarding quality of life and survival, in addition to the possible effects of the diet. These influences might approximately double the length of survival, which is the same rate reported by a number of mind-body interventions (see Chapters 4–7)

Lawrence Kushi has stated that it is not a macrobiotic diet per se that has an anti-cancer effect but any healthy vegetarian diet that does not contain substantial amounts of dairy products. It is surprising that the macrobiotic community has produced so little in the way of definitive research on the effects of macrobiotics on cancer. The available evidence is suggestive that macrobiotics may be of modest help in certain people with some types of cancer. However if we consider the biologic adaptation of the human organism (Chapter 8) it would be somewhat surprising to find a diet so heavily based on grains (relative latecomers to human dietary history) to be particularly healthy. The effect of the "hard fibers" in grains might also be found to promote cellular division in the gastrointestinal tract and not inhibit cancer, for example. On the whole, a health professional might be reluctant to endorse macrobiotics in the prevention or management of cancer based upon current evidence and understanding of nutrition and cancer.

# Gerson Diet

Gerson diet therapy was, for many years, the best known alternative nutritional therapy for cancer in the United States. Today, thousands of cancer patients practice diets based on Gerson's regimen. The Gerson Institute in Bonita, California (directed by Charlotte Gerson, Max Gerson's daughter), and the Gerson Clinic in Tijuana, Mexico, continue this work. Derived from a combination of research by German physician Max B. Gerson and European folk medical traditions, these therapies require a raw vegetarian diet for a prolonged period. Cooked foods and some animal products may be added later. A patient drinks specific freshly prepared vegetable and fruit juices every hour, takes four types of enemas, including coffee enemas, and also consumes two to three glasses of fresh calf's liver juice each day.

The Gerson regimen involves a significant level of personal commitment. It requires a full-time effort by a reasonably mobile and energetic person who does not have to work and who has access to the requisite fresh organic produce year-round. It works best when undertaken jointly by a cancer patient and a spouse or friend, and even then it is close to a full-time project for both people. The psychologic consequences of making and sustaining such a full-time commitment to physical recovery are potentially a significant element in the Gerson program (see Chapters 4–7).

*The U.S. Congressional Office of Technology on the Gerson Diet (1988)*

It is one of the least edifying facts of recent American medical history that the profession's leadership so long rejected as quackish the idea that nutrition affects health. Ignoring both the empirical dietary wisdom that pervaded western medicine from the pre-Christian Hippocratic era until the late nineteenth century and a persuasive body of modern research in nutritional biochemistry, the politically-minded spokesmen of organized medicine in the U.S. remained long committed to surgery and radiation as the sole acceptable treatments of cancer. . . .

The historical record shows that progress lagged especially in cancer immuno-therapy including nutrition and hyperthermia—because power over professional affiliations and publication (and hence over practice and research) rested with men who were neither scholars nor practitioners nor researchers themselves, and who were often unequipped to grasp the rapidly evolving complexities of the sciences underlying mid-twentieth-century medicine.

Nowhere is this maladaptation of professional structure to medicine's chang-ing scientific content more tragically illustrated than in the American experience of Max B. Gerson (1881–1959), founder of the best-known nutritional treatment for cancer of the premacrobiotic era. A scholar's scholar and a superlative observer of clinical phenomena, Gerson was a product of the German medical education which Americans in the late $19^{th}$ and early $20^{th}$ centuries considered so supe-rior to our own that all who could afford it went to Germany to perfect their training. . . .

## History

Gerson graduated from the University of Freiburg in 1901, having studied with leading specialists in internal medicine, physiologic chemistry, and neurology. By 1919 he had set up a practice and devised an effective dietary treatment for migraine, from which he himself suffered. In 1920, while treating migraine patients with a salt-free diet, he discovered it was also effective in lupus vulgaris [tuberculosis (TB) of the skin, then considered incurable] and, later, in arthritis as well.

His success with tuberculosis of the skin brought Gerson an opportunity to test the diet with larger numbers of TB patients at a special Bavarian government-sponsored clinic. He also served as a member of the State Board of Health in Prussia and as a consultant on how to restore depleted soils for agriculture. He learned that modern farming methods often rob plants of their natural mineral vitamin riches while increasing their sodium content.

## Cancer Cases

Gerson first used his diet for cancer in 1928, when a woman with bile duct cancer metastatic to the liver insisted that he put her on the diet, despite his reluctance to do so. The patient introduced him to a special soup that, according to German folk medicine,

Hippocrates had used for "cancer" and that Gerson later adopted for his own therapy. Gerson observed that this patient seemed fully recovered within 6 months. He had the same results with two patients with inoperable stomach cancer.

After the rise of Hitler, Gerson moved to Vienna, where he reported that the diet had failed with six cancer patients as a result of poor dietary supervision at the institution where he worked, in his view. He then moved to Paris, where he reported that the diet produced positive results in three of seven cases. He emigrated to the United States in 1938, where he continued to develop his diet therapy.

At a subsequent U.S. Senate hearing that was hostile to conventional approaches to cancer therapy, Gerson presented patients of his who had failed on conventional therapies. He received strong testimony of support from the medical director of Gotham Hospital, who also reported the results of a study that found that patients who received no treatment for cancer lived longer than conventionally treated patients. Another witness called Gerson's successes "miracles" and urged the senators to protect their further investigations against control by any existing medical organization.

## Opposition

Historically, this time was the period when the allopathic medical approach, through AMA, had recently established its hegemony over American medicine. The AMA advocated against promoters of unconventional cancer therapies with attacks on Gerson, Hoxsey (see Chapter 13), and other advocates of unconventional therapies. When faced with congressional hearings hostile to conventional cancer treatment, the AMA went on the attack. The AMA eventually destroyed Gerson's professional reputation, and Gerson lost his hospital affiliation and was denied malpractice insurance.

## Complementary Care

Regardless of the possible merits of the Gerson therapy, mainstream medical opinion at that time firmly held the view that nutritional therapies had nothing to offer for cancer treatment. To this day the evidence for definitive positive results from Gerson therapy remains highly questionable. In contemporary observations, the Gerson program emerges as a potentially useful *adjunct* to conventional cancer therapies. Gerson had allowed himself to become part of a very public critique of the medical establishment of this time, and he did not disassociate himself from testimony by others that his cases were "miracles." The AMA did not attack Gerson before he participated in this hearing before Congress. Prior to that time, he was able to develop a thriving medical practice using an alternative therapy for cancer and was affiliated with a New York hospital. The view of some advocates that Gerson discovered a "cure" for cancer and was therefore made an innocent victim of an unprovoked attack by the AMA does not stand up to scrutiny.

History cannot tell what would have happened if Gerson had quietly continued his practice, strengthened his contacts with the medical profession, and continued to publish a stream of professional reports in which he made it clear that his nutritional therapy for cancer was not a cure but deserved further evaluation as a useful adjunctive cancer treatment. It is common, among some of the best known practitioners of unconventional cancer therapies, to have a sense of mission that is sometimes accompanied by a sense of personal invincibility and self-confidence that can appear grandiose. Nor are charismatic leaders in mainstream medicine any more exempt from these particular characteristics.

---

*Elements in Gerson Diet Therapy*

- Salt and water management through sodium restriction and potassium supplementation
- High doses of micronutrients through frequent administration of raw fruit and vegetable juices
- Extreme fat restriction
- Temporary protein restriction through a basic vegetarian diet
- Thyroid administration
- Frequent coffee enemas

Raw calf's liver juice, an iodine solution, thyroid extract, extra potassium, pancreatin, and vitamin C were later added to the regimen.

In October 1989, the Gerson Institute issued instructions to all patients to substitute carrot juice obtained from growers in the United States instead of calf's liver juice. This decision was based on multiple outbreaks of bacterial infections at the Hospital de Baja California, where liver juice was part of the therapy. Liver juice had been added to the therapy by Gerson in 1950 since the nutritional quality of fruits and vegetables was declining because of modern farming practices. According to the Gerson Institute, the rise of modern organic farming holds out the promise of higher quality fruits and vegetables than were available during Gerson's lifetime.

---

# Other Perspectives

Gerson's therapy was long considered one of the prototypical "quack" cancer therapies. Later, as the nutritional research literature on cancer developed (see Chapter 9), an increasing number of physicians and researchers have been asking whether Gerson may have had something to contribute.

In 1971 it was suggested that a more favorable sodium/potassium ratio (such as that theoretically created by the Gerson therapy) might affect the cancer process. A series of studies, found evidence that the level of electrical polarization found in the membranes of healthy cells was significantly higher than that found in the membranes of proliferating cancer cells.

## Low-Sodium Diet

In 1980 it was suggested that Gerson's low-sodium diet, with its coffee enemas and thyroid supplementation, altered the cancer process with occasional clinical results in those patients with the stamina to undertake it.

In 1983, Ling wrote an article exploring the clinical implications of this emerging work and its possible theoretical basis. This line of research was seized on by Cope, in an article entitled "A Medical Application of the Ling Association-Induction Hypothesis: The High Potassium, Low-Sodium Diet of the Gerson Cancer Therapy" (Cope, 1978).

In a 1983 a Hungarian team performed x-ray microanalyses of intraoperative biopsy material from human thyroid cancers and compared these cells with normal human epithelial cells. They then compared the levels of sodium and potassium in the malignant and normal cells and found that increasing levels of sodium in relation to potassium were associated with increasing malignancy in the human thyroid, thereby supporting Cone's original theories.

## High Potassium

In 1985 it was reported that high concentrations of potassium altered the shape and growth of rat kidney cells infected with a sarcoma virus. High concentrations of potassium returned the cells to their normal structure. Other researchers noted positive effects of high potassium concentrations on cellular differentiation.

# Adjunctive Treatment

Lechner and colleagues (1987) at the Second Surgical Department of the Landeskranken-haus in Graz used a modified Gerson treatment for 4 years. They excluded the liver juice and routine thyroid supplementation. Patients did not take more than two coffee enemas a day no later than 5 p.m. to avoid disturbances of sleep. Four enemas a day led to colitis in three patients at the beginning of therapy. They used the Gerson therapy not as an alternative but as an adjunctive treatment, often combined with chemo and/or radio-therapies and with patients who had surgery. Diagnosis was verified by tissue biopsy. The 60 patients were both male and female, 23 to 74 years of age, with many types of cancer and many kinds of prior treatment. The Gerson program was given on an outpatient ba-sis, so the level of compliance could not be carefully assessed. Lechner found only a small percentage of patients willing to follow the modified but still restrictive Gerson program.

The Gerson patients showed markedly better tolerance for radiotherapy and es-pecially chemotherapy. They did not show alterations in liver or kidney function or depressions of red or white blood cell count. Clinical side effects such as nausea, vom-iting, loss of appetite and weight, and loss of hair were seen three times less frequently on the Gerson diet. In no case did the Gerson therapy lead to a complete remission, but two Gerson patients survived at least twice as long. An observation of improved *weight gain* in Gerson patients was intriguing.

Overall, Lechner found significant advantages for Gerson patients. Some lived longer. Others were healthier and had better responses to conventional therapies and fewer side effects, less pain, and better quality of life. Some of these advantages seemed directly related to the Gerson regimen. The psychological and physical characteristics that enabled these people to undertake the regimen may have played a part in the results (see Chapters 4–7).

## Contemporary Concerns

These findings are far from the dramatic results claimed by Gerson or claimed in his name by colleagues and admirers while he was alive, as well as leaders of the Gerson Institute after his death. At the same time, Lechner did use a reduced Gerson therapy, also combined with chemotherapy and radiation, both of which are immuno-suppressive. Any immune enhancement brought about by the Gerson program as an alternative therapy may therefore have been compromised by its use as complementary therapy.

Gar Hildenbrand, as director of the Gerson Institute, stated that the recent results obtained by the Gerson Institute are analogous to those Gerson himself achieved. Neither he nor other long-time observers of the Gerson program suggest that they achieve anything approaching cure in advanced cancer patients.

Albert Schweitzer said, "I see in Dr. Max Gerson one of the most eminent geniuses in medical history." In Gerson's writings, and writings about him, it is not difficult to see why he inspired admiration. He was a profoundly ethical man who helped redis-cover the healing potential of nutritional medicine based on the conventional scientific understanding of his time and on his own empirical experience. He sought to modernize and understand nutritional therapy in the context of a commitment to science and to his patients with cancer.

## Livingston–Wheeler Diet

Virginia C. Livingston, a physician who died in her late eighties in 1990, developed a multifaceted nutritional, medical, and immunosupportive program, which can be traced back in part to the German naturopathic tradition applied by Max Gerson. Livingston was an observer of the methods of others, including the Gerson program and other nutritional/metabolic programs in the San Diego/Tijuana area, one of the centers of alternative cancer therapies in North America. She was also a good friend of Josef Issels, a pioneering nutritional/metabolic practitioner from Germany, and also drew on his work. She can therefore be considered a "second-generation" nutritional cancer thera-pist, especially because fully half of her program is nutritional in content. Livingston's treatment has been offered at the Livingston Clinic in San Diego.

### History

Virginia Livingston was one of four women to receive her MD from New York University in 1936 and was appointed the first woman resident physician at a New York hospital—the prison hospital for venereally infected prostitutes.

In 1950, she and Alexander Jackson published an article in the *American Journal of Medical Sciences*, coauthored by four others, including James Hillier, developer of the electron microscope and head of electron microscopy at RCA Victor Laboratories in Princeton. They described how Koch's postulates could be satisfied in the case of *P. cryptocides* and that she had isolated a microorganism that caused cancer in both animals and humans.

In 1965, a friend convinced Livingston to try to help her husband, Wheeler, a physician with a malignant lymphoma of the thymus gland. She treated him with a vaccine cultured from his own blood as nonspecific immune stimulation, mild antibiotics, and diet. He died of a heart attack, after living almost 20 years longer.

In 1968 she founded what was to become the Livingston-Wheeler Medical Clinic. Over the 22 years from 1968 until Dr. Livingston's own death in 1990, the Livingston-Wheeler Clinic became one of the landmark alternative therapy clinics in the United States and one of the treatment centers of choice for many cancer patients seeking other options. It still provides the treatment originally designed by Livingston.

---

*"Dr. Livingston's Treatment, I Presume"*
- A primarily vegetarian whole-foods diet, with elimination of poultry products and prohibition on smoking, alcohol, coffee, refined sugars, and processed foods. Microbes thrive on sugar, iron and copper. Iron deficiency in a cancer patient is seen as a defense mechanism and a sign that something else is wrong, not a disease in itself.
- Fresh, whole-blood transfusion from a young, healthy person—preferably a family member—and gamma globulin (often of placental origin) as a source of antibodies.
- Splenic extract to increase the white blood count [and] enhance immunogenic systems.
- A variety of vaccines, including an autogenous vaccine prepared from the patient's own blood, BCG vaccine (Bacille Calmet-Guerin and attenuated bovine tuberculosis bacillus) to stimulate immune function, and other vaccines.
- A supplement program that includes vitamin $B_6$, $B_{12}$, liver, multiple vitamins, A, C, and E as effective anticancer agents. Trace minerals, especially organic iodine (such as that found in kelp), are prescribed. Additional thyroid is also given when tolerated.
- Antibiotics, which Livingston reports can sometimes shrink tumors but which more generally reduce the number of the reputed cancer microbial organisms circulating in the blood.
- A program to acidify the blood, because an imbalance toward the alkaline is observed in cancer patients. Hydrochloric acid in various forms can be given.
- Attention to dental hygiene with a view to eliminating dental, tonsillar, and sinus infections that may diminish immune function (an emphasis shared with the German cancer therapist Josef Issels).
- A program of frequent baths in a hot tub with one cup of white vinegar to help eliminate toxins through the skin, along with purging and enemas, which Livingston believed reduced the *P. cryptocides* population and contributed to detoxification.
- Enemas, including coffee enemas, and sometimes high colonics, for detoxification.

## Treatment Recommendations and Research

To affect the course of the disease, Livingston postulated, two courses of action are possible: One is to destroy the cancer cells and the other is to build immunity in the host to resist the infecting agent. The well-known destructive route is to employ surgery, radiation, and chemotherapy. Surgery is considered the most useful of the three methods because it physically removes as many cancer cells as possible so that the immunologic drain on the patient is lessened.

Livingston believed that radiation destroys immunity but had limited usefulness for localized lesions. She thought radiation was also useful in early treatment of some solitary cancers, in some metastatic lesions, and in some early lymphomas. The role of chemotherapy, she maintained, was difficult to evaluate but generally ran counter to the immunologic treatment of the disease. She viewed acute leukemia, premenopausal breast cancer, lymphoma, multiple myeloma, Wilm's tumor in children, and chorioepithelioma as cancers in which chemotherapy had a role, though often a restricted one. Even when chemotherapy is used, immunization should also be instituted at the same time or at intervals between short courses of chemotherapy. However, it was understood that the patient eventually survived only because of the stimulation of a potentially intact immune system. Everything else was of secondary importance. Livingston devised three diets for her patients: one for acutely ill patients, one for recuperating patients, and one for patients on a maintenance program.

## Three Diets

The strict diet (for acutely ill patients) included at least 50% raw foods (some patients were given completely raw foods diets for up to a year) and included up to a quart of fresh carrot juice a day, other fresh vegetable juices, whole-grain breads, whole-grain cereals, fresh fruits, nuts, baked or boiled potatoes, salad, homemade soups, and raw or freshly cooked vegetables. The diet was based on fresh juices, which, in addition to pure carrot juice, included carrot juice mixed with apple juice, spinach juice, cabbage juice, cucumber juice, beet juice, or tomato juice. The Livingston diet is similar to Gerson's diet, but more permissive.

In *The Conquest of Cancer*, Livingston presented cases that she said were selected "at random" from the clinic files. Livingston claimed that an examination of 62 "random" cases showed the success rate had been 82%. This claimed 82% success rate is not credible and is similar in its exaggeration to Gerson's claim of a 50% success rate with advanced cancers, as well as the claims made by many of the other alternative cancer clinics in the San Diego/Tijuana area. Grossly overstated claims of success are endemic among alternative cancer therapists. These claims greatly diminish their credibility and contribute to marginalization in the scientific and medical communities.

In subsequent work autogenous vaccine made according to Livingston's instructions is useful in reversing immunosuppression in cancer patients. Livingston's vaccine bears a resemblance to the Maruyama vaccine from Japan, which is perhaps the most widely used Japanese alternative cancer therapy. The Maruyama vaccine is similar to BCG, but derived from human tuberculosis rather than bovine tuberculosis.

## Quality of Life

It might be the opinion that Livingston probably did about as well as oncologists in the treatment of advanced metastatic cancer. It was found that there was no difference in survival between a group of patients with metastatic cancer and poor prognoses who were treated at the Livingston Clinic and a similar group treated with conventional therapy at the University of Pennsylvania Cancer Center. Quality of life was judged to be lower for those at the Livingston-Wheeler Clinic than for those at the University of Pennsylvania (see Chapter 19).

For patients with extensive disease and for this particular unorthodox treatment regimen, conventional and unorthodox treatments produced similar results. One way to interpret this observation is that patients should not waste their time and money on this alternative treatment. Another way to interpret this finding is that conventional treatments are equally doubtful.

The hypothesis that quality of life would be better in patients at the Livingston-Wheeler Clinic was based on the benefits that patients are thought to receive from the various aspects of unorthodox therapy, especially its self-care components, and on the absence of the toxicity often associated with chemotherapy. Popular media reports suggested that the surprise observation was that quality of life was worse for Livingston's patients, suggesting evidence for no dramatic benefit from the nutritionally based unconventional cancer treatments for patients with advanced metastatic cancer.

# Issel's Whole Body Therapy

Joseph Issels, MD, of Germany came to the conclusion that the only way to heal cancer was not to attack the local tumor as most conventional therapies do, but to strengthen the entire body. He developed "Ganzheitstherapie," or whole body therapy, combining many different modalities in a single protocol. Issel's program employed oxygen therapies such as hematogenic oxidation therapy. He shared many principles with the Gerson and Livingstone-Wheeler therapies, as above.

# Kelley–Gonzalez Diet

Some investigators have suggested that digestive enzymes may be useful in treating cancer patients. Based on early work by Beard and by Kelley, Nicholas Gonzalez suggested that digestive enzymes may be used as anticancer agents. The Gonzalez program consists of high doses of multiple proteolytic enzymes, although the program also includes patient-specific dietary modifications and vitamin and mineral supplementation. Gonzales presented a series of case studies to the National Cancer Institute, who encouraged him to pursue further study. With supervision from the National Cancer Institute (NCI), Gonzalez attempted a clinical trial in New York on patients with pancreatic cancer.

## The Kelley Program

In Kelley's program, patients receive a protease/amylase mixture orally, in incremental doses. The effects are often severe and can include flulike symptoms, fever, perspiration, shivering, headache, and nausea. Inflammation commonly appears at known tumor sites and other locations. At this point treatment is suspended until the patient's condition stabilizes and is then resumed. Coffee enemas are advised to stimulate the release of bile from the liver, thereby facilitating the transport of waste metabolites into the intestines for excretion.

## Case Reports

Evidence put forward by individuals identified strongly with particular treatments has generally been of a type not acceptable to the mainstream medical community. A common format is a series of individual case histories, described in narrative. The end points are often "longer than expected" survival times, sometimes with claims of tumor regression. In mainstream research, case reports of unexpected outcomes are useful and have a place, but they do not provide definite evidence of a treatment's effectiveness.

A series of case reports of 50 patients treated by Kelley with his nutritional program were described by Gonzalez in his book about Kelley, *One Man Alone: An Investigation of Nutrition, Cancer, and William Donald Kelley*. This series has been singled out by unconventional treatment proponents as one of the best of its kind that has been ignored by mainstream medicine. In 1990, the U.S. Congress Office of Technology Assessment carried out a review of Gonzalez' material by six members of an advisory panel consisting of three physicians generally supportive of unconventional treatments (none associated directly with the Kelley program) and three mainstream oncologists. Each case was assigned randomly to one unconventional and one mainstream physician.

Fifteen cases were judged by the unconventional reviewers as definitely showing a positive effect of the Kelley program, whereas the mainstream reviewers of each case found 13 of these unconvincing and 2 unusual. Nine cases were judged unusual or suggestive by the unconventional reviewers, whereas the mainstream reviewers found these cases unconvincing. Fourteen cases were judged by the unconventional reviewers to have been helped by a combination of mainstream plus Kelley treatment; the mainstream reviewers found 12 of these cases unconvincing and 2 unusual. Twelve cases were considered unconvincing to both the unconventional and mainstream reviewers.

The mainstream reviewers had similar general comments about the cases. The general conclusion, based on the material presented, was that it was not possible to relate results to particular treatments. Nearly all patients had mainstream treatment, which, along with the natural variability of the disease, might have been sufficient to account for the observed outcome. One reviewer commented as follows: "Those of us who have worked over the years with cancer patients have come to respect the vagaries of human biology wherein there are cancer patients who for unclear reasons fare better than we would have expected."

Another common criticism was that comparing an individual patient's survival with average group statistics is misleading and an invalid use of data. General comments of the unconventional reviewers were significantly different, and in general, positive about the Kelley treatment. One reviewer commented as follows: ". . . I would judge that the patients under my review appear probably, but not certainly, to have presented for the most part an unusual course, that the outcome exceeded normal management and that the effect of the Kelley treatment contributed significantly, although not necessarily exclusively, to the outcome."

What this review demonstrates most clearly is that some of Gonzalez's cases may be convincing to physicians already supportive of unconventional treatment but are not convincing to the mainstream physicians who participated in the OTA review and probably would not be to most other mainstream physicians. Key issues appear to be lack of adequate documentation of the course of disease and reliance on longer survival rather than documented tumor regression as an outcome in most cases.


## Clinical Trial

A Phase III study of the Kelley–Gonzalez diet was initially designed to randomize 90 pancreatic cancer patients to one of two treatment arms. The first arm was the standard treatment for advanced pancreatic cancer that cannot be surgically resected. It consisted of a drug called gemcitabine given intravenously for 30 minutes once weekly for 7 weeks. The second arm was called the nutritional arm in which patients received pancreatic enzymes orally every 4 hours and at mealtime for 16 days. Patients also received up to 150 pills daily in the form of dietary supplements such as magnesium citrate, papaya plus, vitamins, minerals, trace elements, and animal glandular products. Coffee enemas were also administered daily.

Only a few patients enrolled in the randomized trial and the design was changed to a single-armed, nonrandomized case-cohort study where patients only enrolled in what was the nutritional arm. Researchers planned to compare patients on the Gonzalez regimen to an accrued group of patients treated with gemcitabine, although such comparisons are difficult because patients selected for the newer or older treatments may not be entirely comparable.

In 1993 Gonzalez had submitted selected results of treatment with his nutritional therapy to the NCI. He had treated 11 patients with diverse cancers but the benefits from his therapy were not clear-cut. NCI felt that to determine whether the treatment was beneficial, a prospective study should be undertaken. Dr. Gonzalez chose to study pancreatic cancer patients because he had an impression that patients with this type of cancer benefited from his therapy. Five of 11 patients in the initial series, which was sponsored by the Nestle Corporation, survived for 2 years or more and the results were published in the journal *Nutrition and Cancer*.

Patients on the Gonzalez regimen lived an average of 17 months, which is nearly three times the usual survival period for patients with advanced pancreatic cancer. The patients who received his therapy may have had less aggressive tumors or may have been in better condition at the beginning of the study. However, observed survival seen in this series was sufficient for a group at Columbia Presbyterian Hospital in conjunction with the National Institutes of Health to attempt a prospective, randomized Phase III trial.

# Other Enzymatic Diets

Others have used multienzyme formulas to treat cancer patients. For example, in the 1960s, Shively treated patients using a combination of chymotrypsin, trypsin, amylase, pepsinogen, and desoxyribonuclease, administered intravenously. According to Shively, many of these patients responded favorably. In many cases, the tumors apparently became necrotic, detached from their surrounding tissue, and were easily removed by surgery. The most commonly treated tumors were carcinomas of the breast, gastrointestinal tract, and genital tract.

# Other Alternative Nutritional Treatments

Although not as extensively documented as the forgoing accounts, other selected alternative cancer therapies are mentioned below to illustrate the range of different alternative approaches that have been taken in attempts to address the problem of cancer.

### Coenzyme Q10

Coenzyme Q10 has been observed to prevent cancer and to reduce the size and metastasis of induced cancer. It improves the ratios of lymphocytes and immune function in experimental models.

### Monoterpenes

In the mid–1980s, it was observed that lovastatin, a compound that had been developed to lower cholesterol, appeared to inhibit cancer. Lovastatin ultimately failed to show significant activity against several tumors in human clinical trials. However, these findings led researchers to look for other compounds called monoterpenes, a family of chemicals that includes limonene, an oil found in citrus fruit peels. Certain food constituents may protect cells from attack by carcinogens. Monoterpenes appear to reverse the process of malignant transformation. Fruits and vegetables are likely to contain other as yet unproven, cancer-fighting compounds that could serve in prevention or treatment for cancer (Chapter 10).

### Revici Therapy

Emmanuel Revici, MD, based his treatment on correcting an imbalance between fatty acids and sterols in the cancer patient as part of a therapy he called "biological dualism." Revici was a dedicated physician and developer of selenium compounds as anticancer agent in clinical practice (see Chapter 10).

A variety of alternative cancer diets and dietary therapies have been advanced over the years and described largely in anecdotal and narrative reports. The available evidence for specific dietary regimens does not approach the level of evidence for individual nutrients and for specific foods.

## REFERENCES AND RESOURCES

Cassileth, B. (1991). Survival and quality of life among patients receiving unproven as compared with conventional cancer therapy. *New England Journal of Medicine, 325*, 1180–1185.

Cone, C. D. (1971). The role of the surface electrical transmembrane potential in normal and malignant mitogenesis. *Annals of the New York Academy of Sciences, 420*, 32.

Cope, F. W. (1978). A medical application of the Ling Association-induction hypothesis: The high potassium, low sodium diet of the Gerson Cancer Therapy. *Physiological Chemistry and Physics, 10*, 465–468.

Gerson, M. (1949). Effects of a combined dietary regime on patients with malignant tumors. *Experimental Medicine and Surgery, 7*(4), 299–317.

Gerson, M. (1954). Cancer, a problem of metabolism. *Medizinische Klinik, 49*(26), 1028–1032.

Gerson, M. (1977). *A cancer therapy: Results of fifty cases* (pp. 7–10). Del Mar, CA: Totality Books.

Gerson, M. (1978). The cure of advanced cancer by diet therapy: A summary of 30 years of clinical experimentation. *Physiological Chemistry and Physics, 10*, 449–464.

Hirayama, T. (1982). Relationship of soybean paste soup to gastric cancer. *Nutrition and Cancer, 3*, 223–233.

Kushi, M., with Jack, A. (1983). *The cancer prevention diet: Michio Kushi's nutritional blueprint for the relief and prevention of disease* (p. 17). New York: St. Martin's Press.

Lechner, P., et al. (1987). *The role of a modified Gerson Therapy in the treatment of cancer.* Unpublished manuscript, Second Department of Surgery, Landeskrankenhaus, Graz, Austria.

Ling, G. N. (1983). The association-induction hypothesis: A theoretical foundation provided for the possible beneficial effects of a low sodium, high potassium diet and other similar regimens in the treatment of patients suffering from debilitating illnesses. *Agressologie, 24*(7), 293–302.

Livingston-Wheeler, V. (1980). *Physician's handbook: The Livingston-Wheeler Medical Clinic.* San Diego, CA: Livingston-Wheeler Clinic.

Livingston-Wheeler, V. (1984). *The conquest of cancer: Vaccines and diet* (pp. 55–56). New York: Franklin Watts.

Newbold, V. (1988). Macrobiotics: An approach to the achievement of health, happiness and harmony. In Edward Esko (Ed.), *Doctors look at macrobiotics.* New York: Japan.

Regelson, W. (1980). The 'grand conspiracy' against the cancer cure. *Journal of the American Medical Association, 243*(4), 337–339.

Sattilaro, A. (1982). *Recalled by life.* New York: Avon Books.

Spain Ward, P. (1988). *History of Gerson Therapy.* Contract report for the U.S. Congress Office of Technology Assessment. (OTA), revised June 1988.

Teas, J., Harbison, M. L., & Gelman, R. S. (1984). Dietary seaweed (laminaria) and mammary carcinogenesis in rats. *Cancer Research, 44*, 2758–2761.

U.S. Congress Office of Technology Assessment. (1990). *Unconventional cancer treatments.* Washington, DC: U.S. Government Printing Office.

Zs-Nagy, M. (1983). Correlation of malignancy with intracellular Na-K ratio in human thyroid tumors. *Cancer Research, 43*, 5395–5397.

## 13

Marc S. Micozzi

## Introduction

As with nutrients, plants have figured prominently in complementary care of cancer. Some medicinal plants are used in isolation (e.g., Iscador and green tea) or in combinations (e.g., Essiac and Hoxsey). Some plants that we consider as foods (e.g., garlic) are here used medicinally.

A long list of herbs and other natural products has been considered with various mechanisms of action ascribed. In alphabetic order, they are aloe vera, arsenic, berberine, bromelain, *Bufo bufo* (toad), cartilage (bovine and shark), Chinese herbs (see Chapter 15), coenzyme Q10, cysteine, dimethyl sulfoxide, echinacea, feverfew, flax, garlic, genistein, ginseng, glutathione, horse chestnut (see Figure 13.1), limonene, melatonin, quercetin, and soy (see Chapter 9). They are thought to have anticancer properties variously through effects on anticarcinogenesis (e.g., horse chestnut and cartilage), cytotoxicity, cell differentiation, hormonal balance (soy), immune stimulation (echinacea), and various combinations. A selective review of the most clinically observed herbs and herbal combinations is provided.

## Iscador (Mistletoe)

Iscador is the trade name of the most commonly available brand and extract of *Viscum album*, a European species of mistletoe—a variety of mistletoe that differs from the North American species. Mistletoe was considered to be sacred in ancient times by certain Germanic tribes as well as by the Celts and Druids in Britain. It has been used in Europe as a treatment for a variety of both acute and chronic health conditions for centuries.

Figure
13.1

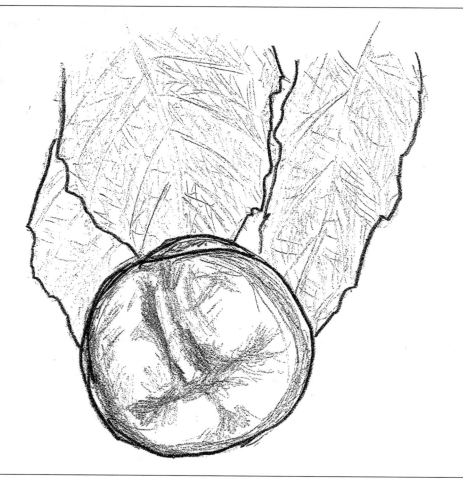

**Horse Chestnut** (*Aesculus hippocastannum*).

The use of mistletoe as a cancer therapy was popularized in the early 20th century by Rudolf Steiner, PhD (1861–1925). Dr. Steiner founded anthroposophy—a blend of spiritual and scientific concepts—and applied these principles to the practice of medicine with a particular focus on the treatment of cancer. Dr. Steiner theorized that the human body was subject to certain forces, some of which result in cell growth and multiplication ("lower organizing forces") and some of which control and organize cell growth to form tissues and organs in an orderly fashion ("higher organizing forces"). He believed that the balance between these forces determined an individual's susceptibility to cancer and that serious imbalance in these forces resulted in cancer.

Dr. Steiner studied the folk remedy mistletoe, a semiparasitic plant that lives symbiotically (in a mutually beneficial relationship) with several tree species. His observations of the biologic properties of mistletoe led him to propose the use of mistletoe extracts as a key component of cancer therapy. He observed that the overall shape of mistletoe is spherical when most other plants are vertical; its growth is not influenced by gravity, it has no direct contact with the Earth because, unlike most other plants, it has no roots. It produces berries all year long and flowers in the winter (thereby explaining its popularity in support of amorous pursuits in winter). Steiner considered these features to indicate that mistletoe exhibits more independence from natural, gravitational, and magnetic forces; shows "strong antagonism towards regular organization" and that it would stimulate the "higher organizing forces" that he believed were needed by cancer patients.

Iscador is prepared by fermenting an aqueous (water-based) extract of the whole mistletoe plant with the bacterium *Lactobacillus plantarum*. Following fermentation the product is mixed and filtered to remove bacteria before being packaged in ampoules for injection. The ampoules contain the active ingredient in specified concentrations ranging from 0.0001 mg mistletoe extract/ampoule to 50.0 mg mistletoe extract/ampoule.

Iscador and other mistletoe preparations are subclassified according to the host tree on which the mistletoe was growing and from which it was harvested. Some of these preparations are recommended for both men and women [e.g., Iscador P (from pine trees) and Iscador U (from elm trees)], whereas others are recommended for women only [e.g., Iscador M (from apple trees)] or men only [e.g., Iscador Qu (from oak trees) or Quercus].

Today, mistletoe preparations are principally advocated and used by physicians practicing in special anthroposophic medical clinics in Switzerland and Germany that have been operating since the 1920s and where in excess of 80,000 patients have been treated with Iscador. In several European countries and in South Africa Iscador is registered for commercial purposes and can be legally prescribed. It is not commonly used in North America but can be obtained from the manufacturer (Waleda AG) in Germany or Switzerland. Some North American patients travel to European clinics for this treatment, and there are several practitioners of anthroposophic medicine who prescribe mistletoe preparations in the United States and Canada.

As is the case with many alternative therapies, proponents of Iscador recommend it be administered as one component of several "holistic" therapies. Thus, at anthroposophic clinics Iscador is given in conjunction with selected artistic, movement, and dietary therapies all intended to strengthen "higher organizing forces" and enhance natural cancer-fighting abilities. These clinics recommend concurrent administration of required conventional therapies. Iscador is most commonly administered as complementary therapy prior to surgery or following completion of chemotherapy and/or radiation.

Some Iscador preparations may be modified by the addition of very dilute concentrations of various metals. These are claimed to enhance the action of Iscador on particular body organs and systems. For example, proponents recommend the addition of silver for the treatment of diseases of the breast and urogenital system; copper for diseases of the liver, gallbladder, stomach and kidneys; and mercury for diseases of the intestine and lymphatic systems. For cancers of the tongue, oral cavity, esophagus, nasopharynx, thyroid, larynx and extremities, Iscador without added metals is utilized.

Iscador is usually administered by subcutaneous injection. It may be injected into the abdominal wall or near the tumor site, if possible. In the case of cancer of the bladder, prostate, or esophagus, anthroposophic practitioners may inject these preparations directly into the tumor. Proponents state that in some cases (for example, in patients with tumors of the brain and spinal cord), Iscador may be administered orally, although a rationale for this difference in treatment protocol is apparently not established.

Proponents recommend that Iscador be used early in the course of the disease. Although Iscador may be administered to patients whose tumors are advanced and/or inoperable, the dosage and treatment regimen should be adjusted to take into consideration the general condition of the patient. Considering the possibility that Iscador is a cytotoxic agent and an immunomodulatory agent, close observation with appropriate lab work, including a complete blood count and standard chemistry panels, are appropriate for patients on this treatment.

A typical course of treatment requires that Iscador be administered daily early in the morning when the body temperature normally rises. However, some proponents recommend only three injections per week. Iscador is administered at gradually increasing concentrations in accordance with Steiner's protocol. In some cases it is recommended that a maintenance dose (which may often be quite high) be continued for many years depending on the individual's health and tumor status.

In the case of patients whose cancer is to be treated surgically, proponents recommend a course of injections 10 to 14 days prior to surgery followed by a maintenance dose of Iscador for a period of several years. Again, the dose and frequency of injection are determined by the general health and tumor status of the patient.

It should be noted that proponents of Iscador also recommend its use in patients who have certain conditions that may place them at increased risk of cancer such as ulcerative colitis, cervical dysplasia, leukopenia, Crohn's disease, papilloma of the bladder or colon, and senile keratoses.

Proponents claim that Iscador stimulates the immune system, causes cancerous cells to revert to more normal forms, improves general well-being and may improve survival especially in patients with cancers of the cervix, ovary, breast, stomach, colon, and lung. It is rarely claimed to reduce the size of solid tumors and is said to be less effective for nonsolid tumors, such as leukemia.

Following injections of Iscador, there is usually local inflammation (redness and swelling) at the injection site and an increase in body temperature that may be accompanied by headache and/or chills. No other evidence of toxicity has been reported. However, proponents note that the recommended dosages must be carefully followed as high concentrations may be dangerous. Several investigators have advocated the use of purified preparations of mistletoe lectins as a way of reducing the frequency of toxic effects.

## Evidence

Review of the literature to assess the effectiveness of Iscador includes review of the information available on all mistletoe preparations because many do not focus specifically on the preparation marketed specifically as Iscador.

Mistletoe preparations contain a number of biologically active constituents but these vary widely depending on whether the extract is crude or fermented, on the host species (variety of tree) from which the mistletoe has been obtained, and on the season in which it was harvested. These variations make it difficult to predict the likely effects of nonstandardized mistletoe preparations, including Iscador. Despite these difficulties, research over several decades studying biologic activity of mistletoe preparations in cell cultures, a variety of animals and among patients with cancer has identified two key components of mistletoe preparations as viscumin (also known as mistletoe lectin I) and viscotoxin.

Viscumin is a lectin (a complex protein/sugar compound that binds to cell surfaces) that can interfere with intracellular protein synthesis. Viscumin also stimulates the production of substances known as interleukins that in turn increase the number of white blood cells, which may help combat cancer.

Viscotoxin is similar to viscumin but has a different molecular structure and is cytotoxic and can cause cellular death. In addition to viscumin and viscotoxin, extracts of mistletoe contain a variety of other polysaccharides and alkaloids, some of which have been shown to have biologic activity.

## Laboratory Experiments

Several in vitro experiments have confirmed the biologic activity of Iscador and of other mistletoe extracts (which may not be bacterially fermented). Iscador appears to enhance the resistance of cells to damage caused by cancer causing substances. Its use is also associated with increases in immune function. The extent to which these effects are of clinical significance in humans is unknown. The use of mistletoe lectins as a component of cancer immunotherapy is currently under evaluation. At higher concentrations mistletoe lectins appear to have the ability to kill cancer cells. Mistletoe viscotoxins have been shown to increase natural killer-cell-mediated cytotoxicity (Tabiasco et al., 2002).

## Clinical Studies

In studies of patients taking Iscador there are several anecdotal reports of beneficial responses, including improvement in quality of life, pain relief, improved appetite, and higher white blood cell counts in patients exposed to chemotherapy or radiotherapy. Stabilization or reduction of tumor size, as well as increased survival, has also been reported anecdotally.

There are reports of some small case series and a few clinical trials. Results from the clinical trials have been mixed—some have suggested a beneficial effect (such as increased survival or improved quality of life) and some have shown no effect. However, all of the trials had significant design limitations, which make them difficult to interpret and seriously limit the value of their findings. Multicentered, controlled clinical studies evaluating the potential anticancer activity of Iscador have been underway in Germany. A cohort study recently evaluated the effects of Iscador mistletoe extract in cancer treatment (Grossarth-Maticek et al., 2001).

Iscador has been used in many thousands of cancer patients since the early 1930s. Although there is some evidence of biologic activity that might be expected to be beneficial to cancer patients, the evidence from human studies remains inconclusive. There is, therefore, no current scientific basis for the widespread use of mistletoe preparations. The absence of serious side effects combined with limited evidence that this agent may offer some therapeutic advantage, particularly in the area of quality of life, suggests further research is warranted (American Cancer Society, 1983; Becker, 1986; Berger & Schmahl, 1983; Beuth, et al., 1992; Bradley & Clover, 1989; Dixon et al., 1994; Gabius et al., 1992; Gawlik et al., 1992; Grossarth-Maticek et al., 2001; Hall et al., 1986; Harvey

& Colin-Jones, 1981; Holtskog et al., 1988; Jung et al., 1990; Kjaer, 1989; Kleijnen & Knipschild, 1994; Kovacs et al., 1991; Stipe et al., 1982; Wagner et al., 1986).

# Green Tea

Tea is a familiar drink that we may not consider as an herb, let alone as an herbal remedy. In many parts of Asia it has been used medicinally as a "tonic" (stimulant and digestive remedy) for 5,000 years.

Tea remains popular throughout the world and is still the most frequently consumed beverage after water. The term *tea*, although commonly used to describe the infusion that results when the dried leaves and leaf buds of the shrub *Camellia sinensis* are steeped in boiling water for 5–15 min, can also be used as a generic term for any infusion made from other plants, such as herbal teas, red tea, and so on. Green tea is one of the three main types of tea prepared from *Camellia sinensis*.

Throughout the world, approximately 2.5 million tons of tea are manufactured annually. Black tea accounts for nearly 80% of production and is prepared by drying and fermenting the leaves. This is the type of tea most widely consumed in Europe, India, and North America. Oolong tea is a specialty tea and comprises only 2% of production. It is only partly fermented and is consumed mostly in southeastern China and Japan.

Green tea accounts for nearly 20% of production and is consumed mostly in China and Japan. The leaves are steamed or pan-fried and dried without fermentation. Approximately 36%, by dry weight of green tea leaves is composed of polyphenols, principally flavonols (mostly catechins), flavonoids, and flavondiols. About 4% is composed of plant alkaloids, including caffeine, theobromine, and theophylline. Other constituents include proteins, carbohydrates, phenolic acids, minerals (including fluoride and aluminum), and fibers. The precise composition of green tea (and all teas) varies with the geographic origin of the leaf, the time of harvest and the manufacturing process. It should be noted that the constituents of black tea are different from those of green tea because of the oxidation process that is part of fermentation. In black tea there are fewer polyphenols and catechins are altered.

When green tea is taken for medicinal purposes, 1–2 teaspoons of the dried herb are steeped in a cup of boiling water for about 15 minutes. Up to 3 cups a day are consumed without the addition of milk or sugar, although recent research shows that the addition of milk to the tea apparently does not alter its medicinal properties.

The medicinal use of green tea has not been reported to have adverse side effects. A cup of black or green tea contains between 10 and 80 mg of caffeine depending on the type of tea and method of preparation. Excess caffeine may cause nervousness, insomnia, and irregularities in heart rate. Herbal handbooks advise that pregnant women, nursing mothers, and patients with cardiac problems should limit their intake to no more than 2 cups daily.

A possible relation between tea consumption and cancer risk has been explored by several researchers and reports of both increased and decreased risk of cancer associated with tea drinking among populations of tea drinkers have been published. There has also been a suggestion that the consumption of very hot or highly salted beverages, including tea, may increase the risk of cancer of the esophagus. However, when the International Agency for Research on Cancer reviewed the available information in 1989 it concluded that there was inadequate evidence to conclude that tea drinking itself presented a carcinogenic risk.

There have been a number of epidemiological studies suggesting that the regular consumption of tea, particularly green tea, decreases the risk of cancer, especially cancers of the upper digestive system. A chemopreventive effect for other cancers in humans remains controversial.

In lab studies, the effects of green tea have been contradictory and inconclusive showing both pro- and anticancer effects. However, a large number of animal studies, mostly using mice and rats, have demonstrated an anticancer effect of green tea given by mouth, by injection, or applied topically. Specifically, the application of extracts of green tea to mouse skin have been shown to inhibit the development of skin cancer in response to known skin carcinogens. Oral and intraperitoneal administration of green tea and green tea extracts have also been shown to reduce the incidence of tumors in animals exposed to carcinogenic agents.

Studies using extracts of green tea have suggested that the polyphenols present are responsible for this chemopreventive effect. Specifically the polyphenols have been shown to decrease the frequency of genetic damage in response to exposure to known carcinogens. Polyphenols are also seen to inhibit cellular proteins that may permit development of cancer (Leone et al., 2003). A particular polyphenol of interest is a flavonoid known as epigallocatechin gallate. This constituent is undergoing further research testing to determine the nature and the extent of its anticarcinogenic activity in humans.

The possible mechanism of action of the tea polyphenols against cancer is uncertain but there is some data to suggest that they function in several ways: as antioxidants decreasing the carcinogenicity of known carcinogens (e.g., UVB light and nitrosamines), by inhibiting enzymes involved in cell multiplication and DNA synthesis, and by interfering with cell to cell adhesion and by inhibiting some of the intracellular communication pathways required for cell division.

There is little research investigating the possible role of green tea in treatment of cancer. Some animal studies have shown that extracts of tea catechins injected intraperitoneally cause previously implanted breast and prostatic tumors to decrease. Several other studies have reported that green tea and green tea extracts reduce the metastatic potential of cancer cells. The capacity of cancer cells to spread to other parts of the body (i.e., their metastatic potential) results in most of the disability and death caused by cancer. The evidence that green tea extracts interfere with both the processes of cancer initiation and cancer promotion, and that they suppress chromosomal abnormalities induced by carcinogens, suggests that green tea could play a role in delaying the cumulative damage necessary for a cell to evolve from normal to cancer.

In summary, moderate consumption of green tea appears safe. There is some evidence that green tea may prevent the occurrence of some forms of cancer. There is preliminary evidence of the potential effectiveness of green tea as a supportive treatment for cancer and early studies suggest that further research would be warranted (Gao et al., 1994; Graham, 1992; He & Kies, 1994; Imanishi et al., 1991; Ito et al., 1989; Junshi, 1992; Kapadia et al., 1976; Kinlen et al., 1988; Komori et al., 1993; Lee et al., 1995; Leone et al., 2003; Oguni et al., 1988; Tewes et al., 1990; Weisberger, 1992; Yang & Wang, 1993).

# Red Tea

The consumption of teas (infusions) made from the African red bush (*Aspalathus linearis*) has long been a popular pastime in South Africa. The Afrikaans name for red bush is *rooibos*. This is the name that is becoming increasingly familiar to consumers in the United States. It is a replacement for regular teas and for green tea because it is caffeine free and lower in tannins, yet has an antioxidant profile similar to that of green tea.

The science on rooibos is increasing. Studies are demonstrating that rooibos is high in many of the ingredients that are proving of interest to cancer prevention, among them the natural constituents of plants that protect the body against oxidants. Many scientists increasingly feel it is important that antioxidants come from rich mixtures of biologically active compounds in plants rather than from isolated synthetic antioxidants. For example, studies on the isolated synthetic antioxidant beta-carotene did not show it to be protective against cancer (Chapter 10). Studies of mixtures of herbal constituents, as found in teas, appear promising.

Red tea specifically contains significant levels of antioxidants that are a possible explanation for its apparent health-promoting properties. Red tea has comparable amounts of the polyphenol antioxidants, such as flavonoids, that are present in green tea. It is thought that the antioxidant effect of green tea is partially because of these phenolic components.

Studies comparing rooibos with other teas found rooibos to have similar levels of the known antioxidants associated with green tea, for example. However, rooibos appears to contain additional active antioxidant components that are not present in green and other teas. Unlike green and black tea, for example, rooibos tea also contains additional polyphenols, such as certain flavonols, flavones, and other antioxidants. These antioxidants may account for the association of teas with anticancer and other beneficial effects. These effects persist over long periods of tea consumption. In addition, rooibos is reported to act immediately, most likely because of the presence of other active plant compounds in this tea. Botanically, as a legume, rooibos contains other plant chemicals that may account for its observed short-term effects in calming the nervous system and the gastrointestinal system and other widely reported effects.

The methods of preparation of rooibos can influence its activity, and the water-soluble component of rooibos also appears active therapeutically. As rooibos has no caffeine, unlike green tea and other teas, higher consumption of rooibos can be comfortably taken without known unwanted side effects. Red tea is more appropriate for children and others who should limit caffeine intake. Studies on red tea indicate this source is an effective way to get the benefits of many of the plant chemicals that appear to help protect against cancer (Marnewick et al., 2000).

# Pacific Yew and Hazelnut

In the late 1950s the National Cancer Institute (NCI) organized a nationwide search and screening program aimed at finding botanical sources with anticancer properties. To help accomplish this goal, the NCI turned to the U.S. Department of Agriculture (USDA), who agreed to send botanical experts into the fields and forests of North America to collect a large variety of plant samples for medical research. In 1962, during the search for medicinal plant samples, members of the USDA botanical team came upon the Pacific yew tree (*Taxus brevifolia*) in the state of Washington, where the small, bushy, needle-bearing trees grow in the wild among dense canopies of old growth forests (U.S. Office of Technology Assessment 1990).

USDA botanists collected and dried samples of the Pacific yew tree bark and needles and sent them to the National Cancer Institute, where research into yew's anticancer properties began. The cancer research on the Pacific yew tree spanned 30 years, leading to a specific anticancer ingredient extracted from the yew tree bark called *paclitaxel*. In 1992, Bristol-Myers Squibb introduced paclitaxel in drug form to the market under the trademark name Taxol, with significant success. Taxol is now semisynthesized and paclitaxel from the Pacific yew tree bark is no longer used as a source or constituent of the drug.

The Pacific yew tree contains many different types of natural anticancer plant chemicals called taxanes. Paclitaxel itself is a taxane, but it is only one of many taxanes that Pacific yew contains. The primary reason that the paclitaxel taxane was selected for cancer research was that it was molecularly less complex and could be isolated and studied. Taxol stabilizes microtubular formation, which inhibits depolymerization of tubulin subunits, resulting in the cessation of cell replication during metaphase. Pacific yew (*Taxus brevefolia*) has been analyzed for its anticancer activity and has also historically been used in its natural form as tea for treating kidney problems, tuberculosis, liver dysfunction, ulcers, and digestion problems.

Historically, Native Americans crushed Pacific yew tree needles to make salves for skin cancer, skin disease, and chest poultices for bronchitis. Needles and bark were brewed as tea to relieve headaches, dizziness, colds, fever, arthritis, rheumatism, wounds, internal injuries, and scurvy, as well as for stomach, kidney, and lung problems. People in the Pacific Northwest have been brewing tea from Pacific yew tree needles for many years as a natural remedy for health problems such as colds, flu, bronchitis, arthritis, rheumatism, and fungal infections, as well as skin problems, and various types of tumors, skin lesions, or cancer.

Recently, Pacific yew has been used as a dietary supplement for thousands of patients at the Bio-Medical Cancer Clinic (Mexico). Over 2,000 cancer patients have included Pacific yew tea capsules and salves in their treatments. Patients are advised to continue the yew in their diets for 1 year. Improvement has been reported with lung cancer patients who mist their lungs with the Pacific yew tea in nebulizers. The use of Pacific yew tree salve on a 63-year-old man with basal cell carcinoma was said to eliminate irritation and produce a 70% decrease in the size of his skin lesions that had not responded to allopathic treatment.

Obvious notes of caution exist for such remedies. Given the crude delivery of such substances, practitioners have limited information about the pharmacokinetics, serum levels, dosing, and toxicity as well as long-term consequences of use of the Pacific yew tree.

## Other Sources of "Taxol"

While trying to find ways to combat eastern filbert blight that was attacking hazelnut trees, researchers in Oregon "found something that looked like Taxol." The Pacific yew (*Taxus brevifolia*) and the needles of other *Taxus* species were the main sources of paclitaxel, and it was not generally known that the substance could be found outside the Taxaceae.

In her presentation to the American Chemical Society in San Francisco on March 29, 2000, Sister Angela Hoffman announced that she had found quantities of paclitaxel in at least 12 species of hazelnut trees and at least 8 species of fungus associated with hazelnut trees. Botanically interesting is the fact that the hazelnut is a flowering tree while the yew is a conifer, which are far apart in the plant world (Meserole, 2006).

This is potentially good news for cancer patients, because hazelnut trees are now known to provide another source for the drug, and it could become less expensive and more available. The research team found paclitaxel in the nuts, shells, leaves, limbs, and bark of the hazelnut tree. The hazelnuts themselves contain very low levels of paclitaxel. There is no evidence that eating hazelnuts regularly would be clinically relevant.

# Garlic

Garlic is a biologically active food with presumed medicinal properties, including possible anticancer effect (Figure 13.2). It is used as a whole food and as an herbal remedy or a natural product. In this context, garlic is covered in this chapter on natural products. Clinical studies of garlic as an herbal remedy or natural supplement in humans address three areas: (1) effect on cardiovascular-related disease and risk factors such as lipids, blood pressure, glucose, atherosclerosis, and thrombosis; (2) protective associations with cancer; and (3) clinical adverse effects. There are multiple clinical studies with promising but conflicting results. High consumer usage of garlic as a health supplement has persisted.

Scant data, primarily from case-control studies, suggest dietary garlic consumption is associated with decreased risk of laryngeal, gastric, colorectal, and endometrial cancer and adenomatous colorectal polyps. Single case-control studies suggest that dietary garlic consumption is not associated with breast or prostate cancer. No epidemiological study has assessed whether using particular types of garlic supplements is associated with reduction in cancer incidence. Preliminary evidence from a large cohort study suggest consumption of any garlic supplement does not reduce risk of breast, lung, colon, or

| Table 13.1 | Research Questions on Garlic |
|---|---|

- Whether oral ingestion of garlic (fresh, cooked, or supplements) compared with no garlic, other oral supplements, or drugs lowers lipids, blood pressure, glucose, and cardiovascular morbidity and mortality
- Whether garlic increases insulin sensitivity and antithrombotic activity
- Associations between garlic and precancerous lesions, cancer, or cancer-related morbidity and mortality
- Types and frequency of adverse effects of oral, topical, and inhaled garlic dust
- Interactions between garlic and commonly used medications

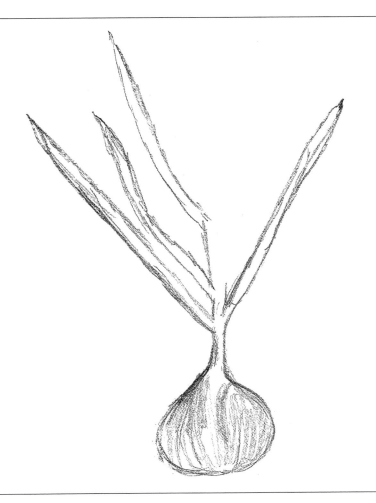

Garlic (*Allium sp.*).

gastric cancer. This study had not reported associations relevant to consumption of fresh or raw garlic, and its data about supplements are limited because information is not available about different types and brands of garlic supplementations.

Cholesterol levels have been related to risk of cancer as well as heart disease. Thirty-seven randomized trials, all but one in adults, consistently showed that compared with placebo, various garlic preparations led to small, statistically significant reductions in total cholesterol at 1 month (range of average pooled reductions 1.2 to 17.3 mg per deciliter [mg/dL]). Garlic preparations studied included standardized dehydrated tablets, "aged garlic extract," oil macerates, distillates, raw garlic, and combination tablets. Statistically significant reductions in low-density lipoprotein levels (0–13.5 mg/dl) and in triglycerides (7.6–34.0 mg/dL) also were found. One multicenter trial involving 100 adults with hyperlipidemia found no difference in lipid outcomes at 3 months between persons who were given an antilipidemic agent and persons who were given a standardized dehydrated garlic preparation.

Garlic has a range of biologic activities. Twenty-seven small, randomized, placebo-controlled trials, all but one in adults and of short duration, reported mixed but never large effects of various garlic preparations on blood pressure outcomes. Most studies did not find significant differences between persons randomized to garlic compared with those randomized to placebo.

Twelve small, randomized trials, all in adults, suggested that various garlic preparations had no clinically significant effect on glucose in persons with or without diabetes. Two small short trials, both in adults, reported no statistically significant effects of garlic compared with placebo on serum insulin or C peptide levels. There are insufficient data to confirm or refute effects of garlic on clinical outcomes such as heart attack.

Adverse effects of oral ingestion of garlic are "smelly" breath and body odor. Other possible, but not proven, adverse effects include flatulence, esophageal and abdominal pain, small intestinal obstruction, contact dermatitis, rhinitis, asthma, bleeding, and heart attack. The frequency of adverse effects with oral ingestion of garlic and whether they vary by particular preparations are not established. Adverse effects of inhaled garlic dust include allergic reactions such as asthma, rhinitis, urticaria, angioedema, and anaphylaxis. Adverse effects of topical exposure to raw garlic include contact dermatitis, skin blisters, and ulcerative lesions. The frequency of reactions to inhaled garlic dust or topical exposures of garlic is not established.

## Long-Term Use

Using any garlic supplement for less than 3 to 5 years was not associated with decreased risks of breast, lung, gastric, colon, or rectal cancer. Some case-control studies suggest that high dietary garlic consumption may be associated with deceased risks of laryngeal, gastric, colorectal, and endometrial cancers, and adenomatous colorectal polyps.

Notable limitations in findings from garlic research include the substantial variability in types of garlic and garlic preparations that have been studied and an inadequate definition of the active, biologically available constituents in the various preparations. In addition, many trials that evaluated the effects of garlic are limited by short durations, inadequate procedures, and lack of clear specification of contents of garlic preparations.

For the studies on associations between garlic consumption and cancer, some pertinent observations may be missed because they address associations with multiple foods and either did not report or analyze findings specific to garlic. Studies sometimes failed to distinguish the type of garlic exposure (raw, cooked, or specific supplement). Adverse effects in general are frequently underreported or reported in ways that do not allow causality and frequency to be determined.

Future studies to evaluate the effect of garlic on cancer and the main constituents of various garlic preparations must be established. Placebos designed to stimulate garlic odor should be assessed in trials. Trials that are longer than 6 months in duration and can assess cancer morbidity and mortality outcomes, as well as lipid outcomes, are needed.

Additional cohort and case-control studies that assess associations between garlic and precancerous and cancerous lesions are likely to be helpful if the frequency, types, and formulations of garlic that are consumed are specified clearly. Such studies should use sampling techniques that allow multiple levels of garlic consumption to be represented.

Consideration should be given to mounting more studies as in China, that evaluate the protective effects of different garlic preparations in persons with very high risk of cancer or precancerous lesions. Reviews in this area should search more broadly for diet-related population studies and aim to place findings specific to garlic in a broader context that takes into account findings regarding other allium-containing vegetables, as well as other foods.

The frequency and severity of adverse effects related to garlic should be quantified. Whether adverse effects are specific to particular preparations, constituents, or doses should be elucidated. In particular, adverse effects related to bleeding and interactions with other drugs such as aspirin and anticoagulants warrant study. Garlic is a common and widely consumed herb for which the evidence regarding its anticancer activities merit serious consideration (Junshi, 1992)

# Camphor

A camphor preparation called 714-X is an unconventional cancer therapy developed in Canada by Gaston Naessens, a French-born scientist and researcher, who worked out of a privately financed laboratory in Quebec for more than 30 years. Early in his career he developed a specialized microscope, which he called a *somatoscope*, that was said to enable one to examine fresh, unstained human blood and study the structure of blood cells at a significantly higher magnification than was possible at the time with ordinary light microscopes. When cells or tissues are examined under the microscope, they are usually preheated with various dyes or stains that help the observer to see the various components of the cells or tissues more clearly. However, this pretreatment process may distort cell structures. The later development of the electron microscope, which allows even higher magnification (although it does not allow the examination of fresh, unstained tissues), displaced interest in the somatoscope and other similar microscopes that used a technique known as dark-field microscopy. Using his somatoscope to examine fresh blood from healthy individuals and those with various diseases, Naessens reported that he could identify entities that he called *somatids* in the blood of individuals with serious disease, including cancer. He believed somatids to be live organisms distinct from bacteria and viruses and he described a life cycle for these organisms—the *somatidian cycle*. Specifically, he identified two distinct life cycles for the somatids—a *microcycle* consisting of three forms, which he observed in healthy individuals, and a more complex *macrocycle* consisting of 16 forms, in which somatids occur in a wide variety of shapes, some resembling bacteria, yeasts, and fungi. He stated that he usually observed this more complex life cycle in individuals with degenerative diseases, including cancer, and claimed to be able to diagnose and monitor disease processes by observing the number and forms of somatids in the blood.

Based on his own research studies, he developed the theory that the complex life cycle of the somatid only occurred when disease processes had damaged the immune system and altered the nature of the intercellular fluids. He considered that when stress or some other environmental factor initiated the somatid macrocycle the somatids secrete "toxic" substances and growth hormones (that he called *trephones*) that disrupt normal cell metabolism and cell division. He stated that under these circumstances cells become more primitive, derive their energy anaerobically, and may become cancerous. Rapidly growing cells also deplete the body of nitrogen and could be thought of as acting as "nitrogen traps." He also believed that the metabolic disruption of immune cells caused by the somatidian macrocycle incapacitates them from effectively fighting disease and thus allows the disease to progress more rapidly.

This theory of disease in which somatids play a central role is not consistent with current thinking about the causes of diseases in general or cancer in particular. However, a number of researchers have long believed that certain bacteria, viruses, and other organisms, such as cell wall-deficient bacteria, play a more important role in the development of cancer than is generally accepted (see Chapters 1 and 2). These are bacteria that assume a variety of shapes or forms because their cell walls or boundaries are deficient in their structure. Cell wall-deficient bacteria are also sometimes known as pleomorphic organisms. Although Naessens did not hold that somatids cause cancer (or other degenerative disease), he considered their presence to be associated with degenerative diseases and regarded them as indicators of disease progression.

Although Naessens, over the years, developed a number of substances (ISO 142, Pacikom, Anablast, and 714-X) for use in the management of cancer and other conditions, this chapter focuses on so-called 714-X, the agent that is made available to cancer patients. He considered that the agent 714-X interferes with the somatidian cycle, permits recovery of the immune system and allows diseases, such as cancer, to regress. He also claimed that 714-X administered to cancer patients can decrease tumor size and the discomfort sometimes associated with cancer while improving appetite and the individual's overall sense of well-being.

The name of this agent (714-X) reflects a proprietor's ample pride in its creation. The numbers 7 and 14 stand for G and N ( Naessens's initials), which are the 7th and 14th letters of the alphabet, respectively. The X stands for 1924, the year of Naessens's birth, X being the 24th letter in the alphabet.

The base of 714-X is a camphor compound that has been chemically combined with nitrogen as well as ammonium salts, sodium chloride, and ethanol. Camphor is a natural product derived from the shrub *Cinnamomum camphora*. Naessens selected camphor as the base of 714-X because he believed it has a special affinity for cancer cells. He added nitrogen because of his observation that cancer cells were "nitrogen traps" and considered that, if their needs for nitrogen were met by 714-X, the immune cells would avoid nitrogen depletion and recover to fight disease again. He also considered that nitrogen-enriched camphor decreases the cancer cells' secretion of "cocancerogenic K factor" (CKF), a substance that he believed inhibits the immune functions that would normally control cancer. Proponents state that they have isolated "CKF" but they have not provided information on its biochemical structure, and thus, other researchers have not been able to evaluate its presence and activity. Naessens also believed that the lymphatic fluid of patients with cancer becomes thickened and creates blockages in the lymphatic system. He included ammonium sulfate salts in 714-X because he believed these serve to liquefy the lymph and allow it to flow through the lymphatic system more easily. He also considered that the ammonium salts in 714-X activate certain substances released by the immune system that inhibit abnormal cell growth and enhance the healthy functioning of the immune system. 714-X is prepared as a sterile solution with the same pH as the blood.

The principle proponent of 714-X has been Gaston Naessens, assisted by his stepsons, Stephan and Daniel Sdicu, and his research associate, Jacinthe Levesque. 714-X is available by prescription under the Emergency Drug Release Program of Health Canada when prescribed for a specific patient on compassionate grounds. The Canadian Health Protection Branch has not received the documentation of safety and efficacy required to approve 714-X for general therapeutic use. 714-X is also available in Mexico and Western Europe (distributed by the Centre D'Orthobiologie Somatidienne de l'Estrie, Inc., a Naessens enterprise) but not in the United States, where it has been under investigation by the Food and Drug Administration (FDA).

714-X is administered by injection, usually into the lymph nodes in the groin. This is a very unusual route of administration for a drug and most health care providers require special instruction to enable them to do it safely and effectively. The proponents have developed training materials (videos and printed matter) to allow caregivers to administer the agent or to allow a patient to self-administer. The area surrounding the injection site is cooled with ice packs prior to and following the injection to minimize discomfort. More recently, proponents have suggested that 714-X can be administered by nasal inhalation. In this case, 714-X is administered using a "nebulizer" similar to that used by patients with asthma. The solution consists of 0.6cc 714-X and 1.9cc saline and is recommended for patients with lung or oral cancer. Naessens does not recommend that 714-X be administered intravenously or by mouth.

Naessens and his colleagues advise that 714-X be administered each morning by injection for a least three cycles of 21 days each. A rest period of 3 days should follow each 21-day treatment cycle. Seven to 12 treatment cycles are recommended for patients with advanced cancer.

Naessens and his colleagues recommend that 714-X be used by patients with several diseases, including cancer and AIDS. They state that it can be given in conjunction with conventional therapies. Although they recommend that it be given as early as possible in the course of disease, they consider that 714-X is more likely to be beneficial in patients who have not received chemotherapy or radiation therapy. They further advise that 714-X not be administered to patients receiving vitamin B or vitamin E supplements and that no alcohol be consumed during treatment.

714-X appears to cause few side effects, although local redness, tenderness, and swelling are common at the injection site, particularly when the injection process has been difficult. There have been no published reports of infection, local or systemic, associated with the use of 714-X. An animal study found that 714-X was well tolerated and there were no noticeable side effects.

Many individuals have provided anecdotal reports of success with the use of 714-X for cancer and other disease, including AIDS. Although these testimonials are of interest, they are not reliable evidence of the effectiveness of 714-X. It is very difficult, when evaluating testimonials, to confirm the diagnosis and the stage of disease at the outset and end of treatment; assess the impact of other therapies (conventional and unconventional) that might have been used; formally evaluate outcomes such as survival, tumor growth, tumor spread or quality of life; or to compare the reported results with those of similar patients who did not use 714-X. Nonetheless, many individuals remain convinced that 714-X has helped them survive longer or better. Many of these individuals have felt so strongly about the benefits of 714-X that they have incurred significant cost and inconvenience to support Naessens in court and elsewhere when his practices have been challenged.

Naessens and his colleagues have tried to maintain appropriate follow-up of individuals who have received 714-X but they have found the data difficult to obtain from patients and their caregivers. Accordingly, their information is incomplete. There have been very few published animal studies of the safety and/or effectiveness of 714-X and those that have been conducted have shown no beneficial effect. However, it should be noted that in these studies 714-X was administered intraperitoneally or intratumorally (directly into the tumor) rather than intralymphatically (into the lymphatic system), which is the route recommended by Naessens. At the recommended dosage, toxic effects have been minor.

A few animal studies using camphor have demonstrated some anticancer activity, specifically a positive effect on some measures of immune function, on enzymes that breakdown carcinogens, and on increasing the susceptibility of cells to radiation. This latter effect may offer some advantage if radiotherapy is employed. However, research into the effects of camphor remains at an early stage.

There is one unpublished study involving administration of 714-X to dogs and cows that developed spontaneous lymphoma. The investigators encountered several difficulties in the course of the study but were not able to demonstrate any benefit associated with the administration of 714-X in animals with this type of cancer. Clinical studies, case series, or clinical trials of the safety and effectiveness of 714-X have not been done. A "best case series," the complete data collection and follow-up on a limited number of cases considered by proponents to be their most convincing examples of success has been considered but not completed.

In summary, 714-X is a Canadian alternative cancer therapy whose use has been increasing over the past 30 years, particularly among patients with breast and prostate cancer. Its formulation and administration are based on unconventional views about the causes of cancer that are not substantiated by mainstream researchers. There are many anecdotal reports of successful outcomes among patients who have used 714-X, although there are no formal clinical studies, animal studies, or in vitro studies documenting its effectiveness.

To further evaluate 714-X, additional laboratory research in parallel with a best case series may be helpful. New information yielded by such studies would likely help in designing a future clinical trial. Proponents of 714-X have expressed an interest in a willingness to participate in research designed to assess its safety and effectiveness. Theories of cancer etiology that incorporate a role for organisms such as bacteria, viruses, and cell wall-deficient organisms may also merit further investigation.

Finally, further exploration of the potential of Naessens's somatoscope (and/or the adaptor he developed in 1991 for standard light microscopes) as a tool to assist in the diagnosis, treatment monitoring, and understanding of cancer may be justified. It is possible that the effects of 714-X are primarily related to the natural product camphor (Banerjee, 1995; Bird, 1991; Gibson et al., 1989; Goel & Rao, 1998).

# Essiac

Essiac, a mixture of a least four different herbs, has been used widely since the 1920s. The original recipe is said to have been formulated in northern Ontario by an Ojibwa healer "to purify the body and place it back in balance with the great spirit." The four main herbs in Essiac, burdock root (*Arctium lappa*), Indian rhubarb (*Rheum palmatum*), also known as turkey rhubarb, sheep sorrel (*Rumex acetosella*), and the inner bark of slippery elm (*Ulmus fulva* or *Ulmus rubra*), have also been used individually in North America among immigrants from Britain and Europe since the early 18th century. Burdock root is also a component of another unconventional therapy—the Hoxsey dietary regimen (see Hoxsey Method in this chapter)

Proponents of Essiac claim that it strengthens the immune system, improves appetite, relieves pain, and improves overall "quality of life" of cancer patients. They also claim that it may reduce tumor size and may prolong the lives of people with many types of cancer.

In the 1920s, the recipe was given to Rene Caisse, a nurse working in Bracebridge, Ontario, by a woman who believed to have been cured of breast cancer many years earlier. She had received the recipe for the herbal tea from an Ojibwa healer. Mrs. Caisse named the herbal mixture *Essiac* (her surname spelled backwards), and she prepared and administered it to several hundred cancer patients over a 40-year period. She modified the formula and reportedly administered one herb by injection, in or near the tumor site when this was possible, and the other three herbs as a tea. The recipe was further modified in the 1950s through 1970s by Rene Caisse working in partnership with an American physician, Dr. Charles Brusch. Four additional herbs (watercress, blessed thistle, red clover, and kelp) were included on the basis of a number of experiments to enhance the action of Essiac, improve its taste, and allow all herbs to be administered orally.

In Canada, Essiac was manufactured by Resperin Corporation, who obtained a formula for Essiac from Mrs. Caisse shortly before her death in 1978. It is now manufactured by Essiac Products in Brunswick and is available directly from the manufacturer or through the Emergency Drug Release program of Health Canada. Another product, Flor-Essence, manufactured in British Columbia, is said to be based on recipes provided by Rene Caisse and Dr. Charles Brusch to Mrs. Elaine Alexander and is widely available through health food stores. The proponents and manufacturers of Flor-Essence are careful not to make claims that it is useful as a cancer therapy. Rather, they promote it as a health enhancing herbal tea.

Different information sources recommend different methods of preparation and dosage. For example, some formulations require spring or nonfluoridated water, and most require refrigeration after brewing. Manufacturers usually recommend that the tea be taken one to three times a day. Because Essiac may cause nausea, vomiting, and diarrhea if taken with food or soon after meals, proponents recommend that it be taken 2 or 3 hours after meals or a least 1 hour before meals.

Most individuals trying Essiac today use it as an addition to conventional treatments or as a component of care for terminal disease after the completion of conventional chemotherapy and radiotherapy. Proponents advise the Essiac is compatible with all other cancer treatment modalities, including chemotherapy and radiation.

There are many anecdotal or testimonial reports describing positive outcomes associated with the use of Essiac in individual patients, some of which have been corroborated by physicians. However, the fact that these reports rarely classify patients by diagnosis or by the stage of their disease as a measure of extent to which the cancer is advanced makes comparison with the results of conventional treatment difficult. In addition, most reports do not provide information on a complete series of patients treated with Essiac, including those who did and those who did not experience benefits in terms of survival. For this reason, the clinical value of Essiac as compared to conventional treatments has not been clearly established.

There is some evidence from laboratory research that each of the main herbs found in the Essiac formula have some biologic activity. However, herbalists believe that the synergistic interaction of herbal ingredients (i.e., the combined effect of the constituent herbs) is critical to their beneficial treatment effects and to the control of side effects. The proponents of Essiac also claim that its effect is dependent on the herbs being present in the correct proportions, in accordance with approved recipes. They caution that laboratory tests of single compounds, isolated from a complex formula, fail to detect possible synergistic effects resulting from the interaction of the components in a living organism. Laboratory evidence of effectiveness is established by applying an agent directly to cancer cells; it will not necessarily have the same effect when the agent is injected or ingested and metabolized in the body. Laboratory studies, using cells or animals, provide a useful indication, but not a guarantee, of the effectiveness of an agent when administered to people.

Some plant constituents found in Essiac herbs, specifically polyphenols, flavones, and polysaccharides, present in all four of the constituent herbs of Essiac, have been shown to have some antitumor and immunomodulatory activity in preliminary studies.

Studies of the four major herbs in Essiac have shown preliminary evidence of biologic activity:

### Burdock root (*Arctium lappa*)

A purified extract of burdock injected into mice with transplanted solid tumors has been reported to result in tumor inhibition, slowing the growth or spread of tumor. In another study burdock was shown to reduce the ability of an agent to cause changes in the DNA of chromosomes in cell systems. Other laboratory studies have been negative.

There have been some unconfirmed reports of possible burdock toxicity. The most common side effects are those characteristic of the plant alkaloid atropine—disorientation, flushing of the skin, and the enlargement of the pupils. However, it is not clear whether these symptoms were because of burdock root toxicity or contaminants in the preparation of the specific mixtures administered to the patients.

### Indian or turkey rhubarb (*Rheum palmatum*)

Extracts of rheum palmatum have been shown to cause significant tumor necrosis in a mouse study.

Another constituent of plants in the rhubarb family—aloe emodin, a naturally occurring anthraquione (a class of chemicals already used as drugs)—has been tested in mice lymphocytic leukemia and shown to have tumor inhibition properties. The activity of aloe emodin in this study varied with the extraction method used to remove and concentrate aloe emodin for testing purposes. This emphasizes the need to consider the extraction methods used, as well as the strength and potency of herbal extracts when evaluating and interpreting experiments on these agents. Some studies have suggested that emodin itself, at high doses, is a carcinogen; however, other studies have shown that it has anticancer properties when taken orally. The role of aloe emodin and indeed most other anthraquinones as anticancer agents remains uncertain and controversial.

Slippery Elm (*Ulmus fulva or Ulmus rubra*)
This plant is known to contain a number of fatty acids and fatty acid esters.
Although the specific fatty acids and fatty acid esters in slippery elm have not been tested, similar fatty acids and fatty acid esters have been shown to have toxic activity in cell systems and in mouse studies.

Sheep Sorrel (*Rumex acetosella*)
Caisse considered this herb to be the most potent herb in the Essiac mixture. It has been used for centuries by healers in many countries and is known to contain a number of biologically active constituents. However, no cancer-related laboratory studies investigating this herb were found.

## Essiac as an Herbal Mixture

There are a number of unpublished papers and letters reporting on laboratory tests using Essiac. Rene Caisse and Charles Brusch claim to have conducted studies in their efforts to refine the formula for Essiac. Unfortunately, the results of these studies have not been published. However, in a letter Dr. Brusch reported that the herbs had to be used together rather than separately to achieve an effect. Some of the other reports have yielded positive results but none of the available studies can be considered definitive Laboratory studies of Essiac conducted by Memorial Sloan-Kettering (MSK) laboratories were carried out in 1959 and from 1973 to 1976. However, the researchers encountered difficulties with their test systems, as well as with the necessary collaboration and information-sharing between Rene Caisse and MSK. Therefore they were unable to ensure that the tests of the herbal mixtures or individual herbs were appropriate or to reach any definite conclusions. Other reports are incorporated into unpublished personal correspondence and provide preliminary evidence of effectiveness. For instance, in one study mice injected with human carcinoma cells and then treated with intravenous Essiac showed more tumor necrosis and degradation than control mice. Unfortunately, these studies were never completed or published.

An unpublished Canadian study, in the late 1970s, using an oral Essiac preparation found no evidence of an effect on the cancer process but some subjective improvements in quality of life. No formal clinical studies demonstrating any observed positive outcomes in cancer patients can be attributed to the use of Essiac rather than to other therapies or to the natural history of the disease. Health Canada gave permission for Essiac to be tested for its safety and effectiveness in 1978 but withdrew this permission in 1982 when it became clear that the research was not proceeding according to plan. At the time they reviewed available, but incomplete, data derived from patients who had received Essiac during 1978–1982, they were unable to find clear evidence of improved survival. They did not evaluate other outcomes such as pain control and quality of life. However, because there was no evidence of harm, Health Canada continues to permit the release of this agent on compassionate grounds and it continues to be available in Canada as it has since the 1920s. There is weak evidence of effectiveness and little evidence of harm, and. although Essiac is a widely used agent, it remains incompletely studied (Bryson 1978, Bryson et al 1978, Caisse 1938, Rhoads et al 1985).

# Hoxsey Method

A similar herbal mixture to Essiac is the Hoxsey treatment. Harry Hoxsey (1901–1974) popularized his great-grandfather's herbal formula, which had reputedly cured horses of cancer. His formula included bloodroot, burdock, buckthorn, cascara, barberry, licorice, red clover, pokeroot, zinc chloride, and antimony trisulfide. Hoxsey's controversial style led to many encounters with federal officials and the American Medical Association. At one time, Hoxsey had thousands of cancer patients going to 17 clinics across the country. With continued pressure from officials, Hoxsey was forced to close his Dallas clinic in the late 1950s and moved to Mexico to continue practicing. Hoxsey's general formula has appeared in topical ointments used to "burn away" surface skin cancers. The use of red clover in the Hoxsey mixture is of particular interest in light of recent research.

# Red Clover (*Trifolium pratense*)

Red clover has been used since antiquity as a treatment for skin disorders and minor respiratory ailments. The National Formulary listed red clover as a skin remedy until the mid-1900s. In the 1940s, the flower heads found their way into Harry Hoxey's controversial anticancer formula, together with numerous other plants. Red clover contains formononetin, biochanin A, daidzein, genistein, and coumestrol, substances that act as weak estrogens in the body (see Chapter 10). Constituents within red clover have been shown to alter vaginal cytology, increase follicle stimulating hormone, and reduce luteinizing hormone in animal models. Sheep in Australia grazing on a related clover (*T. subterraneum*) developed "clover disease," a condition associated with abnormal lactation, infertility, and prolapsed uterus. These adverse effects were thought to be the result of estrogenic substances in the clover. Consumption of large amounts of red clover is associated with infertility in livestock. It is because of these "estrogenic" activities in animals that some researchers and herbal manufacturers began to explore and promote the use of red clover for relief of menopausal symptoms.

Human trials have been small and conflict with the data generated by animal studies. The largest and most recent randomized, double-blind, placebo-controlled trial of 252 menopausal women failed to find any significant benefit for two different strengths of red clover. Women who were recently postmenopausal (mean = 3.3 years since menopause) experiencing 8 hot flashes per day were included in the trial. Exclusion criteria included vegetarianism, consumption of soy products more than once per week, or ingestion of medications that would affect isoflavone absorption. After a 2-week placebo run-in, participants were randomly assigned to Promensil (82 mg of total isoflavones per day), Rimostil (57 mg of total isoflavones per day), or an identical placebo and followed-up for 12 weeks. Two hundred forty-six women (98%) completed the 12-week protocol. The reductions in mean daily hot flash count at 12 weeks were similar for the Promensil (5.1), Rimostil (5.4), and placebo (5.0) groups. However, women in the Promensil group, but not in the Rimostil group, had faster relief of hot flashes than women in the placebo group. Quality-of-life improvements and adverse events were comparable in the three groups.

A 1999 double-blind, placebo-controlled, cross-over trial was conducted with 51 menopausal women who had been at least 6 months without menses and were experiencing at least three hot flashes per day. They received placebo or red clover extract Promensil (40 mg of total isoflavones; genistein 4 mg, daidzein 3.5 mg, biochanin 24.5 mg, formononetin 8 mg). The first phase lasted 3 months followed by a 4-week wash-out period. The second phase lasted 14 weeks. The Greene Menopause Score was used to evaluate symptoms in a diary kept by participants. At the beginning and conclusion of each phase of the trial, participants were evaluated by blood work that included a complete blood cell count, liver function tests, follicle stimulating hormone, estradiol, and sex hormone binding globulin; a 24-hour urine to test for isoflavone levels; vaginal cytology; and transvaginal ultrasound to evaluate endometrial thickness. Forty-three women completed the study. There were no significant differences between groups in Green Scores, blood work, vaginal cytology, endometrial thickness, or body weight. Hot flashes were reduced by 18% in the placebo group and by 20% in the treatment group.

Another randomized, placebo-controlled study enrolled 37 postmenopausal women who were having at least three hot flashes per day. Participants received placebo, Promesil (40 mg total isoflavones), or Promensil (160 mg total isoflavones) per day for 12 weeks. Evaluation was similar to the trial mentioned above. There were no significant differences between the three groups in blood work or vaginal cytology. Urinary isoflavone levels rose in both of the groups taking Promensil. A small but insignificant rise in urinary isoflavones was noted in the placebo group. Though not adequately confirmed, this small rise was thought to be because of the consumption of alfalfa (a phytoestrogen also included in herbal mixtures) by one participant.

These three studies are in contrast to a small randomized, double-blind, placebo-controlled trial of 30 women with more than 12 months amenorrhea and experiencing more than five hot flashes per day that showed a beneficial effect with 80 mg/d isoflavones (Promensil). After a single-blind placebo run-in for 4 weeks, the women were randomized to either 80 mg isoflavones or placebo for 12 weeks. Efficacy was measured by the decrease in number of hot flashes per day and changes in Greene Climacteric Scale Score. During the first 4 weeks of placebo the frequency of hot flashes decreased by 16%. During the subsequent double-blind phase, a further, statistically significant decrease of 44% was seen in isoflavones group, whereas no further reduction occurred within the placebo group. The Greene Score decreased in the active group by 13% and remained unchanged in the placebo group. The small sample size and low placebo response challenge the results of this study.

Safety for women who have had an estrogen receptor positive cancer is unclear. Although red clover is a prominent ingredient in the Hoxsey cancer formula, an in vitro study found that the herb was equipotent to estradiol in its ability to stimulate cell proliferation in estrogen receptor positive breast cancer cell. Other researchers found that methanol extracts of red clover showed significant competitive binding to estrogen receptors alpha (ER alpha) and beta (ER beta) and exhibited estrogenic activity in cultured endometrial cells. Until further research is available, it would seem wise to avoid prolonged use of red clover in women with a history of breast cancer. This is especially true given the fact that three of four trials, including the largest and best done study, fail to show any clinically significant benefit for relieving menopausal symptoms.

**Figure 13.3**

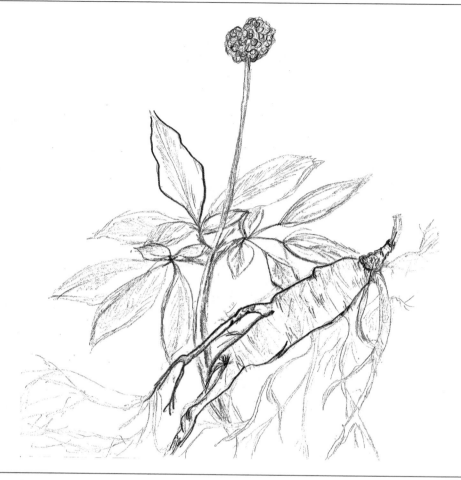

Ginseng (*Panax sp.*).

## Chinese Herbal Mixtures

### PC–SPES Chinese Herbal Mixture

PC-SPES is a traditional Chinese herbal preparation used for the treatment of prostate cancer. Commercially available since November 1996, PC-SPES consists of extracts from the following eight distinct herbs: *Dendrantherma morifolium, Tzvel; Ganoderma lucidium, Karst; Glycyrrhiza glabra* L.; *Isatis indigotica, Fort; Panax pseudo-ginseng, Wall; Robdosia rubescens; Scutellaria baicalensis, Georgi;* and *Serenoa repens* (Figure 13.3; Table 13.2). Three studies evaluating PC-SPES have been published in peer-reviewed journals.

A joint study conducted by the UCSF Comprehensive Cancer Center and Memorial Sloan-Kettering Cancer Center used PC-SPES to treat 32 patients with androgen-dependent or -independent prostate cancer. After treatment with PC-SPES, all those in the androgen-dependent group had a PSA decline of more than 80%. In the androgen-independent group, 54% of patients had a PSA decline of more than 50%.

Two other studies indicated PC-SPES is effective in alleviating symptoms of advanced prostate cancer in patients, including those who have failed conventional therapy. Researchers at the Brander Cancer Institute propose that this complex composition of herbal material could "target many signal transduction and metabolic pathways simultaneously thereby eliminating the back-up and redundant mechanisms that otherwise promote cell survival when single-target agents are used."

Workers at Columbia University, in collaboration with French researchers, demonstrated that PC-SPES can induce apoptosis of cancer cells in vitro. PC-SPES was also effective in suppressing the growth rate of hormone insensitive prostate cancer cells in human volunteers.

All three studies agreed that PC-SPES appeared to stabilize the disease and improve quality of life in patients suffering from advanced prostate cancer. With the exception of a low incidence of deep venous thrombosis or thromboembolic events, side effects of PC-SPES are relatively mild and comparable to those associated with estrogen treatment.

The Brander study suggests that because of its complex make-up, PC-SPES is potentially able to eliminate back-up mechanisms that otherwise promote cell survival. Among major concerns associated with both single herb commodities and multiherb patents are herb/herb and herb/drug interactions. Complex preparations, such as PC-SPES, represent a challenge from the standpoint of authentication, quality control, and standardization. Recently, an National Institutes of Health-sponsored study of PC-SPES ran into difficulty when it was discovered that the PC-SPES source was adulterated (as may often be the case with herbs from China). Controversy ensued about halting the study because many of the enrolled subjects nonetheless experienced benefits and wanted to continue the treatments.

# Safety and Herb/Drug Interactions

Herb safety and herb/drug interactions are complex and controversial issues. With the increasing use of herbs by Westerners has come legitimate concern for potential abuse and toxicity. The safety of a drug, herb, or food is always relative and contextual. Safety

| Table 13.2 | PC-SPES Formula Composed of Eight Herbs |
|---|---|
| | • Chrysanthemum flowers (*Chrysanthemum morifolium*) |
| | • Reishi mushroom (*Ganoderma lucidum*) (see Mushrooms in this chapter) |
| | • Licorice root (*Glycyrrhiza glabra*) |
| | • Dyer's woad (*Isatis indigotica*) |
| | • Sanchi ginseng (*Panax pseudoginseng*) |
| | • *Huang qui* or Baikal skullcap root (*Scutellaria baicalensis*) |
| | • *Radhosia rubescens*, Lamiaceae [D1] |
| | • Saw Palmetto fruit (*Serenoa repens*) |

is determined by defining the conditions under which a substance is considered to be safe or dangerous and weighing potential benefits against possible short and long-term adverse effects. Herb/drug interaction is a similar puzzle: All substances that enter the body interact with each other, ultimately affecting all body processes. The issue, again, is determining the benefit or detriment of such interactions.

Compared to the record of approved pharmaceutical drugs, with a few well-known exceptions such as *Aconitum carmichaelii* (*fu zi*), Cinnabaris (*zhu sha*), *Aristolochia fangchi* (*guang fang ji*), and *Ephedra sinica* (*ma huang*), Chinese medicinal herbs are safer. Aconite contains aconitine, a recognized poison that is traditionally detoxified by boiling and then combined with other herbs such as *Zingiberis officinale* (*jiang*) (Figure 13.3), *Ziziphus jujuba* (*da zao*), and *Glycyrrhiza uralensis* (*gan cao*) that further mitigate its toxicity, yielding important therapeutic benefits. For example, treated Aconite is combined with *Panax ginseng* in the treatment of acute cardiac failure. Cinnabaris, a crude ore, contains mercuric oxide and although considered unsafe by American standards, it is still utilized in small doses in China for the short-term treatment of acute mental agitation without negative consequences. Many *Aristolochia* species have recently been shown to exert carcinogenic effects when used continuously for longer than 6 months, yet these species continue to be used in China with good results in the treatment of cancer and nephropathy, the very conditions for which they have been considered causative agents in the West. *Ephedra sinica* (*ma huang*) has appropriately been used as an antiasthmatic, antitussive diaphoretic, and vasodilating component of numerous pulmonary and antiarthritic formulas for centuries. In the United States since the late 1970s, *Ephedra* has been inappropriately marketed over the counter as a natural energy and weight loss stimulant, resulting in incidences of high blood pressure, palpitations, agitation, and insomnia. It is unfortunate that abuse and misuse have caused herbs such as these to become less available to professional health care providers and have cast a dark shadow over the credibility and safety of Chinese medicinal herbs in general.

The hundreds of herbs that are in common use in China and the West are rarely associated with adverse effects that are not easily reversible. These effects are seldom serious and include such transient reactions as nausea, indigestion, diarrhea, headache, dizziness, hot flashes, chills, and rashes that are rapidly abated by discontinued use or dose reduction. The preponderance of evidence shows that when used as an adjunct to conventional medicine, Chinese herbs both enhance the desired effects and mitigate the harmful ones.

Sophisticated monitoring with biologic testing, sterilization, and spectrographic analyses by manufacturers in the United States is ensuring that herbal products are free of chemical contaminants, adulterants, pathogens, and substitutions. This heightened awareness along with stringent standards is encouraging Chinese manufacturers to adopt the good manufacturing practices required by the Food and Drug Administration and the Federal Trade Commission.

There is a paucity of data that describe the interactions between pharmaceutical agents and even less between herbs and drugs. A few herbs and foods have well-understood interactions with drugs. Tetracycline absorption can be impeded by milk-based foods, whereas grapefruit juice increases the blood volume of certain drugs (e.g., antidepressants, antihistamines, and antihypertensives) by inhibiting a drug-metabolizing enzyme (cytochrome P-450). *Hypericum perforatum* (St. John's Wort; *tian ji huang*) reduces blood

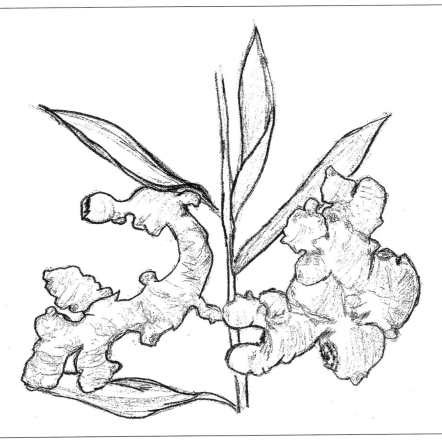

**Ginger** (*Zingiber officinale*).

levels of protease inhibitors by increasing their metabolism while potentiating the effects of monoamine oxidase and selective serotonin reuptake inhibitor antidepressants by elevating seratonin levels. Green vegetables high in vitamin K can oppose the blood-thinning action of drugs such as heparin, Coumadin or warfarin. Because *Gingko biloba* (*yin guo ye*), *Salvia miltiorrhiza* (*dan shen*), and *Angelica sinensis* (*dang gui*) promote microcirculation and inhibit platelet aggregation, they can potentiate the effects of anticoagulants, as can *Allium sativum* (garlic; *da suan*) (Figure 13.2) and *Zingiberis officinale* (ginger; *jiang*) (Figure 13.4). *Astragalus membranaceus* (*huang qi*), because of its immunostimulating properties, may counter the immunosuppressive action of antirejection drugs such as cyclosporin. In high doses, *Glycyrrhiza uralensis* (licorice; *gan cao*) can mimic the action of cortisol, elevating blood pressure and increasing fluid retention. These findings are based on the use of these herbs as single agents.

When *Angelica sinensis* is incorporated into a formula such as *Shi Quan Da Bu Tang*, which supplements *qi* and *blood* and activates circulation, its hematopoietic properties are enhanced and its anticoagulant properties are reduced by the inclusion of herbs such as *Rehmannia glutinosa* (*di huang*) and *Peonia lactiiflora* (*bai shao*), making it an effective treatment for the anemia, bruising, and bleeding caused by radiation and chemotherapy. One of the side effects of standard anticoagulant therapy is anemia. To solve this problem with Chinese medicine, the herbs *Panax pseudoginseng* (*tian qi*) and *Millettia reticulata* (*ji xue teng*) are used because of their triple hematopoietic, circulation-activating, and antihemorrhagic properties. *Glycyrrhiza uralensis* is ubiquitous, appearing in countless formulas in part because of its ability to modulate adrenal function. For example, the decoction of *Bupleurum chinense* (*chai hu*) and *Poria cocos* (*fu ling*) (*Chai Ling Tang*) contains many herbs, including *Glycyrrhiza uralensis*, and is used to aid in the withdrawal from corticosteroid dependence.

Rather than suggesting that people stop eating grapefruit or green vegetables, new information is broadening our understanding of the complexity of drug/food and drug/herb combinations, enhancing our ability to make prudent choices. Biologist Subhuti Dharmananda, PhD, suggests,

> Herb-drug interactions may be minimized by having patients take the herbs and drugs at different times (one hour apart to avoid direct interaction in the digestive tract; 1.5 hours to avoid maximum blood levels of drug and herb at the same time). The dosage of herbs that are aimed therapeutically at the same function as the drugs (e.g. both are sedatives; both are hypoglycemics; both are anti-coagulants) should be reduced to alleviate concerns about additive or synergistic effects that are too great. A certain level of additive effects might be desired in cases where the drug therapy is not producing the desired response.

## Anecdotal Report

From 1984 to 1997 William Fair was the Chairman of the Department of Urology at Memorial Sloan-Kettering Cancer Center in Manhattan, directing surgical oncology research projects. Oncologist Jerome Groopman recorded his story in a *New Yorker* article appearing in 1998. In 1994 Dr. Fair was diagnosed with colon cancer, and during surgery he was found to have two lymph nodes adjacent to the tumor site with signs of metastatic disease. His statistical chances of 5-year survival were 40%, and his cancer type was particularly resistant to both radiation and chemotherapy. He underwent adjuvant chemotherapy initially for 3 months and then for another 12-month period. In 1997 a mass was found in a lymph node near his liver. Suddenly his 5-year survival chances had reduced to 1 in 10, with no viable conventional treatment options. Research associates of Dr. Fair harvested cells from his tumor and proceeded to grow his cell line in mice. Because Fair's tumor was found to have a p53 mutation, he was determined to be a good candidate for the Chinese herbal preparation SPES, the parent formula for PC SPES developed for prostate cancer by Dr. Xu-Hui Wang at Shanghai Medical University in conjunction with Sophie Chen at New York Medical College. First the herbal preparation was tested on Fair's tumor-bearing mice. Within several weeks, the tumors in the SPES-fed mice regressed by 50%, whereas the masses in the control group grew. Then Dr. Fair began ingesting large doses of the formula for more than a year, and his tumors shrunk, with no evidence of new tumor growth. By 2002, Dr. Fair continued to enjoy the benefits of his personal experiment with Chinese herbal medicine before eventually succumbing to the disease.

# Mushrooms and Mushroom Extracts

Although there has been relatively little clinical research and few clinical observations in the United States, interest has developed over the years in the potential anticancer effects of certain mushrooms and their constituents. Since the early 1970s, reports of possible anticancer activities have been coming to light, primarily from Asia. Historically, herbalists and other healers have ascribed various healing properties to mushrooms. There have been many attempts to market various mushrooms by elements of the natural products industry without any research to substantiate the claimed attributes. Patients should be cautioned against the common claims for mushrooms made in marketing materials.

There has been strong interest and experience in medical practice with various toxic mushrooms and the effects of and treatments for mushroom poisoning. These biologic properties may point to the potential for other potent activities of mushrooms against cancer. Many of the most effective chemotherapeutic drugs have cytotoxic activities against cancer cells that are also quite toxic to the patient (see Chapter 1).

Sun soup is a traditional Chinese herbal mixture that contains Chinese mushrooms (see Chapter 15). Some studies have been conducted in China on traditional Chinese medicine combined with radiation and chemotherapy for cancer. In Japan, interest has centered on the shiitake and maitake mushrooms. In addition, extracts of the *Coriolus versicolor* (Turkey tail) mushroom have been studied in the laboratory.

As part of their metabolic activity, mushrooms produce a variety of polysaccharides. Polysaccharides form components of cellular walls in plants and cellular membranes in animals and appear to play a role in cellular communication. As a result of these properties, specific polysaccharides are known to stimulate the immune system. The immune system may recognize certain polysaccharides on cells as foreign. This characteristic is one mechanism by which the immune system may recognize and attack a cancer cell.

The immune system cells involved in recognizing and killing cancer cells are known as natural killer (NK) cells. Some of the mushrooms used for cancer in traditional Asian medicine appear to contain polysaccharides that activate these immune system NK cells. In addition, some mushroom extracts are able to directly kill cancer cells in vitro but are not harmful to normal cells.

These observations have been made with mushrooms that are edible, such as shiitake, maitake, and gandoderma. Other polysaccharides have been extracted from mushrooms that are not edible, or poisonous. Some polysaccharides from mushrooms may also help protect the bone marrow from the harmful effects of chemotherapy and may ultimately find clinical application in complementary cancer care.

Phase I, II, and III clinical trials are under way in Japan to evaluate the use of mushrooms as adjunctive therapy to chemotherapy. The National Cancer Center Research Institute of Japan demonstrated in a 15-year epidemiological study from 1972 to 1986 whereby among close to 175,000 individuals, farmers of the edible mushroom *Flammulina velutipes* had overall lower cancer death rates when compared to those of nonfarmer populations (160.1 per 100,000 compared to 97.1 per 100,000).

A case-control study from Korea evaluating 272 patients adjusted for sex, age, socioeconomic status, family history of gastric cancer, and duration of refrigerator use found an odds ratio of 0.38 for medium intake and high intake of mushrooms and prevalence of gastric cancer.

The only randomized, placebo–controlled, double–blind study known by these authors was conducted using a polysaccharide peptide isolate of *Coriolus versicolor* in a total of 68 patients with advanced nonsmall cell lung cancer. Leukocyte and immunoglobulin levels were found to be increased in the intervention group, but no complete or partial responders were noted. More patients withdrew from the study in the placebo group, possibly indicating a reduced rate of deterioration from the intervention.

# Essential Oils Therapy

Essential oils therapy (often called aromatherapy) is the therapeutic use of essential oils extracted from plants and is often applied to supportive care of the cancer patient. Food and perfume industries are the largest users of essential oils. Some confusion about the therapeutic potential of aromatherapy may be because of this link with the cosmetic industry. Essential oils are described as oils forming the odiferous part of plants and are ethereal, suggesting not only a chemical constituent but also a spiritlike or airy quality. Aromatherapy treatment uses a range of organic compounds of which the odor or fragrance play an important part.

Essential oils are extracted from different parts of plants such as the roots, bark, stalks, flowers, or leaves. These extracts are mostly distilled, although other methods might be used. Essential oils might be applied to the body via massage with a vegetable oil, inhaled, used as a compress, mixed into an ointment, or inserted internally through the rectum, vagina, or mouth. The latter method is used chiefly by the medical profession in France.

Modern–day aromatherapy is one of the fastest growing complementary therapies. This growth includes not only training and practice of aromatherapy but also production of essential oils. Aromatherapy gradually is becoming more accepted in the orthodox medical field as a treatment to enhance both physical and psychologic aspects of cancer patient care.

## Essential Oils

Essential oils are volatile, fragrant, organic constituents that are obtained from plants either by distillation, which is most common, or by cold pressing, which is used for the extraction of citrus oils. Oils may be extracted from leaves (e.g., eucalyptus and peppermint), flowers (e.g., lavender and rose), blossoms (e.g., orange blossom or neroli), fruits (e.g., lemon and mandarin), grasses (e.g., lemongrass), wood (e.g., camphor and sandalwood), barks (e.g., cinnamon), gum (e.g., frankincense), bulbs (e.g., garlic and onion), roots (e.g., calamus), or dried flower buds (e.g., clove). Varying amounts of essential oil can be extracted from a particular plant; 220 pounds of rose petals will yield less than 2 ounces of the essential oil, whereas other plants, such as lavender, lemon, or eucalyptus, yield a much greater proportion. This accounts for the variation in price among essential oils. Essential oils come from sources worldwide, such as lavender from France, eucalyptus from Australia, and sandalwood from India.

Essential oils are commonly a mixture of more than 100 organic compounds, which may include esters, alcohols, aldehydes, terpenes, ketones, coumarins, lactones, phenols, oxides, acids, and ethers. Within the oils there might be more of some active constituents than others, which gives the oil its particular therapeutic value. For example, oils containing large amounts of esters (50%–70%), such as neroli (*Citrus aurantium aurantium*), are thought to be calming, whereas other oils, such as tea tree (*Melaleuca alternifolia terpineol-4*), are regarded as antibacterial, antiviral, and immune system boosters because of the large amounts of alcohol (45%–50%) in their composition (Franchomme & Pénoel, 1990). Critics may say that the idea of an active ingredient goes against the desire for a whole natural substance. There is a question of the naturalness of any oil removed from a plant because immediately after the flower is cut, chemical changes occur; other chemicals may appear in the oil that were not original in the plant (Dodd, 1991).

Aromatherapy is used for a wide range of physical, mental, and emotional conditions in cancer patients, and in those suffering burns, severe bacterial infections, insomnia, depression, hypertension, or arrhythmias. Potential side effects of essential oils include neurotoxic and abortive qualities, as well as dermal toxicity, photosensitivity, allergic reactions, problems with internal use, and liver sensitivity.

## Treatment and Administration

Essential oils are taken into the body through the oral, dermal, rectal, or vaginal routes or simply by olfaction. The cutaneous administration of essential oils mixed in a vegetable carrier oil in the form of an aromatherapy massage is a common method of administration. Benefits can be gained not only from the oils through the skin but also from inhalation of the vapor and from physical therapy in the form of massage. Once the oil reaches the upper dermis, it enters the capillary circulation, where the oil can be transported throughout the body. A massage oil can penetrate the skin after approximately 10 minutes. Blood samples taken at intervals after massage showed that two major constituents of lavender oil, for example, reached maximal concentrations 20 minutes after the massage, although traces had been evident at 5 minutes. Levels returned to baseline after 90 minutes, indicating elimination of lavender oil from the bloodstream. Other studies support the passage of aromatic compounds through the skin of humans.

Oral administration of essential oils carries more potential risks of poisoning or irritation to the gastric mucosa if administered by unqualified persons. It might be useful for qualified medical practitioners to get larger doses of essential oils into the body for the treatment of serious infections. A more detailed knowledge of essential oil toxicology is required for administration via this route.

A significantly smaller dose is administered to the body through the skin than when given orally. Rectal administration of oils in the form of suppositories may be useful for local problems and to avoid the hepatic-portal system of the body, thus allowing higher systemic concentration of the oils to be absorbed. Vaginal administration in the form of pessaries or douches also is used for local problems. However, it should be noted that for patients undergoing standard chemotherapy, rectal administration is often discouraged, and even expressly prohibited, especially when white blood counts are low and seeding of bacteria highly likely through rectal routes.

Simple inhalation of the oils is a method used for respiratory conditions, insomnia, and mood elevation and enhancement or simply for making an environment more pleasant. It is not surprising that essential oils are absorbed through inhalation, considering that conventional medications such as those for asthma are administered in this way. Steam inhalers can be used for respiratory infections, and a variety of electrical and fan-assisted apparatus may be used to scent a room. Overexposure to oils absorbed can result in headaches, fatigue, or allergic reactions such as streaming eyes and skin problems.

## Touch

The influence of touch in the form of massage is a major aspect of aromatherapy treatment when the oils are administered cutaneously. One study was able to show additional psychologic benefit, including reduction in anxiety, to patients who had aromatherapy massage with the essential oil of neroli (*citrus aurantium ssp. aurantium*) compared with those who had massage with a plain vegetable oil. Other studies have shown positive psychologic benefits from massage, including positive subjective response, relaxation, pleasurable feelings, and reduction in the level of anxiety. Massage for both relaxation and release of physical and psychologic stress can be of benefit in the administration of essential oils.

## Central Nervous System

It is suggested that aromatherapy would not have gained its rapid increase in popularity if the oils were not fragrant, thus affecting mood and emotions. Several references have been made to the links between human biology, the sense of smell, and the importance of aromas. Sigmund Freud developed the idea of "organic repression" of the sense of smell. He attributed this to upright gait, which elevates the nose from the ground, where it had enjoyed pleasurable sensations previously. This repression may not be complete but many people have a diminished sense of smell, which is now more vital to the survival of animals than to humans. The emotional and psychologic benefit of aromatherapy is important in many clinical situations, including chronic, life-threatening conditions such as cancer, heart disease, and acquired immunodeficiency syndrome.

## Clinical Applications

Aromatherapy is used in many clinical settings for cancer patients and others. These settings include clinics run by private aromatherapists, clinics attached to general medical practices, and orthodox health care settings used by aromatherapists or other health care professionals who have been trained in aromatherapy.

Aromatherapists who work in practices with general medical practitioners generally do so on a session-by-session basis. The physician often maintains clinical responsibility for the patient who is referred to the aromatherapist. Aromatherapy in orthodox health care settings is being provided by lay aromatherapists and increasingly by trained nurses or other health care professionals such as physical therapists and massage therapists with aromatherapy training.

Settings where aromatherapy has been adopted are included in Table 13.3. The reasons for the use of aromatherapy in these settings are diverse and may include the reasons mentioned in Table 13.4.

## Table 13.3  Chemical Component of Essential Oils and Their Therapeutic Actions

| Chemical Component | Therapeutic Action |
| --- | --- |
| Aldehydes | Anti-infectious, litholitic, calming |
| Ketones | Mucolitic, litholitic, cicatrising, calming |
| Esters | Antispasmodic, calming |
| Sesquiterpenes | Antihistamines, anti-allergic |
| Coumarins, lactones | Balancing, calming |
| C15 and C20 alcohols | Estrogen-like action |
| Acids, aromatic aldehydes | Anti-infectious, immunostimulants |
| Phenols, C10 alcohols | Anti-infectious, immunostimulants |
| Oxides | Expectorant, antisparasitic |
| Phenyl methyl ethers | Anti-infectious, antispasmodic |
| C10 terpenes | Antiseptic, cortisone-like action |

(From Franchomme P., Pénoël D., 1990. L'aromatherapie Exactement. Roger Jallois. Limoges, with permission.)

## Research

### Antimicrobial Effects

The effect of essential oils on a wide variety of pathogens is well known. Their chemical constituents of alcohols and aldehydes, terpenes, and phenyl methyl ethers help explain this action. The antimicrobial aspects of essential oils have been the most widely investigated. Janssen et al. (1987) concluded that many essential oils have antimicrobial effects but found this difficult to qualify because of the variation in test methods and insufficient description of essential oils and microorganisms in some studies. From the different chemical subgroups of *Thymus vulgaris* (common thyme), the strongest antifungal constituent chemical had eight times the effect of the weakest.

Other investigations have reported antibacterial activity of a number of oils, including *Artemisia dracunculus* (tarragon), *Salvia officinalis* L. (sage), *Salvia sclarea* (clary sage),

## Table 13.4  Utilization of Aromatherapy for Medical Purposes

**Relaxation**
Stress and anxiety relief
Pain and discomfort relief
Insomnia and restlessness
Infections and wound healing
Burns
Enhancing self-image
Stimulating immune function
Treatment for constipation

and *Thymus vulgaris*. The alcohols geraniol, eugenol, menthol, and citral all show high antibacterial activity.

## Sedation

Buchbauer et al. (1991) performed perhaps the most extensive research on essential oils in animal models. After 1 hr of inhaling an essential oil or fragrance compound, mice became sedated by sandalwood, rose, neroli, and lavender. Some of the constituent compounds found to have a sedative effect on inhalation were anethole, bornyl salicylate, coumarin, 2-phenylethyl acetate, benaldehyde, citronell, and geranyl acetate. Compounds that resulted in stimulation after inhalation include geraniol, isoborneol, isoeugenol, nerol, methylsalicylate, alpha–pinene, and thymol. Lavender oil was found to be a more effective sedative than either of its major constituents (linalool and linalyl acetate) in isolation. This observation supports claims of synergy between essential oils.

## Digestion

Peppermint, commonly known for its benefit in digestive disorders, has been found to inhibit gastrointestinal smooth muscle in tissue models and affects the flow of calcium across the cell wall of the gastrointestinal smooth muscle (see Chapter 10). Large doses of peppermint might have been found to induce spasm. This idea would support findings that large doses in essential oils may produce opposite effects from the usual smaller doses, as seen in other areas of complementary therapies.

## Analgesia

Analgesic properties are attributed to some oils. One study demonstrated that lemongrass leaves produced a dose–dependent analgesia in rats. Both subplantar and oral doses of the constituent myrcene were administered with similar effect. Myrcene is a common constituent of oils, including rosemary, lavender, juniper, and lemongrass. Undiluted lavender oil is well known as a first-aid remedy for minor burns, both reducing pain and promoting healing.

## Intensive and Palliative Care

A number of studies have been performed in the intensive care setting, palliative care, and care of the elderly. Some of these trials found psychologic benefits to the patients from aromatherapy, in addition to massage. In a randomized controlled trial, 100 cardiac surgery patients in intensive care received the aromatherapy oil of neroli citrus (*aurantium ssp. aurantium*) in foot massage and found anxiety in particular to be further reduced than in patients who were massaged with a plain vegetable oil after 4 days. Both groups who had the massage with or without the neroli oil scored significantly better on an anxiety questionnaire than did the control groups on the day of massage. In one study, patients were massaged with two different lavender essential oils, *Lavandula angustifolia* and *Lavandula latifoli*, following open heart surgery. There was some difference between the two oils, somewhat supporting the conclusion that massage with essential oils proved more beneficial than massage without essential oils. In an unpublished study Dunn (1992) used intensive care as a setting in a randomized trial to measure the effects of massage with lavender oil compared with plain oil massage and rest in 122 patients. Positive psychologic changes were noted for those massaged with essential oil than for those who received the plain oil massage or the period of rest.

In a study of 51 patients attending a center for palliative care, the effects of three aromatherapy massages given weekly were examined with or without the essential oil of Roman chamomile, *Chamemalum nobile*. All patients improved in the aromatherapy group on physical symptoms, quality-of-life, and anxiety scale. In a small study on a long-term elderly care ward, researchers assessed sleep over three consecutive 2-week periods—the first period with night sedation, the second without, and the third with lavender diffused into the air at set intervals. Sleep was poorer in the second period, and in the third period sleep was as good as in the first. These research findings indicate that essential oils therapy can have an appropriate role in care of the patient with cancer (Buckle, 1993; Buchbauer et al., 1991; Dale & Cornwall, 1994; Janssen et al., 1987; Kovar et al., 1987; Moleyar & Narasimhan, 1992; Reed & Held, 1988; Steele, 1992; Stevensen, 1994; Taylor et al., 1983, 1984).

Although research continues on most of the herbal treatments that have been applied to the treatment of cancer, options for the use of these alternatives remain available to many, although not all, who might desire them. The cancer patient who has been told he or she has an incurable disease may feel there is "nothing in lose" in pursuing alternative remedies. A familiarity with these alternatives will be helpful to the practitioner in counseling and guiding their patients about their possible interest in the use of these remedies.

# REFERENCES

American Cancer Society. (1983). Unproven methods of cancer management: Iscador. *CA: A Cancer Journal for Clinicians, 33*(3), 186–188.

Banerjee, S., Welsch, C. W., & Rao, A. R. (1995). Modulatory influence of camphor on the activities of hepatic carcinogen metabolizing enzymes and the levels of hepatic and extrahepatic reduced glutathione in mice. *Cancer Letter, 88*, 163–169.

Balick, M., Duke, J., Kaptchuk, T., McCaleb, R. S., Pavek, R., Pellerin, C., et al. (1994). Herbal medicine. In *Alternative medicine: Expanding medical horizons: A report to the National Institutes of Health on alternative medical systems and practices in the United States* (NIH Publication No. 94-066) (pp. 183–206). Washington, DC: U.S. Government Printing Office.

Becker, H. (1986). Botany of European mistletoe (*Viscum album* L.). *Oncology, 43*(1 Suppl.), 2–7.

Belkin, M., & Fitzgerald, D. B. (1952). Tumor-damaging capacity of plant materials. I. Plants used as cathartics. *Journal of the National Cancer Institute, 13*, 139–155.

Berger, M., & Schmahl, D. (1983). Studies on the tumor-inhibiting efficacy of Iscador in experimental animal tumors. *Journal of Cancer Research and Clinical Oncology, 105*, 262–265.

Beuth, J., Ko, H. L., Gabius, H. J., Burrichter, H., Oette, K., & Pulverer, G. (1992). Behavior of lymphocyte subsets and expression of activation markers in response to immunotherapy with galactoside-specific lectin from mistletoe in breast cancer patients. *Clinical Investigator, 60*, 658–661.

Bird, C. (1991). *The persecution and trial of Gaston Naessens: The true story of the efforts to suppress an alternative treatment for cancer, AIDS, and other immunologically based diseases.* Tiburon, CA: H. J. Kramer.

Bradley, G. W., & Clover, A. (1989). Apparent response of small cell lung cancer to an extract of mistletoe and homeopathic treatment. *Thorax, 44*, 1047–1048.

Bryson, P. D. (1978). Burdock root tea poisoning. *Journal of the American Medical Association, 240*(15), 1586.

Bryson, P. D., Watanabe, A. S., & Rumack, B. H., & Murphy, R. C. (1978). Burdock root tea poisoning: Case report involving a commercial preparation. *Journal of the American Medical Association, 239*(20), 2157.

Buckle, J. (1993). Aromatherapy: Does it matter which lavender oil is used? *Nursing Times, 89*(20), 32–35.

Buchbauer, G., et al. (1991). Aromatherapy: Evidence for sedative effects of the essential oil of lavender after inhalation. *Zeitschrift für Naturforschung A, 46*, 1067–1072.

Caisse, R. (1938). *"Essiac": A treatment for cancer: Report of patients presented to The Royal Cancer Commission of Ontario (Canada)*. Toronto: Royal Cancer Commission of Ontario.

Centre d'Orthobiologie Somatidienne de l'Estrie, Inc. (C.O.S.E). (1995). *Protocol for 714-X*. Quebec: Author.

Chaudhury, R. R. (1992). *Herbal medicine for human health* (SEARO No. 20). Geneva: World Health Organization.

Crellin, J. K., & Philpott, J. (Eds.). (1990). *Herbal medicine past and present: Vol. II. A reference guide to medicinal plants*. Durham, NC: Duke University Press.

Dale, A., & Cornwall, S. (1994). The role of lavender oil in relieving perineal discomfort following childbirth: A blind randomized clinical trial. *Journal of Advanced Nursing, 19*, 89–96.

Dixon, A., Schumacher, U., Pfüller, U., & Taylor, I. (1994). Is the binding of mistletoe lectins I and III a useful prognostic indicator in colorectal carcinoma? *European Journal of Surgical Oncology, 20*, 648–652.

Duke, J. A. (1987). *CRC handbook of medicinal herbs* (4th ed., pp. 53–54, 106–107, 200, 404, 414–416, 495–496, 512–513, 517–523, 552, 568). Boca Raton, FL: CRC Press.

Franz, G. (1993). The senna drug and its chemistry. *Pharmacology, 47*(Suppl. 1), 2–6.

Gabius, H. J., Walzel, H., Joshi, S. S., Kruip, J., Kojima, S., Gerke, V., et al. (1992). The immunomodulatory Beta-galactoside-specific lectin from mistletoe: Partial sequence analysis, cell and tissue binding, and impact on intracellular biosignalling of monocytic leukemia cells. *Anticancer Research, 12*, 669–672.

Gao, Y. T., McLaughlin, J. K., Blot, W. J., Ji, B. T., Dai, Q., Fraumeni, J. F., Jr. (1994). Reduced risk of esophageal cancer associated with green tea consumption. *Journal of the National Cancer Institute, 86*(11), 855–858.

Gawlik, C., Versteeg, R., Engel, E., Arps, H., & Kleeberg, U. R. (1992). Antiproliferative effect of mistletoe-extracts in melanoma cell lines. *Anticancer Research, 12*(6A), 1882.

Graham, H. N. (1992). Green tea composition, consumption, and polyphnol chemistry. *Preventive Medicine, 21*, 334–350.

Gibson, D. E., Moore, G. P., & Pfaff, J. A. (1989). Camphor ingestion. *American Journal of Emergency Medicine, 7*(1), 41–43.

Goel, H. C., & Roa, A. R. (1998). Radiosensitizing effect of camphor on transplantable mammary adenocarcinoma in mice. *Cancer Letter, 43*(102), 21–27.

Grimminger, W., & Witthohn, K. (1993). Analytics of senna drugs with regard to the toxicological discussion of athranoids. *Pharmacology, 47*(Suppl. 1), 98–109.

Grossarth-Maticek, R., Kiene, H., Baumgartner, S., & Ziegler, R. (2001). Use of Iscador, an extract of Mistletoe, in cancer treatment: Prospective nonrandomized and randomized matched-pair studies nested with a cohort study. *Alternative Therapies in Health Medicine, 7*, 62–79.

Hall, A. H., Spoerke, D. G., & Rumack, B. H. (1986). Assessing mistletoe toxicity. *Annals of Emergency Medicine, 15*(11), 1320–1323.

Harvey, J., & Colin-Jones, D. G. (1981). Mistletoe hepatitis. *British Medical Journal, 282*, 186–187.

Hauser, S. P. (1991). Unproven methods in oncology. *European Journal of Cancer, 27*(12), 1549–1551.

Hauser, S. P. (1993). Unproven methods in cancer treatment. *Current Opinion in Oncology, 5*(4), 646–654.

He, Y. H., & Kies, C. (1994). Green and black tea consumption by humans: Impact of polyphenol concentration in feces, blood and urine. *Plant Foods for Human Nutrition, 46*(3), 221–229.

Hill, M. J. (1980). Bacterial metabolism and human carcinogenesis. *British Medical Bulletin, 36*(1), 89–94.

Holtskog, R., Sandvig, K., & Olsnes, S. (1988). Characterization of a toxic lectin in Iscador, a mistletoe preparation with alleged cancerostatic properties. *Oncology, 45*, 172–179.

Huang, M. T., Ho, C. T., Wang, Z. Y., Ferraro, T., Finnegan-Olive, T., Lou, Y. R., et al. Inhibitory effect of topical application of a green tea polyphenol fraction on tumor initiation and promotion in mouse skin. *Carcinogenesis, 13*(6), 947–954.

Imanishi, H., Sasaki, Y.F., Ohta, T., Watanabe, M., Kato, T., & Shirasu, Y. (1991). Tea tannin components modify the induction of sister-chromatid exchanges and chromosome aberration in mutagen-treated cultured mammalian cells and mice. *Mutation Research, 259*, 79–87.

Isemura, M., Suzuki, Y., Satoh, K., Narumi, K., & Motomiya, M. (1993). Effects of catechins on the mouse lung carcinoma cell adhesion to endothelial cells. *Cell Biology International, 17*(6), 559–564.

Ito, Y., Maeda, S., & Sugiyama, T. (1986). Suppression of 7,12-dimethylebenz[a]anthracene-induced chromosome aberrations in rat bone marrow cells by vegetable juices. *Mutation Research, 172*, 55–60.

Ito, Y., Ohnishi, S., & Fujie, K. (1989). Chromosome aberrations induced by aflatoxin $B_1$ in rat bone marrow cells in *vivo* and their suppression by green tea. *Mutation Research, 222*, 253–261.

Janssen, A. M., Scheffer, J. J., & Baerheim Svendsen, A. (1987). Antimicrobial activity of essential oils: 1976–1986 literature review. *Planta Medica, 53*(5), 395–398.

Jung, M. L., Baudino, S., Ribereau-Gayon, G., & Beck, J. P. (1990). Characterization of cytotoxic proteins from mistletoe (*Viscum album* L). *Cancer Letters, 51*, 103–108.

Junshi, C. (1992). The antimutagenic and anticarcinogenic effects of tea, garlic and other natural foods in China: A review. *Biomedical and Environmental Sciences, 5*(1), 1–17.

Kapadia, G. J., Paul, B. D., Chung, E. B., Ghosh, B., & Pradhan, S. N. (1976). Carcinogenicity of *Camellia sinensis* (tea) and some tannin-containing folk medicinal herbs administered subcutaneously in rats. *Journal of the National Cancer Institute, 57*(1), 207–209.

Kinlen, L. J., Willows, A. N., Goldblatt, P., & Yudkin, J. (1988). Tea consumption and cancer. *British Journal of Cancer, 58*(3), 397–401.

Kjaer, M. (1989). Mistletoe (Iscador) therapy in stage IV renal adenocarcinoma: A phase II study in patients with measurable lung metastases. *Acta Oncologica, 28*(4), 489–494.

Kleijnen, J., & Knipschild, P. (1994). Mistletoe treatment for cancer: Review of controlled trials in humans. *Phytomedicine, 1*, 255–260.

Komori, A., Yatsunami, J., Okabe, S., Abe, S., Hara, K., Suganuma, M., et al. (1993). Anticarcinogenic activity of green tea polyphenols. *Japanese Journal of Clinical Oncology, 23*, 186–190.

Kovacs, E., Hajto, T., & Hostanska, K. (1991). Improvement of DNA repair in Lymphocytes of breast cancer patients treated with *Viscum album* extract (Iscador). *European Journal of Cancer, 27*(12), 1672–1676.

Kovar, K. A., Gropper, B., Friess, D., & Ammon, H. P. (1987). Blood levels of 1,8-cineole and locomotor activity of mice after inhalation and oral administration of rosemary oil. *Planta Medica, 53*(4), 315–318.

Kupchan, S. M., & Karim, A. (1977). Tumor inhibitors: 114. Aloe emodin: Antileukemic principle isolated from *Rhamnus frangula* L. *Lloydia, 39*(4), 223–224.

Lee, H., & Tsai, S. J. (1991). Effect of emodin on cooked-food mutagen activation. *Food Chemistry and Toxicology, 29*(11), 765–770.

Lee, M. J., Wang, Z. Y., Li, H., Chen, L., Sun, Y., Gobbo, S., et al. (1995), Analysis of plasma and urinary tea polyphenols in human subjects. *Cancer Epidemiology, Biomarkers and Prevention, 4*(4), 393–399.

Leone, M., et al. (2003). Cancer prevention by tea polyphenols is linked to their direct inhibition of antiapoptotic Bcl-2-family proteins. *Cancer Research, 63*, 8118–8121.

Lorenzetti, B. E., Souza, G. E., Sarti, S. J., et al. (1991). Myrcene mimics the peripheral analgesic activity of lemongrass tea. *Journal of Ethnopharmacology, 34*(1), 43–48.

Marnewick, J. L., et al. (2000). An investigation of the antimutagenic properties of South African herbal teas. *Mutation Research, 471*, 157–166.

Meserole, L. (2006). Western herbalism, In M. S. Micozzi (ed.) *Fundamentals of complementary and integrative medicine* (3rd ed.). St Louis: Elsevier.

Moleyar, V., & Narasimham, P. (1992). Antibacterial activity of essential oil components. *International Journal of Food Microbiology, 16*(4), 337–342.

Moss, R. W., Silversmith, L., Standish, L., & Wievel, F. (1994). Pharmacological and biological treatments. In *Alternative medicine: Expanding medical horizons: A report to the National Institutes of Health of alternative medicine systems and practices in the United States* (NIH Publication No. 94-066) (pp. 159–182). Washington, DC: U.S. Government Printing Office.

Nakagami, T., Nanaumi-Tamura, N., Toyomura, K., Nakamura, T., & Shigehisa, T. (1995). Dietary flavonoids as potential natural biological response modifiers affecting the autoimmune system. *Journal of Food Science, 60*(4), 653–656.

Oguni, I., Nasu, K., Yamamoto, S., & Nomura T. (1988). On the antitumor activity of fresh green tea leaf. *Agricultural & Biological Chemistry, 52*(7), 1879–1880.

Panizzi, L., Flamini, G., Cioni, F. L., & Morelli, I. (1993). Composition and antimicrobial properties of essential oils of four Mediterranean Lamiacease. *Journal of Ethnopharmacology, 39*(3), 167–170.

Parkins, T. (1994). Anti-cancer drug origins: Truth is stranger than fiction. *Journal of the National Cancer Institute, 86*(3), 173–175.

Parmiani, G., & Rivoltini, L. (1991). Biologic agents as modifiers of chemotherapeutic effects. *Current Opinion in Oncology, 3*, 1078–1086.

Perdue, R. E., Jr., & Hartwell, J. L. (1969). The search for plant sources of anticancer drugs. *Morris Arboretum Bulletin, 20*, 35–53.

Reed, B. V., & Held, J. M. (1988). Effects of sequential tissue massage on autonomic nervous system of middle aged and elderly adults. *Physical Therapy, 68*(8), 1231–1234.

Rhoads, P. M., Tong, T. G., Banner, W., & Anderson, R. (1985). Anticholinergic poisoning associated with commercial burdock root tea. *Clinical Toxicology, 22*(6), 581–584.

Risberg, T., Lund, E., Wist, E., Dahl, O., Sundstrom, S., Andersen, O. K., et al. (1995). The use of non-proven therapy among patients treated in Norwegian oncological departments: A cross-sectional national multicenter study. *European Journal of Cancer, 31A*(11), 1785–1789.

Steele, J. J. (1992). The anthropology of smell and scent in ancient Egypt and South American Shamanism. In S. Van Toller & G. H. Dodd (eds.), *Fragrance: The psychology and biology of perfume*. New York: Elsevier.

Sterling, K. (1991). Old Canadian remedies: 1922: Rene Caisse: Essiac. *Canadian Journal of Herbalism, xi*(iii), 1–4.

Stevensen, C. J. (1994). The psychophysiological effects of aromatherapy massage following cardiac surgery. *Complementary Therapies in Medicine, 2*, 27–35.

Stripe, F., Sandwig, K., Olsens, S., & Pihl, A. (1982). Action of viscumin, a toxic lectin from mistletoe, on cells in culture. *Journal of Biological Chemistry, 257*(22), 13271–13277.

Tabiasco, J., Pont, F., Fournie, J. J., & Vercellone, A. (2002). Mistletoe viscotoxins increase natural killer cell-mediated cytotoxicity. *European Journal of Biochemistry, 269*, 2591–2600.

Taylor, B. A., Luscombe, C. K., & Duthie, H. L. (1983). Inhibitory effect of peppermint oil on gastrointestinal smooth muscle. *Gut, 24*, A992.

Taylor, B. A., Luscombe, C. K., & Duthie, H. L. (1984). Inhibitory effect of peppermint and menthol on human isolated coli. *Gut, 25*, A1168.

Tewes, F. J., Koo, L. C., Meisgen, T. J., & Rylander, R. (1990). Lung cancer risk and mutagenicity of tea. *Environmental Research, 52*(1), 23–33.

United States Office of Technology Assessment. (1990a). *Herbal treatments*. In Unconventional Cancer Treatments (pp. 60–87). Washington, DC: U.S. Government Printing Office.

Wade, A. E., Holl, J. E., Hilliard, C. C., Molton, E., & Greene, F. E. (1986). Alteration of drug metabolism in rats and mice by an environment of cedarwood. *Pharmacology, 1*, 317–328.

Wagner, H., Jordan, E., & Feil, B. (1986). Studies on the standardization of mistletoe preparations. *Oncology, 43*(1 Suppl.), 16–22.

Weisburger, J. H. (1992). Introduction: Physiological and pharmacological effects of *Camellia* sinensis (tea): First international symposium. *Preventive Medicine, 21*, 329–330.

World Health Organization. (1989). *In vitro* screening of traditional medicines for anti-HIV activity: Memorandum from a WHO meeting. *Bulletin of the World Health Organization* (Switzerland), *67*, 613–618.

Yanagihara, K., Ito, A., Toge, T., & Numoto, M. (1993). Antiproliferative effects of isoflavones on human cancer cell lines established from the gastrointestinal tract. *Cancer Research, 53*, 5815–5821.

Yang, C. S., & Wang, Z. Y. (1993). Tea and cancer. *Journal of the National Cancer Institute, 85*(13), 1038–1049.

# 4

# Alternative Systems of Medicine

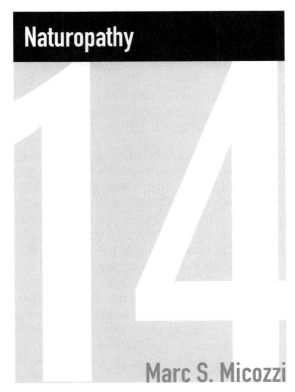

# Naturopathy

## Introduction

Naturopathic medicine as a model for integrative medicine is presently undergoing a resurgence. With its integration of vitalistic, scientific, academic, and clinical training, the naturopathic medical model is a contributing factor to contemporary health care (Zeff, Snider, & Myers, 2006). Many traditional naturopathic theories, principles, and practices are related to the avoidance of unhealthy habits, elimination of unhealthy substances from the body, and detoxification (Standish, Snider, Calabrese, & NMRA Core Team, 2004). These approaches can now be seen in light of contemporary science as related to the prevention of cancer and, in some cases, treatment and alleviation of its symptoms.

Naturopathic medicine traces its philosophical roots to many traditional world medicines. Its body of knowledge derives from a heritage of writings and practices of Western and non-Western doctors since Hippocrates (circa 400 B.C.). Modern naturopathic medicine grew out of healing systems of the 18th and 19th centuries. The term *naturopathy* was coined in 1895 by Dr. John Scheel of New York City to describe his method of health care. However, earlier forerunners of these concepts already existed in the history of natural healing, both in America and in the Austro-Germanic European core. Naturopathy became a formal profession after its creation by Benedict Lust in 1896. Over the centuries, natural medicine and biomedicine have alternately diverged and converged, shaping themselves, often in reaction to each other. Since the early 1900s, the practice has progressed through several fairly distinct phases (see Table 14.1).

In 1892, at the age of 23, Lust came from Germany as a disciple of Father Kneipp (the practitioner of hydrotherapy) to bring Kneipp's hydrotherapy practices to America. Exposure into the United States to a wide range of practitioners and practices of natural healing broadened Lust's perspective. After a decade of study, he purchased the term naturopathy from Scheel in 1902 to describe the eclectic complication of doctrines of natural healing that he envisioned was to be the future of natural medicines. Naturopathy,

Marc S. Micozzi

or "nature cure," was defined by Lust as both a way of life and a concept of healing that used various natural means of treating human infirmities and disease states. The earliest therapies associated with the term involved a combination of American hygienics and Austro-Germanic nature cure and hydrotherapy.

In January 1902, Lust, who had been publishing the *Kneipp Water-Cure Monthly* and its German language counterpart in New York since 1896, changed the name of the journal to *The Naturopathic and Herald of Health* and began promoting a new way of thinking of health care with the following editorial:

> We believe in strong, pure, beautiful bodies ... of radiating health. We want every man, woman and child in this great land to know and embody and feel the truths of right living that mean conscious mastery. We plead for the renouncing of poisons from the coffee, white flour, glucose, fat, and like venom of the American table to patent medicines, tobacco, liquor and the other inevitable recourses of perverted appetite. We long for the time when an eight-hour day may enable every worker to stop existing long enough to live; when the spirit of universal brotherhood shall animate business and society and the church; when every American may have a little cottage of his own, and a bit of ground where he may combine Aerthotherapy, Heliotherapy, Geotherapy, Aristophagey and nature's other forces with home and peace and happiness and things forbidden to flat-dwellers; when people may stop doing and thinking and being for others and be for themselves, when true lover and divine marriage and prenatal culture and controlled parenthood may fill this world with germ-gods instead of humanized animals. In a word, Naturopathy stands for the reconciling, harmonizing and unifying of nature, humanity and God. Fundamentally, therapeutic because men need healing; elementally educational because men need teaching; ultimately inspirational because men need empowering. (Lust, 1896)

In this statement, many of the ideas relevant to complementary and alternative medicine for the prevention and care of cancer one century later are apparent.

| Phases of Naturopathy |
| --- |
| Late 19th Century: Founded by Benedict Lust; origin in the Germanic hydrotherapy and nature cure traditions. |
| 1900 to 1917: Formative years; convergence of the American dietetic, hygenic, physical culture, spinal manipulation, mental and emotional healing, Thompsonian/electric, and homeopathic systems. |
| 1918 to 1937: Halcyon days; during a period of great public interest and support, the philosophical basis and scope of therapies diversified to encompass botanical, homeopathic, and environmental medicine. |
| 1938 to 1970: Suppression and decline; growing political and social dominance of the American Medical Association, lack of internal political unity, and lack of unifying standards, combined with the American love affair with technology and the emergence of "miracle" drugs and effective modern surgical techniques perfected in two world wars resulted in legal and economic suppression. |
| 1971 to present: Naturopathic medicine reemerges; reawakened awareness of the American public of the importance of health promotion, prevention of disease, and concern for the environment and naturopathic medicine, resulting in rapid resurgence. Current projections predict a continuing increase in naturopathic physicians. |

# History of Natural Medicine

According to his published personal history, Lust had a debilitating condition in his late teens while growing up in Michelbach, Barden, Germany, and had been sent by his father to undergo the Kneipp cure at Woerishofen. He stayed there from mid-1890 to early 1892. Not only was he "cured" of his condition, but he became a protégé of Father Kneipp. He emigrated to America to proselytize the principle of the Kneipp Water-Cure.

By making contact in New York with other German Americans who were also becoming aware of the Kneipp principles, Lust participated in the founding of the first Kneipp Society, which was organized in Jersey City, New Jersey, in 1896. Subsequently, through Lust's organization and contracts, Kneipp Societies were also founded in Brooklyn, Boston, Chicago, Cleveland, Denver, Cincinnati, Philadelphia, Columbus, Buffalo, Rochester, New Haven, San Francisco, the state of New Mexico, and Mineola on Long Island. The members of these organizations were provided with copies of the *Kneipp Blatter* and a companion English publication Lust began to put out, called *The Kneipp Water-Cure Monthly*. In 1895 Lust opened the Kneipp Water-Cure Institute on 59th Street in New York City.

Father Kneipp died in Germany, at Woerishofen, on June 17, 1897. With his passing, Lust no longer bound himself strictly to the principles of the Kneipp Water-Cure. He had begun to associate earlier with other German American physicians, principally Dr. Hugo R. Wendel (a German-trained "Naturarzt"), who began, in 1897, to practice in New York and New Jersey as a licensed osteopathic physician. In 1896 Lust entered the Universal Osteopathic College of New York and became licensed as an osteopathic physician in 1898.

Once he was licensed to practice as a health care physician in his own right, Lust began the transition toward the concept of "naturopathy." Between 1898 and 1902, when he adopted the term *naturopath*, Lust acquired a chiropractic education. He changed the name of his Kneipp Store (which he had opened in 1895) to Health Food Store (the first facility to use that name and concept in this country). The store specialized in providing organically grown foods and the materials necessary for drugless cures. At this time, Lust also founded the New York School of Massage (in 1896) and the American School of Chiropractic.

In 1902, he also began to operate the American School of Naturopathy, all at the same 59th Street address. By 1907 Lust's enterprises had grown sufficiently large that he moved them to a 55-room building. It housed the Naturopathic Institute, Clinic, and Hospital; the American Schools of Naturopathy and Chiropractic; the now-entitled Original Health Food Store; Lust's publishing enterprises; and New York School of Massage. The operation remained in this four-story building, roughly twice the size of the original facility, from 1907 to 1915.

In the period of 1912 through 1914, Lust took a sabbatical from his operations to further his education. By this time he had founded his large, estatelike sanitarium at Butler, New Jersey, known as "Yung-born," after the German sanitarium operation of Adolph Just. In 1912 he attended the Homeopathic Medical College in New York, which in 1913 granted him a degree in homeopathic medicine and, in 1914, a degree in eclectic medicine. In early 1914 Lust traveled to Florida and obtained a medical doctor's license on the basis of his graduation from the Homeopathic Medical College.

From 1902, when he began to use the term *naturopathy*, until 1918, Lust replaced the Kneipp Societies with the Naturopathic Society of America. When, in December 1919, the Naturopathic Society of America was formally dissolved because of insolvency, Lust founded the American Naturopathic Association. Thereafter, the association was incorporated in some additional 18 states. Lust claimed to at one time have 40,000 adherents practicing naturopathy. In 1918, as part of this effort to replace the Naturopathic Society of America with the American Naturopathic Association, Lust published the first *Yearbook of Drugless Therapy*. Annual supplements were published in either *The Naturopath and the Herald of Health* or its companion publication, *Nature's Path* (which began publication in 1925). The *Naturopath and Herald of Health*, sometimes printed with the two phrases reversed, was published from 1902 through 1927 and from 1934 until after Lust's death in 1945.

Benedict Lust's principles of health are found in the introduction to the first volume of the *Universal Naturopathic Directory and Buyer's Guide*, a portion of which is reproduced here:

*The Seven Healthy Principles*
1 Healing power of nature
2 First do no harm
3 Find the cause
4 Treat the whole person
5 Preventive "medicine"
6 Wellness
7 Doctors as teacher

Although the terminology is almost a century old, the concepts Lust proposed have provided a powerful foundation that has endured despite almost a century of active political suppression. Many of its recommendations are now seen in light of universally accepted recommendations for the avoidance of chronic diseases such as cancer.

## Medical Eclecticism

Because of its eclectic nature, the history of naturopathic medicine is complex. Although the following discussion is divided into distinct schools of thought, this is somewhat artificial because those who founded and practiced these arts (especially the Americans) were often trained in, influenced by, and practiced several therapeutic modalities. However, it was not until Benedict Lust that the many threads were woven together into a unified professional practice, making naturopathic medicine a Western system of full-scope integrative natural medicine. The following presents the formative schools of Western thought in natural healing and some of their leading adherents. Although the therapies differ, the philosophical thread of promoting health and supporting the body's own healing processes runs through them. These threads are derived from centuries of medical scholarship, both Western and non-Western, concerning the self-healing process. After a brief overview of Hippocrates' seminal contributions to the basic themes are presented in order: healthful living; natural diet; detoxification; exercise, mechanotherapy and physical therapy; mental, emotional, and spiritual healing; and natural therapeutic agents. Hippocrates and centuries of nature doctors' writings remain empirically rich repositories of observations for future reference.

## Hippocrates

Some ancient peoples believed that disease could be caused by magic or supernatural forces, such as devils or angry gods. Hippocrates, breaking with this superstitious belief, became an early naturalistic doctor in recorded Western history. Hippocrates regarded the body as a whole and instructed his students to prescribe only beneficial treatments and refrain from causing harm or hurt.

Hippocratic practitioners assumed that everything in nature had a rational basis; therefore the physician's role was to understand and follow the laws of the intelligible universe. They viewed disease as an effect and looked for its cause in natural phenomena: air, water, food, and so forth. They first used the term *vis medicatrix naturae*, the healing power of nature, to denote the body's homeostatic ability and tendency to heal itself. One central tenet is that "there is an order to the process of healing which requires certain things to be done before other things to maximize the effectiveness of the therapeutics."

## Hydrotherapy

The earliest philosophical origins of naturopathy were clearly in the Germanic hydrotherapy movement: the use of hot and cold water for the maintenance of health and the treatment of disease. One of the oldest known therapies (water was used therapeutically by the Romans and Greeks), the modern history of hydrotherapy is notable for the publication of *The History of Cold Bathing* in 1697 by Sir John Floyer. Probably the strongest impetus for its use came next from Central Europe, where it was advocated by such well-known hydropaths as Priessnitz, Schroth, and Father Kneipp. They were able to popularize specific water treatments that quickly became the vogue in Europe during the 19th century. Vincent Preissnitz (1799–1851), of Graefenberg, Silesia, was a pioneer natural healer. He was prosecuted by the medical authorities of his day and was convicted of using witchcraft because he cured his patients by the use of water, air, diet, and exercise. He took his patients back to nature—to the woods, the streams, the open fields—treated them with nature's own forces, and fed them on natural foods. His patients numbered by the thousands, and his fame spread over Europe. Father Sebastian Kneipp (1821–1897) became the most famous of the hydropaths, with Pope Leo XIII and Ferdinand of Austria (whom he had walking barefoot in new-fallen snow for purposes of hardening his constitution) among his many famous patients. He standardized the practice that was widely emulated through the establishment of health spas or sanitariums. The first sanitarium in this country, the Kneipp and Nature Cure Sanitarium, was opened in Newark, New Jersey, in 1891.

The best known American hydropath was J. H. Kellogg, a medical doctor who approached hydrotherapy scientifically and performed many experiments trying to understand the physiologic effects of hot and cold water. In 1900 he published *Rational Hydrotherapy*, which is still considered a definitive treatise on the physiologic and therapeutic effects of water, along with an extensive discussion of hydrotherapeutic techniques (Figure 14.1).

## Nature Cure

Natural living, a vegetarian diet, and the use of light and air formed the basis of the Nature Cure movement founded by Dr. Arnold Rickli (1823–1926). In 1848 he established at Veldes Krain, Austria, the first institution of light and air cure or, as it was called in Europe,

Figure
14.1

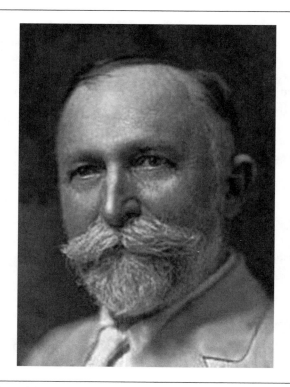

Dr. John Harvey Kellogg, brother of the Kellogg of the breakfast cereal company.

the *atmospheric cure*. He was an ardent disciple of the vegetarian diet and the founder, and, for more than 50 years, president, of the National Austrian Vegetarian Association. In 1891 Louis Kuhne (circa 1823–1907) wrote the *New Science of Healing*, which presented the basic principles of "drugless methods." Dr. Henry Lahman (circa 1823–1907), who founded the largest Nature Cure institution in the world at Weisser Hirsch, near Dresden, Saxony, constructed the first appliances for the administration of electric light treatment and baths. He was the author of several books on diet, nature cure, and heliotherapy. Professor F. E. Bilz (1823–1903) authored the first natural medicine encyclopedia, *The Natural Method of Healing*, which was translated into a dozen languages. The German edition alone ran into 150 editions.

Nature Cure became popular in America through the efforts of Henry Lindlahr, MD, ND, of Chicago, Illinois. Originally a rising businessman in Chicago indulging in all the unhealthy habits of the Gay Nineties era, he became chronically ill while only in his 30s. After receiving no relief from the orthodox practitioners of his day, he learned of Nature Cure, which improved his health. Subsequently, he went to Germany to stay in a sanitarium to be cured and to learn Nature Cure. He went back to Chicago and earned his degrees from the Homeopathic/Eclectic College of Illinois. In 1903 he opened a sanitarium in Elmhurst, Illinois, Lindlahr's Health Food Store, and shortly thereafter founded the Lindlahr College of Natural Therapeutic. In 1908 he began to publish *Nature Cure Magazine* (Lindlahr, 1914a) and began publishing his six-volume series of *Philosophy of Natural Therapeutics* (Lindlahr, 1914b).

One of the chief advantages of training in the early 1900s was the marvelous inpatient facilities that flourished during this time. These facilities provided in-depth training in clinical nature cure and natural hygiene in inpatient settings. Nature cure and natural hygiene are still at the heart of naturopathic medicine's fundamental principles and approach to health care and disease prevention.

## The Hygienic System

Another forerunner of American naturopathy, the "hygienic" school, amalgamated the hydrotherapy and nature cure movements with vegetarianism. It originated as a lay movement of the 19th century and had its genesis in the popular teachings of Sylvester Graham and William Alcott. Graham began preaching the doctrines of temperance and hygiene in 1830, and published, in 1839, *Lectures on the Science of Human Life*; two hefty volumes that prescribed healthy dietary habits. He emphasized a moderate lifestyle, a flesh-free diet, and bran bread as an alternative to bolted or white bread.

The earliest physician to have a significant impact on the hygienic movement and the later philosophical growth of naturopathy was Russell Trall, MD. Trall founded the first school of natural healing arts in this country to have a 4-year curriculum and the authorization to confer the degree of medical doctor. It was founded in 1852 as a "Hydropathic and Physiological School" and was chartered by the New York State Legislature in 1857 under the name New York Hygio-Therapeutic College. He eventually published more than 25 books on the subjects of physiology, hydropathy, hygiene, vegetarianism, and temperance, among many others. The most valuable and enduring of these was his 1851 *Hydropathic Encyclopedia*, a volume of nearly 1,000 pages that covered the theory and practice of hydropathy and the philosophy and treatment of disease advanced by older schools of medicine. The encyclopedia sold more than 40,000 copies.

Martin Luther Holbrook expanded on the work of Graham, Alcott, and Trall and, working with an awareness of the European concepts developed by Pressnitz and Kneipp, laid further groundwork for the concepts later advanced by Lust, Lindlahr, and others.

Holbrook and Trall both advanced the idea that physicians should teach the maintenance of health rather than simply provide a last resort in times of health crisis. In addition to providing a strong editorial voice denouncing the evils of tobacco and drugs, they strongly advanced the value of vegetarianism, bathing and exercise, dietetics, and nutrition along with personal hygiene. This emphasis on prevention would precede the recognition in medicine of the importance of limiting disease by controlling their risk factors, especially for diseases such as cancer, where the problems of treatments impose significant limitations.

John Harvey Kellogg, MD, another medically trained doctor who turned to more nutritionally based natural healing concepts, also greatly influenced Lust. Kellogg was renowned through his connection, beginning in 1876, with the Battle Creek, which was founded in the 1860s as a Seventh-Day Adventist institution designed to perpetuate the Grahamite philosophies. Kellogg, born in 1852, was a "sickly child" who, at age 14 after reading the works of Graham, converted to vegetarianism. At the age of 20, he studied for a term at Trall's Hygio-Therapeutic College and then earned a medical degree at New York's Bellevue Medical School. He maintained an affiliation with the regular schools of medicine during his lifetime because of his practice of surgery.

Kellogg designated his concepts, which were basically the hygienic system of healthful living, as "biologic living." Kellogg expounded vegetarianism, attacked sexual misconduct and the evils of alcohol, and was a prolific writer through the late 19th and early 20th centuries. He produced a popular periodical, *Good Health*, which continued in existence until 1955. When Kellogg died in 1943 at the age of 91, he had had more than 300,000 patients through the Battle Creek Sanitarium, including many celebrities, and the "San" became nationally well known.

Kellogg was also extremely interested in hydrotherapy. In the 1890s he established a laboratory at the San to study the clinical applications of hydrotherapy. This led to his writing of *Rational Hydrotherapy* in 1902. The preface espoused a philosophy of drugless healing that came to be one of the bases of the hydrotherapy school of medical thought in early 20th-century America.

## Autotoxicity

Lust was also greatly influenced by the writing of John H. Tilden, MD, who published between 1915 and 1925. The concept of autotoxicity can be seen to be related to contemporary ideas of cancer causation through the accumulation of internally generated carcinogenic substances in the colon, breast, and other glandular organs (see Chapter 8). Tilden became disenchanted with orthodox medicine and began to rely heavily on dietetics and nutrition, formulating his theories of "autointoxication" (the effect of fecal matter remaining too long in the digestive process) and "toxemia." The term *toxemia* is carried down to this day to describe a dangerous condition of pregnancy. He provided the natural health care literature with a 200-plus-page dissertation entitled *Constipation*, which flowed freely, with a whole chapter devoted to the evils of not responding promptly when nature called.

Elie Metchnikoff (director of the prestigious Pasteur Institute and winner of the 1908 Nobel Prize for contributions to immunology) and Kellogg wrote prolifically on the theory of autointoxication. Kellogg, in particular, believed that humans, in the process of digesting meat, produced a variety of intestinal self-poisons that contributed to autointoxication. These theories remain similar to some contemporary ideas about the possible cause and nutritional prevention of intestinal cancer (see Chapter 10). Kellogg widely proselytized that people must return to a more healthy natural state by facilitating the naturally designed physiology of the colon. He believed that the average modern colon was devitalized by the combination of a low-fiber diet, sedentary living, the custom of sitting rather than squatting to defecate, and the modern civilized habit of ignoring "nature's call" out of an undue concern for politeness.

All naturopathic students are presented with these concepts. Some of that presentation relies on outdated materials, such as the naturopathic tests of the early 1900s—Lindlahr, Tilden, and so forth. However, modern research and textbooks are beginning to investigate these phenomena. Drasar and Hill's *Human Intestinal Flora* (1974) demonstrates some of the biochemical pathways of the generation of metabolic toxins in the gut through bacterial action on poorly digested food. (These concepts in turn are familiar to students of Ayurveda, the traditional medicine of India, presented in Chapter 16.)

Since the early 1980s, understanding of the concept of autotoxicity has been significantly updated by practitioners in the newly emerging field of functional medicine, a health care approach that focuses attention on biochemical individuality, metabolic balance, ecologic context, and unique personal experience in the dynamics of health.

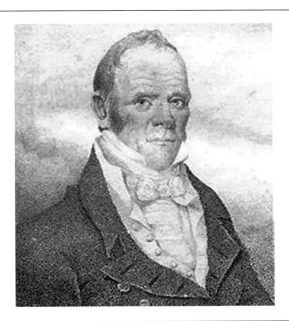

Samuel Thomson (1769-1843).

Maldigestion, malabsorption, and abnormal gut flora and ecology are often found to be primary contributing factors not only to gastrointestinal disorders but also to a wide variety of chronic, systemic illnesses and in some theories are suspected to contribute to cancer. Laboratory assessment tools have been developed that are capable of evaluating the status of many organs, including the gastrointestinal tract. These cutting-edge diagnostic tools provide physicians with an analysis of numerous functional parameters of the individual's digestion and absorption and may precisely identify what in the colonic environment represents imbalance.

## Thomsonianism

In 1822 Samuel Thomson published his *New Guide to Health*, a compilation of his personal view of medical theory and American Indian herbal and medical botanical lore. Thomson espoused a belief that disease had one general cause—derangement of the vital fluids from "cold" influences on the human body—and that disease therefore had one general remedy: animal warmth or "heat." The name of the complaint depended on the part of the body that was affected. Unlike the conventional American "heroic" medical tradition that advocated bloodletting, leeching, and the substantial use of mineral-based purgatives, such as antimony and mercury, Thomson believed that minerals were sources of "cold" because they come from the ground and that vegetation, which grew toward the sun, represented "heat" (see Figure 14.2).

Thomson's view was that individuals could self-treat if they had an adequate understanding of his philosophy and a copy of *New Guide to Health*. The right to sell "family franchises" for use of the Thomsonian method of healing was the basis of a profound popular movement between 1822 and 1843, the year of Thomson's death. Thomson adamantly believed that no professional medical class should exist and that democratic medicine was best practiced by laypersons within a Thomsonian family unit. By 1839 Thomson claimed to have sold some 100,000 of these family franchises, called *friendly botanic societies*. These ideas fit well with the new Jacksonian democracy ushered in by the election of president Andrew Jackson in 1828, as well as the tenets and realities of frontier medicine, where there was no regular physician.

Despite his criticism of the early medical movement for their "heroic" tendencies, Thomson's medical theories were "heroic" in their own fashion. He did not advocate bloodletting or heavy metal poisoning and leeching but rather botanic purgatives— particularly *Lobelia inflata* (Indian tobacco) was a substantial part of the therapy.

## Eclectic Medicine

Some of the doctors practicing Thomsonian medicine, called *botanics*, decided to separate themselves from the lay movement. They established a broader range of therapeutic applications of botanical medicines and founded a medical college in Cincinnati. These Thomsonian doctors were later absorbed into the Eclectic School, which originated with Wooster Beach of New York.

Wooster Beach, from a well-established New England family, started his medical studies at an early age, apprenticing under an old German herbal doctor, Jacob Tidd, until Tidd died. Beach then enrolled in the Barclay Street Medical University in New York. After opening his own practice in New York, Beach set out to win over fellow members of the New York Medical Society (into which he had been warmly introduced by the screening committee) to his point of view that heroic medicine was inherently dangerous and should be reduced to the gentler theories of herbal medicine. He was summarily ostracized from the medial society. He soon founded his own school in New York, calling the clinic and educational facility *The United States Infirmary*. However, because of political pressure from the medial society, he was unable to obtain charter authority to issue legitimate diplomas. He then located a financially ailing but legally chartered school, Worthington College, in Worthington, Ohio. There he opened a full-scale medical college, creating the Eclectic School of medical theory based on the European, Native American, and American traditions. The most enduring eclectic herbal textbook is *King's American Dispensary* by Harvey Wickes Felter and John Uri Lloyd. Published in 1898, this two-volume, 2,500-page treatise provided the definitive identification, preparation, pharmacognosy, history of use, and clinical application of more than 1,000 botanical medicines. The eclectic herbal lore formed an integral core of the therapeutic armamentarium of the naturopathic doctor.

## Homeopathic Medicine

Homeopathy, the creation of an early German physician, Samuel Hahnemann (1755–1843), had four central doctrines: (1) the "law of similars," that likes cures like; (2) the effect of a medication could be heightened by its administration in minute doses (the more diluted the dose, the greater the "dynamic" effect); (3) nearly all diseases were the result of a suppressed itch or "psora"; and (4) Hering's law: healing proceeds from within outward, above downward, from more vital to less vital organs, and in the reverse order of the appearance of symptoms (pathobiography).

Originally, most homeopaths in this country were converted orthodox medical doctors, or *allophaths* (a term coined by Hahnemann). The high rate of conversion made this particular medical sect the archenemy of the rising orthodox medical profession. The first American homeopathic medical school was founded in 1848 in Philadelphia; the last purely homeopathic medical school, based in Philadelphia, survived into the early 1930s (see Chapter 17).

## Manipulative Therapies

In Missouri, Andrew Taylor Still, originally trained as an orthodox practitioner, founded the school of medical thought known as *osteopathy*. He conceived a system of healing that emphasized the primary importance of the structural integrity of the body, especially as it affects the vascular system, in the maintenance of health. In 1892 he opened the American School of Osteopathy in Kirksville, Missouri.

In 1895 Daniel David Palmer, originally a magnetic healer from Davenport, Iowa, performed the first spinal manipulation, which gave rise to the school he termed *chiropractic*. His philosophy was similar to Still's except for a greater emphasis on the importance of proper neurological function. He formally published his findings in 1910, after having founded a chiropractic school in Davenport.

Less well known is Zone Therapy, originated by Joe Shelby Riley, DC, a chiropractor based in Washington, DC. Zone therapy was an early forerunner of acupressure as it related "pressures and manipulations of the fingers and tongue, and percussion on the spinal column, according to the relation of the fingers to certain zones of the body."

## Spirituality

Christian Science, formulated by Mary Baker Eddy in 1879, comprises a profound belief in the role of systematic religious study (which led to the widespread Christian Science Reading Rooms), spirituality, and prayer in the treatment of disease. She published *Science and Health with Key to the Scriptures* (Eddy, 1875), the definitive textbook for the study of Christian Science.

Lust was also influenced by the works of Sidney Weltmer, the founder of Suggestive Therapeutics. Weltmer's work dealt specifically with the psychologic process of desiring to be healthy. The theory behind Professor Weltmer's work was that whether it was the mind or the body that first lost its grip on health, the two were inseparably related. When the problem originated in the body, the mind nonetheless lost its ability and desire to overcome the disease because the patient "felt sick" and consequently slid further into the diseased state. Alternatively, if the mind first lost its ability and desire to "be healthy" and some physical infirmity followed, the patient was susceptible to being overcome by disease.

## Physical Culture

Bernarr McFadden, a close friend of Lust's, founded the "Physical Culture" school of health and healing, also known as *physcultopathy*. This school of healing gave birth across the country to gymnasiums at which exercise programs, designed to allow the individual man and woman to establish and maintain optimal physical health, were developed and taught.

Many theories exist to explain the rapid dissolution of these diverse healing arts (which at one time made up more than 25% of health care practitioners in the United States). In the early part of the 20th century, low ratings in the Flexner Report (which rated all these schools among the lowest), the application of term *scientific* to allopathic medicine, and the growing political sophistication of the AMA clearly played significant roles.

All of these healing systems and modalities were naturally unified in the field of naturopathic medicine because they shared one common tenet: respect for and inquiry into the self-healing process and what was necessary to establish health.

# Naturopathy and Cancer

The naturopathic journals of the 1920s and 1930s provided valuable insight into the prevention of disease and the promotion of health. Much of the dietary advice focused on correcting poor eating habits, including the lack of fiber in the diet and an overreliance on red meat as a protein source. Today the recommendations of the American Cancer Society, the American Medical Association, the U.S. Surgeon General, the National Institutes of Health, and the National Cancer Institute generally substantiate the early assertions of the naturopaths that poor dietary habits lead to degenerative diseases, including cancers associated with the digestive tract and the colon.

The December 1928 volume of *Nature's Path* was the first American publication of the works of Herman J. DeWolff, a Dutch epidemiologist. He was one of the first researchers to identify, on the basis of studies of the incidence of cancer in the Netherlands, a correlation between exposure to petrochemicals and various types of cancerous conditions. He saw a connection between chemical fertilizers and their use in some soils (principally clay) that led to their remaining in vegetables after they had arrived at the market and were purchased for consumption. Almost 50 years later, orthodox medicine began to see the importance of such observations in helping to control cancer and other chronic diseases.

## Recent Influences

It is now well established that nutritional factors are important in the pathogenesis of both atherosclerosis and cancer, the two leading causes of death in Western countries. Studies validating their importance in the pathogenesis of many other diseases continue to be published. A tremendous amount of scientific support for the principles of naturopathic medicine has been gathered through mainstream research. In fact, mainstream medicine is increasingly turning to the use of naturopathic methods in the search for effective preventive strategies against today's intractable and expensive diseases, such as cancer (Werbach, 1996).

Naturopaths were astute clinical observers, and a century ago, began to recognize many of the concepts that are now gaining popularity with the support of scientific data. The scientific tools of the time were inadequate to assess the validity of their concepts. In addition, as a group, they seemed to have little inclination toward the application of laboratory research, especially because "science" was a weapon used by the AMA to suppress the profession. This situation has now changed. In the past few decades a considerable amount of research is now providing the scientific documentation of many of the concepts of naturopathic medicine. A new generation of scientifically trained naturopaths is using this research to continue development of the profession. The following section describes some of the most important trends.

## Therapeutic Nutrition

Since 1929, when Eijkman and Hopkins shared the Nobel Prize in medicine and physiology for the discovery of vitamins, the role of these trace substances in clinical nutrition has been a matter of scientific investigation. The discovery that enzyme systems depended on essential nutrients provided the naturopathic profession with great insights into why and how diet is important for health. In 1955, nutritional biochemist Roger Williams's formulation of the concept of "biochemical individuality" further developed these ideas and provided great insights into the unique nutritional needs of each individual, how to correct inborn errors of metabolism, and even treat specific diseases through the use of nutrient-rich foods or large doses of specific nutrients.

Linus Pauling, the two-time Nobel Prize winner, coined the concept of orthomolecular medicine and provided further theoretical substantiation for the use of nutrients as therapeutic agents. Functional medicine is a recent development in the use of therapeutic nutrition in the prevention of illness and promotion of health. Focusing on biochemical individuality, metabolic balance, and the ecologic context, functional medicine practitioners avail themselves of recently developed laboratory tests to pinpoint imbalances in an individual's biochemistry that can set into motion a cascade of biologic triggers, paving the way to suboptimal function, chronic illness, and degenerative disease. A broad range of functional laboratory assessment tools in the areas of digestion (gastrointestinal), nutrition, detoxification/oxidative stress, immunology/allergy, production and regulation of hormones (endocrinology), and heart and blood vessels (cardiovascular ) provide physicians with the information needed to recommend nutritional interventions specific to the individual's needs and to precisely monitor their efficacy.

## Environmental Medicine/Clinical Ecology

Although recognition of the clinical impact of environmental toxicity and endogenous toxicity has existed since the earliest days of naturopathy, it was not until the environmental movement that a scientific basis was established. Clinical research and the development of laboratory methods for assessing toxic load have provided objective tools to increase the sophistication of clinical practice. Clinical and laboratory methods have been developed for the assessment of idiosyncratic reactions to environmental factors and foods.

## Psychoneuroimmunology

Naturopathic medicine's philosophy of treating the whole person and enhancing the individual's inherent healing ability is closely aligned with its mission of integrating spirituality into the healing process. Scientific evidence is growing on how spirituality can play a part in healing. Since Descartes separated mind from body in the 17th century, medical science has attempted to explain disease independently of mind, in terms of germs, environmental agents, or wayward genes. Today, however, the evidence is not just from clinical observation but is biochemically based. An explosion of research in the new and rapidly expanding field of psychoneuroimmunology is revealing physical evidence of the mind/body connection that is changing our understanding of disease.

Scientists no longer question whether, but how, our minds have an impact on our health. The implications of these connections uncovered since the early 1980s are significant in the care of cancer (see Chapters 4–7).

## Laboratory Methods

A significant influence has been the development of laboratory methods for the objective assessment of nutritional statues, methabolic dysfunction, digestive function, bowel flora, endogenous and exogenous toxic load, and liver detoxification. Each of these has provided ever more effective tools for accurate assessment of patient health status and effective application of naturopathic principles.

# Naturopathic Principles in Practice

Naturopathic medicine is a distinct system of health-oriented medicine that stresses promotion of health, prevention of disease, patient education, and self-responsibility. However, naturopathic medicine symbolizes more than simply health practices; it is a way of life. Naturopathy is not identified with any particular therapy but rather a way of thinking about life, health, and disease. It is defined not just by the therapies it uses but by the philosophical principles that guide the practitioner in the application of these therapies.

Seven concepts provide the foundation that defines naturopathic medicine: (1) the healing power of nature (*vis medicatrix naturae*), (2) first do no harm (*primum non nocere*), (3) find the cause (*tolle causam*), (4) treat the whole person (*holism*), (5) preventive medicine, (6) wellness (*proposed*), and (7) doctor as teacher (*docere*).

## The Healing Power of Nature (vis medicatrix naturae)

Belief in the ability of the body to heal itself—the *vis medicatrix naturae* (the healing power of nature)—if given the proper opportunity, and the importance of living within the laws of nature are the foundation of naturopathic medicine. The healing power of nature was also a concept of regular medical practitioners during the colonial era in America, as physicians of the time often had little else to offer, for example, during epidemics of infectious disease for which there was no cure. Although the term *naturopathy* was coined in the late 19th century, its philosophical roots are popularly traced back to Hippocrates. It all derives from a common wellspring with traditional world medicines: belief in the healing power of nature.

Medicine has long grappled with the question of the *vis medicatrix naturae*. As Neuberger stated in 1932, "the problem of the healing power of nature is a great, perhaps the greatest of all problems which has occupied the physician for thousands of years. Indeed, the aims and limits of therapeutics are determined by its solution." The fundamental reality of the healing power of nature was a basic tenant of the Hippocratic school of medicine, and "every important medical author since has had to take a position for or against it." Naturopathic medicine is "vitalistic" in its approach (i.e., life is viewed as more than just the sum of biochemical processes), and the body is believed to have an innate intelligence or process that is always striving toward health. Vitalism maintains that the symptoms accompanying disease are not typically caused by the pathogenic agent (e.g., bacteria); rather, they are the result of the organism's intrinsic response or reaction to the agent and the organism's attempt to defend and heal itself. Symptoms are part of a constructive phenomenon that is the best "choice" the organism can make, given the circumstances. In this construct the physician's role is to understand and aid the body's efforts and not to take over or manipulate the functions of the body, unless the self-healing process has become weak or insufficient.

Although the context of naturopathic medicine is its vitalistic core, both vitalistic and mechanistic approaches are applicable to modern naturopathic medicine. Vitalism has reemerged in today's terms in the body/mind/spirit connection. Matter, mind, energy, and spirit are each part of nature and therefore are part of a medicine that observes, respects, and works with nature. Much of modern biomedicine and related research is based on the application of the theory of mechanism (defined in Webster's dictionary as the "theory that everything in the universe is produced by matter in motion; materialism") in a highly reductionistic, single-agent, pathology-based, disease-care model. Applied in a vitalistic context, mechanistic and reductionistic interventions provide useful techniques and tools to naturopathic physicians. Naturopathic medicine provides clinical guidance for integrating both approaches.

## First Do No Harm (primum non nocere)

Naturopathic physicians prefer noninvasive treatments that minimize the risks of harmful side effects. They are trained to use the lowest force and lowest risk strategies for preventive, diagnostic, and therapeutic purposes. They are trained to know which patients they can safely treat and which ones they need to refer to other health care practitioners. Naturopathic physicians follow three precepts to avoid harming the patient: (1) use methods and medicinal substances that minimize the risk of harmful effects and apply the least possible force or intervention necessary to diagnose illness and restore health; (2) when possible, the suppression of symptoms is avoided because suppression generally interferes with the healing process; and (3) respect and work with the healing power of nature in diagnosis, treatment, and counseling because if the self-healing process in not respected, the patient may be harmed.

## Find the Cause (tolle causam)

Every illness has an underlying cause or causes, often in aspects of the lifestyle, diet, or habits of the individual. A naturopathic physician is trained to find and remove the underlying cause(s) of disease. The therapeutic order helps the physician remove them in the correct "healing order" for the body. As the new science of psychoneuroimmunology demonstrates, the body is a seamless web with a multiplicity of brain/immune system/gut/liver connections. Not surprisingly, chronic disease typically involves a number of systems, with the most prominent or acute symptoms being those chronologically last in appearance. As the healing process progresses and these symptoms are alleviated, further symptoms then resurface that must then be addressed to restore health (many of these ideas are also found in the practice of Chinese medicine; see Chapter 15).

## Treat the Whole Person (holism)

Health or disease comes from a complex interaction of mental, emotional, spiritual, physical, dietary, genetic, environmental, lifestyle, and other factors. Naturopathic physicians treat the whole person, taking all of these factors into account (Grumbach, 2003). Naturopathically, the body is viewed as a whole. Naturopathy also represents a *holistic medicine* in reference to the term *holism*, coined by philosopher Jan Christian Smuts in 1926 to describe the whole of a system as greater than the sum of its parts. A change in one part causes a change in every part; therefore the study of one part must be integrated into the whole, including the community and biosphere.

Naturopathic medicine asserts that one cannot be healthy in an unhealthy environment and is committed to the creation of a world in which humanity may thrive. In contrast to the high degree of specialization in the present medical system, which reflects a mechanistic orientation to single organs, the holistic model places specialists in an ancillary role. Emphasis is placed on the physical, emotional, social, and spiritual integration of the whole person, including awareness of the impact of the environment on health.

## Preventive Medicine and Wellness

The naturopathic approach to health care helps prevent disease and keeps minor illnesses from developing into more serious or chronic degenerative diseases. Patients are taught the principles with which to live a healthful life, and by following these principles, they can help prevent major illness. Health is viewed as more than just the absence of disease; it is considered a dynamic state that enables a person to thrive in, or adapt to, a wide range of environments and stresses. Health and disease are points on a continuum, with death at one end and optimal function at the other. The naturopathic physician believes that a person who goes through life living an unhealthful lifestyle will drift away from optimal function and move relentlessly toward progressively greater dysfunction. Genotype, constitution, maternal influences, and environmental factors all influence individual susceptibility to deterioration and the organs and physiologic systems affected. The virulence of pathogenic agents or insults also plays a central role in disturbance, causing decreasing function and ultimately serious disease.

In our society, although our life span at birth has increased, our health span has not, nor has our health expectancy at age 65. We are living longer but often as disabled individuals. Although such deterioration is accepted by our society as the normal expectation of aging, it is not common in animals in the wild or among those rare peoples who live in an optimal environment (i.e., no pollution, low stress, regular exercise, and abundant natural, nutritious food).

In the naturopathic model death is inevitable; progressive disability is not. This belief underscores a fundamental difference in philosophy and expectation between the conventional and naturopathic models of health and disease. In contrast to the disease-treatment focus of allopathic medicine, the health-promotion focus of naturopathic medicine emphasizes the means of maximizing health span.

## Doctor as Teacher (docere)

The original meaning of the word *docere* is teacher. A principle objective of naturopathic medicine is to educate the patient and emphasize self-responsibility for health. Naturopathic physicians also recognize the therapeutic potential of the doctor/patient relationship. The patient is engaged and respected as an ally and a member of her or his own health care team. Adequate time is spent with patients to thoroughly diagnose, treat, and educate them.

## Therapeutic Modalities

Naturopathic medicine uses natural medicines and interventionist therapies as needed. Natural medicines and therapies, when properly used, generally have low invasiveness and rarely cause suppression or side effects. This is because, when used properly, they generally support the body's healing mechanisms rather than taking over the body's processes. The ND determines when, why, and with what patient more invasive therapies are needed based on the therapeutic order and appropriate diagnostic measures. He or she also recognizes that the use of natural, low-force therapies; lifestyle changes; and early functional diagnosis and treatment of nonspecific conditions is a form of prevention. This approach offers one viable solution for cost containment in primary health care. Traditional health care disciplines such as traditional Chinese medicine (TCM), Unani medicine, and homeopathic medicine each have a philosophy, principles of practice, and clinical theory that form a system for diagnosis, treatment, and case management. A philosophy of medicine is, in essence, the rational investigation of the truth and principles of that medicine. The principles of practice form an outline or guidelines to the main precepts or fundamental tenets of a system of medicine. Clinical theory provides a system of rules or principles explaining that medicine, and applying that system to the patient by means of diagnosis, treatment, and management. The specific substances and techniques, as well as when, why, and to whom they are applied and for how long, depend on the system. Modalities (e.g., botanical medicine and physical medicine) are not systems but rather therapeutic approaches used within these systems. One modality may be used by many systems but in different ways.

It is the system used by each of these disciplines that makes it a uniquely effective field of medicine rather than a vague compendium of complementary and alternative medicine (CAM) modalities. Techniques from many systems are used within naturopathic medicine because of its primary care integrative approach and strong philosophical orientation.

### Clinical Nutrition

The use of diet as a therapy serves as a therapeutic foundation of naturopathic medicine. A rapidly increasing body of knowledge supports the use of whole foods, fasting, natural hygiene, and nutritional supplements in the maintenance of health and treatment of disease. The recognition of unique nutritional requirements caused by biochemical individuality has provided a theoretical and practical basis for the appropriate use of megavitamin therapy. Controlled fasting is also used clinically.

### Botanical Medicines

Plants have been used as medicines since antiquity. The technology now exists to understand the physiologic activities of herbs and a tremendous amount of research worldwide, especially in Europe, is demonstrating clinical efficacy. Botanical medicines are used for both vitalistic and pharmacologic actions. Pharmacologic effects and contraindication, as well as synergetic, energetic, and dilutional uses, are fundamental knowledge in naturopathic medicine.

## Homeopathic Medicine

Derives etymologically from the Greek word *homeos*, meaning "similar," and *pathos*, meaning "disease." Homeopathy is a system of medicine that treats a patient and his or her condition with a dilute, potentiated agent, or drug, that will produce the same symptoms as the disease when given to a healthy individual; the fundamental principle being that like cures like. This principle was actually first recognized by Hippocrates, who noticed that herbs and other substances given in small doses tended to cure the same symptoms they produced when given in toxic doses. Prescriptions are based on the totality of all of the patient's symptoms and matched to "proving" of homeopathic medicines. Provings are symptoms produced in healthy people who are unaware of the specific remedy they have received. Large numbers of people are tested, and these symptoms documented. The symptoms are then added to toxicology, symptomatology, and data from cured cases to form the homeopathic materia medica. Homeopathic medicines are derived from a variety of plant, mineral, and animal substances and are prepared according to the specifications of the *Homeopathic Pharmacopoeia of the United States*. Over 100 clinical studies have demonstrated the clinical efficacy of homeopathic therapies (see Chapter 17).

## Acupuncture

Acupuncture is an ancient Chinese system of medicine involving the stimulation of certain specific points on the body to enhance the flow of vital energy (*qi*) along pathways called *meridians*. Acupuncture points can be stimulated by the insertion and withdrawing of needles, the application of heat (moxibustion), massage, laser, electrical, or a combination of these methods. Traditional Chinese acupuncture implies a very specific acupuncture technique and knowledge of the Chinese system of medicine, including yin/yang, the five elements, acupuncture points and meridians, and a method of diagnosis and differentiation of syndromes quite different from that of Western medicine. Although most research in this country has focused on its use for the pain relief and the treatment of addictions, it is a complete system of medicine effective for many diseases (see Chapter 15).

## Hydrotherapy

Hydrotherapy is the use of water in any of its forms (e.g., hot, cold, ice, and steam) and methods of application (e.g., sitz bath, douche, spa and hot tub, whirlpool, sauna, shower, immersion bath, pack, poultice, foot bath, fomentation, wrap, and colonic irrigations) in the maintenance of health or treatment disease. It is one of the most ancient methods of treatment and has been part of naturopathic medicine since its inception. Nature doctors before and since Sebastian Kneipp have used hydrotherapy as a central part of clinical practice. Hydrotherapy has been used to treat disease and injury by many different cultures, including the Egyptians, Assyrians, Persians, Greeks, Hebrews, Hindus, and Chinese. Its most sophisticated applications were developed in 18th-century Germany. Naturopathic physicians today use hydrotherapy to stimulate and support healing, for detoxification, and to strengthen immune function for many chronic and acute conditions.

## Physical Medicine

Physical medicine refers to the therapeutic use of touch, heat, cold, electricity, and sound. This includes the use of physiotherapy equipment such as ultrasound, diathermy, and other electromagnetic energy agents; therapeutic exercise; massage; massage energy techniques, joint mobilization (manipulative), and immobilization techniques; and hydrotherapy. In the therapeutic order, correction of structural integrity is a key factor; the hands-on approach of naturopathic physicians through physical medicine is important in care.

## Detoxification

Detoxification is the recognition and correction of endogenous and exogenous toxicity, is an important theme in naturopathic medicine that involves liver and bowel detoxification, elimination of environmental toxins, and correction of the metabolic dysfunction(s) that cause the buildup of non-end-product metabolites. These techniques all are important ways of decreasing toxic load that have direct relevance in the development of cancer. Spiritual and emotional toxicity are also recognized as important factors in restoring health and these problems are also now seen as having direct chemical consequences through psychoneuroimmunologic mechanisms.

## Spirituality

Spirituality and health issues are central to naturopathic practice and based on the individual patient's belief and/or spiritual orientation, what moves the patient toward life and a higher purpose than himself or herself. Because total health also includes spiritual health, naturopathic physicians encourage individuals to pursue their personal spiritual development. As number of studies demonstrate in the newly emerging field of psychoneuroimmunology that the body is not a mere collection of organs, but a body, mind, and spirit in which the mind/spirit part of the equation marshals tremendous forces promoting health or disease (see Chapter 7).

## Counseling Techniques

Counseling, health psychology, and lifestyle modification techniques are essential modalities for the naturopathic physician. An ND is formally trained in mental, emotional, and family counseling. Various treatment measures include hypnosis and guided imagery, counseling techniques, correcting underlying organic factors, and family systems therapy.

# Clinical Approach

The therapeutic approach of the naturopathic doctor is basically twofold: to help patients heal themselves and to use the opportunity to guide and educate the patient in developing a more healthful lifestyle. Many supposedly incurable conditions respond very well to naturopathic approaches.

A typical first office visit with an ND takes 1 hour. The goal is to learn as much as possible about the patient using thorough history and review of systems, physical examination, laboratory tests, radiology, and other standard diagnostic procedures. Moreover, the patient's diet, environment, toxic load, exercise, stress, and other aspect of lifestyle are evaluated, and laboratory tests are used to determine physiologic function. Once a good understanding of the patient's health and disease status is established (making a diagnosis of a disease is only one part of this process), the ND and patient work together to establish a treatment and health promotion program.

# Management of Preneoplastic Conditions

The naturopathic approach to the management of preneoplastic conditions can be illustrated by the case of cervical dysplasia. The traditional medical approach to treating cervical dysplasia, a precancerous condition of the cervix, is surgical resection. The typical naturopathic treatment would include the following:

1 *Education:* Specifically about factors that increase the risk of cervical cancer, such as smoking (risk = 3.0), multiple sex partners (risk = 3.4), and the use of oral contraceptives (risk = 3.6).

2 *Prevention:* Because many patients with cervical cancer are deficient in one or more nutrients, the woman's nutritional status would be optimized (through diet, especially by increasing intake of fruits and vegetables) and with regard to those nutrients known to be deficient (often a result of oral contraceptive use) in women with cervical dysplasia and the deficiencies of which may promote cellular abnormalities: folic acid, beta-carotene, vitamin C, vitamin $B_6$, and selenium.

3 *Treatment:* The vaginal depletion pack (a traditional mixture of botanical medicines placed against the cervix) would be used to promote sloughing of the abnormal cells.

The advantages of this approach are as follows: the causes of the cervical dysplasia have been identified and addressed (obviously, changing the woman's high-risk lifestyle is a complicated matter and not one easily solved but nonetheless attempts to educate have been made); no surgery is used, thus no scar tissue is formed (it is duly recognized that standard medicine may also use exfoliative regimens and not resect as well); and the cost, particularly considering that many women with cervical dysplasia have recurrences when treated with standard surgery, is reasonable. More important, however, is that the woman's general health has been improved, and other conditions that could have been caused by the identified nutritional deficiencies have now been helped.

The disadvantages, however, are that the results are undependable and unproven empirically. Therefore, it should be noted that women take ownership over their ultimate outcome by disassociating themselves from traditional mainstream medicine, and failure of naturopathic therapies may lead to poorer outcomes should they fail. Furthermore, many insurance companies will not reimburse ND care, and cost may paradoxically be higher than that of traditional care. Of course, education and prevention and care of the woman's general health are of concern to both naturopathic and mainstream practitioners.

Lifestyle modification is crucial to the successful implementation of naturopathic techniques—health does not come from a doctor, pills, or surgery but rather from the patients' own efforts to take proper care of themselves. Our society expends considerable resources to encourage lifestyles that we now know include disease-promoting habits. Although it is relatively easy to tell a patient to stop smoking, get more exercise, and reduce his or her stress, such lifestyle changes are difficult in the context of peers, habits, and commercial pressures. The ND is specifically trained to assist the patient in making the needed changes. This involves many aspects: helping the patient acknowledge the need; setting realistic, progressive goals; identifying and working through barriers; establishing a support group of family and friends or of others with similar problems; identifying the stimuli that reinforce the unhealthy behavior; and giving the patient positive reinforcement for his or her gains.

# Summary

The problem of cancer continues to grow in modern society. Attempts to control recognized risk factors are difficult and there are inherent limitations to many of the available cancer therapies. Naturopathic approaches to prevention of cancer and care of the patient offer a model for effective integration of the various complementary and alternative modalities shown to have benefit. In this way, the modern eclectic approach of naturopathy may provide one path for the practice of integrative medicine in the care of the cancer patient.

## REFERENCES AND RESOURCES

Blois, M. (1988). Medicine and the nature of vertical reasoning. *New England Journal of Medicine, 318*(13), 847–851.

Clarke, E., Hatcher, J., McKeown-Essyen, G., & Liekrish, G. (1985). Cervical dyplasia: Association with sexual behavior, smoking, and oral contraceptive use. *American Journal of Obstetrics and Gynecology, 151*, 612–616.

Cooper, R., & Stoflet, S. (1996). Trends in the education and practice of alternative medicine clinicians. *Health Affairs, 15*(3), 226 and 233.

Dawson, E., Nosovitch, J., & Hannigan, E. (1984). Serum vitamin and selenium changes in cervical dysplasia. *Federal Proceedings, 46*, 612.

Grumbach, K. (2003). Chronic illness, comorbidities, and the need for medical generalism. *Annals of Family Medicine, 1*, 4–7.

Lindlahr, H. (1914). Philosophy of natural therapeutics: Vols. I, II, and III. *Dietetics*. Maidstone, UK: Maidstone Osteopathic.

Lust, B. (1918). *Universal naturopathic directory and buyer's guide*. Butler, NJ: Lust.

Lust, B. (1945). Program of the 49th Congress of the American Naturopathy Association.

Pellegrino, E. (1979). Medicine, science, art: An old controversy revisited. *Man and Medicine, 4*, 43–52.

Standish, L., Snider, P., Calabrese, C., & NMRA Core Team. (2004). *The future and foundations of naturopathic medical science: Report to the NIHCCAM on naturopathic medical research agenda (NMRA)*. Bethesda, MD: National Institutes of Health.

Werbach, M. (1996). *The American Holistic Health Association complete guide to alternative medicine* (pp. 118 and 123). New York: Werner Books.

Whorton, J. (1982). *Crusaders for fitness*. Princeton, NJ: Princeton University Press.

Zeff, J. (1997). The process of healing: A unifying theory of naturopathic medicine. *Journal of Naturopathic Medicine, 7*(1), 122.

Zeff, J., Snider, P., & Myers, A. (2006). A hierarchy of healing: The therapeutic order—The unifying theory of naturopathic medicine. In J. Pizzorno & M. Murray (Eds.), *Textbook of natural medicine*. St Louis, MO: Churchill Livingstone.

# Chinese Medicine and Cancer Care

*Activity is closer to the essence of life than struc-
ture, since structure exists for the sake of activity.
The key to the living thing is the excellence of its
agency. An organism can change itself.*
— Robert Augros and George
Stanciu in *The New Biology*

## Harriet Beinfield
## Efrem Korngold
## Marc S. Micozzi

Every medicine emerges from the interaction between biology and culture. Medical
practices are the product of a social, political, and economic milieu, shaped by customary
habits and traditions, many having little to do with science, evidence, or even medicine
itself (Beinfield & Beinfield, 1997). Chinese traditional medicine has been shaped through
continuous use by what is now one-quarter of the world's population. For more than
23 centuries the people of China have used it to diagnose, treat, and prevent disease as
well as to foster health.

All medicines seek to explain why people fall sick in the service of crafting therapies
that will make those people well. These explanations predictably vary. The Chinese traditional medical system is both a heterogeneous and comprehensive body of knowledge,
organized by explanatory models that significantly diverge from those of modern Western medicine.[1] Differing worldviews are represented by distinct conceptual vocabularies.
What is conventional in one time and place is alternative in another.

Chinese traditional medicine might even view Western medicine as experimental
from the vantage point of its comparative maturity. Yet common to the medicines of
diverse traditions is the intention to relieve discomfort, pain, and suffering, to protect
life, and to promote happiness.

In modern Western medicine, the mechanistic, quantitative constructs of science prevail, whereas in the traditional medicine of China, organismic,[2] qualitative
schemata describe individuals as resilient, dynamic ecosystems. Whereas the focus of
medical science is on the pathologic entity, Chinese traditional medicine draws on a

nature-centered cosmology that emphasizes the relationship between the seed and the soil: what is it about the terrain that permits cancer, or any disease, to take root?

Since the time of its origins 3,000 years ago, Chinese medicine (*Zhong Yi*) has been used for the treatment of tumors, identified in antiquity as *liu yan,* meaning "lumps as hard as a rock," or as *zhong yang,* meaning "inflamed ulcers." Over the course of these millennia, various strategies have developed, ranging from:

- Reducing pain, swelling, inflammation, and tumor mass
- Improving host resistance through the use of *Fuzheng Gu Ben* therapy, meaning to "strengthen what is correct and secure the root," which in modern language means to preserve immune competence and enhance the function of the internal organs to counter chemotherapy-induced immune or myelosuppression
- Potentiating the effects of conventional radiation and chemotherapies
- Preventing, controlling, and treating the adverse effects of conventional treatment, including fatigue, weakness, gastrointestinal distress, loss of appetite, nausea, emesis, and leucopenia

In 1999, a San Francisco population-based study indicated that 72% of women with breast cancer used at least one form of complementary or alternative medicine (CAM) (Adler, 1999). Although few abandoned conventional treatment, only half reported the use of CAM to their physicians (Cassileth et al., 1984). An understanding and appreciation of Chinese medicine may lead to greater comfort on the part of providers ill at ease with the use of therapies about which they have neither training nor experience. This in turn may lead to improved doctor/patient communication and cooperation. Oncologist Debu Tripathy comments, "Conventional cancer treatment is only partially or minimally effective in many settings. Most common epithelial (solid) tumors in adults are not curable at the advanced stages. Although many therapies may induce transient responses, often resistance will develop. Furthermore, side effects of therapy can require discontinuation or, in some cases, patient refusal of therapy altogether. Even newer biologically targeted therapies tend to be effective only in a minority of treated patients, and resistance to these novel agents eventually develops as it does with conventional cancer drugs. Given the clear limitations of standard cancer treatment, many patients with cancer will opt to add CAM to their plan with the attitude that it cannot hurt and might help."[3] Cancer levels the playing field in medicine: no one knows how to prevent or solve this epidemic problem. It is with humility that health care providers of all types seek, to the best of their ability, to be helpful.

Because Chinese medicine appears to protect against the damaging effects of chemotherapy and radiation, it increases the likelihood that patients will suffer less during and recover their health after completing these therapies, enhancing quality of life. Chinese medicine treats the patient as well as the disease.

There are various approaches to the subject of how Chinese medicine treats cancer, and there is also an equivalent number of languages. One language expresses how Chinese medicine understands the body and thinks about what we call cancer, using its own traditional vocabulary that has endured over centuries; another is scientific, reporting research findings on the use of acupuncture and Chinese herbal medicine, describing them in modern neurophysiologic and biochemical terms; and the third is the universal cross-cultural medium of story, anecdotes describing the experience of the patient.

# Historical Origins

There are mythic Chinese heroes who were simultaneously the progenitors of Chinese civilization and medicine. Fu Xi invented picture symbols, the rules of marriage, the arts of cooking, music, and the *ba gua* or eight trigrams, on which the *Yi Jing* (*Book of Changes*) is based. The originator of herbal medicine is Shen Nong, the Divine Husbandman and legendary founder of agriculture. Believed to have lived 4,600 years ago, he taught the Chinese people how to cultivate plants and identify their healing virtues as well as how to raise livestock. The *Shen Nong Ben Cao Jing* (*Divine Husbandman's Classic of the Materia Medica*) is attributed to Shen Nong but was written during the latter Han Dynasty between 200 and 500 A.C.E. (Unschuld, 1986). This text, still in use, describes the medicinal properties of 252 botanical herbs, 45 minerals, and 67 animal substances (Bensky & Gamble, 1993). Although there are more than 13,000 substances currently catalogued in the *Chinese Materia Medica*, physicians routinely use about 500 to 700 of them.

About 2,000 years ago, the mythic Yellow Emperor, Huang Di, is said to have produced the *Huang-di Nei-jing* (*Inner Classic of the Yellow Emperor*), written over the course of 200 years as a dialogue between himself and his minister, Qi Bo, setting forth the systematic theories of Chinese medicine. The *Nei Jing* describes human harmony with the seasons, advising doctors how to guide patients toward an accord with the natural world. It is divided into two texts: the *Su Wen* (*Fundamental Questions*) elaborates basic medical concepts, including *yin-yang*, five phases, anatomy, physiology, pathology, and treatment; and the *Ling Shu* (*Spiritual Axis*) explains the principles of acupuncture. In addition to medicine, Huang Di is said to have taught humankind how to build with wood, weave with silk, and craft boats, wheeled carts, bows, and arrows. Disease from this time forth was not simply regarded as a natural cataclysm about which to seek supernatural aid— medicine became a human endeavor, and environmental and behavioral vectors were seen as causes of disease (Birch & Felt, 1999).

# Why History Matters

According to the preeminent historical scholar of Chinese medicine Paul Unschuld,[4] although science and medicine arose simultaneously in both Greece and China, European medical ideas differed dramatically from those in China. In both places people were clever and thoughtful, shared the same biology, and complained about similar maladies—the differences lay in the realm of cultural interpretation. Unique social, economic, and political conditions within each culture generated unique explanatory models.

Unschuld notes that the Ancient Greeks originated the notion of democracy, the pillar of which was one person/one vote. New rules were needed to make self-governance work. Because even natural laws are human constructs, the ideas underlying the organization of the state were transposed onto the body, and the image of the human body was modeled on the political body (*polis*). Just as the state was composed of individual citizens, the body was reduced to an aggregate of discrete structural components forming larger entities. To understand the whole, it was necessary to dissect it into smaller parts.

In China, chaos reigned during the warring states period when approximately 1,500 small kingdoms remained in constant combat for generations. This situation shifted during the 3rd century B.C.E., when smaller states were consolidated and unified as the Chinese Empire. Lo and behold the image of the body was similarly consolidated and integrated. Only after the birth of the empire did the idea of the human body as a coherent organism emerge. The visceral organs were assigned roles that corresponded to the political structure of the state: the heart was the emperor, the spleen the minister of agriculture, the stomach the granary, the liver the general, and the gall bladder the judge. The body became a mutually interacting set of organized bureaucracies. Just as canals, rivers, and irrigation agriculture enabled the production and transport of goods and resources throughout the empire, a matrix of channels were presumed to transport *qi* and blood throughout the body.

Where the Greeks saw individuals, the Chinese saw interdependent networks. Although Western science demands analysis of the composition of structures (organs, tissues, cells, molecules, atoms, subatomic particles), the Eastern tradition sees dynamic functional processes interacting within a complex whole. Western logic is reductive and quantitative; Eastern logic is contextual and qualitative. Whereas in the West authority is derived from the latest research, in China it is derived from classic texts. In Chinese medicine it is often necessary to clothe a new idea in the language of ancient authors to gain acceptance. History matters.

Kim Taylor (2005) documents the origins of traditional Chinese medicine in postrevolutionary China. In the 1950s, Mao knew there were not enough Western-trained doctors to meet China's needs, so he mandated that traditional medicine be "rehabilitated" to fill the gap. Committees of Western-trained physicians, with a few traditional doctors as advisors, were formed to carve a logical, internally consistent, standardized, homogenous medical system from the vast heterogeneous legacy of traditional knowledge. This neat, *new* system also had to conform to the ideologies of dialectical materialism and modern science. What we now know as traditional Chinese medicine (TCM) was the work product of these committees that were hardly representative of the ancient pluralistic medical traditions of China. We now recognize that TCM is a Westernized version, constructed over the years since the mid-1950s, and that it excises what was deemed antithetical to Maoist doctrines, associated with either *elitist* (Mandarin) schools of thought or, alternatively, *backward* folk traditions. For that reason, many have adopted the broader term Chinese traditional medicine (CTM), or the traditional medicine of China (TMC), or even China's traditional medicine, rather than the politically charged TCM.

# Western References

References to acupuncture in the West can be traced back to the year 1700 in Germany, Holland, and England. In 1755, the Dutch physician Gerhard van Swieten speculated that acupuncture triggered neurologic phenomena, and its use was primarily for pain. Louis Berlioz wrote a book on acupuncture in France in 1816, and another Frenchman,

George Soulie de Morant, wrote a major compendium text in the early part of the 20th century. In 1892 William Osler of the John Hopkins School of Medicine described the use of acupuncture for low back pain in a book circulated in the United States (Birch & Felt, 1999). And Chinese-born traditional physicians provided acupuncture for the Chinese laborers building the railroads in the West, with evidence of herbal pharmacies in Idaho in the early part of the 20th century (Muench, 1984).

For the past several centuries in China, traditional medicine has evolved yet remained rooted in the contending, sometimes conflicting, theories of the preceding millennia. After the 1949 revolution, a decision was made to revive China's native medicine in addition to developing the Western medicine that had seeded itself there in the 1800s. Before this time, indigenous medical knowledge was transmitted less formally through apprenticeship and family lineage, and officially recorded in thousands of texts from a succession of imperial courts. In both cases, differences have abounded.

Traditional Chinese medicine was introduced into the United States when President Nixon lifted the Bamboo Curtain. *New York Times* journalist James Reston traveled to China in 1971 and was treated with acupuncture there for postsurgical pain following an appendectomy. He sent back front-page headlines claiming, "I've seen the past, and it works." Since that time, the popularity of acupuncture and Chinese herbal medicine has mushroomed in the Western world.

In 1973 the U.S. Food and Drug Administration classified acupuncture needles as experimental, and the American Medical Association echoed that this modality should be restricted to use by physicians in research protocols. Yet schools of acupuncture were formed, and state licensing initiatives were undertaken in the mid-1970s. In states such as Nevada and California, acupuncturists were licensed as primary care providers by 1976. In 1980, a Texas judge ruled on limiting the practice of acupuncture to physicians, stating that acupuncture "is no more experimental as a mode of medical treatment than is the Chinese language as a mode of communication. What is experimental is not acupuncture, but Westerners' understanding of it and their ability to use it properly" (Birch & Felt, 1999). Acupuncture needles were reclassified as safe and effective more than 20 years after the Food and Drug Administration (FDA) conducted their initial review (Birch & Felt, 1999). There is now growing cooperation and collaboration between the established conventional medical community and those who practice Chinese medicine.

# Current Utilization

Safety, effectiveness, and low cost appear to drive the utilization of Chinese medicine in the West. It is one of the fastest growing forms of health care in the United States (Fass, 2001). The National Institutes of Health Consensus Conference (1997) stated, "The data in support of acupuncture are as strong as those for many accepted Western medical therapies. One of the advantages of acupuncture is that the incidence of adverse effects is substantially lower than that of many drugs and other accepted medical procedures used for the same conditions."

As of the year 2000, there are more than 1 million acupuncture practitioners worldwide.[5] As of 2005, there are over 15,000 state-licensed or board–certified acupuncturists practicing in the United States, and approximately 9,000 who are medical doctors. There are projected estimates that there will be 40,000 practitioners by the year 2015.[6]

Fifty states have recognized the practice of acupuncture, many issuing state licenses. There are more than 56 schools of acupuncture that are either accredited or in candidacy status.[7] These schools graduate hundreds of students from 3- and 4-year programs. In 1993 the Food and Drug Administration estimated that Americans logged between 9 and 12 million yearly acupuncture visits. By 2002, it was estimated that 20 million Americans, or 1 in 10, had experienced an acupuncture treatment (Lytle, 1993). It is estimated that $1 billion is spent annually by Americans on Chinese medicine.

The *Western Journal of Medicine* reported on a study undertaken by the Kaiser Health Maintenance Organization that found 57.2% of primary care physicians in northern California used or recommended acupuncture within a 12-month period in 1996 (Gordon, Sobel, & Tarazona, 1998). Controlled clinical trials evaluating acupuncture added to standard protocols in the treatment of stroke-induced paralysis found that 80% of the patients receiving acupuncture had beneficial results at an average cost saving of $26,000 per patient (Johansson, Lindgren, Widner, Wiklund, & Johansson, 1993).

A study in six Chinese medicine clinics in five states within the United States supported findings of cost savings and effectiveness of acupuncture for a variety of complaints and diseases: of patients treated, 91.5% reported disappearance or improvement of symptoms, 84% said they saw their physicians less, and 79% said they used fewer prescription drugs (Cassidy, 1998).

# Chinese Traditional Medicine on Its Own Terms

Chinese medicine is based on particular modes of knowing (epistemology), beliefs about the nature of reality (metaphysics), theories about the nature of human behavior (physiology and psychology), as well as instrumental means of being helpful (methods of therapeutic intervention). Because the concepts of Chinese medicine differ from Western pathophysiologic categories of disease, familiarity with its unique vocabulary is a stepping stone to the theoretical framework within which health and disease are understood.[8]

The human body is a microcosm, a universe in miniature. Just as nature includes air, sea, and land, so the body is a matrix composed of *qi, moisture, blood, jing,* and *shen.* Life is characterized by a coherent, transformative dynamism known as *qi* (pronounced "chee") *Qi* is responsible for and manifest by movement, rhythm, and warmth. Everything that pulsates, wiggles, changes, cogitates, and radiates is *qi. Blood (xue)* is more than red fluid—it is the material from which the body grows itself. Although tissue arises from *blood,* the distribution and transformation of substance are governed by *qi.* Together *qi* and *blood* maintain the body's form and composition. *Qi* and *blood* in turn arise from *jing,* translated as *essence,* the original primal substrate responsible for and manifested by growth, development, and maturation. *Jing* is the body's reproductive and regenerative substance, whereas *shen* is *mind,* responsible for perception, sensation, expression, and self-awareness. An integrated sense of identity that coheres in space and endures over time is conveyed by the concept of *shen-jing,* the inextricable unity of psyche and soma, mind and body. Together the three treasures known as *qi, jing,* and *shen* maintain shape, function, and identity—the self-transforming, self-making, and self-actualizing human capacity.

The five constituents—*jing, blood, moisture, qi,* and *shen*—exist on a continuum of greater and lesser density and materiality. *Qi* is unseen and insubstantial, *moisture (jin ye)* (body fluid) is more dense than *qi*, but less so than *blood*, and *blood* is more substantial still. Relative to each other, *qi* is more dynamic, whereas *blood* is more stable. Yet of greater density than *blood* is *essence*, from which *blood* itself is formed; and *shen (mind)*, ephemeral and entirely lacking in substantiality, arises as personhood emerges from the body's life.

*Qi* is also an overarching concept—it is everything that exists and occurs. In the body, it is both a single constituent as well as the aggregate of all constituents. Scholar Nathan Sivin writes that in early manuscripts about nature, *qi* meant *basic stuff*, simultaneously "what makes thing happen in stuff" and "stuff that makes things happen. . . . *Qi* is often the material basis of activity, but the activity itself is often also described as *Qi*" (Sivin, 1987).

All substances and functions are part of a continuum called *yin-yang*. The dynamism known as *qi* is the emanation of the unceasing interplay and cogeneration of polar and complementary forces known as *yin-yang*. The light *qi* of heaven rose upward to become heaven (*yang*), and the heavy *qi* bore down to become earth (*yin*). Between heaven and earth, human beings appear as the fruit of this union. *Yin-yang* represents dynamic balance, intrinsic relativity, and the tension of duality: contraction/expansion, visible/invisible, dark/light, cold/hot, wet/dry, internal/external, empty/full, depleted/congested, lower/upper, deep/superficial, weak/strong, slow/fast, dense/porous, concentrated/dilute, inhibited/excited, quiescent/active, chronic/acute, hypoactive/hyperactive. The constituents and functions of the body can be delineated along the *yin-yang* continuum: *essence, blood,* and *moisture* (*yin*) are relatively dense and tangible compared to *qi* and *shen* (*yang*), which are relatively light and intangible. The storage of *blood* and *moisture* is *yin*, whereas their circulation is *yang*. The process of digestion and assimilation is *yang*, whereas the acquisition of flesh and the deposition of fat is *yin*. Whereas catabolism is *yang*, anabolism is *yin*. *Yin* and *yang* inextricably depend on one another: where the *mind* leads, the *qi* follows, where *qi* goes, *blood* flows, and *blood* is the mother of *qi*.

The body is governed by five organ networks (*zang fu*)—the *heart, kidney, liver, spleen,* and *lung*—whose function is to organize, regulate, store, and distribute the five constituents (*shen, jing, blood, moisture,* and *qi*). These *zang fu* assume primary responsibility for the tasks of the organism. Although these organs bear Western anatomical names, their meaning differs. In Chinese medicine these organs represent broad functional networks rather than strictly distinct physical structures. Each organ network governs visceral organs, associated structures, tissues, and functions, as well as the pathways of *qi*, known as the acupuncture channels (*jing luo*). A blueprint of the relationship between these networks and the life processes of the organism is like a map charting the relationship between the oceans and the continents. Currents and land masses meet and flow together, yet each occupies its own territory. Similarly, the body is seen as a structural and functional whole with mutually engendering patterns of interconnectedness.

For example, the *kidney* stores the *jing* (*essence*), whereas the *heart* houses the *shen* (*mind*). The *kidney* includes but extends beyond the job of managing fluid metabolism—it governs the will, growth, development, reproduction and regeneration, the bones and marrow (the brain being considered the *sea of marrow*), the lumbar region, ears, and teeth. Problems such as retarded growth, ringing in the ears, infertility, low back pain, apathy, or despair are viewed as dysfunctions of the *kidney network*. In addition to propelling the blood, the *heart* sustains the higher functions of the central nervous system, including internal and external perception and communication. The *liver* stores and governs the *blood*, tendons, and nerves, the volume, pressure, and evenness of circulating *qi* and *blood*, temperament, and judgment. The *lung* governs respiration, circulation, and distribution of *moisture* and *qi*, maintaining the skin and other defensive boundaries of the body. The *spleen* assumes responsibility for digestion, assimilation, distribution of fluids; maintains stability, density, and viscosity of tissue and fluid; generates muscle and flesh; and holds the *blood* within the vessels.

Pathologic conditions are *adverse climates* within the body ecosystem. *Heat* is a condition of excess *yang* characterized by subjective and objective sensations, as well as by the coloration of fluids, secretions, and tissue. Symptoms of *heat* behave like heat—red, hot, dry, and overactive. *Heat* can be produced externally by hot weather or internally by hyperactivity because of emotional and physical stresses such as anxiety, rage, excitement, infection, trauma, poisoning, allergic reaction, and loss of body fluids. Signs of *heat* include fever, burning, inflammation, thick yellow to green secretions, darkened urine, rashes, fast pulse, and a dry, bright red tongue. *Cold* is an abnormal *yin* condition characterized by subjective and objective sensations of chilliness as well as by the coloration of fluids, secretions, and tissue. Symptoms of *cold* act like cold: slowing of circulation and chilliness cause contractions and pain. Signs of *cold* include feeling chilled and numb; pallor of the skin and eyes; profuse, odorless, colorless urine; excessive, bland secretions and discharges; a slow pulse; and a pale, wet, purplish tongue. *Cold* can result from exposure to frigid weather, immersion in cold water, overwork, lack of rest or food, loss of blood, prolonged diarrhea, raw or refrigerated foods, iced liquids, shock or grief, all of which can retard circulation and depress metabolic activity. *Phlegm* is more than the sticky mucus that collects in sinus cavities or the nasopharynx; it is the accumulation and thickening of any secretion or fluid that manifests as a swelling, nodule, or cyst. Examples of *phlegm* include fatty tumors, atherosclerotic or neural plaque, enlarged or hardened lymph nodes, swollen joints, cystic acne, and hydroceles. A *toxin* is an externally or internally generated substance that degrades a healthy body constituent or transforms less serious entities such as *phlegm* or stagnant *blood* into more virulent pathogens such as *hot phlegm, or blood heat*. *Blood heat* or *blood toxicity* is the result of the *blood* becoming contaminated with external or internal pathogens (e.g., *heat, damp-heat*, metabolic waste, and food toxins). Severe *blood heat* can become a principal factor leading to severe *blood* stagnation and may result from prolonged obstruction of *qi, moisture*, or *blood*. It is an example of *entanglement (hunluan)*, a condition in which a healthy body constituent (*blood*) becomes enmeshed with a pathogen to form a more complex pathogenic entity.

Unresolved emotional suffering affects the *qi*: whereas anger and anxiety raise the *qi*, terror pushes it down; whereas grief scatters the *qi* so that it loses cohesion, ruminating thoughts bind the *qi*. Whereas fright causes *qi* to become chaotic, joy modulates and relaxes the *qi*. Just as anger can generate *heat*, so depression, worry, and grief can lead to the binding of the *qi*, inhibited movement, and stasis of *qi* that can produce blood stagnation.

*Qi, moisture*, and *blood* circulate within the web of channels and vessels called *jing luo* that link all parts of the organism to each other. Health is the product of the equitable distribution of body constituents and the smooth and coordinated interaction of the organ networks. Dysfunction and disease are always the consequence of attrition and impaired circulation of *qi* and *blood*, resulting in a progression from congestion to stagnation to accumulation to obstruction. The key words associated with health are *circulation, harmony, coherence,* and *integration.*

Diagnosis is based on an analysis of the relationship between harmonious and inharmonious activities of the five constituents and organ networks, the goal being to grasp the unique character of the patient's body, mind, and circumstances, as well as the nature of the illness. Neither health nor disease is a static condition; rather, both are processes that occur simultaneously and in relationship to each other. For example, loss of blood can be normal and healthy or abnormal and pathologic. Normal menstruation is a healthy cyclical process in which the body first generates a surplus of blood and then discharges it, whereas prolonged or excessive bleeding leads to a condition of depletion in which the loss exceeds the body's ability to replenish itself. The signs and symptoms characterizing this diagnostic pattern known as deficiency of *blood* might include restless fatigue, chilliness, dryness, irritability, insomnia, and palpitations. Healthy physical and mental activity includes periods of focused or sustained effort, alternating with relaxation and rest. Overwork and prolonged mental strain result in the weakening of the body's ability to recover from stress. This is described as a condition of *qi* deficiency, characterized by persistent fatigue, lethargy, sleepiness, sensitivity to weather changes, vulnerability to infection, diminished stamina, flaccidity of muscles and organs, diminished sensory acuity, long recovery from illness, reduced pulmonary capacity, and vague feelings of depression and disinterest.

# Chinese Medicine and Cancer: Ancient and Modern Concepts

Derived from the word *malign*, meaning "harmful or malevolent," malignant means that which may cause mortal damage. In Chinese medicine, mortal damage is a consequence of the disorganization and separation of *yin-yang* (*jing-shen, blood-qi*)—a threshold beyond which the organism is unable to sustain harmony and integrity. Cancerous masses, lumps, and tumors are the consequence of unmitigated accumulations of *qi, moisture,* and *blood* that have become *toxic*, transforming what is healthy into morbid tissue, simultaneously obstructing and usurping normal circulation. Prolonged stagnation eventually leads to depletion of *qi* and *blood* and ultimately *essence*. Because *essence* governs growth and maturation, loss of or damage to it can result in a disregulation of growth typical of cancer, a process of uncontrolled proliferation of immature, undifferentiated, malformed cells. Therefore, treatment that supplements *qi, moisture,* and *blood*; restores circulation and eliminates stasis; removes *toxins*; replenishes *essence*; and dissolves masses is critical in the treatment of cancer.

As early as the 11th century B.C.E., descriptions of tumors were inscribed on oracle bones and turtle shells. Certain doctors specialized in the treatment of these lesions, referred to as *liu*, meaning "tumor," derived from a word meaning "stuck." Around 200 B.C.E., during the Han Dynasty, tumors became known as hard lumps or ulcerated lesions. Both benign and malignant masses were further differentiated anatomically as ulcers or abscesses that arise between the muscle and bone (*yen, ai, chu*), carbuncles (*yung*) that appear on the surface of muscles and skin, and hard obstructions (*cheng chia*) that arise in the internal organs. In the 12th century, the term *ai*, another expression for *inflamed ulcers*, became synonymous with that for cancer. Comparable to identifying contemporary *early warning signs*, traditional doctors noted the severity of swellings, lumps, and masses; their depth (skin, muscle, bone, viscera), density, and firmness; mobility; color; heat; presence of fluid or pus; and the severity, quality and variability of pain and other sensations such as itching and burning in formulating the diagnosis of malignancy (Hsu, 1982).

Classic and modern writings regard the etiology of most serious disorders, including benign and malignant tumors, as stemming from internal injuries, emotional trauma, invasion of pathogenic factors such as *heat*, *cold*, *dampness*, *dryness*, or the accumulation of *toxins*, often because of improper digestion and poor elimination of metabolic wastes. Jia Kun, a Chinese traditional medicine oncologist writing in 1980, says that whatever upsets normal body function can lead to tumor formation, causing cancer. Tumors are the end result of a prolonged process of accumulation and densification of tissue because of the persistent stagnation of *qi* and *blood,* which, if unrelieved, becomes *toxic*, critically damaging the healthy function of the organ systems (Hsu, 1982).

C. S. Cheung explains the relationship between generating *blood* and circulating it, preventing both deficiency and stagnation:

> The essence of fluid and grain [nourishment from food and drink] infuses into the meridians and forms *ying qi.* It then circulates to the *heart* and enters the *blood.* The *blood* flows to every part of the body and moistens and lubricates all the tissues. When there is insufficiency of *ying qi,* the distribution of *qi* is endangered. Thus, the *blood* does not flow smoothly, encouraging the formation of *blood* stasis and ecchymosis [*blood* that congeals outside the vessels]. New *blood* is unable to be generated when obstructed by stasis and ecchymosis. Consequently, therapeutic measures are taken to remove the obstruction and generate new *blood.*

Cheung recommends that herbs such as angelica, salvia, and millettia be used, explaining that the herb millettia treats both deficiency and stasis because it both engenders and circulates *blood* (Cheung & Hirano, 1982).

As discussed, the circulation of *qi* and *blood* can be impeded by physical or psychologic disturbances. Just as thermal *cold* constricts blood vessels, causing inhibition of movement and depressed metabolism, so can prolonged sadness. *Heat* dries the *blood*, and emotions such as anxiety, anger, and anguish that produce *heat* can be as harmful as prolonged exposure to intense summer sun. Congestion of *blood* and *moisture* can generate emotional discomfort, and unresolved suffering can cause *qi* and *blood* stasis. An osteoma could be the outcome of accumulated *heat* (regardless of its source) in the *kidney* (the *kidney* governs bone and marrow) that dries and erodes the moist, spongy substances in bone, causing the formation of a hard and immobile mass. Additional factors such as the effects of environmental pollution, chemical contamination of food, fungi, viruses, and bacteria can also produce stagnation of *qi* and *blood*. The traditional view does not give greater emphasis to either the poisonous effects of entrenched negative emotions or spoiled food: *toxins*, regardless of their origin, are identified by their pernicious effects. Tumors in the breast may result from *toxic* accumulation and stagnation of *qi* and *blood* in the channels that pass through the breast, eventually producing a lump.

The following sequence outlines a likely etiology of malignancy: adverse pathogenic factors initiate the stagnation and depletion of *qi, moisture,* and *blood*; the persistence

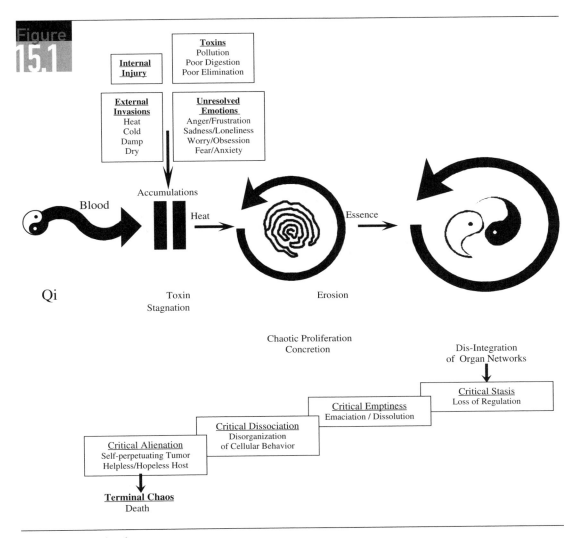

The pathogenesis of cancer.

of deficiency and stasis impairs the coordinated function of the organ networks, which leads to further weakness, obstruction, and attrition of *essence*, the original source (*yuan*) of *qi* and *blood*. The malignant process is characterized by extreme disorder. When *qi*, *blood*, and *essence* become depleted enough, *yin-yang* begins to disintegrate or separate and chaos ensues. Disorganization of cellular behavior is a manifestation of the loss of coherence—failure of the body to govern differentiation and proliferation.

The development of cancer is a progression from extreme stagnation to emptiness to dissociation to alienation, and finally, to anarchy and death. Critical stasis means that a region of tissue is no longer governable by the ordinary circulatory and regulatory mechanisms of *qi*, leading eventually to a degeneration of coordinated activity. Critical emptiness means that the region sequestered by the malignant process consumes the physiologic resources of the organism but contributes nothing in return, engendering an accelerating process of attrition. Critical alienation is manifested in the attitude of

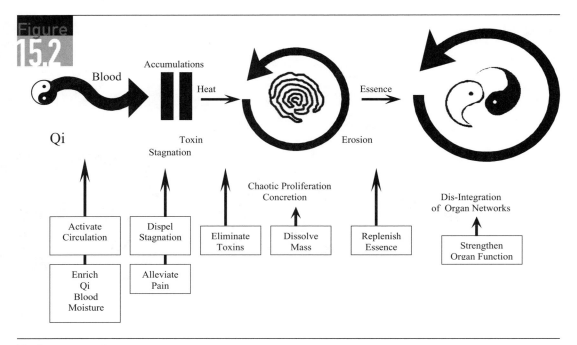

**The treatment of cancer.**

hopelessness and helplessness that a person experiences when a nonresponsive and insensate entity—the cancer—arising from the organism's own sacred terrain, expropriates its vital resources while ceasing to be subject to its ontological influence. Cancer is a condition of functional chaos, representing one of the most advanced stages of disorganization—*wild qi*—requiring intensive and aggressive strategies to restore integrity. This condition known as *wild qi* prefigures the fatal *separation of yin-yang* (Hammer, 1998, 2001).

## Cancer Types: Diagnostic Patterns

Cancer patterns typically involve *phlegm, toxins*, deficient *qi* and *blood*, and *blood* stagnation. The same cancer (e.g., stomach cancer) may result from a variety of patterns, such as *liver qi* invading the *stomach, stomach yang* deficiency, *phlegm* stagnation and food retention, *blood* stagnation because of *qi* stagnation, *stomach yin* deficiency because of *stomach heat*, or *qi* and *blood* deficiency. For colon cancer, the patterns may be *damp heat* in the large intestine, *toxins, spleen* and *kidney yang* deficiency, *liver* and *kidney yin* deficiency, and *qi* and *blood* deficiency. Breast cancer patterns include *liver qi* stagnation, *blood* stagnation and accumulation of *toxins, qi* and *blood* deficiency, and *spleen qi* deficiency with *phlegm* accumulation. Brain tumors may result from *phlegm* accumulation and *kidney qi* or *yin* deficiency (Boik, 1995).

There are two diagnostic categories that interact: one is called *bian zheng*, meaning the "constitutional pattern of the person," and the other is *bian bing*, meaning the "pattern of the disease." Depending on these patterns, acupuncture treatment and herbal therapy are tailored to fit—individualized according to the pathologic pattern and the nature of the patient. Acupuncture relieves stagnation and deficiency by mobilizing the *qi* of particular organ networks. Herbal formulas relieve stagnation by using *qi* and *blood* activating herbs, clear *heat* via cooling herbs, dispel *dampness* with *drying* herbs, and antidote *toxins* or dissolve *phlegm* with herbs that remove or dissolve these pathogenic entities. *Cold* is relieved through the use of warming herbs, and overall strength is restored with tonic herbs. Some patterns may serve as markers for enhanced survival as well. For example, in a study of 254 women with cervical cancer treated with radiotherapy and followed for 3 years, those diagnosed with *qi* stagnation exhibited a significantly reduced survival compared to those diagnosed with *liver* and *kidney yin* deficiency (Yu, Zhang, Yang, Qian, & Peng, 1991).

There are many treatment protocols that combine acupuncture and medicinal herbs to reduce swelling and eliminate the pain caused by tumors as well as the adverse effects of surgery, radiation, and chemotherapy. In particular, herbal prescriptions that invigorate the *qi*, nourish the *blood*, clear *heat* and *toxins*, and eliminate *blood* stasis can strengthen the body, enhance adaptation to stress, increase host resistance to infection, inflammation, and proliferation of tissue, and retard the progression of tumors, promoting long-term survival. These are primary therapeutic strategies for shrinking tumors that have been applied since the 17th century (Mingji, 1992). Although surgery, radiation, and chemotherapy are welcomed as viable treatments for cancer in modern China, Japan, and other Asian countries, acupuncture and Chinese herbal medicine represent complementary or adjunctive therapies that sometimes improve the capacity of conventional Western medicine to achieve desired outcomes (Hsu, 1982).

# Chemotherapy and Radiation: A *Yin–Yang* Perspective[9]

Radiation is a form of extreme *yang* that produces heat and inflammation, *cooking* the *yin*, damaging the *blood* and *moisture*. The drying of *blood* and *moisture* leads to coagulation (static *blood*) and congelation (*phlegm*). Stagnant *blood* and *phlegm* further impair the circulation of *qi*, *moisture*, and *blood*, resulting in more deficiency and weakening of the organ networks. Radiation often penetrates deep into the bones, drying the marrow and eroding *essence*.

Chemotherapy is a form of extreme *yin*, a poison that damages the *yang*, the ability of *qi* to move the *blood* and *moisture*, warm the body, and transform food into *qi* and *blood*. When the *qi* fails to move *blood* and fluids, *blood* stagnation and *dampness* arise. When circulation is retarded, it becomes difficult for the body to stay warm. Internal *cold* can transform *dampness* into *phlegm* and cause *blood* to coagulate. When digestion is impaired, the *stomach* and *spleen* fail to generate adequate *qi* and *blood*, and deficiency ensues. When *qi* is depleted, blood and fluids easily leak from the blood vessels and body membranes. Prolonged deficiency leads to the attrition of marrow and *essence*. The adverse effects of radiation and chemotherapy parallel the signs and symptoms of severe deficiencies of *qi*, *moisture*, *blood*, and *essence*: weakness, fatigue, pallor, susceptibility to infection, edema, dehydration, hair loss, restlessness, irritability, depression, hot flashes, night sweats, thirst, dry skin, infertility, lack of libido, amenorrhea, indigestion, anorexia, weight loss, diarrhea, ulcerations, bruising, bleeding, flaccidity, joint and muscle pain, anemia, leukopenia, shortness of breath, congestive heart failure, inability to concentrate, memory loss, heartburn, and headache. Just when there is a demand for adequate *qi* and *blood*, the capacity to generate these resources is undermined. The conditions that produce cancer, namely stagnation, deficiency, and disharmony, are further aggravated by radiation and chemotherapy, neither of which discriminates between healthy and abnormal tissue. The vicious cycle of attrition caused by the disease is paralleled by the treatment. Although Western medicine aggressively attacks the cancer, Chinese traditional medicine supports and restores the healthy function that enables patients to tolerate and recover from conventional therapies, surviving with an improved quality of life.

# Acupuncture

The National Institutes of Health Consensus Development Conference (1997) declared that there is clear evidence that acupuncture is an effective modality, particularly for nausea and vomiting induced by chemotherapy and for the relief of pain. The American Cancer Society informs consumers that, "Acupuncture is simple, and often works. It has few side effects or complications, and the cost is low. For these reasons, it can be a good choice for some problems."

Acupuncture is based on the assumption that *qi* courses through a network of channels (*jing luo*), just as streams and rivers flow under and across the surface of the Earth. This lattice of channels forms a *web of qi* that unites all parts of the organism. Within the Chinese traditional model, acupuncture works by regulating the movement of *qi*. By restoring healthy circulation of *qi* and *blood*, stagnation resolves. By optimizing the function of the five organ networks, vulnerability to disease is reduced. In modern language, acupuncture modulates fundamental homeodynamic mechanisms that govern hematopoeisis, cellular and humoral immunity, temperature and pressure, respiration, metabolism, hormonal secretion and sensitity, neuromuscular coordination, and diurnal rhythms. Microcirculation in the capillary beds that surround internal organs is encouraged, thereby supporting processes of healthy nutrition and detoxification. Acupuncture also stimulates the central nervous system, activating mechanisms of repair and regeneration. In traditional language, acupuncture harmonizes *yin-yang* and the organ networks responsible for regulating growth, proliferation, and dynamic harmony. Pain signals the stagnation of *qi*, *blood*, and *phlegm* within the channels. Slender stainless steel needles inserted in particular points located along these channels near the surface of the skin (acupoints) can clear stagnation, reinvigorating the function of the internal organs. Within the modern scientific model, the mechanism of action of acupuncture has only been partially described, mostly in the area of pain relief. Through the use of functional magnetic resonance imaging, descriptive studies have documented that sensory-related acupoints have brain cortical correspondences that may point toward an explanation of how acupuncture has effects beyond analgesia, namely on homeostatic regulatory mechanisms not yet understood by Western physiology or medicine (Cho et al., 2001). Normalizing of the physiologic processes of the cardiovascular (Ballegaard et al.,

1993), immunologic (Yang, Ng, Zeng, & Kwok, 1989) and gastrointestinal (Iwa & Sakita, 1994) systems, as well as an anti-inflammatory (Lao, Bergman, Hamilton, Langenberg, & Berman, 1999) modulatory effects have been also been documented in preliminary studies.

## Acupuncture Analgesia

Since the early 1970s, neurophysiologist Bruce Pomeranz has studied the effectiveness of acupuncture on pain, nerve regeneration, and cutaneous wound healing. In 1976 Pomeranz used naloxone, an endorphin antagonist, to successfully block acupuncture analgesia, suggesting a physiologic mechanism of action. He showed that acupuncture relieved chronic pain in 55%–85% of patients, compared to a 30% relief of pain by placebo, demonstrating that acupuncture is as effective as many potent drugs (Pomeranz & Stux, 1989). Pomeranz (2001) comments, "It should be apparent that we know more about acupuncture analgesia than about many chemical drugs in routine use. For example, we know very little about the mechanisms of most anesthetic gases but still use them regularly." Acupuncture analgesia is initiated by the stimulation of small afferent sensory nerve fibers embedded in musculature that send impulses to the spinal cord to affect the three centers: spinal cord, midbrain, and hypothalamic-pituitary. When these centers are activated, neurotransmitters release endorphins, enkephalins, monoamines, and cortisol to block the pain messages (Pomeranz, 2001). Increases in serum beta-endorphin, met-enkephalin, and leu-enkephalin with acupuncture have also been documented (Han, 1989).

Needles placed near the pain site, either on an acupoint or at a tender spot (trigger point), activate segmental circuits to the spinal cord as well as all three centers. Local needling usually provides a more intensive analgesic effect than distal needling that activates the midbrain and pituitary without benefit to the local segmental circuit to the spinal cord. In practice, both local and distal needling enhances the overall analgesic effect. The Chinese experience with the use of acupuncture analgesia as an adjunct or alternative to chemical anesthesia during surgery reveals that, in addition to effectively inhibiting the pain response, acupuncture also maintains normalized blood pressure, visceral reflexes (prevents collapse of the mediastinum and diaphragm and preserves gut motility), and body temperature while markedly reducing the risk of hemorrhage, accelerating wound repair, and shortening postoperative recovery time.[10]

Because pain medications can cause nausea, constipation, and fatigue, as well as require escalating doses that place patients at risk for cardiopulmonary depression and hepatic or renal toxicity, acupuncture pain relief may prove to be of significant benefit (Perneger, 1994; Whitcomb & Block, 1994). In a study of 286 patients experiencing metastatic bone pain, use of an electroacupuncture apparatus resulted in 74% significant pain relief in addition to a much lower need for long-term narcotic analgesics (Guo et al., 1995). In a randomized study of 48 gastric carcinoma patients receiving chemotherapy, acupuncture was compared to pharmacologic pain management with narcotics and nonsteroidal anti-inflammatory agents. Although immediate (12 hour) control was better with pharmacologic therapy, after 2 months, long-term pain control was similar. Only in the acupuncture group was plasma leu-enkephalin increased at 2 months, along with improvement in other side effects of chemotherapy and overall quality of life measures (Dang & Yang, 1998). Acupuncture has also been reported to relieve the pain of herpes zoster, a typical chemotherapeutic side effect (Zhang & Zhang, 1999), as well as aid in the regeneration of nerve tissue as evidenced by improved nerve conduction in patients suffering from peripheral neuropathy (Shan & Shao, 1999). Both pain and edema were reduced in a study of 122 patients with late-onset edema because of radiation therapy (Bardychev, Guseva, & Zubova, 1988).

## Acupuncture for Nausea and Vomiting

There is reliable, compelling data for the effectiveness of acupuncture in relieving nausea and vomiting. The NIH Consensus Panel on Acupuncture in 1997 concluded, "there is clear evidence that needle acupuncture is efficacious for adult postoperative and chemotherapy nausea and vomiting" (National Institutes of Health Consensus Panel, 1997). A systematic review of randomized controlled trials showed consistent, positive results (Vickers, 1996). Of 29 trials in which acupuncture was used when patients were awake, and not under anesthesia, 27 supported acupuncture. More than 2,000 patients showed positive results in a review of the trials that were of the best methodologic quality. A 1989 study by J. W. Dundee from Queen's University in Belfast showed acupuncture to significantly relieve postoperative nausea and vomiting: 78% of patients treated with acupuncture were free of sickness compared to 32% of the nontreated control group (Dundee et al., 1989). Dundee's initial comparative studies examined the antiemetic effect of the acupoint known as Pericardium 6 (Pc6 is located on the medial aspect of the arm above the wrist) in 105 patients with a history of nausea and vomiting in a previous round of chemotherapy. This study reported a 63% antiemetic benefit from the acupuncture (Dundee et al., 1986; Dundee & McMillan, 1991, 1992; Dundee & Yang, 1990). Thirty percent to 40% of women with early stage breast cancer still experience nausea and vomiting within 1 week of chemotherapy administration, even with the use of seratonin receptor antagonists (The Italian Group for Antiemetic Research, 1995). Subsequent well-controlled studies have similarly shown acupressure or acupuncture applied to Pc6 provides a treatment benefit in 60%–70% of patients compared to a 30% benefit with sham treatment (Lewis & Vincent, 1996). At Duke University, a study of 75 women showed that acupuncture was more effective than the commonly used antiemetic, ondansetron (Zofran), in reducing postoperative nausea, vomiting, and pain (Gan et al., 2001).

## Acupuncture Effects on Myelosuppression and Hormonal Markers

In a study of 386 patients with medium and advanced-stage cancer with chemotherapy-induced leukocytopenia, acupuncture and moxibustion (heat produced by burning the herb *Artemesia vulgaris* on acupoints) increased the leukocyte count in 38% of the patients (Chen & Huang, 1991). Among 48 patients with persistent leukopenia, stimulation of the acupoint known as Stomach 36, located laterally below the knee, led to an increased white blood cell count in more than 90% of those treated (Wei, 1998). In another study of 121 patients with leukopenia during radiation and chemotherapy, after five daily acupuncture and moxibustion treatments, white blood cell counts markedly increased (Zhou, Li, & Jin, 1999).

The immune modulatory effects of acupuncture on patients undergoing chemotherapy and radiation are summarized in a review article that shows an increase in peripheral blood counts of $CD_3^+$, $CD_4^+$, and NK cells, as well as an elevation in the $CD_4^+/CD_8^+$ ratio. Macrophage activity is also increased by both acupuncture and moxibustion (Wu, Zhow, & He, 1999). In a study of premenopausal women that compared normal subjects to those with benign mammary hyperplasia, measuring immune and hormonal markers, levels of $CD_8^+$ cells rose significantly after acupuncture, and the $CD_4^+/CD_8^+$ ratio was reduced to match the control group. Serum estrogen $E_2$ and prolactin levels declined following acupuncture, whereas levels of follicle stimulating hormone increased. More than 50% of the women with hyperplasia had complete resolution of their nodules, whereas the others had a significant reduction (Xu et al., 1998). Women with climacteric symptoms because of chemotherapy-induced menopause or treatment with agents such as Tamoxifen experience hot flashes, night sweats, dry skin and vaginal dryness, and insomnia. Studies have indicated that acupuncture can help to control these symptoms in over 90% of the women treated (Zhang, Zheng, & Wang, 1999).

# Modern Chinese Herbal Research

With the renaissance of traditional Chinese medicine in the 1950s, clinical researchers in China and Japan began searching for ways to improve outcomes for cancer patients undergoing chemotherapy and radiation. Over the last decades, this approach has become known as *Fuzheng Gu Ben* therapy, meaning "to strengthen what is correct and secure the root." *Fuzheng* herbs support nonspecific resistance and are known as biologic response modifiers or adaptogens. In a monograph in 1981 on the use of *fuzheng* herbs with cancer patients, Tu Gouri commented as follows:

> the treatment of malignant tumors with combined methods of traditional Chinese medicine and western medicine has made much progress,... patients with advanced malignant tumors usually have the symptoms of deficiency in qi and blood, deficiency of *liver* and *kidney*; and dysfunction of spleen and stomach. Tonics may improve the general condition and the immune function of the patients, enhance resistance against disease, and prolong their survival period. Furthermore, tonics also have protective effects against immune suppression, lowering of leukocyte count, suppression of bone marrow, and decrease of plasma cortisol levels induced by radiotherapy and chemotherapy. All this benefits the treatment of malignant tumors. (Guorui, 1981)

Researchers from the University of California, San Francisco (UCSF) have commented that *Fuzheng* therapy produces possible diverse biologic effects that include the following:

> reduce the tumor load; prevent recurrence or formation of a new primary cancer; bolster the immune system; enhance the regulatory function of the endocrine system; protect the structure and function of internal organs and glands; strengthen the digestive system by improving absorption and metabolism; protect bone marrow and hematopoietic function; and prevent, control, and treat adverse side effects caused by conventional treatments for cancer. (Tagliaferri, Cohen, & Tripathy, 2001)

Excellent resources for the use of Chinese herbal medicine in cancer can be found in Hanks (2000), and the relevant monographs written by Subhuti Dharmananda, PhD, of the Institute for Traditional Medicine in Portland, Oregon (1998).

## Treatment Strategies

Clinically, Chinese herbs are usually administered not as single agents, but in multi-ingredient formulas. Formulas are designed to address various aspects of the disease pattern, as well as the constitutional needs of the individual patient. For example, a given formula might use herbs that supplement *qi, blood,* and *essence* combined with other ingredients to eliminate stagnation, *toxins,* and reduce tumor mass. Crude herbs are decocted in teas; ingested as powders; compressed into tablets; or extracted in alcohol, water, or both and in China they may be prepared for injection or intravenous administration.

Five principles organize the formulation of many herbal prescriptions for the treatment of cancer: supplement the *qi* and *blood* to strengthen host resistance; activate circulation to dispel *blood* stasis and ecchymosis; relieve pain; eliminate *heat* and eliminate *toxins;* and soften lumps and dissolve masses (Pan, 1992).

Herbal formulas may contain anywhere from 6 to 20 ingredients and emphasize one or all of the five therapeutic principles. The clinical application of these principles might best be illustrated by describing the known pharmacologic properties and actions as well as the traditional characteristics, indications, and effects of several individual herbs and multi-ingredient formulas that are currently being investigated and used clinically in China, Japan, and the United States.

# Individual Herbs

The preponderance of herbs used for cancer has been an integral part of traditional practice for centuries. Although recently identified as adaptogenic, immune enhancing, anticoagulant and fibrinolytic, detoxifying, and tumor resolving, agents such as *Astragalus membranaceus (huang qi), Panax ginseng (ren shen), Atractylodes macrocephala (bai zhu), Glycyrrhiza uralensis (gan cao), Poria cocos (fu ling), Ganoderma lucidum (ling zhi cao), Polyporus umbellatus (zhu ling), Cordyceps sinensis (dong chong xia cao), Coix lachryma-jobi (yi yi ren), Angelica sinensis (dang gui), Salvia miltiorrhiza (dan shen), Rheum palmatum (da huang), Coptis chinensis (huang lian), Scutellaria baicalensis (huang qin), Isatis tinctoria (ban lan gen), Chrysanthemum morifolium (ju hua), Bupleurum chinense (chai hu), Artemesia capillaries (yin chen hao), Sophora subprostrata (shan dou gen),* and *Oldenlandia diffusa (bai hua she she cao)* have 1,800 years of clinical use.

In addition to these venerable medicines, new herbs have been discovered and old ones have been put to new uses. Through modern research *Eleutherococcus senticosus (ci wu jia)* and *Gynostemma pentaphyllum (jiao gu lan)* were discovered to contain saponin glycosides similar to those found in *Panax ginseng (ren shen)* and to exert similar adaptogenic and anticancer effects with the added advantage of being easier to cultivate and therefore cheaper and easier to supply. *Astragalus membranaceus (huang qi), Eleutherococcus senticosus (ci wu jia),* and *Angelica sinensis (dang gui)* were also found to contain immune-modulating polysaccharides similar to those occurring in *Ganoderma lucidum (ling zhi cao),*

*Polyporus umbellatus* (*zhu ling*), *Poria cocos* (*fu ling*), *Cordyceps sinensis* (*dong chong xia cao*), and *Lentinus edodes* (*xiang gu*). *Salvia miltiorrhiza* (*dan shen*), *Angelica sinensis* (*dang gui*), and *Rheum palamatum* (*da huang*) have demonstrated effects on microcirculation, including normalization of fibrin, platelet adhesion, and significant antiangiogenic properties. *Coptis chinensis* (*huang lian*), *Scutellaria baicalensis* (*huang qin*), *Isatis tinctoria* (*ban lan gen*), *Chrysanthemum morifolium* (*ju hua*), *Glycyrrhiza uralensis* (*gan cao*), *Bupleurum chinense* (*chai hu*), *Artemesia capillaris* (*qing hao*), *Sophora subprostrata* (*shan dou gen*), and *Oldenlandia doffisa* (*bai hua she she cao*), traditionally used to treat poisoning, infection, inflammation, and ulceration, have proven to have a broad range of actions, including antitumor, antihistamine, antithrombic, antiproliferative, antiangiogenic, cytotoxic, and immune stimulating activity.

Because modern investigators are in the habit of analyzing single agents and identifying active compounds, considerable research has focused on celebrity herbs such as *Astragalus membranaceus* (*huang qi*-astragalin polysaccharides), *Panax ginseng* (*ren shen*-saponin ginsenosides), *Glycyrrhiza uralensis* (*gan cao*-saponin glycyrrhizin), *Eleutherococcus senticosus* (*ci wu jia*-polysaccharides and saponin eleutherosides), *Angelica sinensis* (polysaccharides), *Curcuma zedoaria* (*e zhu*-curcumin), *Ganoderma lucidum* (*ling zhi cao*-beta glucan polysaccharides), *Lentinus* (*xiang gu*-beta glucan polysaccharides), *Coriolus versicolor* (PSK and PSP-beta glucan polysaccharides), *Sophora subprostrata* (*shan dou gen*-matrine and oxymatrine alkaloids), and *Isatis tinctoria* (*ban lan gen*-indirubin alkaloid). A single herb is biologically more complex than an isolated organic compound and in traditional thinking confers a better result because of the natural synergism of all the constituents. Similarly, a multiherb formula is exponentially more complex than a single herb, delivering even more therapeutic benefits than one herb alone (see Table 15.1).

## Herbal Formulas

Many of the herbal formulas used in modern cancer therapy and research in China are part of the traditional pharmacopoeia. *Shi Quan Da Bu Tang* (All Inclusive Great Tonifying Decoction), *Jian Pi Tang* (Decoction For Tonifying The Spleen And Stomach), *Si Jun Zi Tang* (Four Gentleman Decoction), *Bu Zhong Yi Qi Tang* (Decoction For Tonifying The Middle And Augmenting The Qi), *Ren Shen Yang Rong Tang* (Ginseng Decoction To Nourish The Nutritive Qi), *Xiao Chai Hu Tang* (Minor Bupleurum Decoction) are classic (pre-19th-century) prescriptions that belong to the category of tonifying and harmonizing formulas that generally improve health, strengthen resistance to stress and disease, and facilitate recovery from the debilitating effects of chronic illness. Because the adverse effects of modern cancer treatments mimic the consequences of chronic illness—weakness, fatigue, decreased resistance, reduced appetite, weight loss, diminished libido, cognitive decline, and musculoskeletal stiffness and soreness—tonic prescriptions treat these conditions and maintain healthy function. Such formulas share many of the promising anticancer agents mentioned above.

Modern herbal protocols often use classic formulas as a foundation and then additional ingredients that have anticancer effects. For example, the formula *Fu Zheng Shengjin Tang* for treating the side effects of radiotherapy is based on *Si Jun Zi Tang*

**Table 15.1** Debu Tripathy Herbal Examples Diagram

| Pinyin Transliteration | Botanical Name and Family | Traditional Indications | Biological Effects | Chemical Constituents |
|---|---|---|---|---|
| *Prevention* Chai hu | Radix *Bupleurum chinensis* DC. (Umbelliferae) | Reducing fever, soothing the liver and upper GI, cures organ ptosis. | CNS effects (Antipyretic effect, sedative effect, analgesic and antitussive effect.). Anti-inflammatory effect. GI effect (hepato-protective and choleretic effect, prevents gastric ulcer.). Hypolipemic effect, antimicrobial effect, protects from renal damage. | Triterpene saponins: saikos-aponins a, $b_1$–$b_4$, c, d, e, and f. Essential oil:bupleurmol, spinasterol, stigmasterol. |
| Dang kui | Radix *Angelica sinensis* (Oliv.) Diels (Umbelliferae) | Enriching the blood and activating blood circulation. Regulating menstruation and relieving menstrual pain. Used for constipation. | Different fractions can both inhibit and stimulate uterine contractions. Endometrial proliferation without direct estrogenic effect was found. Decrease contraction magnitude and frequency of heart muscle. Significantly dilates and increases coronary flow. Decreases artery pressure while reducing arterial resistance and increasing | Essential oil: ligustilide, ferulic acid, n-butylidenephthalide, n-valerophenone-O-carboxylic acid. Novolatile: brefeldin A, sitosterol, stigmasterol, sitosterol-D-glucoside, vitamin A, $B_{12}$ and E. |

| | | | | |
|---|---|---|---|---|
| Bai shao | Radix *Paeonia lactiflora* Pall. (Ranunculaceae) | Supplements blood, controls pain, alleviates sudden onset of disease, subdues hyperactive liver, controls excessive sweating. | arterial flow. Inhibits platelet aggregation and serotonin release. Decreases blood lipids and reduces arteriosclerosis. Analgesic effect Antiasthmatic effect. Antispasmodic and analgesic effect by lowering muscle tonicity. Sedative effect, inhibits gastric secretions and inhibits gastric ulceration. Antibacterial effect. Protects from myocardial ischemia and from platelet aggregation. Causes coronary and peripheral vasodialation. | Paeoniflorin, paeonol, paeonin, albiflorin, oxypaeoniflorin, benzoylpaeoniflorin, and paeoniflorigenone. Benzoic acid, sitosterol, gallotannin, pedunculagin. Polysaccharide: peonan SA. Acidic polysaccharide: peonan SB, peonan PA, and Triterpenoids. |
| Chen pi | Pericarpium *Citrus reticulata* blanco. (Rutaceae) | Regulating the flow of qi and invigorating digestive function. Eliminating damp and resolving phlegm. | Inhibits GI smooth muscle movement. Inhibits gastric ulceration without inhibition of gastric secretions. Expectorant and antitussive effect. Anti-inflammatory and antiallergic effect. Relaxes uterine muscle contraction. | Essential oil: d-limonene, citrol. Monoterpenes: pinene, pinene, camphene, myrcene, 3-carene, phellandrene, phellandrene, terpinene, terpinene. Flavones, alkaloids, synephrine, and N-methyltyramine. |
| Wang bu liu xing | Semen *Vaccariae pyramidata* Medic. (Caryophyllacea) | Moves blood, regulates menses, increases lactation, disperses swelling carbuncles, promotes healing of incised wounds. | Stimulates uterine contraction. | Saponins: vacasegoside, isosaponarin. Starch, fat, alkaloids, cyclic peptides. |

Table
15.1

## Debu Tripathy Herbal Examples Diagram (Continued)

| Pinyin Transliteration | Botanical Name and Family | Traditional Indications | Biological Effects | Chemical Constituents |
|---|---|---|---|---|
| *Commonly prescribed herbs with chemotherapy* | | | | |
| Huang qi | Radix *Astragalus membranaceus* (Fisch.) Bge. (Leguminosae) | Supplements qi, increases yang, consolidates surface, increases resistance to diseases, controls sweating, delivers fluids, disperses swelling, discharges pus. | Increased $CD_4/CD_8$ ratio and phagocytic activity in patients with gastric cancer undergoing chemotherapy. Stimulation of lymphocyte IL-2, IL-3, IL-6, TNF-$\alpha$ and IFN-$\gamma$. Diuretic effect and anti-nephrotoxic effect. Anti-inflammatory effect. Hepatoprotective effect. | Saponins: astragalosides I-VIII, acetylastragalosidel I. Flavones: kaempferol, quercitin, isorhamnetin, rhamnocitin, formononetin, calycosin. Polysaccharides: astragalans I,II,III. Glucans: AG-1 and AG-2. |
| Bai zhu | Rhizoma *Atractylodis macrocephalae* Koidz. (Compositae) | Replenishing qi and reinforcing the spleen. Harmonizes spleen and stomach, relieves fatigue. Induces diuresis and eliminate damp. Arresting excessive perspiration and spontaneous sweating. | Increased phagocytosis, lymphocyte transformation, rosette formation, and serum Ig G post chemotherapy. Increases body weight and endurance. Potentiates reticuloendothelial system. Diuretic effect, antiulcerative effect, hypoglycemic effect. Anticuagulant effect. Hepatoprotective effect. Lowers blood pressure and dilates blood vessels. | Essential oil: atractylon. Lactones: atractylenolides II,III. Vitamin A. Sesquiterpene and furfural. |

| Ling zhi | *Ganoderma lucidum* (Leyss. Ex Fr.) Karst. (Basidiomycetes) | Nourishes, tonifies, supplements qi and blood. Removes toxin, astringes essence and disperses accumulations. Relieves fatigue and subdues deficiency insomnia. | Antitussive effect. Expectorant effect. Hypotensive effect. Hepatoprotective effect. Antibacterial effect. Sensitizes radiation effect. Protects from radiation damage. Immune stimulating effect. | Ergosterol, coumarin, mannitol, polysaccharides, organic acids, resins. |
|---|---|---|---|---|
| Dang shen | Radix *Codonopsis pilosula* (Franch.) Nannf. (Campanulaceae) | Tonify qi, increases body resistance, promotes digestion, absorption of nutrients. Increases secretion of body fluids. | Promotes digestion and metabolism. Stimulates the CNS: decrease monoxidase-B (MAO-B) activity in the brain. Hematopeiteic, Hypotensive effect. Significantly decrease erythrocyte electrophoretic time and fibrinogen. Enhance cardiac function and increases tolerance to cold without increasing body weight and it elevates activity of superoxide dismutase (SOD). Increases phagocytosis, promotes leukocyte production. Increases hemoglobin levels, antagonizes insulin-induced hypoglycemia, but was ineffective with phagocytosis and the transformation of lymphocytes. It also inhibited type II allergic reactions and stimulated the adrenal cortex. Inhibits transplanted sarcoma 180 in mice. | Phytosterols and triterpenes: spinasterol and D-glucopyranoside, 7-stigmasterol, 5,22-stigmasterol, taraxerol, taraxeryl acetate, and friedelin. Phenols: syringaldehyde, vanillic acid, syringin, tangshenoside I. Essential oil: methyl palmitate, octadecane, nonadecane, heptadecane, carboxylic acid3. |

*(Continued)*

Table
15.1

## Debu Tripathy Herbal Examples Diagram (Continued)

| Pinyin Transliteration | Botanical Name and Family | Traditional Indications | Biological Effects | Chemical Constituents |
|---|---|---|---|---|
| Fu ling | Sclerotium *Poria cocos* (Schw.) Wolf (Polyporaceae) | Induces diuresis and excreting dampness. Invigorating the spleen function. Tranquilizing the mind. | Increased monocyte GM-CSF production. Enhanced recovery of myelosuppression in mice after radiation. Increased spontaneous rosette formation, lymphocyte transformation, and serum IgG. Diuretic effect. Sedative effect. Antitumor promotion effect. Increases cardiac contractility. | Polysaccharide: -pachyman. Triterpene: pachymic acid, tumulosic acid, eburicoic acid, pinicolic acid. |
| *Antineoplastic agents*<br>Pu gong ying | Herba *Taraxacum mongolicum* Hand.-Mazz. (Compositae) | Removes toxic heat. Removes swelling and nodulation. Relieves dysuria. | Antimicrobial effect. Immune stimulating effect: increases peripheral lymphoblast transformation rate. Choleretic effect and hepatoprotective effect. | Taraxasterol, taraxacerin, taraxicin, choline, inulin, and pectins. |
| Jin yin hua | Flos *Lonicera japonica* Thunb. (Caprifoliaceae) | Removes toxic heat. Dispels wind heat. | Antimicrobial effect. Anti-inflammatory effect, antilipemic effect. Decreases pregnancy rate after mating. Antispasmodic effect. Diuretic effect. | Chlorogenic acid. Inositol and flavonone. Essential oil: 2,6,6-trimethyl-2-vinyl-5-hydroxytetrahydropyran and linalool. |

| | | | | |
|---|---|---|---|---|
| Shan ci gu | Bulbus *Cremastra variabilis* (Blume) Nakai (Orichidaceae) | Reduces heat. Removes toxin, disperses accumulation, dissipates swelling. | Antineoplastic effect. Cardiotonic effect. Antiviral effect. | Tulipine, colchicines. |
| Huang yao zi | Rhizoma *Dioscorea bulbifera* L. (Dioscoreaceae) | Resolves phlegm. Controls cough. Disperses goiter and controls bleeding. | Antibacterial effect. Antifungal effect. Increases uterine contraction. | Terpenoids: diosbulbin A,B,C,D. 2,4,6,7-tetrahydroxy-9,10-dihydrophenanthrene, 2,4,5,6-tetrahydroxy-phenanthrene. Tannin. |
| Bai hua she she cao | Herba *Oldenladia diffusa* (Willd.) Roxb. (Rubiaceae) | Removes toxic damp heat, clears abscesses, infections with fever. | Increases phagocytosis, lowers fever, arrests growth of spermatogonia and empties convoluted seminiferous tubules. | Iridoid glycosides: oldenlandosides A and B, hentriacontane, stigmasterol, ursolic acid, oleanolic acid, $\beta$ sitosterol, sitosterol-D-glucoside, p-coumaric acid, and flavonoid glycosides. |

Used with permission from Debu Tripathy, a Professor of Medicine and Director of the Komen Breast Cancer Research Program at the University of Texas Southwestern Medical Center in Dallas, Texas.

(Four Gentleman Decoction) with the addition of ingredients to supplement *yin* (*blood* and *moisture*) and eliminate *heat* (*yang*) and *toxins*: *Codonopsis pilolusa* (*dang shen*) (a substitute for *Panax ginseng*), *Atractylodes macrocephala* (*bai zhu*), and *Poria cocos* (*fu ling*), *Glycyrrhiza uralensis* (*gan* cao) are the base formula for supplementing *qi* to which are added *Ophiopogon japonicus* (*mai men dong*), *Asparagus cochinchinensis* (*tian men dong*), *Glehnia littoralis* (*sha shen*), *Rehmannia glutinosa* (*di huang*), *Anemarrhena asphodeloides* (*zhi mu*), and *Polygonatum odoratum* (*yu zhu*) for supplementing *yin*; *Scrophularia ningpoensis* (*xuan shen*), *Imperata imperitae* (*bai mao gen*), *Lonicera japonica* (*jin yin hua*), *Solanum lyratum* (*shu yuan quan*), and *Oldenlandia diffusa* (*bai hua she she cao*) for eliminating *heat* and *toxins*; and, finally, *Salvia miltiorrhiza* (*dan shen*) for activating *blood* and removing stagnation. The objectives of the formula are not only to relieve the *blood* deficiency (anemia), *moisture* deficiency (dehydration), *heat* (due to radiation), and *toxins* (waste products and dead tissue because of tumor necrosis) but also to enhance the anticancer effects of the radiation via the antitumor activity of *Salvia miltiorrhiza* (*dan shen*), *Oldenlandia diffusa* (*bai hua she she cao*), *Glycyrrhiza uralensis* (*gan cao*), and *Solanum lyratum* (*shu yuan quan*) (Pan, 1992).

The same formula, *Si Jun Zi Tang* (Four Gentleman Decoction), can be used as the core of a prescription to treat the side effects of chemotherapy. Chemotherapy damages the *qi* and weakens the *spleen* and *stomach*, ultimately depleting the *essence* and undermining the *kidney*. Adding *Astragalus membranaceus* (*huang qi*), *Polygonatum odoratum* (*yu zhu*), *Pseudostellaria heterophylla* (*tai zi shen*), *Euryale ferox* (*qian shi*), *Nelumbo nucifera* (*lian zi*), and *Dioscorea opposita* (*shan yao*) augment the *qi* supplementing and *stomach* and *spleen* strengthening properties of the formula. Three more herbs, *Ligustrum lucidi* (*nu zhen zi*), *Rehmannia glutinosa* (*shu di huang*), and *Lycium barbarum* (*gou qi zi*), replenish *essence* and strengthen the *kidney*. This formula called *Bu Shen Jian Pi Tang* alleviates fatigue, weakness, chilliness, anorexia, anemia, leukopenia, and hair loss and increases resistance to infection (Pan, 1992).

In 1983, Jia Kun created a formula called *Ping Xiao Dan*, containing *Citrus aurantium* (*zhi ke*), *Curcuma longa* (*yu jin*), Niter (*xiao shi*), *Lacca sinica exsiccata* (*gan qi*), Alumen (*ming fan*), *Strychnos nux-vomica* (*ma qian zi*), *Trogopterus xanthipes* (*wu ling zhi*), and *Agrimonia pilosa* (*xian he cao*). Dr. Kun recommends *Ping Xiao Dan* as a general formula for the prevention and treatment of cancer combined with additional formulas that are specific for particular types of cancer. *Ping Xiao Dan* has multiple effects: *Lacca sinica exsiccata* (*gan qi*), *Trogopterus xanthipes* (*wu ling zhi*), *Curcuma longa* (*yu jin*), *Citrus aurantium* (*zhi ke*), *Strychnos nux-vomicus* (*ma qian zi*), and *Agrimonia pilosa* (*xian he cao*) eliminate stagnation of *qi* and *blood*, promote the normal function of the liver and intestines, relieve pain, promote tissue regeneration, and dissolve lumps and masses. Niter (*xiao shi*) and Alumen (*ming fan*) neutralize *toxins* and reduce fever and inflammation. Moreover, even though the major thrust of the formula appears to be antipathogenic, *Curcuma longa* (*yu jin*), *Agrimonia pilosa* (*xian he cao*), and *Citrus aurantium* (*zhi ke*) also have a tonic effect on the body as a whole: "The combination of all these ingredients... controls and palliates solid neoplasms and manages the corrosion. It also has the function of a tonic, antidote, analgesic and appetizer, revives vigor, nourishes the nerves, encourages recovery, increases the capacity of organs to resist disease, nourishes *qi*, and causes cancer cells to degenerate, change shape, reduce in size, and melt" (Kun, 1985).

# Research Investigations

A literature review performed in 1998 by the University of Texas Center for Alternative Medicine Research in Cancer summarized many Chinese studies, including controlled trials with human subjects and animal and in vitro laboratory experiments (DeGuzman & Nanney, 1998). The studies showed the impact of medicinal herbs on disease response, survival outcome, immune response, reduction in adverse effects from chemotherapy and radiation, improved recovery from surgery, better quality of life, and alleviation of pain. This review indicated that some patients who received Chinese herbal medicine combined with conventional Western treatment demonstrated significantly better survival and/or disease response than patients receiving Western treatment alone. But often research design has involved inadequate methodology, including the absence of randomized, placebo, or blinded controls. Although the examples that follow hardly constitute proof of efficacy, they are suggestive of benefit, indicating that further research is desirable and necessary.

For example, in a study of 76 patients with second-stage primary liver cancer there were no 5-year survivors in the groups treated with chemotherapy or radiation alone, whereas there was 10% survival in the group treated with a combination of *Fu Zheng* herbs and radiation and 16.7% survival in those treated with both herbs and chemotherapy (Li & Lien, 1986). Five-year survival rates in another study of patients with liver cancer who received chemotherapy alone were 6%, whereas when combined with the herb formula *Si Jun Zi Tang* (*Panax ginseng*, *Atractylodes macrocephala*, *Poria cocos*, *Glycyrrhiza uralensis*), 5-year survival rose to 43% (Zhang, 1988). In another study of patients with Stage II liver cancer treated with chemotherapy alone, the 1-year survival rate was 30%, and the 5-year survival was only 5%. When combined with herbal therapy, the 1-year survival rate rose to 70%, and the 5-year survival rate increased to between 10% and 20%.[11] A review of 39 studies concluded that combined treatment of traditional Chinese medicine with conventional therapies improved the clinical outcomes and prolonged survival in patients with advanced primary liver cancer (Zho–Qing, 1998). Another meta-analysis of 26 randomized controlled trials representing 2,079 patients also showed improved survival (Xiaojuan, McCullough, & Broffman, 2005).

Strengthening the *spleen* and replenishing *qi* has been effective in hindering tumor growth, decreasing tumor size, and improving the health of the host while strengthening the function of T lymphocytes and adjusting NK cells (Yu & Lu, 1987). Herbs that are *qi* and *yang* tonifying, that warm and strengthen the *spleen* and *kidney*, are thought to ameliorate the adverse effects of chemotherapy and radiation. Zhang Xinqi comments, "The leukopenia caused by chemo- or radiotherapy is classified as a deficiency type of illness which is referred to as the morbid condition showing deficiency of genuine *qi*, lowered body resistance, and declining of function. Then, supplementing *qi* and nourishing the *blood*, warming and invigorating the *spleen* and *kidney*, are the essential therapeutic principles for remitting toxic side effects" (Xinqi et al., 1996).

Two of the important toxin-removing herbs used in cancer therapy are *Sophora flavescens (ku shen*, meaning "bitter root of miraculous effect") and *Sophora subprostrata* (*shan dou gen*), containing matrine and oxymatrine series alkaloids that show cytotoxic activity in vitro and antitumor activity in vivo (inhibit the growth of sarcoma-180 in lab mice). Oxymatrine itself is 7.8 times stronger than the chemotherapeutic agent mitomycin C in its tumor-inhibiting effects, without suppressing the immune system (Kojima et al., 1970). *Sophora flavescens* (or subprostrata) also increases leukocytes and promotes peripheral immune responses. *Scutellaria baicalensis* (*huang qin*) is another potent heat- and toxin-clearing herb with antitumor and immune-stimulating properties in vivo and in vitro that inhibits platelet aggregation and induces apoptosis (Chang & But, 1986). And another herb, *Isatis tinctoria* (*ban lan gen*), contains the compound indirubin, observed by Chinese scientists to exert an effect against chronic myelocytic leukemia (CML). It inhibits DNA synthesis in neoplastic cells, particularly immature leukemic cells in bone marrow, while simultaneously stimulating immune response (Chang & But, 1987).

*Angelica sinensis* (*dang gui*) is a *blood*-supplementing and -activating herb with antitumor, immune-stimulating, and antiangiogenic properties that reduces vascular permeability in vitro (Yamada et al., 1990). Other potent herbs in the *blood* activating category with direct cancer-inhibiting properties are *Curcuma zedoaria* (*e zhu*), *Salvia miltiorrhiza* (*dan shen*), and *Panax pseudoginseng* (*tian qi*). These herbs are fibrinolytic, antithrombic, and anti-inflammatory. People with cancer often have elevated fibrinogen levels, increasing the stickiness of the blood so that it is more likely to coagulate. Because the "sticky" factors in blood facilitate the adherence of metastatic cells to healthy tissue, and because tumors are often encapsulated within a tough fibrin coating difficult for antineoplastic drugs or immune cells to penetrate, herbs that increase microcirculation, make the blood less viscous the fibrin coating more permeable, and help soften and disperse tumorous masses. When extracts of curcuma are injected in mice with tumors, the tumors shrink (Shi, 1981).

# Enhancing Conventional Protocols

To overcome the adverse effects while at the same time potentiating the desired effects of conventional treatment, a popular biologic response modifying formula called All Inclusive Great Tonifying Decoction (*Shi Quan Da Bu Tang*) is often used. It appears to restore hematopoeitic function to improve peripheral blood counts and increase interleukin production along with NK cells. This formula contains *Panax ginseng* (*ren shen*), *Angelica sinensis* (*dang gui*), *Poria cocos* (*fu ing*), *Atractylodes macrocephala* (*bai zhu*), *Astragalus membranaceus* (*huang qi*), *Ligusticum wallichii* (*chuan xiong*), *Peonia lactiflora* (*bai shao*), prepared *Rehmannia glutinosa* (*shu di huang*), *Cinnamomum cassia* (*rou gui*), and prepared *Glycyrrhiza uralensis* (*zhi gan cao*). It was found to potentiate the therapeutic activity of chemotherapy (mitomycin, cisplatin, cyclophosphamide, fluorouracil) and radiotherapy, inhibit recurrence, prolong survival, and prevent or ameliorate adverse treatment effects such as: anorexia, nausea, vomiting, hematotoxicity, immuno-suppression, leukopenia, thrombocytopenia, anemia, and nephropathy. In traditional terms, the herbs *Panax ginseng* (*ren shen*), prepared *Glycyrrhiza uralensis* (*gan cao*), *Poria cocos* (*fu ling*), and *Atractylodes macrocephala* (*bai zhu*) tonify *qi*; *Angelica sinensis* (*dang gui*), *Ligustici wallichii* (*chuan xiong*), *Peonia lactiflora* (*bai shao*), and prepared *Rehmannia glutinosa* (*shu di huang*) nourish the *blood*; and *Astragalus membranaceus* (*huang qi*) and *Cinnamomum cassia* (*rou gui*) further invigorate *qi* and *yang* (Zee-Cheng, 1992). In another study to determine effects of this formula on white blood cell counts, 134 patients with cancer who had previously undergone chemotherapy and radiation therapy that resulted in leukopenia were given the formula, and 113 patients experienced an increase of white blood counts to normal levels (Shen & Zhan, 1997). In a study of 58 patients with osteogenic sarcoma who were receiving either cisplatin and dexamethasone (CD) or high-dose methotrexate and vincristine (MV), patients were randomly assigned to the herbal arm or observation. Those using the herb formula in the MV group experienced improvements in white blood cell and platelet counts and there was less transaminase enzyme elevation. Both the CD and MV groups showed improvement in posttherapy cardiac function, less nausea and vomiting, and fewer rashes than those in the control group (Liu & Wu, 1993).

Whereas tumor recurrence for postsurgical patients with bladder cancer was 65% with conventional treatment alone, this was reduced to 33% when patients added the use of the Chinese medicinal mushroom *Polyporus umbellatus* (*zhu ling*) (*maitake* in Japanese) (Yang, Li, & Li, 1994). In another study, those receiving radiation alone suffered from low white blood cell and platelet counts, but this was reversed in subjects who received Chinese herbs: 40 patients recovered from 3450/c.mm to 5425/c.mm, whereas in the control group without herbs, white blood cell counts dropped significantly (Zhang, Qian, Yang, Wang, & Wen, 1990).

Five-year survival for advanced nose and throat cancer patients receiving radiation alone was 24%, whereas adding the herbal formula *Yi Qi Yang Yin Tang* to the conventional protocol produced a 5-year survival rate of 52% (Li, Chen, & Li, 1992). In a study of 197 patients with Stages III and IV nose and throat cancers, half received radiation in combination with the formula *Yi Qi Yang Yin Tang* and half received only radiotherapy. After 3 years the survival rates were 67 and 33%, respectively. This formula is targeted to nourish the *qi* and fluids as well as clear *heat* and *toxins* and eliminate *blood* stagnation (Sun, 1988). In yet another study of this formula for nasopharyngeal cancer, 272 patients were treated with radiation, half of whom received the formula. In the herb-treated group, 5-year relapse was 68% lower (12% versus 38%), and survival rates were also significantly improved (67% versus 48% at 5 years) (Li et al., 1992).

In 285 patients with lymph node metastases, one group received only chemotherapy with no significant tumor shrinkage, whereas another received only herbal medicine with only 12% showing significant shrinkage. In the group that received chemo, radiation, and herbs, or radiation plus herbs, 75% showed significant tumor shrinkage (Cui & Li, 1995). When 70 patients with chronic gastritis and dysplasia were divided in groups according to traditional Chinese pattern diagnosis (hyperactive *liver qi*, deficiency *cold* of the *spleen* and *stomach*, deficiency of *stomach yin*, and *damp heat* in the *spleen* and *stomach*) and treated accordingly, 84% markedly improved, 4% responded partially, and 11% were unresponsive (Zhang, Shen, Xu, Wang, & Xu, 1989).

A study at Drew University in Los Angeles investigated the effects of medicinal mushrooms on patients with advanced malignancies: in two weeks there were marked decreases in tumor associated antigens and marked increases in natural killer (NK) cell activity in 8 of 11 subjects (Ghoneum, 1998). In another study, patients with primary liver carcinoma who received herbs in combination with chemotherapy had increased numbers of NK cells (Ling, Wang, & Zhu, 1989).

A study of 176 patients compared half the subjects who received injections of *Astragalus membranaceus* (*huang qi*) and *Panax ginseng* (*ren shen*) while undergoing chemotherapy for colon cancer to a control group that was not administered herbal injections. Those receiving the herbal injections had higher white blood cell counts, greater macrophage activity, and increased body weight (Li, 1992). A study of the herb *Astragalus* at MD Anderson Hospital and Tumor Institute in Houston, Texas, confirmed earlier reports by the same authors that this herb possesses immunopotentiating activity, correcting in vitro T-cell function deficiency found in many cancer patients. Decades of pharmacologic research have revealed that the polysaccharides and other compounds in *Astragalus membranaceus* promote cellular (intensifies phagocytosis) and humoral (increases function of B lymphocytes) immune function and have in vitro antitumor effects on cancer cell lines (Sun et al., 1983). Research at MD Anderson Hospital in Houston reproduced these results in a 1983 study, demonstrating that aqueous extracts of *Astragalus membranaceus* in vitro and in vivo enhanced levels of circulating lymphocytes. A second study in 1988 confirmed and expanded the previous findings that extracts of Chinese herbs possess potent immune restorative activity. A polysaccharide fraction of *Astragalus membranaceus* (fraction 3, F-3) was isolated as most potent. The data indicated that extracts of *Astragalus* could restore T cells from immunocompromised cancer patients to normal levels of function (Chu, Wong, & Mavligit, 1988). In a human trial, *Astragalus membranaceus* was found to potentiate IL-2 10-fold, permitting a smaller, less toxic effective dose, restoring T-cell function in 9 of 10 cancer patients (Chu, 1994). Whereas the common dose of *Astragalus membranaceus* is 9 to 30 g of dried herb for noncancerous conditions, doses as high as 60 g/day may be administered as an immunostimulant. Although toxicity is low at high doses, occasionally symptoms of overstimulation such as insomnia, increased heart rate, palpitations, or hypertension can occur at these high doses (Boik, 2001).

Multiple studies on patients with stomach cancer were conducted using the formula *Pishen Fang* (aka *Jian Pi Yi Shen*), supplements *qi* and *yang*, which has immunostimulating properties, and contains *Codonopsis pilolusa* (*dang shen*), *Atractylodes macrocephala* (*bai zhu*), *Lycium barbarum* (*gou qi zi*), *Ligustrum lucidum* (*nu zhen zi*), *Cuscuta chinensis* (*tu si zi*), and *Psoralea corylifolia* (*bu gu zhi*). One study examined 81 patients with Stage III gastric cancer who received chemotherapy. Those who also took the herbal formula experienced improved digestive and bone marrow function, as well as increased survival. In the herbal group, 5-year survival was 46% compared to 20% in the chemotherapy-only group (Pan, 1992). In another study, 669 late-stage gastric cancer patients who were receiving chemotherapy were randomly divided into the herbal group and the control group. Improvements in body weight, appetite, and reduced nausea and vomiting were observed in the group that received the formula. White blood cell counts were 7% in the herb-treated group compared to 33% in the control group. Macrophage activity was 21% greater in the treated group, and 5-year survival rates among 303 Stage III and 63 Stage IV patients who received follow-up were 53 and 10%, respectively. After 10 years, 47% of the Stage III patients remained alive (Yu et al., 1993). Another study examined 216 postoperative stomach cancer patients at Stage III, and 110 patients at Stage IV, showing that of the half who did not receive the herbal formula, 75% were able to finish the complete chemotherapy course, compared to 95% who received the herbs. Patients in the herb-treated group gained weight (23% vs. 8%), fewer lost weight (6% vs. 14%), fewer lost their appetite (10% vs. 32%), and fewer had vomiting (4% vs. 12%) (Ning et al., 1988; Zhan, 1992).

In an animal study, mitomycin C showed a stronger antitumor effect when combined with ginseng (Matsuda, 1992). Similarly, when an extract of the mushroom *Polyporous umbellatus* (*zhu ling*) was combined with mitomycin C, the lifespan of tumor-bearing mice was increased by 119.9% compared to 70% in the control group treated with the drug alone (You, 1994). Ginsenosides, the active saponin compounds in the ginsengs, increase phagocytosis, appetite, and blood formation; accelerate the biosynthesis of DNA; and appear to induce cancer cells to change their morphology and become more like healthy cells. The polysaccharides in *Astragalus membranaceus* (*huang qi*) and *Panax ginseng* (*ren shen*) and medicinal mushrooms regulate T cells and stimulate interferon and phagocytosis, producing both immune-restorative and cancer-inhibiting effects.

An herbal formula used to relieve signs of cardiac distress (palpitation, irregular, small and slow pulse, occasional premature systole, lower wall myocardial ischemia) secondary to treatment with adriamycin (doxorubicin) is called *Zhi Gan Cao Tang* (Baked Licorice Decoction), consisting of 20 g *Glycyrrhiza uralensis* (*gan cao*), 30 g *Rehmannia glutinosa* (*di huang*), 30 pieces *Ziziphus jujuba* (*da zao*), 15 g *Zingiberis officinale* (*jiang*), 15 g *Cannabis indica* (*huo ma ren*), 10 g *Panax ginseng* (*ren shen*), and 10 g *Cinnamomum cassia* (*gui zhi*) administered as a decoction. When cardiac function normalized after 6 days, Adriamycin therapy resumed, and administration of the decoction was continued (Ruizhi et al., 1995).

Another prescription developed in modern times is a formula described in 1982 by Dr. Hong-Yen Hsu containing *Wisteria sinensis* (*zi teng*), *Terminalia chebula* (*he zi*), *Trapa bispinosa* (*ling jiao*), and *Coix lachryma-jobi* (*yi yi ren*) (Hsu, 1986). Both *Wisteria sinensis* (*he* zi) and *Trapa bispinosa* (*ling jiao*) have a history of use in China and Japan for the treatment of tumors. *Coix lachryma-jobi* (*yi yi ren*) and *Terminalia chebula* (*he zi*) have been used traditionally to strengthen digestive and respiratory functions as well as to relieve infection and inflammation (Hsu, 1986). *Coix lachryma-jobi* is now considered a general anticancer agent. This prescription conforms to the principles of invigorating *qi* and strengthening resistance (improving digestive and respiratory function) and clearing *heat* and eliminating *toxins* (removing infection and inflammation).

The U.S. Food and Drug Administration approved the first Chinese-made anti-cancer drug for Phase II clinical human trials in 2001, to be conducted by the U.S. biopharmaceutic company Oncoherb. The drug, called Kanglaite injection, is an extract distilled from the seeds of the herb *Coix lachryma-jobi* (yi yi ren). It has demonstrated efficacy against nonlobular *lung* cancer in clinical trials with over 200,000 cancer patients conducted in China. Studies have indicated that it may also be useful in the treatment of other types of cancer, including stomach and cervical cancers and solid tumors. The preliminary findings of research conducted in the U.S. support the Chinese trials. The new drug significantly improves the efficacy of radiation therapy and chemotherapy treatments in late-stage, nonlobular lung cancer patients. It is far less toxic than existing chemotherapeutic agents and is effective in patients for whom existing treatments did not show any improvements.

In the November 2001 issue of the *Life Sciences* journal, Henry Lai from the University of Washington reported on the cytotoxic activity of artemesinin, a compound from *Artemesia annua* (*quing hao*). Artemesinin kills human breast cancer cells in vitro by interfering with their iron metabolism. It was first discovered to be an effective antimalarial agent in chloroquine-resistant cases. Malarial parasites depend on high iron concentrations for reproduction, as do cancer cells. Breast cancer cells have up to 15 times more transferrin receptors than healthy cells. Acute leukemia and pancreatic cancers have also been responsive to this agent in vitro, with no apparent adverse effects on healthy tissue. The Breast Cancer Fund in San Francisco is supporting this research. Earlier studies showed that *Artemesia annua* and capillaries have direct cytotoxic effects in vivo without causing immunosuppression (Mori et al., 1989).

Researchers at UCSF conducted a placebo–controlled randomized trial for women with breast cancer, using a formula containing 21 Chinese herbs to investigate the alleviation of common side effects of chemotherapy, namely nausea, vomiting, fatigue, marrow suppression, risk of infection, and hair loss (Tagliaferri et al., 2001).

# Safety and Herb/Drug Interactions

Herb safety and herb/drug interactions are complex and controversial issues. With the increasing use of herbs by Westerners has come legitimate concern for potential abuse and toxicity. The safety of a drug, herb, or food is always relative and contextual. Safety is determined by defining the conditions under which a substance is considered to be safe or dangerous, and weighing potential benefits against possible short and long-term adverse effects. Herb/drug interaction is a similar puzzle: all substances that enter the body interact with each other, ultimately affecting all body processes. The issue again is determining the benefit or detriment of such interactions.

Compared to the record of approved pharmaceutic drugs, with a few well-known exceptions such as *Aconitum carmichaelii* (*fu zi*), Cinnabaris (*zhu sha*), *Aristolochia fangchi* (*guang fang ji*), and *Ephedra sinica* (*ma huang*), Chinese medicinal herbs are safer (Lazarou, Pomeranz, & Corey, 1998). Aconite contains aconitine, a recognized poison, that is traditionally detoxified by boiling and then combined with other herbs such as *Zingiberis officinale* (*jiang*), *Ziziphus jujuba* (*da zao*), and *Glycyrrhiza uralensis* (*gan cao*) that further mitigate its toxicity, yielding important therapeutic benefits. For example, treated Aconite is combined with *Panax ginseng* in the treatment of acute cardiac failure. Cinnabaris, a crude ore, contains mercuric oxide and although considered unsafe by American standards, is still utilized in small doses in China for the short-term treatment of acute mental agitation without negative consequences. Many *Aristolochia* species have recently been shown to exert carcinogenic effects when used continuously for longer than 6 months, yet these species continue to be used in China with good results in the treatment of cancer and nephropathy, the very conditions for which they have been considered causative agents in the West. *Ephedra sinica* (*ma huang*) has appropriately been used for centuries as an antiasthmatic, antitussive diaphoretic, and vasodilating component of numerous pulmonary and antiarthritic formulas. In the United States over the past 2 decades, *Ephedra* has been inappropriately marketed over the counter as a natural energy and weight loss stimulant, resulting in incidences of high blood pressure, palpitations, agitation, and insomnia. It is unfortunate that abuse and misuse have caused herbs such as these to become less available to professional health care providers and have cast a dark shadow over the credibility and safety of Chinese medicinal herbs in general.

The hundreds of herbs that are in common use in China and the West are rarely associated with adverse effects that are not easily reversible. These effects are seldom serious and include such transient reactions as nausea, indigestion, diarrhea, headache, dizziness, hot flashes, chills, and rashes that are rapidly abated by discontinued use or dose reduction. The preponderance of evidence shows that when used as an adjunct to conventional medicine, Chinese herbs both enhance the desired effects and mitigate the harmful ones.

Sophisticated monitoring with biologic testing, sterilization, and spectrographic analyses by manufacturers in the United States is insuring that herbal products are free of chemical contaminants, adulterants, pathogens, and substitutions. This heightened awareness along with stringent standards is encouraging Chinese manufacturers to adopt the good manufacturing practices required by the FDA and the Federal Trade Commission.

There is a paucity of data that describe the interactions between pharmaceutic agents and even less between herbs and drugs. A few herbs and foods have well understood interactions with drugs. Tetracycline absorption can be impeded by milk-based foods, whereas grapefruit juice increases the blood volume of certain drugs (antidepressants, antihistamines, antihypertensive) by inhibiting a drug-metabolizing enzyme (cytochrome P-450). *Hypericum perforatum* (St. John's Wort)(*tian ji huang*) reduces blood levels of protease inhibitors by increasing their metabolism, while potentiating the effects of monoamine oxidase and selective serotonin reuptake inhibitor antidepressants by elevating seratonin levels. Green vegetables high in vitamin K can oppose the blood-thinning action of drugs such as heparin, Coumadin, or warfarin. Because *Gingko biloba* (*yin guo ye*), *Salvia miltiorrhiza* (*dan shen*) and *Angelica sinensis* (*dang gui*) promote microcirculation and inhibit platelet aggregation, they can potentiate the effects of anti-coagulants, as can *Allium sativum* (garlic)(*da suan*) and *Zingiberis officinale* (ginger)(*jiang*). *Astragalus membranaceus* (*huang qi*), because of its immunostimulating properties, may counter the immunosuppressive action of antirejection drugs such as cyclosporin. In high doses, *Glycyrrhiza uralensis* (licorice)(*gan cao*) can mimic the action of cortisol, elevating blood pressure and increasing fluid retention (Dharmananda, 2001). These findings are based on the use of these herbs as single agents.

When *Angelica sinensis* is incorporated into a formula such as *Shi Quan Da Bu Tang*, which supplements *qi* and *blood* and activates circulation, its hematopoietic properties are enhanced and its anticoagulant properties are reduced by the inclusion of herbs such as *Rehmannia glutinosa* (*di huang*) and *Peonia lactiiflora* (*bai shao*), making it an effective treatment for the anemia, bruising, and bleeding caused by radiation and chemotherapy. One of the side effects of standard anticoagulant therapy is anemia. To solve this problem with Chinese medicine, the herbs *Panax pseudoginseng* (*tian qi*) and *Millettia reticulata* (*ji xue teng*) are used because of their triple hematopoietic, circulation-activating, and antihemorrhagic properties. *Glycyrrhiza uralensis* (licorice)(*gan cao*) is ubiquitous, appearing in countless formulas in part because of its ability to modulate adrenal function. For example, the decoction of *Bupleurum chinense* (*chai hu*) and *Poria cocos* (*fu ling*) (*Chai Ling Tang*) contains many herbs, including *Glycyrrhiza uralensis* (*gan cao*), and is used to aid in the withdrawal from corticosteroid dependence (Shizuo et al., 1983).

Rather than suggesting that people stop eating grapefruit or green vegetables, new information is broadening our understanding of the complexity of drug/food and drug/herb combinations, enhancing our ability to make prudent choices. Biologist Subhuti Dharmananda, PhD, suggests, "Herb/drug interactions may be minimized by having patients take the herbs and drugs at different times (one hour apart to avoid direct interaction in the digestive tract; 1.5 hours to avoid maximum blood levels of drug and herb at the same time). The dosage of herbs that are aimed therapeutically at the same function as the drugs (e.g. both are sedatives; both are hypoglycemics; both are anti-coagulants) should be reduced to alleviate concerns about additive or synergistic effects that are too great. A certain level of additive effects might be desired in cases where the drug therapy is not producing the desired response" (Dharmananda, 2001).

## Anecdotal Reports

The following stories illustrate how Chinese medicine is currently used clinically in the United States.

Lori is a 38-year-old woman diagnosed 5 years ago with breast cancer and metastatic liver tumors. Since the time of her diagnosis, she had undergone multiple, nearly continuous, courses of chemotherapy. At the time of her first visit, 3 months following her mastectomy, an angry, weeping crevice in her chest wound refused to heal. Lori used the formula known as *Yunnan Bai Yao*, an herbal powder packed in gelatin caps, prescribed to improve microcirculation and relieve bruising, swelling, and nonhealing injuries. Lori was advised to apply the powder topically and ingest two pills internally twice daily, along with weekly acupuncture. After 2 weeks, the chest wound was 50% healed, and after 4 weeks, it was completely healed. After months of intensive chemotherapy, Lori fell prey to afternoon fevers. These fevers are understood as the consequence of eroded *yin*—*moisture, blood*, and *essence* are damaged by chemotherapy, producing an upsurge of *empty yang*, in this case, afternoon fevers. Herbs that nourish the *yin* restore the *blood* and *essence*, moisturizing and supplementing the body successfully treated her afternoon fevers. Acupuncture reliably provides Lori with an elevation of her mood—it makes her feel happier and more tranquil—as well as relieving fatigue, headaches, and muscle and emotional tension.

In January 1992, Barbara was 38 years old and sought help from Chinese medicine after 6 years of surgery, radiation, and chemotherapy for what was then Stage IV endometrial cancer. At that time, her disease was not well controlled, plus she had developed mild congestive heart failure, secondary to cardiomyopathy induced by adriamycin, and renal insufficiency as evidenced by a creatinine level of 4.9 mg/dl, which disqualified her for further chemotherapy. She had constant shortness of breath, preventing her from lying flat on the treatment table. After a month of weekly acupuncture and daily herbs, she was no longer short of breath, her creatinine had decreased to 2.3, the lowest it had been in 3 years, and she was able to tolerate more chemotherapy. With the combination of Chinese medicine and conventional therapy, macroscopic measure of disease was not evident for a year, at which time she moved away to live with her sister, a level of health she had not been able to achieve in 6 years of conventional treatment.

Barbara continued to take hydrocortisone, Captopril, Lasix, allopurinol, colchicine, and Megace for Addison's disease, heart failure, gout, and menopausal symptoms. Her creatinine continued to rise with chemotherapy, and the acupuncture and herbal medicine continued to bring it down. She discontinued chemotherapy because "it was clearly not working and I realized that the doctors had given up." In June her general health improved considerably, and by the middle of August a CT scan demonstrated no visible signs of cancer. Barbara went through a period of crisis in which she reorganized her life around continued survival rather than the prospect of an imminent demise. She wrote, "I still have cancer in my body, but it should not cause me problems for some time. I don't know what has brought about my healing, but among other things I am aggressively doing Chinese medicine and acupuncture." She died a year later, in August 1993. Acupuncture and herbs seem to promote a sense of integration.

Meredith requested acupuncture to be administered to her at home when she was too weak to move. She was in the final stages of cervical cancer, with an inoperable tumor that had metastasized to her bones. Unable to eat or drink, and in substantial pain, she fiercely wanted to be at home, and preferably off the morphine, which made her groggy. She complained that her upper body felt disconnected from her lower body. *Yin* and *yang* were beginning to separate, a sign that death was near. Acupuncture every 6 hours enabled her to discontinue morphine, sip herbal broth, and eat bits of rice porridge. Minutes after the needles were in place she felt as if her chest and abdomen were rejoining her lower limbs. She reported a sense of calm, connectedness, and imbued with more clarity, feeling *more herself.*

Shirley was 46 years old when she was diagnosed with nodular lymphoma in 1987. After a year of chemotherapy that was accompanied by compromised kidney function, she went into remission for 6 months. Then she was treated with adriamycin and cytoxin for a recurrence. At that time she began receiving weekly acupuncture and daily herbal medicine. Within 3 months, her overall health strikingly improved, evidenced in part by CBC counts within normal limits and no compromised kidney function, but her lymph nodes remained enlarged. In June she began receiving nitrogen mustard in a more aggressive effort to suppress the disease, and by September the size of her lymph nodes was diminished. Throughout the chemotherapy, she managed well, with minimal hair loss, a normal appetite and digestion and moderate activity. Her general health continued to improve through March 1990, when she decided to take a break from acupuncture and herbal therapy. She returned for further treatment in June 1991 to prepare for yet another course of chemotherapy triggered by splenomegaly. In July, she underwent a splenectomy after which the cancer appeared to become more aggressive. This was followed by another course of chemotherapy (prednisone, vincristine, cytoxin, and VP-16). Her blood counts plummeted and she developed a serious case of thrush that required a 4-day hospitalization. Despite of everything, her energy, digestion, and elimination remained adequate.

In January 1992, Shirley's condition worsened again: her left leg was edematous, she had many prominent and painful nodes, and her abdomen was quite enlarged. By February, she had discontinued chemotherapy and her course began to reverse: the size of her nodes and her leg edema diminished. In May, she was feeling better than she had in the previous year: she had good energy and stamina, blood levels were holding, and the edema and nodes had significantly reduced. In August 1992 her oncologist referred to her as "a case of spontaneous remission," one of only two such lymphoma cases he had observed in 20 years. Her general health was good. She continued to receive acupuncture once a month and use Chinese herbal medicine. In June 1994, her lymphoma became active again and she received radiation treatment for a large node in her groin. Her oncologist prescribed VP-16. By October, she had resumed an intensive program of acupuncture and herbal medicine along with vitamin and nutritional supplements. Shirley was last seen for acupuncture in December 1994, 6 years later almost to the day. She gained 2 good years during which she began a new career, healed her personal and family relationships, and deepened her emotional and spiritual life. She died comfortably in January 1995, grateful that she had accomplished more with her life than she had expected.

Hugh is a 56-year-old man recently treated with brachytherapy for early-stage prostate cancer confined within the capsule. The usual side effects of embedded radioactive pellets can include swelling, inflammation, and pain of the urinary tract requiring catheterization, fatigue, erectile dysfunction, decreased libido, diarrhea, and incontinence. Hugh began acupuncture and Chinese herbal therapy before beginning brachytherapy. Although he required Vioxx for pain management, the only other adverse effect he experienced was intermittent mild fatigue. His urologist commented that Hugh was tolerating his treatment markedly better than any other patient.

## Summary

Fundamentally, Chinese medicine is concerned with the behavior of *qi*. Consequently, all of the major modalities of Chinese medicine (acupuncture, herbal medicine, dietetics, and *qi* gong) are employed to provoke the *qi* to reorder itself once a pathologic process has begun and, ideally, before it has become clinically manifest. And although Chinese medicine has developed its own sophisticated repertoire of treatments for specific diseases, its primary emphasis is ultimately on restoring and preserving the healthy function of the body.

Several oncologists refer scores of patients to Manhattan physician/acupuncturist Frank Lipman, who comments, "Using acupuncture during chemotherapy decreases nausea, gastrointestinal disturbances, fatigue, and increases appetite, white blood cell counts, and a generalized sense of well-being. My colleagues began sending me their patients after noticing that they tolerated their chemotherapy treatment better" (F. Lipman, personal communication, November 27, 2001). Oncologist and clinical researchers in Chinese medicine at the UCSF comment that, "Some empirically derived observations may be clinically useful, even if the physiologic basis remains unclear" (Tagliaferri et al., 2001).

Fundamentally, Chinese medicine is concerned with behavior, not only at the gross level that can be observed with the senses but also at the deepest level of organization, that of the behavior of *qi*. Consequently, all the major modalities of Chinese medicine (acupuncture, herbal medicine, diet, massage, *qi gong*) are employed to provoke the body to reorder itself once a pathologic process has begun and, ideally, before it has become clinically manifest. Although Chinese medicine has developed its own sophisticated repertoire of treatments for specific diseases, its primary emphasis is ultimately on restoring and preserving the healthy function of the body.

## Acknowledgments

The authors thank Stephen Cowan, John Boik, Subhuti Dharmananda, Larry Baskind, and Ken Rose for their contributions to this chapter.

### NOTES

1. Historically, over the span of millennia, many competing and contradictory logics produce internal inconsistencies in Chinese medicine—it cannot be regarded as one coherent system but rather as a syncretic compendium of contending theories and practices.

2. "The organicist conception in which every phenomenon was connected with every other according to a hierarchical order was universal amongst Chinese thinkers. . . . In other words, the Chinese were *a priori* inclined to field theories" (Needham, 1982).
3. Lecture to medical students, UCSF Medical Center, November 2001.
4. Paul Unschuld, seminar organized by Beinfield and Korngold in Northern California, August 25, 2003.
5. The National Certification Commission for Acupuncture and Oriental Medicine (NCCAOM) was established by the profession in 1982 to develop and implement nationally recognized standards of competence.
6. Estimates are based on presentations from the Workshop on Acupuncture sponsored by the Office of Alternative Medicine and the FDA reported in the *Journal of Alternative and Complementary Medicine*, 2(1), 1996, and presentations at the Consensus Development Conference on Acupuncture at the National Institutes of Health, November 3–5, 1997. Web site: http://www.NCCAOM. org
7. The Accreditation Commission for Acupuncture and Oriental Medicine (ACAOM) is a peer-review group formed in 1982 and recognized by the Department of Education Council for Higher Education Accreditation and the Commission on Recognition of Postsecondary Accreditation to develop clinical guidelines and core curriculum requirements for master's and doctoral level programs in acupuncture and Oriental medicine. The Council of Colleges of Acupuncture and Oriental Medicine (CCAOM) provides a list of accredited training programs. Web site: http://www.CCAOM. org
8. For a more thorough explanation of basic concepts, read Beinfield and Korngold (1991), Kaptchuk (2000), and Maciocia (1989).
9. This section is an original rendering by the authors of the logic of conventional therapies within the model of Chinese traditional medical thinking.
10. Observations by the author of a lung dissection using acupuncture analgesia in Yunnan, People's Republic of China, 1980.
11. Adverse drug reactions (ADR) have become the United States' fourth biggest killer. The results of 39 studies of adverse drug reactions suggest that they could affect as many as 2.2 million hospital patients a year, causing 106,000 deaths. This is equivalent to 4.6% of all recorded deaths. These figures are probably conservative, the researchers add, because their ADR definition did not include patient outcomes linked to errors in drug administration, overdoses, drug abuse, and therapeutic failures.

# REFERENCES AND RESOURCES

Adler, S. (1999). Complementary and alternative medicine use among women with breast cancer. *Medical Anthropology Quarterly, 13*, 214–222.

Ballegaard, S., Muteki, T., Harada, H., Ueda, N., Tsuda, H., Tayama, F., et al. (1993). Modulatory effect of acupuncture on the cardiovascular system: A crossover study. *Acupuncture and Electrotherapy Research, 18*, 103–115.

Bardychev, M. S., Guseva, L. I., & Zubova, N. D. (1988). Acupuncture in edema of the extremities following radiation or combination therapy of cancer of the breast and uterus. *Voprosy Onkologii, 34*(3), 19–22.

Beinfield, H., & Beinfield, M. (1997). Revisiting accepted wisdom in the management of breast cancer. *Alternative Therapies in Health and Medicine, 3*(5):117–123.

Beinfield, H., & Korngold, E. (1991). *Between heaven and earth.* New York: Ballantine.

Bensky, D., & Gamble, A. (1986). *Chinese herbal medicine: Materia medica.* Seattle: Eastland.

Birch, S. J., & Felt, R. L. (1999). *Understanding acupuncture.* London: Churchill Livingstone.

Boik, J. (1995). *Cancer and natural medicine: A textbook of basic science and clinical research.* Princeton, MN: Oregon Medical Press.

Boik, J. (2001). *Natural compounds in cancer therapy.* Princeton, MN: Oregon Medical Press.

Cassidy, C. M. (1998). Chinese medicine users in the United States. Part I. Utilization, satisfaction, medical plurality. *Journal of Alternative and Complementary Medicine. 4*(1), 17–27.

Cassileth, B. R., Lusk, E. J., Strouse, T. B., et al. (1984). Contemporary unorthodox treatments in cancer medicine: A study of patients, treatments, and practitioners. *Annals of Internal Medicine, 101*, 105–112.

Chang, H. M., & But, P. P. H. (1986). *Pharmacology and applications of Chinese materia medica* (Vol. 1). Teaneck, NJ: World Scientific.

Chang, H. M., & But, P. P. H. (1987). *Pharmacology and applications of Chinese materia medica* (Vol. 2). Teaneck, NJ: World Scientific.

Chang, M. (1992). *Anticancer medicinal herbs*. Changsha, China: Hunan Science and Technology.

Chen, H. L., & Huang, X. M. (1991). Treatment of chemotherapy-induced leukocytopenia with acupuncture and moxibustion. *Chung Hsi I Chieh Ho Tsa Chih, 11*(6), 350–352.

Cheung, C. S., & Hirano, M. (Eds.). (1982). Blood stasis—Ecchymosis entity. *Journal of the American College of Traditional Chinese Medicine, 2,* 22–32.

Cho, Z. H., Na, C. S., Wang, E. K., et al. (2001). Functional magnetic resonance imaging of the brain in the investigation of acupuncture. In G. Stux & R. Hammerschlag (Eds.), *Clinical acupuncture: Scientific basis* (pp. 83–95). Berlin: Springer-Verlag.

Chu, D. T. (1994). The in vitro potentiation of LAK cell cytotoxicity in cancer and AIDS patients induced by F3—a fractionated extract of astragalus membranaceus. *Chung Hua Chung Liu Tsa Chih, 16*(3), 167–171.

Chu, D.-T., Wong, W. L., & Mavligit, G. M. (1988). Immunotherapy with Chinese medicinal herbs. I. Immune restoration of local xenogenic graft-versus-host reaction in cancer patients by fractionated *astragalus membranaceus* in vitro. *Journal of Clinical & Laboratory Immunology, 25,* 119–123.

Cui, H., & Li, P. (1995). Therapeutic effects of the combined Chinese and Western medicine on metastatic carcinoma in the supraclavicular lymph nodes—An analysis of 285 cases. *Journal of Traditional Chinese Medicine, 15,* 87–89.

Dang, W., & Yang, J. (1998). Clinical study on acupuncture treatment of stomach carcinoma pain. *Journal of Traditional Chinese Medicine, 18,* 31–38.

Dharmananda, S. (1997). *The treatment of gastro-intestinal cancers with Chinese medicine*. Portland, OR: Institute for Traditional Medicine.

Dharmananda, S. (1998). *Countering the side effects of modern medical therapies with Chinese herbs*. Portland, OR: Institute for Traditional Medicine.

Dharmananda, S. (1998a). *Oriental perspectives on cancer and its treatment*. Portland, OR: Institute for Traditional Medicine.

Dharmananda, S. (1999). *The physiological responses to immunologically-active polysaccharides*. Portland, OR: Institute for Traditional Medicine.

Dharmananda, S. (2001). *The interactions of herbs and drugs*. Portland, OR: Institute for Traditional Medicine.

Dundee, J. W., Chestnut, W. N., Ghaly, R. G., et al, (1986). Traditional Chinese acupuncture: A potentially useful antiemetic? *British Medical Journal, 293,* 583–584.

Dundee, J. W., Ghaly, R. G., Fitzpatrick, K. T., et al. (1989). Acupuncture prophylaxis of cancer chemotherapy-induced sickness. *Journal of the Royal Society of Medicine, 82,* 268–271.

Dundee, J. W., & McMillan, C. (1991). Positive evidence for P6 acupuncture antiemesis. *Postgraduate Medical Journal, 67,* 417–422.

Dundee, J. W., & McMillan, C. (1992). Some problems encountered in the scientific evaluation of acupuncture antiemesis. *Acupuncture in Medicine, 10,* 2–8.

Dundee, J. W., & Yang, J. (1990). Prolongation of the antiemetic action of P6 acupuncture by acupressure in patients having cancer chemotherapy. *Journal of the Royal Society of Medicine, 83,* 360–362.

Fass, N. (Ed.). (2001). *Integrating complementary medicine into health systems*. Gaithersburg, MD: Aspen.

Ghoneum, M. (1998). Enhancement of human natural killer cell activity by modified arabinoxylane from rice bran (MGN-3). *International Journal of Immunotherapy, XIV*(2), 89–99.

Gordon, N. P., Sobel, D. S., & Tarazona, E. Z. (1988). Use of and interest in alternative therapies among adult primary-care clinicians and adult members in a large health maintenance organization. *Western Journal of Medicine, 169*(3), 153–161.

Guo, R., Zhang, L., Gong, Y., et al. (1995). The treatment of pain in bone metastasis of cancer with the analgesic decoction of cancer and the acupoint therapeutic apparatus. *Journal of Traditional Chinese Medicine, 15,* 262–264.

Guorui, T. (1981). *The use of tonics in China—Past, present, and future*. Beijing: Academy of Traditional Chinese Medicine.

Hammer, L. (1998). The unified field theory of chronic disease, with regard to the separation of *Yin* and *Yang* and the "*Qi* wild" pulse. *Oriental Medicine Journal, 6*(3&4), 15–49.

Hammer, L. (2001). *Contemporary pulse diagnosis.* Seattle: Eastland Press.

Han, J. (1989). Central neurotransmitters and acupuncture analgesia. In B. Pomeranz & G. Stux (Eds.), *Scientific bases of acupuncture* (pp. 7–33). Berlin: Springer-Verlag.

Hanks, A. (2000). *Cancer and traditional Chinese medicine.* Seattle, WA: Eastland Press.

Hsu, H.-Y. (1982). *Treating cancer with Chinese herbs.* Taiwan: Oriental Healing Arts Institute.

Hsu, H.-Y. (1986). *Oriental materia medica: A concise guide.* Long Beach, CA: Oriental Healing Arts Institute.

Iwa, M., & Sakita, M. (1994). Effects of acupuncture and moxibustion on intestinal motility in mice. *American Journal of Chinese Medicine, 22,* 119–125.

Johansson, K., Lindgren, I., Widner, H., Wiklund, I., & Johansson B. B. (1993). Can sensory stimulation improve the functional outcome in stroke patients? *Neurology, 43,* 2189–2192.

Kaptchuk, T. (2000). *The web that has no weaver.* Chicago: NTC/Contemporary.

Kojima, R., Fukushima, S., Ueno, A., et al. (1970). Anti tumor activity of leguminosae plants constituents. I. Anti-tumor activity of constituents of sophora subprostrata. *Chemical & Pharmaceutical Bulletin, 18*(12), 2555–2563.

Kun, J. (1985). *Prevention and treatment of carcinoma in traditional Chinese medicine* (Rev. ed.). Hong Kong: The Commercial Press Ltd.

Lao, L., Bergman, S., & Hamilton, G. R., Langenberg, P., & Berman, B. (1999). Evaluation of acupuncture for pain control after oral surgery: A placebo-controlled trial. *Archives of Otolaryngology—Head & Neck Surgery, 125,* 567–572.

Lazarou, J., Pomeranz, B. H., & Corey, P. N. (1998). Incidence of adverse drug reactions in hospitalized patients: A meta-analysis of prospective studies. *Journal of the American Medical Association, 279*(15), 1200–1205.

Lewith, G. T., & Vincent, C. (1996). On the evaluation of the clinical effects of acupuncture: A problem reassessed and a framework for future research. *Journal of Alternative and Complementary Medicine, 2,* 79–90.

Li, L., Chen, X., & Li, J. (1992). Observations on the long-term effects of "yi *qi yang yin* decoction" combined with radiotherapy in the treatment of nasopharyngeal carcinoma. *Journal of Traditional Chinese Medicine, 12,* 263–266.

Li, N. Q. (1992). Clinical and experimental study on *shen-qi* injection with chemotherapy in the treatment of malignant tumor of digestive tract. *Chung Kuo Chung Hsi I Chieh Ho Tsa Chih, 12*(10), 588–592.

Li, W., & Lien, E. J. (1986). Fu-zhen herbs in the treatment of cancer. *Oriental Healing Arts International Bulletin, 11*(1), 1–8.

Ling, H. Y., Wang, N. Z., Zhu, H. Z. (1989). Preliminary study of traditional Chinese medicine-Western medicine treatment of patients with primary *liver* carcinoma. *Chung Hsi i Chieh Ho Tsa Chih (Chinese Journal of Modern Developments in Traditional Medicine), 9,* 325, 348–349.

Liu, J. Q., & Wu, D. W. (1993). Fifty-eight cases of postoperative osteogenic sarcoma treated by chemotherapy combined with Chinese medicinal herbs (translated by Amy Hanks). *Zhong guo zhong xi yi jie he za zhi, 13,* 150–152.

Lytle, C. D. (1993). *An overview of acupuncture.* Washington, DC: United States Department of Health and Human Services, Health Sciences Branch, Division of Life Sciences, Office of Science and Technology, Center for Devices and Radiological Health, Food and Drug Administration.

Maciocia, G. (1989). *The foundations of Chinese medicine.* New York: Churchill Livingstone.

Matsuda, H. (1992). Pharmacological study on *Panax ginseng* C.A.Meyer.XIV: Effect of 70% methanolic extract from red ginseng on the cytocidal effect of mitomycin c against rat ascites hepatoma AH 130. *Yakugaku Zasshi, 112*(11), 846–855.

Minji, P. (1992). *Cancer treatment with Fu Zheng Pei Ben Principle.* Fujian PRC: Fujian Science and Technology Publishing House.

Mori, H., et al. (1989). Mechanisms of anti-tumor activity of aqueous extracts from Chinese herbs: Their immunopharmacological properties. *Japanese Journal of Pharmacology, 49*(3), 423–431.

Muench, C. (1984). One hundred years of medicine: The Ah-Fong physicians of Idaho. In H. G. Schwarz (Ed), *Chinese medicine on the golden mountain: An interpretative guide* (pp. 51–80). Seattle: Washington Commission for the Humanities.

National Institutes of Health Consensus Panel. (1997). Acupuncture. *National Institutes of Health Consensus Development Statement, Bethesda, MD, November 3–5. Sponsors: Office of Alternative Medicine and Office of Medical Applications of Research.* Bethesda, MD: National Institutes of Health.

Needham, J. (1982). *Science in traditional China.* Cambridge, MA: Harvard University Press.

Ning, C. H., Wang, G. M., Zhao, T. Y., et al. (1988). Therapeutical effects of jian pi yi shen prescription on the toxicity reactions of postoperative chemotherapy in patients with advanced gastric carcinoma. *Journal of Traditional Chinese Medicine, 8*(2), 113–116.

Pan, M. (1992). *Cancer treatment with Fu Zheng Pei Ben Principle* (pp. 48–51). Fujian, China: Fujian: Science and Technology Institute.

Perneger, T. V., et al. (1994). Risk of kidney failure associated with the use of acetaminophen, aspirin, and nonsteroidal anti-inflammatory drugs. *New England Journal of Medicine, 331*, 1675–1679.

Pomeranz, B. (2001). Acupuncture analgesia—Basic research. In G. Stux & R. Hammerschlag (Eds.), *Clinical acupuncture: Scientific basis* (pp. 1–29). Berlin: Springer-Verlag.

Pomeranz, B., & Stux, G. (1989). *Scientific bases of acupuncture.* Berlin: Springer-Verlag.

Ruizhi, L., et al. (1995). Utilizing Zhigancao Tang to relieve doxorubicin's adverse effects. *Chinese Journal of Chinese Materia Medica, 20*(1), 56–57.

Shan, B., & Shao, S. (1999). The clinical observation on treating peripheral nerve injury by electroacupuncture. *Shanghai Journal of Acupuncture & Moxibustion, 1*, 24–26.

Shen, R, & Zhan, Z. (1997). Clinical study of the use of ginseng and tang-kuei ten combination in the treatment of leukopenia. *International Journal of Oriental Medicine*[PMR90], *22*, 30–31.

Shi, J. (1981). Experimental pharmacological studies on the volatile oil of wen-e-zhu (*Curcuma aromatica* salisb.): Study on the antitumor activity of beta-elemene. *Zhongyao Tongbao, 6*(6), 32–33.

Shizuo, T., et al. (1983). The effect of Chinese formulas on the side effects of glucorticoid hormones. *Bulletin of the Oriental Healing Arts Institute, 8*(3), 1–7.

Sivin, N. (1987). *Traditional medicine in contemporary China.* Ann Arbor: University of Michigan.

Stux, G., & Hammerschlag, R. (Eds.). (2001). *Clinical acupuncture: Scientific basis.* Berlin: Springer-Verlag.

Sun, Y., Hersh, E. M., Lee, S. L., et al. (1983). Preliminary observations on the effects of the Chinese medicinal herbs *Astragalus membranaceus* and *Ligustrum lucidum* on lymphocyte blastogenic responses. *Journal of Biological Response Modifiers, 2*(3), 227–237.

Sun, Y. (1988). The role of traditional Chinese medicine in supportive care of cancer patients. *Recent Results in Cancer Research, 108*, 327–334.

Tagliaferri, M., Cohen, I., & Tripathy, D. (2001). Complementary and alternative medicine in early-stage breast cancer. *Seminars in Oncology, 28*(1), 130.

Taylor, K. (2005). *Chinese medicine in early Communist China 1945–1963: A medicine of revolution.* London/New York: Routledge Curzon.

The Italian Group for Antiemetic Research. (1995). Dexamethasone, granisetron, or both for the prevention of nausea and vomiting during chemotherapy for cancer. *New England Journal of Medicine, 332*, 1–5.

Unschuld, P. (1986). *Medicine in China: A history of pharmaceutics.* Berkeley: University of California Press.

Unschuld, P. (1985). *Medicine in China: A history of ideas.* Berkeley: University of California Press.

Vickers, A. J. (1996). Can acupuncture have specific effects on health?: A systematic review of acupuncture antiemesis trials. *Journal of the Royal Society of Medicine, 89*, 303–311.

Wei, Z. (1998). Clinical observation on therapeutic effect of acupuncture at St 36 for leukopenia. *Journal of Traditional Chinese Medicine, 18*, 94–95.

Whitcomb, D. C., & Block, G. D. (1994). Association of acetaminophen hepatotoxicity with fasting and ethanol use. *Journal of the American Medical Association, 272*, 1845–1850.

Wu, B., Zhow, R., & He, J. (1999). Current situation and prospect of researches on acupuncture mediating immunoresponses. *Shanghai Journal of Acupuncture & Moxibustion, 1*, 73–76.

Wu, L., & Zhou, X. (1998). Menopausal syndrome treated by acupuncture. *Journal of Traditional Chinese Medicine, 18*, 259–262.

Xiaojuan, S., McCullough, M., & Broffman, M. (2005). Chinese herbal medicine and chemotherapy in the treatment of hepatocellular carcinoma: A meta-analysis of randomized controlled trials. *Integrative Cancer Therapies, 4*(3), 219–229.

Xinqi, Z., et al. (1996). Clinical study on treatment of chemotherapy or radiotherapy induced leukopenia with fuzheng compound. *Chinese Journal of Integrated Traditional and Western Medicine, 2*(4), 290–291.

Xu, Z, Liu, L, Xiu, H, et al: The influence of acupuncture on relationship between T lymphocyte subsets and estrogen in patients with mastoplasia. *Shanghai J Acupuncture Moxibustion* 1:13-15, 1998.

Retrieved from http://www.asiabiotech.com.sg/kh-biotech/readmore/vol5/v5n16/fda.html http://www.sciencedaily.com/releases/2004/10/041029104938.html.

Yamada, H., Kmiyama, K., Kiyohara, H., et al. (1990). Structural characterization and antitumor activity of a pectic polysaccharide from the roots of angelica acutiloba. *Planta Medica, 56*, 182–186.

Yang, M. M. P., Ng, K. K. W., Zeng, H. L., & Kwok, J. S. L. (1989). Effect of acupuncture on immunoglobulins of serum, saliva, and gingival sulcus fluids. *American Journal of Chinese Medicine, 17*, 89–94.

Yang, D. A., Li, S. Q., & Li, X. T. (1994). Prophylactic effects of zhuling and BCG on postoperative recurrence of bladder cancer. *Chung Hua Wai Ko Tsa Chih, 32*, 433–434.

You, J. S. (1994). Combined effects of chuling (*Polyporous umbellatus*) extract and mitomycin C on experimental liver cancer, *American Journal of Chinese Medicine, 22*(1), 19–28.

Yu, E. X. (1988). Prolonging long-term therapeutic effect on liver cancer by using the combination of radiotherapy and traditional herbal medicine. *Applied Tumor Journal, 3*(1), 5–7.

Yu, E. X., & Lu, L. N. (1987). Research in treatment and mechanism of primary cancer through strengthening the Spleen and replenishing Qi. *Journal of Traditional Chinese Medicine, 28*(6), 28–30.

Yu, G., Ren, D., Sun, G., et al. (1993). Clinical and experimental studies of JPYS in reducing side effects of chemotherapy in late-stage gastric cancer. *Journal Traditional Chinese Medicine, 13*(1), 31–37.

Yu S. Y., Zhang, L. A., Yang, J. X., Qian, Z. K., & Peng, Y. W. (1991). Dialectic classification of syndrome diagnosis in traditional Chinese medicine used as new criterion for evaluating prognosis of patients with cervical caner. *Journal of Tongji Medical University, 11*(2), 123–125.

Zee- Cheng, R. K. (1992). Shi-quan-da-bu-tang (ten significant tonic decoction), SQT.Quan Da Bu Tang. *Methods and Findings in Experimental and Clinical Pharmacology, 14*(9), 725–736.

Zhang, D. (1989). *Treatment of cancer by integrated Chinese-Western medicine*. Boulder, CO: Blue Poppy Press.

Zhang, D., Zheng, X., & Wang, Q. (1999). Clinical study on climacteric syndrome treated by acupuncture and moxibustion. *Shanghai Journal of Acupuncture & Moxibustion, 3*, 29–32.

Zhang, D. Z. (1988). Prevention and cure by traditional Chinese medicine, of the side effects caused by radio-chemotherapy of cancer patients. *Chung Hsi I Chieh Ho Tsa Chih (Chinese Journal of Modern Developments in Traditional Medicine), 8*(2), 114–116.

Zhang, D. Z. (1992). Effects of traditional Chinese medicine and pharmacology on increasing sensitivity and reducing toxicity in tumor patients undergoing radio-chemical therapy. *Chung Kuo Chung Hsi I Chieh Ho Tsa Chih, 12*(3), 135–138.

Zhang, J., & Zhang, P. (1999). Treatment of 56 cases of shingles by point injection therapy. *Shanghai Journal of Acupuncture & Moxibustion, 1*, 24–26.

Zhang, R. J., Qian, J. K., Yang, G. H., Wang, B. Z., & Wen, X. L. (1990). Medicinal protection with Chinese herb-compound against radiation damage. *Aviation Space & Environmental Medicine, 61*, 729–731.

Zhang, W. Y., Shen, L. H., Xu, H., Wang, X. L., & Xu, Y. R. (1989). Traditional Chinese treatment of chronic gastritis with gastric dysplasia—A clinical analysis of 70 cases. *Journal of Traditional Chinese Medicine, 9*, 79–83.

Zhang, Y. H., & Rose, K. (1999). *Who can ride the dragon?* Brookline, MA: Paradigm.

Zhou, J., Li, Z., & Jin, P. (1999). A clinical study on acupuncture for prevention and treatment of toxic side effects during radiotherapy and chemotherapy. *Journal of Traditional Chinese Medicine, 19*, 16–21.

# Ayurvedic Medicine

**Marc S. Micozzi**

A yurveda, the traditional medicine of India, offers several modalities that may be helpful in cancer prevention and cancer care. These modalities include Transcendental Meditation (TM; through postulated effects on reducing cancer-causing free radicals), Ayurvedic modulation of physiologic processes such as digestion, and the use of complex herbal preparations, called *rasayanas*, among other techniques.

## Free Radicals, Cancer, and Transcendental Meditation

The use of TM in anxiety reduction may have broader health implications. Effects of TM on free radicals and cancer have also emerged in various studies.

Many think of oxygen as the most benign element imaginable, but in fact it has a dark side. Various metabolic processes create highly reactive forms of oxygen and other molecules; these are known as free radicals. These unstable molecules damage other molecules. Although free radicals serve as part of our defense against invading pathogens, they also can cause extensive injury to cells, including DNA, and lead to the development of cancer.

Free-radical damage has been implicated in up to 80% of all human disease, including cancer. More generally, free radicals may cause much of the general deterioration of mind and body associated with aging.

Researchers have identified a number of factors that generate excess free radicals, including mental stress, pollution, excessive sun exposure, overexertion, radiation, chemotherapy, and ingestion of alcohol, tobacco, meat, and smoked, barbecued, or processed foods. Many of these are also regarded as cancer risk factors. Reducing these factors may reduce the level of free radicals, also called oxidants, and thus reduce cancer. Because Transcendental Meditation is effective in reducing stress, it might be expected to influence free radical generation through various mechanisms.

The term *stress* refers not only to environmental challenges but also how the body reacts to them. The stress syndrome, or fight-or-flight response, was designed to deal with prehistoric emergencies, which were of short duration and called for quick reactions. It serves us poorly in the postindustrial age, where most of our emergencies are slow-burn aggravations and anxieties—traffic jams or irate bosses who plague day-to-day existence. The body reacts to these with neurochemical overkill. And many of the specific processes involved—the generation of cortisol and other stress-related chemicals and even the basic increase in energy involved in the stress response—greatly increase free-radical production. In a variety of ways, stress causes the body to produce its own toxic substances, free radicals.

Transcendental Meditation, with its ability to counter stress, reduces free-radical production. A study done by Sharma at Ohio State, with Schneider and other collaborators at Maharishi University of Management, compared elderly long-term meditators to age-matched controls. The researchers examined lipid peroxides, which are cellular constituents that have been damaged by free radicals, and in turn can cause a great deal of damage of their own. They are used to assess free-radical levels, because it is assumed that if lipid peroxide levels are high (the result of free radical damage to lipids), free-radical levels must be high. TM meditators showed significantly lower levels of lipid peroxides. Those between ages 60 and 69 showed 14.5% lower levels, and those between ages 70 and 79 showed 16.5% lower. This magnitude of reduction is significant. A certain level of free radicals is necessary for the body's self-defense, and the body's own antioxidant and repair mechanisms can handle excess free radicals up to a certain point.

A number of studies, using different approaches, have found TM to influence processes associated with cancer and aging. The first study on this topic was done by Wallace et al. (1982), a pioneer of meditation research. He used the Adult Growth Examination, a test derived in part from the United States National Health Survey, standardized using a carefully selected representative cross-sample of several thousand adults, and validated in various studies in North America. The examination measures basic functions—including near-point vision, auditory discrimination, and blood pressure—that typically decline with age. This test helped lead to the concept of biological age as distinct from chronological age. Biologic age measures age in terms of physical function; chronologic age measurers age in terms of years. George Bernard Shaw died at the age of 94 as the result of injuries sustained when he fell from a tree he was pruning. He probably had a biologic age much younger than his chronologic age up until his final days.

Dr Wallace applied the test to 73 people between the ages of 40 and 64 who practice TM. His study statistically controlled for the effects of diet and exercise. As compared to normal values established over many years, those who had practiced TM for up to 5 years had an average biological age 5 years younger than their chronological age. Those who had meditated for more than 5 years had an average biological age 12 years younger.

Wallace's findings have since been corroborated by other studies. In a study published in the *Journal of Behavioral Medicine*, Glaser et al. (1992) looked at hormonal markers of aging, such as a reduction in hormone secretion. Richard Cutler has theorized that reduced hormonal secretions may be because of cell dysdifferentiation (cells "forget" what they are specialized to do and behave in a more general manner) and that this is caused by free-radical damage. A similar process occurs with carcinogens (Cutler, 1985).

Glaser tested this theory by looking at one of the body's most significant hormones—dehydroepiandrosterone sulfate (DHEA-S). In a young adult, DHEA-S is the most abundant hormone in the body, but the levels decline rapidly with age. Men who maintain relatively high levels of DHEA-S have been shown to have less atherosclerosis and heart disease and lower mortality rate from all causes. Women with high levels of DHEA-S are known to have less breast cancer and osteoporosis. Whereas the stress hormone cortisol leads to the breakdown of muscle (to provide fuel for energy), DHEA-S leads to the buildup of muscle tissue. Influenced by DHEA-S, the body continues to build, instead of wasting.

The study compared DHEA-S levels in the blood of 423 people who practiced TM to the levels of 1,253 who did not. The ages ranged from 20 to 81 years. Results were gathered in 5-year age ranges. The effects of diet, obesity, and exercise were statistically ruled out. The results were consistent with Wallace's study. Depending on the age range, people who practiced Transcendental Meditation had levels of DHEA-S that were as high as members of the control group who were 5 to 10 years younger (Glaser et al., 1992).

Also relevant is the finding that TM practitioners had a significantly lower blood erythrocyte sedimentation rate (ESR) than matched controls—which included a large group of vegetarian monks and nuns practicing a meditative lifestyle and a group of Seventh-Day Adventists. ESR rates are correlated with aging and premature mortality.

Another corroboration of Wallace's study came from a Harvard University study of 77 elderly nursing home residents. This study, conducted by psychologists Alexander and Langer, compared three types of meditation and relaxation techniques—TM, mindfulness training, and mental relaxation, a meditation technique loosely modeled on TM. The study, which lasted 3 years altogether, showed that residents in the TM group had the greatest reductions in stress. The TM group also had a significantly higher survival rate: they were the only group in which no one died during the study, although the average mortality rate in nonparticipating residents during those 3 years was more than one-third (Alexander, Langer, Davies, Chandler, & Newman, 1989).

Some years later, the researchers did a follow-up study of the above groups and found that the results held. After 8 years, the TM group's mean survival time was 65% higher than that of the other groups combined; after 15 years, it was 22% higher. Mortality showed a similar pattern: the TM group had distinct decreases compared to the other groups.

# Clinical Results

Studies on specific cancer and other health risk factors—such as cholesterol, cardiovascular disease, and smoking—have shown TM to have significant benefits.

Transcendental Meditation is known to reduce the cancer risk factors of smoking and alcohol as well as other types of substance abuse. A special 1994 double issue of *Alcoholism Treatment Quarterly* contained 17 articles on the effectiveness of TM in this

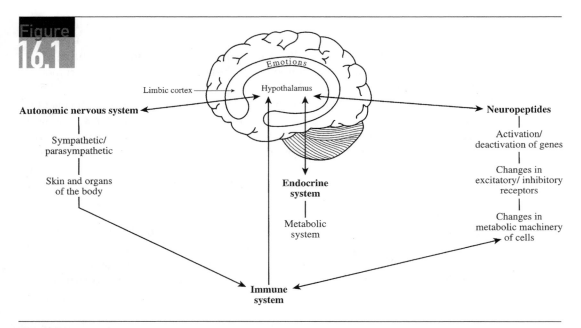

Figure
16.1

The limbic system.

area. One article was a meta-analysis of 19 studies on TM and substance abuse. Among those studies that looked at TM and substance abuse in the general population, this meta-analysis found the effect size for the TM groups to be 0.42 for alcohol and 0.74 for drug abuse (note that an effect size of 0.20 is considered small, one of 0.50 is medium, and one of 0.80 is large). In populations being treated for substance abuse, the effect size for TM was greater: 1.35 for alcohol and 1.16 for illicit drugs. To get a sense of how significant these numbers are, note that a meta-analysis of the popular DARE (Drug Abuse Resistance Education) program, which is used in high schools around the country, found an effect size of only 0.06. A meta-analysis also looked at 143 adolescent drug prevention programs and found their average effect size to be only 0.17 for alcohol and 0.21 for drugs.

TM, which is said to produce a "fourth state" of consciousness, reduces stress and anxiety more effectively than any other techniques tested to date. Many researchers feel that meditation is simply relaxation, but the data indicate that a fourth state of consciousness reduces anxiety two to four times better than physical relaxation techniques. Similarly, the TM group in the Alexander and Langer experiment with the elderly had the highest survival rate of three groups doing meditation techniques, and the greatest reduction of stress.

Ayurvedic practitioners recommend TM as an adjunct to whatever other measures they prescribe. TM is not all one would prescribe in every case and is not necessarily what is needed to cure a specific complaint, but is recommended as a general health measure, both in the preventive and the care stages. The possible influences of transcendental meditation on the limbic system of the brain are shown by the connections illustrated in Figure 16.1.

# Diet and Digestion

Another important factor in Ayurveda is a substance called *ojas*. *Ojas* is the end product of perfect digestion and metabolism, but it has a more profound status. It is also said to stand as a "lamp at the door" between consciousness and matter, connecting them and thus ensuring that the sequence of natural law is expressed properly in the body. It is also said to nourish and sustain the various tissues of the body.

*Ojas* is said to pervade the body. According to Charaka, when the quantity of *ojas* diminishes too much, life itself is threatened (*Charaka Samhita, Sutrasthana*, XVII, 74). When *ojas* is present in abundance, it gives strength, immunity, contentment, and good digestion. It is said to be the most important biochemical substance mediating the influence of consciousness on the body.

All Ayurvedic treatment is designed to increase aspects considered central to avoid reducing *ojas*; both aspects are considered central to restoring health and to preventing cancer and other illness.

Factors said to increase *ojas*, and that are to be maximized, include the following:

- Consciousness. The main factor determining *ojas* production is one's level of consciousness. As the inner Self becomes more and more "awake," one result is said to be that more *ojas* is spontaneously produced. This may in part reflect the principle that growing to enlightenment means growing in inner happiness. Happiness is the most effective means of producing *ojas*.
- Good digestion and balanced diet. MAV (Maharishi Ayur Veda) advise a diet aimed to improve *ojas* production, for *ojas* is held to be the end product of perfect digestion and metabolism.

Two additional points are relevant. The first is that some foods directly increase *ojas*, whereas others decrease it. Charaka describes the qualities of *ojas* and says that foods with those qualities, such as milk, ghee, and rice, increase *ojas*. Foods with the opposite qualities, such as alcohol, decrease the amount and quality of *ojas*. The second point is that for *ojas* production what is important is not only *what* one eats but also *how* one prepares and eats. Food taken in an atmosphere of warmth, uplift, and congeniality increase *ojas*. This reflects the factors said to increase *ojas*:

- Positivity in feelings, speech, and behavior. Love, joy, and appreciation produce more *ojas* and, therefore, better immunity. This ties in well with current findings in mind/body medicine, relative to cancer, and may provide a way of understanding such findings.
- *Panchakarma*, or Ayurvedic purification therapy, which removes impurities from the *shrotas*, the physiological channels in the body. This is said to improve the cells' ability to take up and receive *ojas*, thus helping rejuvenate the body.
- *Rasayanas*, special Ayurvedic herbal and mineral substances. *Rasayanas* have been defined as "that which causes ojas to be produced all over."

Factors that diminish *ojas*, and that should be avoided, are as follows:

- Negative emotions
- Stress
- Hurrying
- *Excessive* exercise (the right amount of exercise varies for different individuals. The weak feeling one gets from too much exercise is said to reflect, in part, the reduction of *ojas*)
- Fasting (moderate fasting is sometimes used in special supervised situations in Ayurveda, but excess fasting can weaken the body by emaciating the bodily tissues and reducing the *ojas* that nourishes them)
- Rough or very light diet
- Overexposure to wind and sun
- Staying awake through much of the night
- Excessive loss of bodily fluids (such as blood)
- Overindulgence in sexual activity
- Injury or trauma to the body
- Alcoholic beverages

*Ojas* is a substance said to have a profound influence on the quality of mental and emotional life as well as physical health. This emphasis is in line with recent understandings of the biochemical meditation of emotion and its effect on the body.

The limbic area of the brain (the physiological seat of emotions), which correlates with deep emotional states, surrounds the hypothalamus, which has often been called the "brain's brain" and is the body's central regulatory switchboard. The hypothalamus regulates temperature, thirst, hunger, blood sugar levels, growth, sleeping, and waking, and emotions such as anger and happiness. Situated just below the hypothalamus is the pituitary gland, the body's master gland, which emits secretions that control the activity of many other glands in the body. Taken together, these three elements—the limbic area, hypothalamus, and pituitary—form the limbic system, which alters with every alteration in emotions, creating a new mix of molecules that transform the functioning of the body.

The hypothalamus is affected by stimuli from a number of sources: the five senses, the immune system, cognitive information, and, above all, emotion. Stimuli coming from the limbic region of the brain cause the hypothalamus to release a wide variety of neuropeptides. These neuropeptides, in turn, stimulate specific hormones from the pituitary gland, and this specific activity in all endocrine glands, including the thymus and adrenal glands. This new combination of chemical messengers changes the operation and makeup of the body, especially the metabolic system and the immune system.

Through the action of the limbic system, particular psychological and emotional states take on molecular form. When you watch an action movie, you may begin to feel a nervous stomach and sweaty palms. Specific chemical messengers have been released. The body has been changed by what it is seeing on the screen. The emotions raised by the movie correlate with activity in the limbic system.

In this sense, the body "metabolizes" the emotional content of every experience it has. Happiness registering in the limbic region stimulates one cascade of chemicals from the hypothalamus and pituitary, with corresponding physiological changes everywhere in the body. Sadness creates another cascade and in turn another physiology.

The hypothalamus can also communicate with the body directly. It modulates the activity of the autonomic nervous system. Neuropeptides produced by the hypothalamus act on the pituitary and other areas. In fact, there are receptors for them on cells throughout the body. An action movie can create a nervous stomach because the digestive tract has receptors for stress/response neuropeptides.

More significantly, these receptors have been found on immune system lymphocytes (fast-reacting immune system cells) throughout the body. Apparently, lymphocytes can tune in to the molecular messages created by thought and feelings. Moreover, chemicals created by the lymphocytes, such as interleukins, have receptors in the hypothalamic region of the brain. Thus, chemical messages from the immune system can modulate nervous system functioning and mental states. There is a two-way communication network between the brain and the immune system. A growing body of data also suggest that neurotransmitters produced by the autonomic nervous system can communicate directly with the immune system and modify its functioning. Is there a more broad analogy between modern findings regarding neuroimmunomodulators and the Ayurveda? One hypothesis is that *ojas* might be equivalent to neuropeptides from the hypothalamus, which has identical effects as described.

We previously discussed TM in terms of stress reduction, brain-wave coherence, free radicals transcendental experience of the unified field. Transcendental Meditation also can be said to have an influence through the limbic system. Instead of metabolizing "stress," the limbic system during TM metabolizes "peace and contentment." This would lead to a better character of neurochemical influence throughout the body, thus producing better health and lower cancer risk.

# Behavioral Rasayanas

Another effect of mind on health is through behavioral *rasayanas*. *Rasayana* is a term for substances that strengthen immunity. But using it to describe certain behavioral patterns seems insightful. It now is clear that the body has its own internal "pharmacological laboratory" in the hypothalamus, pituitary, and so on—which also produce substances that influence immune strength. Neuropeptides affect the whole body: negative emotions such as anger, hate, or fear release a rush of neurochemicals that strain and damage the organs; positive emotions such as love, laughter, and appreciation release health-promoting chemicals. Laughter, for example, reduces levels of such stress hormones as cortisol and epinephrine and increases the activity of immune cells, such as T cells, natural killer cells, and antibodies. A positive mental state correlates with increased survival time for some patients with AIDS and cancer. Severe mental depression, by contrast, has been shown to result in suppression or even loss of immune system functioning.

The behavioral *rasayanas* deal with the mind's influence on the body in a systematic sway: they prescribe behaviors that elicit health-promoting biochemical effects. These are valuable both for prevention and as adjuncts to treatments. They include such traditional virtues as moderation and respect for teachers and elders and emotions such as love and compassion. They exclude such emotions and moods as anger, negativity, and violence, which are said to damage health. One result of practicing the behavioral *rasayanas* is that the limbic system is metabolizing positive emotions far more often and negative ones far less so.

Specific behavioral *rasayanas* are mentioned in the *Charaka Samhita* and other classical Ayurvedic sources. These are traditional teachings in many cultures and reflects the insight of long-lived traditions into the principles upholding human health.

One of the behavior *rasayanas* listed in the Charaka is: "knowing the measure of time and place with propriety." This refers to, among other things, what we now call chronobiology, the study of daily and annual physiological cycles.

## Bedside Manner

Another effect of the mind on health is through what medicine has traditionally called bedside manner. Family doctors were once known for their warm and reassuring bedside manner and every good physician knew that if patients felt comforted and encouraged they would do better. Until recently, however, family doctors have been a disappearing species, and fear of a malpractice suit had led doctors to reverse their style: to tell their patients of every conceivable catastrophe their symptoms might lead to, lest they be accused of incompetence. Ayurveda encourages physicians to resist such pressures: although it is important for the patient to be informed, one should also remember that too much directness can destroy a patient's sense of well-being.

## Active Ingredients, Free Radicals, and Herbal Medicines

Traditional herbal medicines provide another source of substances active against free radicals. Like humans, plants need to protect themselves against toxins and pathogens, which come from both within and without. Like human bodies, plants produce chemicals for that purpose. Not surprisingly, these chemicals can benefit human bodies as well—a fact well-known to both Western and Ayurvedic pharmacology. Ayurvedic pharmacology (called *dravyaguna*) differs from modern pharmacology in a crucial way. *Dravyaguna* uses plants (or plant parts) as they occurred in nature, with all their ingredients, whereas Western pharmacology isolates active ingredients from plants and then (usually) synthesizes them.

A majority of Western medications have been derived, in this way, from natural substances. For example, Western researchers derived acetylsalicylic acid from the pain remedy willow bark and the antihypertensive/antipsychotic drug reserpine from *Rauwolfia serpentina*, an herb prescribed in ancient Ayurvedic texts for mental disorders. Medical science tends to assume that the replacement of natural herbs with synthetic active ingredients is unambiguous progress.

However, the active ingredient approach compromises whatever synergies exist among organic components, which can be significant. Also, many apparently inactive ingredients have turned out to play significant health-giving roles. For example, the medical value of bioflavonoids (a class of molecules found in plants) was often dismissed by early researchers, especially those who favored synthetic vitamins, which they saw as the plants' active ingredients. But many bioflavonoids have since been found to have significant benefits. They act as antioxidant, anti-inflammatory, antiallergic, antitumor, antiulcerogenic, and hepatoprotective agents. What other valuable compounds remain, as yet unidentified, in plants?

Finally, the active ingredient approach relates to the issue of side effects. Western pharmaceuticals frequently create unwanted side effects, sometimes serious. Active ingredients act not only at the site intended but also at other sites and organs; one reason why toxicity may arise. With whole herbs, inactive ingredients are thought to help control the effects at nontarget sites.

This chapter reviews the research that has emerged on certain herbal formulations, and their effect on free-radical formation.

# Herbal Formulations as Anticancer Agents

A decade ago it might have seemed unreasonable to suggest that cataracts, rheumatoid arthritis, and strokes may all have a basic source of damage in common or that the etiology of cancer, heart disease, and dandruff may share a common mechanism. But now the evidence for this unified understanding is growing. For much of aging, cancer, and other diseases the common link is the molecules known as free radicals.

Some regard discovery of the medical role of free radicals as being as big an advance as Pasteur's theory of infectious disease. In a sense, free radicals take medical theory one step deeper. Pasteur's discovery involved microorganisms and cells, whereas free radicals involve a more fundamental level—the subatomic realm of electrons.

Free radicals are molecules, usually of oxygen, that have lost an electron. This makes them unstable (in chemical terms, *reactive*). They begin to powerfully covet their neighboring molecules' electrons. In stealing an electron, they can attack DNA, leading to dysfunction, mutation, and cancer. They can attack enzymes and proteins, disrupting normal cell activities. They can attack cell membranes, producing a chain reaction of destruction. Such membrane damage in the cells that line blood vessels can lead to hardening and thickening of the arteries and may eventually lead to heart attack and strokes. Free-radical attacks on the protein in collagen can cause cross-linking of protein molecules and resulting stiffness in the tissue.

The most dangerous free radicals are the small, mobile, and highly reactive oxy radicals. Other dangerous atomic and molecular varieties of oxygen are known as reactive oxygen species (ROS). These are not technically free radicals, but they are nonetheless unstable and highly reactive with the molecules around them. Research is demonstrating that oxidative stress—the constant attack by oxy radicals and reactive oxygen species—is important in both the initiation and promotion stages of cancer. They help cause the disease in the first place and then add impetus to its spread in the body.

It now appears that the clinical presentation of different diseases—the way the illness appears when a patient comes to the clinic—may not be because of different causal mechanisms but because of variations in the protection provided by the body's antioxidant defenses. Under oxidative stress, the weakest link in the body may give way.

The list of diseases now linked to oxy radicaSl and ROS is long:

- Cancer
- Arteriosclerosis, atherosclerosis
- Heart disease
- Cerebrovascular disease
- Stroke
- Emphysema
- Diabetes mellitus
- Rheumatoid arthritis
- Osteoporosis
- Ulcers
- Sunburn
- Cataracts
- Crohn's disease
- Bechet's disease
- Senility
- Aging

The onslaught of free radicals and ROS also contribute to many of the less serious but still troubling symptoms of aging: not only wrinkled and nonresilient skin but also gray hair, balding, and bodily stiffness. Oxy radicals and ROS have been linked to such minor but bothersome conditions as dandruff and hangovers. The Japanese biochemist Yukie Niwa estimates that a least 85% of chronic and degenerative diseases are the result of oxidative damage.

Despite the lengthy list of problems they cause, free radicals are not all bad. They have vital roles to play in a healthy human body. First, certain types of free radicals are inevitably produced by many chemical reactions that occur in the body. The body can, however, usually keep control over the free radicals that typically result. Second, the body attempts to harness the destructive power of the most dangerous free radicals—the small and highly reactive oxy radicals and ROS—for use in the immune system and inflammatory reactions. Certain cells in these systems engulf bacteria or viruses, taking up oxygen molecules from the bloodstream, creating a flood of oxy radicals and ROS by removing an electron and bombarding the invader with this toxic shower. To an impressive degree, this aggressive use of toxic oxygen species succeeds in protecting the body against infectious organisms.

Unfortunately, the process may go out of control, creating a destructive chain reaction that leads to overproduction of free radicals. Like other formation of free radicals, this can wreak havoc in the body.

Production of free radicals in the body is continuous. The energy-producing process in every cell generates oxy radicals and ROS as toxic waste, continuously and in abundance. Oxygen is used to burn glucose molecules that act as fuel. In this energy-freeing operation, oxy radical are thrown off as destructive by-products. Given the insatiable electron hunger of oxygen, there is no way to have it suffusing the body's energy-producing processes without the constant creation of oxy radicals and ROS.

The cell has a complex structure and function, including a number of metabolic processes. Each of these can produce different free radicals. Thus, even a single cell can produce many different kinds of free radicals. Immune system cells create oxy radicals and ROS deliberately, as weapons.

We are also constantly exposed to external substances that generate free radicals in the body. The food most of us buy and eat contains farm chemicals, including fertilizers and pesticides that, when we ingest the food, produce free radicals as by-products. The same is true for many prescription drugs; side effects may be created by free radicals they generate. Processed foods frequently contain high levels of lipid peroxides, which produce free radicals that damage the cardiovascular system. Cigarette smoke generates high free-radical concentrations; much lung damage associated with smoking is caused by free radicals. The same is true of environmental pollution. Alcohol is a particularly potent free radical generator. In addition, all types of electromagnetic radiation can cause free radicals—including sunlight. When sunlight hits the skin, it generates free radicals that then age the skin, causing roughness and wrinkles. If the exposure is severe and prolonged, skin cancer may be one result.

The fast pace of modern life is also a recipe for free radicals. The constant time pressure experienced by most people in industrialized countries causes them to experience high levels of stress. And the stress response in the body creates free radicals in abundance. It races the body's energy-creating apparatus, increasing the number of free radicals created as toxic waste. Moreover, hormones that mediate the stress reaction in the body—cortisol and catecholamines—themselves degenerate into particularly destructive free radicals. Researchers now know one way in which stress may cause disease. A stressful life produces free radicals.

## Free-Radical Defenses

Given the many sources of free radicals, all aerobic forms of life maintain elaborate anti-free-radical defense systems also known as antioxidant systems (Sharma, 2002). Every cell in the body creates its own "bomb squad"—antioxidant enzymes (complex, machinelike proteins) whose particular job it is to defuse oxy radicals and ROS. One of the most destructive free radicals, for example, is superoxide. The most thoroughly studied defense enzyme, known as superoxide dismutase (SOD), takes hold of superoxide molecules and changes them to much less reactive forms. SOD and other important antioxidant enzymes, the glutathione system, work within the cell. By contrast, circulating biochemicals such as uric acid and ceruloplasmin react with free radicals in the intercellular spaces and bloodstream.

As a second tier, the body makes use of many standard vitamins and other nutrients, including vitamins C and E, beta-carotene, bioflavanoids, and many others, to quench the oxy radicals' thirst for electrons. Many free-radical researchers feel that to quench free radicals effectively the general levels of all these free radical-fighting nutrients need to be much higher than nutritional experts previously thought. This demonstrates how the substances that plants create to fight free radicals can help the human body do the same things.

In addition to using enzymes and nutrients for direct attacks on oxy radicals, the body also has a rapid and thorough system to repair and/or replace damaged building blocks of the cell. For example, the system for repairing damage to DNA and other nucleic acids is particularly elaborate and efficient, involving separate specific enzymes that first locate damaged areas and then snip out ruined bits, replace them with the correct sequences of molecules, and seal up the strand once again. Every aspect of the cell is given similar attention. Most protein constituents in the cell, for example, are completely replaced every few days. Scavenger enzymes break used and damaged proteins into their components parts for reuse by the cell.

# Finding Balance

The body's elaborate biochemical responses to the free radical challenges suggest that it is not necessary to reduce excess free radicals to zero. The body need strike a proper balance between the number of free radicals generated and the defense and repair mechanisms available. The goal is to keep oxidative stress below the level at which normal repair and replacement can maintain 100% cell efficacy. Oxy radicals might slip through the enzyme and nutrient defenses to attack the DNA, for instance. But ideally these attacks would be few enough that the DNA repair mechanisms could fix the damage and maintain the genetic code intact.

How to keep that balance? This is a major topic of research; the results of the above approaches have been mixed. Beta-carotene supplementation to date has had no effect in reducing malignant neoplasms, cardiovascular disease, or death from all causes. One problem may be that active ingredients such as beta-carotene are not "full spectrum" antioxidants: they affect certain free radicals and not others (and each cell can produce a wide variety of free radicals). Two recent studies also suggest that there is another problem. Beta-carotene and vitamin E were found not to prevent lung cancer in male smokers; in fact, beta-carotene was linked with *higher* incidence of lung cancer. Beta-carotene and vitamin A supplements, too, were found to increase risk of lung cancer in smokers and workers expose to asbestos and to have no offsetting benefits. A reason for the harmful effects may be that the vitamins, after quenching free radicals, become oxidized themselves unless they have been given in correct doses or regenerated by additional antioxidants, which must be in proper doses themselves. Beta-carotene, moreover, works as an antioxidant only when oxygen concentrations are low; in high oxygen concentrations, such as those found in the lungs or heart, it becomes an oxidant itself. In addition, large amounts of any one micronutrient may inhibit absorption of other micronutrients needed for proper nutritional balance.

Such problems might be offset if vitamins were taken in their natural condition, surrounded by dozens of apparently inactive ingredients that modulate their effects. This conclusion is suggested by a study that found vitamin E to have no effect in reducing death from coronary heart disease in postmenopausal women when taken in the form of supplements but to have significant benefits when absorbed from food (see Chapter 10).

Even if these problems with vitamin supplements were solved a formidable one remains: the body's natural enzymes are molecule for molecule, much more effective. When a molecule of vitamin C or E sacrifices an electron to appease a free radical, the vitamin molecule becomes damaged and useless. It can reenter the fray only if it is regenerated by a helpful companion. Enzymes, however, can run through thousands of destructive free radicals and ROS without help and without pause.

Yet although internally produced enzymes are far more powerful than vitamins, they cannot be taken by mouth. They are gigantic protein molecules that cannot pass through the walls of the digestive system and into the bloodstream. Digestive juices break them down into their component amino acids. Although SOD has been given by injection directly into inflamed joints, this is not practical for all-purpose home use. This is particularly so because SOD has only a brief half-life in the bloodstream: in less than 5 minutes, 50% of it is gone, broken down by natural bodily processes, and within an hour only 0.1% of it is left. Recently, the Japanese researcher Tatsuya Oda found a way around this: He succeeded in attaching SOD to artificial polymer molecules. Riding on the polymers, the SOD lasts in the bloodstream for at least 5 hours. But this raises questions about the long-term effects of adding an enzyme to the body in large quantities; these are not known as yet, and the question is far from trivial.

In an ideal world, we would find antioxidant substances with (1) low molecular weight, so they can pass from the digestive tract to the bloodstream undamaged; (2) the anti-free-radical ability, weight for weight, of an enzyme like SOD; and (3) the ability to defuse a wide range of free radicals. It may sound too much to hope for. But, if found, such powerful antioxidants might tip the scales against free-radical damage decisively.

# Herbal Rasayanas

Powerful free radical scavengers that appear to fulfill the above criteria have been identified. These natural antioxidants scavenge superoxide as effectively as SOD. Weight for weight, they stop lipid peroxide chain reactions hundreds and even thousands of times better than antioxidant vitamins and a much-researched antioxidant drug. They are not active ingredients, not vitamin pills, but food supplements, and can be eaten and digested easily. As shown below, they combine natural plant products to create synergies, rather than isolating active ingredients.

Ayurvedic substances called *rasayanas* are herbal formulations that stimulate overall health. The term literally means "that which supports *rasa*." Rasa, as we've seen, is the first of the seven *dhatus*; it is equivalent to chyle and blood plasma and is said to nourish all the other bodily tissues. *Rasayanas* are also said to stimulate the production of *ojas*, the substance that sustains all the *dhatus*.

*Rasayanas* can be useful in treating specific illness, but most of them are intended to increase general immune strength (known in Ayurveda as *bala* or life force) and general health and well-being. *Rasayanas* are held to promote general health by increasing resistance to disease, activating tissue repair mechanisms, and arresting or reversing the deterioration associated with aging. According to Charaka, *rasayanas* promote "longevity, memory, intelligence, freedom from disorders, youthfulness, excellence of luster, complexion and voice, optimum strength of physique and sense organs. . . . "

Such claims can be seen to fit with what research has shown about *rasayanas* and their effects on free radicals. They are not artificial drugs isolated in a test tube but natural herbal mixtures from India's Vedic tradition that contain a rich variety of plant substances.

The recipes for these herbal formulations were first discovered thousands of years ago. As with much else in the ancient Vedic tradition, over the course of time knowledge of these herbal supplements was diffused. The herbal formulas were carefully maintained, however, guarded and handed down through generations by a small number of Ayurvedic *vaidyas*.

Balraj Maharshi, leading expert on *dravyaguna*, the identification and utilization of medicinal plants, made a specific suggestion. Many years earlier he had studies with a venerable *vaidya* who had passed on to him the ancient formula for *amrit kalash*— with the admonition that it should be revealed only when the time had come it could be widely used. After saving the formula for many years, Maharshi decided that *amrit kalash* now had the opportunity to be scientifically accepted. He shared the formula with other *vaidyas* to restore the mixture and its preparation to the ancient standards recorded in the classical Ayurvedic texts.

The results of this effort have been available in the West for several years in two separate formulations. One of these, MAK-4 (the herbal preparation Maharish Amrit Kalash, number 4), is an herbal concentrate; the other, MAK-5 is an herbal tablet. Between them they comprise more than 24 different herbs and fruits, each of which is composed of hundreds of substances. MAK-4's ingredients are as follows: *Terminalia chebula, Emblica officinalis, Cinnamomum zuylancium, Eletaria cardamomum, Cyperus rotundus, Curcuma longa, Piper longum, Santalum album,* and *Glycyrrhiza glabra.* These are processed in an extract of *Eragrostis cynosuroides, Premna integrifolia, Desmondium gangeticum, Phaseolus trilobus, Teramnus labialis, Aegle marmelos, Oroxylum indicum, Ipomoea digitata,* and many other herbs.

MAK-5's main ingredients are as follows: *Withania somnifera, Glycyrrhiza glabra, Ipomoea digitata, Asparagus adscendens, Emblica officinalis, Tinosporaa cordifolia, Asparagus racemous, Vitex trifolia, Argyreia speciosa, Curculigo orchioides,* and *Capparis aphylla.*

Preparing the *rasayanas* involves many subtleties. For example, plant chronobiology—choosing the optimum time to harvest an herb—is vital because the presence and levels of phytochemicals (such as bioflavonoids) differ at different times of the year. Further, Ayurvedic herbs were traditionally prepared through a long and careful process of grinding. The goal was to reduce each component of a formula to the finest possible powder, and no effort was spared to reach this highly refined stage. Modern research suggests an explanation for this method of preparation. In complex natural products, many of the important components are tangled together and inassimilable, and the grinding process apparently works to enhance their digestibility.

This whole process of formulation and preparation is unfamiliar to Western scientists, who are used not to taking whole flowers, plants, and roots and grinding them down into an unanalyzable potpourri of various substances but rather to seeking a single active ingredient. They are also accustomed to the protocols of objective investigation—taking isolated substances made of identical molecules, testing them in the laboratory, putting them through human clinical trials, and finally prescribing them as cures for specific diseases.

The ancient herbal food supplements are completely different from modern drugs. They are compilations of intact plants or parts of plants and comprise a profusion of components, a rich stew of molecules intended to enrich the human physiology in it entirety. There is no attempt to isolate individual molecules. Moreover, these formulations are not drugs, but rich herbal foods said to produce overall health and well-being. Although there have been thousands of years of clinical observations and systematic use by Vedic doctors in their practices—there has not been (until recently) the type of lab work and systematic experimentation typical of modern medicine. Nevertheless, recent scientific experiments have shown these formulas to be effective and to have virtually no side effects.

Ayurvedic *vaidyas* assert that the effectiveness of these herbal formulations comes precisely from the richness of their mixtures. They are a deliberate attempt to maximize synergism: the components help each other move through the digestive system, arrive at the correct cells, penetrate the cell membrane, and achieve intracellular effects.

# Synergism

Recent research on vitamins and bioflavonoids had identified simple synergistic effects; for example, *combinations* of antioxidants may do more to stop oxidation damage and cancer cell growth than would the sum effect of the same substances acting alone. One reason suggested is that the sequence of natural complex plant products sets up a cascade effect, which counters the damaging cascades set up among free radicals. But such cascades may well represent just a narrow spectrum of the full range of synergies that plant compounds display.

Assertions about complex synergisms are essentially impossible to check through objective science. The concept of the isolated active ingredient sprang up largely because modern scientific investigation works best in that situation. It must use a fragmentary, reductionist approach. One aim of scientific investigation is to work on the simplest possible isolated systems.

This approach has a logical basis. With only one type of molecules to work with, a scientist can clearly show cause-and-effect relations. If you put one type of molecule into your beaker filled with fluid and the fluid turns from colorless to green, you know what caused the change. If you put in two types of molecules and the fluids turns green, you cannot be sure if it was one molecule or the other or a combination of both. The uncertainty increases exponentially as you add more ingredients. Thus, the objective, scientific approach to knowledge biases the investigators toward uncomplicated, isolated reductionist solutions.

Researchers long schooled in this approach feel uncomfortable when a complex formula such as MAK is shown to produce positive results, because they cannot identify the "ingredient" that causes the effect. Their objective training makes it difficult to think that it might be all the ingredients at once, working together. They know they will never be able to unravel such complication in the lab. And the tendency is to think that if you cannot examine it through reductionist experiment, then it is not significant.

Yet there is no logical reason why substances composed of a single molecular type should be more effective than a carefully chosen combination of ingredients. There is nothing untenable about the idea that a combination of ingredients may produce synergistic effects that enhance effectiveness and reduce side effects. In fact, this view seems to fit naturally with the inconceivably complex operation of the human body and the manner in which the body interacts with the natural environment. To use a musical analogy, the body is not a single instrument, hitting a single note. It is a symphony of thousands of different instruments (biochemicals) varying and combining to countless ways—all at once, all interactively. Just as individual notes produce a harmony with other notes, so every chemical reaction in a healthy body is functioning in harmony with every other reaction.

It seems reasonable that to move this entire symphony in a more harmonious direction, it would be effective to intervene with complex and holistic substances—with supplements that could affect the whole symphony at once. One need some way of knowing what the formula should be in the first place, and reductionist scientific investigation cannot provide that answer. But even if research cannot tease out complex synergistic mechanisms, it *can* assess overall results. The research evidence on Maharishi Amrit Kalash to date is wide ranging, showing marked antioxidant effects and a broad spectrum of specific benefits for specific disease.

# Free-Radical Scavenging Effects

The Niwa Institute in Japan has tested over 500 compounds for free-radical scavenging effects. Much of his research has focused on the excess inflammation often caused by the immune system.

To begin examination of Maharishi Amrit Kalash, Niwa conducted a chemical analysis of herbs in MAK-4 and MAK-5. These analyses revealed a mixture with in low-molecular-weight substances that are well-known antioxidants, including vitamin C, vitamin E, beta-carotene, polyphenols, bioflavonoids, and riboflavin.

Niwa then conducted experiment to measure MAK's antioxidant effect. His investigation involved the immune system's most rapidly reacting defense: the neutrophil. Once inflammation begins, immune system cells such as neutrophils overproduce free radicals and other ROS, causing extensive damage to healthy cells in the vicinity. Chemicals released by damaged cells encourage rapid transit by neutrophils and other immune cells to the inflammation site, quickly worsening the damage.

Niwa's study showed that, in the presence of MAK, this neutrophil "chemotaxis" slowed down significantly. In addition, the multiplication of lymphocytes in their most aggressive form (blastogenesis) was also tempered. He also identified the specific reason why MAK-5 and MAK-5 had this tempering effect on the mechanism of inflammation. Both of them markedly scavenged the neutrophil leakage of their serious free radicals known as superoxide, hydrogen peroxide, and the hydroxy radical. According to Niwa, MAK scavenged free radicals more effectively than any substance he had tested previously.

Fields and colleagues at Loyola University Medical School in Chicago followed Niwa's work. They focused on superoxide because it is the "master radical"—the first produced and precursor of both hydrogen peroxide and the hydroxy radical. Fields' group compared MAK with SOD, the enzyme designed specifically to scavenge superoxide. Human immune system cells (neutrophils) were stimulated to create superoxide, as if to kill an invader. MAK and SOD were used to scavenge the superoxide.

The results showed that both MAK and SOD, separately, were able to scavenge completely the superoxide molecules. MAK proved as potent as SOD. Because MAK has so many components, Fields and his colleagues conducted tests to make sure that, in defusing the superoxide, MAK had not damaged the neutrophils themselves. Results showed the neutrophils still healthy and functioning normally.

The implications were significant. First, the tests indicated that MAK can reduce the random damage caused by neutrophils as they fight invaders. Second, if MAK scavenged superoxide as effectively as the body's own enzyme (SOD), its anti-free-radical effectiveness clearly deserved serious attention.

Further experiments reaffirmed MAK's ability to scavenge superoxide. Also, a separate study by Dr Chandradhar Dwivedi and coworkers at South Dakota State University showed that MAK-4 and MAK-5 were able to scavenge other dangerous molecules: lipid peroxides (Dwivedi, Sharma, Dobrowski, & Engineer, 1991).

Sharma and other researchers at Ohio State University College of Medicine designed and executed another systematic test of MAK, directly comparing MAK-4 and -5 with three individual antioxidants—vitamins C, vitamin E, and the well-researched drug probucol (Sharma et al., 1990; Sharma, Guenther, Abu-Ghazaley, & Dwiviedi, 1994; Sharma, Hanna, Kauffman, & Newman, 1992, 1995).

Sharma et al. (1992) tested a third oxidant, low-density lipoprotein (LDL), which had been oxidatively damaged by free radical attack. LDL is known as the "bad" cholesterol, not owing to its natural state, which is benign, but to its transformed state after free-radical attack. Oxidized LDL (LDL-ox) is capable of causing extensive damage, which is central to the process that scars, thickens, and stiffens arterial walls, narrowing the artery passageway and attracting platelets that can aggregate into clots and block the artery entirely. The research indicated that if LDL-ox could be scavenged effectively, cardiovascular disease could be markedly reduced. Lipophil-mediated reduction of toxidants can be effected by Ayurvedic detoxification procedures (Herron & Fagan, 2002).

Vitamins C and E, probucol, and MAK all prevented the radicalization of LDL. All stopped the ongoing free-radical chain reactions. But the difference in potency was startling. Weight for weight, the aqueous extracts of MAK were several hundred times more potent than vitamins C and E and probucol.

The same study also tested two other MAV herbal formulas. MA-631 is described as similar in purpose to the MAK formulas; Maharishi Coffee Substitute is an herbal beverage. Each scavenged LDL-ox radicals with a relative effectiveness that was close to that of MAK.

The above research indicates that there is now an effective means to protect LDL against free radical attack. If this is true, it means there are natural food supplements that may help keep arteries clear and work adjunctively to prevent cancer, heart disease, stroke, and other disease.

These findings are consistent with a large body of research. Nearly 40 studies have been done on MAK worldwide, research conducted by at least 50 investigators representing a broad range of universities and independent research institutions. These studies have painted a consistent picture.

If MAK is an effective free radical scavenger, it should enhance health in a significant way. Laboratory and animals studies and human trials have given evidence that MAK's antioxidant effects translate into specific benefits for cancer and other diseases. The details give a picture of the possibilities available from synergistic free radical management.

# Enhancing Immunity

A sound immune system is vital to continued health and is thought to help protect against cancer. For this reason, a number of studies have focused on immune function. Both MAK-4 and MAK-5 increase the responsiveness of lymphocytes and MAK-5 increases the responsiveness of macrophages. Both results can be understood in terms of reduced free-radical damage.

Researchers at the University of Kansas Medical Center collaborated with the Indiana University School of Medicine and Ohio State University to conduct a study on the immune system in laboratory animals. (Sharma et al., 2002) Under laboratory conditions, animals fed MAK-5 produced 32%–88% more lymphocytes than the control animals. This capacity for increased lymphocyte generation persisted for 15 days after MAK was removed from the diet.

Two subsequent studies revealed further immunity-enhancing properties of MAK-5, as well as of MAK-4 (Sharma et al., 2002). A follow-up study by the researchers at the University of Kansas Medical Center showed that lymphocytes from mice fed MAK-5 proliferated significantly more than those from mice that were not fed MAK-5. A study by researchers at Gifu University School of Medicine in Japan showed that both MAK-4 and MAK-5 yielded significantly greater proliferation of lymphocytes from mice fed either MAK-4 or MAK-5. This indicates that MAK-4 and MAK-5 may increase the responsiveness of the immune system.

The University of Kansas follow-up study also showed that macrophages from mice fed MAK-5 showed a significantly greater ability to destroy tumor cells when stimulated by two separate biochemical activators (Sharma et al., 2002). In addition, the production of nitric oxide was significantly higher in the activated macrophages from the mice fed MAK-5. Nitric oxide is considered an important mediator in the process used by macrophages to destroy both bacteria and cancer cells.

The effect of MAK-5 on the immune system was also indicated in a study on humans by the Maharishi Ayur-Veda Health Center in Lancaster, Massachusetts. Many common allergic reactions are caused by excessive immune system response. White blood cells react to, say, a particle of pollen as if it were a deadly invading bacteria. The damage sown by these reactions results in inflammation of the nasal passage (hay fever) or the lungs (asthma). To test the effectiveness of MAK-5 on this type of immune system overreaction, Glaser randomly assigned subjects to two groups. One received MAK-5 and the other a placebo pill. Over the next 4 weeks, during peak allergy season, the group receiving MAK-5 showed significantly fewer allergic symptoms (Sharma et al., 2002).

# Controlling Free-Radical Effects on the Immune System

MAK's effectiveness against free radicals can reasonably explain both the increased responsiveness of the immune system and the increased control of its tendency to overact. Immune system cells are uniquely subject to damage. When oxy radicals and ROS released by immune cells damage their own membranes, their functioning is compromised. Cell receptors are damaged, reducing the responsiveness of immune cells and the immune system as a whole. Loss of membrane fluidity and destruction of protein machinery embedded in the cell membrane also cause decreased ability of the immune cells to respond to a challenge. Thus, if free-radical damage can be significantly controlled, increased responsiveness by the immune system should result.

Free radicals may also cause the immune system to spiral out of control. In the inflammatory response, oxy radicals and ROS overact, and the damage feeds on itself by attracting more and more hyperexcited inflammatory cells. Antioxidants can temper this tendency to self-inflicted damage by rapidly scavenging the excess free radicals released by the neutrophils and other cells. The neutrophils, macrophages, and other immune cells can ingest and destroy toxic invaders without causing as much damage to their surroundings—and without attracting an excessive number of their cohorts.

The initial laboratory tests on MAK indicate the presence of both effects (Sharma et al., 2002). The immune system becomes more responsive and more controlled at the same time. This shows promise for the control of both external (infectious) and internal (degenerative and inflammatory) disease. With the rich variety of molecules in MAK, there may be other mechanisms also involved, including the mind/body effects mediated through the limbic system in the brain and other mechanisms. MAK's free radical mediating capabilities may be one explanation for these immune system findings.

# Cancer Prevention and Regression

Cancer may be tied to free-radical damage and thus has been another major area of MAK research. MAK has been observed to have certain antineoplastic properties.

## Prevention and Regression of Breast Cancer

The first cancer studies were on breast carcinoma, carried out as a joint project in laboratories at Ohio State University College of Medicine and South Dakota State University (Sharma et al. 2002).

Carcinogenesis is ordinarily thought of as a two-step process: (1) an apparently irreversible initiation stage, when alterations occur in the DNA of one or more cells, and (2) a promotion stage, in which the population of initiated cells expands. Free radicals are active in both of these phases (see Chapter 9).

The initiation phase may be related to chronic inflammation, an observation that has been made for many years. In chronic inflammation, white blood cells are constantly releasing showers of free radicals. The neutrophils and macrophages release superoxide and hydrogen peroxide in all directions, and both can enter nearby cells and travel to the cell nucleus to damage genetic material. Hydroxy radicals and acids released in intercellular spaces have the same effect indirectly. They attack cell membranes externally, giving rise to a chain reaction of radicalized lipids and the eventual production of aldehydes that can travel inward to the nucleus, where they cross-link DNA and its surrounding proteins.

As for the promotion phase, there is evidence that cancer cells generate free radicals and ROS that speed their metastasis or break through from a local area to distant sites. Cells isolated in the laboratory from various types of tumors have recently been shown to produce copious flows of hydrogen peroxide. There is also indirect evidence that cancerous cells still living in the body produce free radicals and ROS, and aggressive cancer cell populations show increased production of antioxidants, indicating free radicals.

In the first cancer experiment, laboratory animals were fed a diet supplemented with MAK-5. They were also exposed to a potent chemical inducer of breast cancer. An "initiation phase" group of animals received MAK-5 for 1 week before and 1 week after DMBA was administered. A "promotion" group received MAK-5 1 week after DMBA administration until the end of the experiment. After 18 weeks, only 25% of the animals receiving MAK-5 during the promotion phase showed tumors, as compared to 67% of the animals in the control group. However, there did not appear to be comparable protection during the initiation phase.

A second experiment with the same design used diet supplemented with MAK-4. The animals on MAK-4 suffered 60% fewer tumors in the initiation stage and 88% fewer tumors in the promotion phase as compared to controls. In addition, in both studies, control animals that had already developed fully formed tumors were given a MAK diet. In both studies the tumors shrank significantly in 60% of these animals. In roughly half of those with tumor regression, the tumor disappeared completely. The animals experiencing tumor regression were those that initially had tumors under a certain size; animals with tumors over this size did not improve. MAK also reduces the toxicity of chemotherapy in breast cancer patients (Srivastava et al., 2000).

## Reduction of Lung Cancer Metastases

Another study was carried out on lung cancer by Dr. Vimal Patel at Indiana University in collaboration with others. Patel chose Lewis lung carcinoma, known to be a cancer that aggressively metastasizes, spreading rapidly to other organs of the body. Rapidly metastasizing cancer is ordinarily the most life-threatening type. This study began with animals that already had Lewis lung carcinoma. MAK-4 was added to their diet. In 65% of the animals the total number of metastatic nodules decreased, and in 45% the size of the individual nodules also decreased (Patel, Wang, Shen, Sharma, & Brahmi, 1992).

## Increased Cancer Survival

Johnston and his colleagues at Stanford Research Institute studied the effect of MAK on skin tumors, measuring increased survival rather than measuring effects on specific tumors. Animals with skin papilloma were fed MAK-5 in their diet. The survival rate for MAK-fed animals was 75% compared to 31% in the control group (Johnston et al., 1991).

## Prevention of Cell Transformation

In research supported by the National Cancer Institute (NCI), Arnold studied the anticancer effects of MAK with two standardized and frequently used tests. With one test, MAK-4 inhibited tumor cell growth by 51%. With the other, MAK-4 inhibited transformation of normal cells to cancer cells by 27%, and MAK-5 inhibited it by 53%. This was the first study to show specifically that MAK could prevent healthy cells from being transformed into cancerous ones. MAK has also been shown to keep nerve cells healthy (Arnold, Wilkinson, & Korytynski, 1991; Rodella et al., 2004).

## Transformation of Cancer Cells to Normal Cells

The most striking cancer study showed the reverse process: cancerous cells being transformed back into apparently healthy, normal cells—one of the rarest types of reports in the research literature on cancer. It is often said that the initiation stage—damaging alteration to the DNA—is irreversible. This study—by Dr. Kedar Prasad, Director of the Center for Vitamin and Cancer Research at the Health Sciences Center, University of Colorado—challenges that supposition. Prasad et al. (1992) experimented with tissue culture cells of neuroblastoma, an aggressive form of neurological cancer most often found in children and considered extremely difficult to treat. Conventional therapies are known to create severe side effects.

Typical nerve cells are by far the largest cells in the body, with large central bodies and branching dendrites and axons (long, fingerlike projections) that can be several feet long. Malignant neuroblastoma cells usually lose much of this nerve cell-style differentiation. They shrink, become circular, and lose their long projections. Once they have reverted to this small, nonspecific (undifferentiated) form, they begin to multiply uncontrollably. Prasad found that MAK-5 reverses this process. Exposed to MAK-5, approximately 75% of the malignant cells appeared to differentiate again, developing a large cell body and dendrites, and to stop their rampant growth. Their biochemical functioning also appeared to return to normal; they produced enzymes that healthy cells usually produce. MAK-4 and MAK-5 have also been found to positively effect cellular transformation of liver cancer in mice (Mazzoleni et al., 2002). Only a few agents had previously been reported that cause cancer cells to revert to a normal-like state, and most of them are highly toxic.

Of course, a number of preclinical agents have been found to be efficacious in vitro or in vivo nonhuman models but either found not to be efficacious or frequently toxic to humans in Phase I, II, and III testing. Therefore, any definitive statement on their role in cancer care is entirely premature. Much work still needs to be done on both finding effective cancer treatments in humans and reducing the toxicity of chemotherapy.

# Reduced Chemotherapeutic Toxicity

Many chemicals are causes of illness and death. This is also true both of medications and occupational exposure. Much of the damage caused by these chemicals is due to free radical mechanisms. Exploratory studies have shown that MAK may have a significant role to play in this sphere. Chemotherapeutic agents are highly toxic as a principle of therapy (see Chapter 1).

## Preventing Toxicity in Chemotherapy

Chemotherapy often destroys cancer cells by producing free radicals, which are not discriminating in their effects. They can sometimes even cause new cancers. MAK has been shown to be effective in reducing the toxic side effects associated with chemotherapy. A nonrandom, controlled, prospective study on 62 cancer patients showed reduced hepatic toxicity, vomiting, diarrhea, and improved sleep, weight, and overall feeling of well-being. They also showed a significant reduction in lipid peroxides compared to the control group. MAK has been shown to reduce the toxicity of chemotherapy in breast cancer patients (Srivastava et al., 2000). Randomized, placebo-controlled prospective trials should be done to draw conclusions on clinical outcome. It may be, for instance, that although MAK limits the toxicity of chemotherapy, it also limits the effectiveness of this very same therapy.

## Detoxifying Adriamycin

For many cancers, adriamycin has been a particularly effective medication. Adriamycin works by creating free radicals that destroy the DNA of cancer cells. However, these free radicals damage healthy cells as well. The danger is especially great in the heart, where cells have high levels of oxygen owing to their incessant muscular activity.

Dwivedi et al. (1991) at South Dakota State University, together with colleagues designed a dual experiment to investigate whether MAK could reduce adriamycin's toxic side effects. First, in a laboratory test, he checked to see if MAK could inhibit adriamycin's production of free radicals.

The first results showed that even in an already efficient biochemical system for creating free radicals, adriamycin increased the production of free radicals by 50%. Second, MAK again proved highly efficient at reducing free-radical levels. The MAK-5 and MAK-4 reduced lipid peroxidation to essentially zero, even in the face of the added free-radical load created by adriamycin.

An additional test was conducted on animals that were given adriamycin. One group was fed a standard diet, whereas the other groups received either MAK-4 or MAK-5. At the end of 4 weeks, the mortality among the control group was 60%. The MAK-5 group had a mortality rate one-third lower and the MAK-4 group had a mortality rate two-thirds lower. The results of these two experiments indicated that MAK may provide substantial protection against the toxic side effects of adriamycin, if it is shown not to reduce its effectiveness. Again, clinical studies are warranted.

## Protection Against Cisplatin

Cisplatin is a potent chemotherapeutic agent and is used successfully for treating testicular, ovarian, and other cancers, but it is toxic to the kidneys. This may reflect decreases it causes in the activity of the antioxidants glutathione (GSH) and gluthathione-$S$ transferase (GST). Sharma in collaboration with colleagues at South Dakota State University (2002) studied the cisplatin-induced changes in GSH and GST in rat liver and kidneys. Cisplatin treatment significantly decreased GSH and GST activity in both rat livers and kidneys. But for rats that had dietary MAK-4 supplementation in addition to the cisplatin treatment, the effects of cisplatin on liver and kidney GSH and GST activity were reversed. These results indicate that MAK-4 may protect against cisplatin-induced toxicity.

## Protection Against Toluene

The *Charaka Samhita* says of a *rasayana* related to MAK-4 that, when used, "even poison is reduced to non-poison." MAK has in fact been found effective in protecting against such toxicities. In addition to reducing the often serious side effects of chemotherapy and of anticancer drugs, it has been found effective dealing with an industrial toxin. Dr. Stephen Bondy at the University of California, Irvine, has tested MAK against the toxic effects of toluene, a hazardous industrial solvent. More than 2 million American workers are exposed to the dangers of toluene every day—dangers that result from toluene's ability to rapidly create free radicals. First, Bondy's laboratory tests showed that MAK effectively scavenged free radicals created by toluene. Next, a study was done on laboratory animals that were first given MAK-5 for 2 days and then exposed toluene. Examinations revealed a significant reduction of free-radical formation in the MAK-5 group as compared to the control group (Bondy, Hernandez & Mattia, 1994). Two other MAV *rasayanas*, Student Rasayana and MA-631, have also been found to reduce significantly toluene-induced toxicity.

# Aging

Aging is the largest risk factor for most of the common cancers in humans. One of the questions in free-radical research is whether effective free-radical control can slow the aging process and extend life, as well as reduce the risk of cancer. Three preliminary studies on MAK throw light on this.

Dr. Jeremy Fields's team at Loyola conducted two of these experiments. In the first test, MAK was fed as a dietary supplement to laboratory mice, staring at the age of 18 months (roughly 50–60 years of age in human terms). Even starting at this relatively advanced age, 80% of the MAK group survived to 23 months of age, compared to only 48% survival for the control group. To check for effects throughout a life span, Fields turned to an experimental standby, the fruit fly. Fruit flies thrive and breed well in the laboratory, but their natural life span is only weeks long, allowing complete experiments in a short period of time. In this case, fruit flies fed MAK from birth lived 70% longer than controls (Fields, Eftekhari, Hagen, Wichilinski, & Schneider, 1991).

A provocative human test has also been conducted by Dr. Paul Gelderloos and his associates at Maharishi University of Management in Fairfield, Iowa. Gelderloos reasoned that if MAK has a positive effect on aging, it should appear in measurements of age-related functioning. He chose a test combining both visual and mental processing to assess complex functioning of the nervous system. Previous research on such tests had shown that the ability to perform them worsens markedly with age owing to physical deterioration (such as reduced retinal metabolism) and to an age-related deficit in information processing.

The results supported the hypothesis. First, performance on the test both for the MAK and placebo group was strongly correlated with age. The younger men consistently scored the highest. Second, the group that took MAK improved significantly more than the placebo group in all ranges after both 3 and 6 weeks (Gelderloos et al., 1990).

Such statistically significant improvement in a matter of weeks would be difficult to explain were it not for the free-radical theory. Long-range testing is still needed, but Gederloos's work has demonstrated that MAK's free-radical scavenging ability may apparently rejuvenate cell function, thus improving a complex physical/mental process.

# Redifferentiation and Rejuvenation in Cancer

The discussion of TM touched on the dysdifferentiation theory of Richard Cutler of the National Institute on Aging—the idea that cells "forget" what specific type they are supposed to be. All cells in a body share the same DNA, but normally different genes express themselves in different cells. In aging and cancer, the cells regress (dysdifferentiate) to a generic and generally useless form. Cutler speculates that free-radical damage to the DNA causes the dysdifferentiation.

This theory has relevance to the MAK research. Cutler has expressed the possibility that antioxidants might slow the rate of dysdifferentiation. The study by Dr. Prasad on neuroblastoma cells (mentioned above) has shown that, in certain circumstances at least, loss of differentiation may actually be reversed.

In Prasad's study, cancer cells incubated with MAK regained some apparently normal attributes of functioning. His study showed that as long as the newly redifferentiated cells continued to be cultured with MAK, they maintained their healthy, normal status. MAK appeared to help maintain their differentiation. This implies at least the possibility that regular use of MAK could help to maintain proper differentiation of bodily cells. If such differentiation continued in the most important glands of the body, which are Cutler's focus, then proper hormone levels may be maintained in the physiology as a whole and the aging process significantly retarded.

# Complications of Cancer

## Pain

This chapter previously discussed the link between emotions and the body in terms of the limbic system and the neuropeptides it produces. Through this neurochemical system, emotions have a profound influence on the functioning of the body. There is both reason and evidence for thinking that neuropeptides are modulated by MAK. For one thing, Vedic tradition has always maintained that *rasayanas* enhance psychologic well-being. For another, if molecules are what mediate the mind/body interface, these particular molecules might be expected to mediate in a positive way.

To test the effects of MAK on both psychologic mood and biochemical operation in the brain, a much-utilized questionnaire that gauges emotional well-being was given people using MAK. The results of this questionnaire showed marked improvements in psychologic mood—greater happiness, tranquility, mental clarity, and emotional balance.

To check for a molecular connection Sharma and colleagues investigated the interaction of MAK with receptors in the brain known as opioid receptors. Opiate drugs, such as morphine, attach to these receptors. There was much publicity when researchers discovered that the body has natural opioids—endorphins and enkephalins—that also lock into these receptors. These can act as natural painkillers, and they also produce positive emotions, create a more relaxed and stable style of operation in the autonomic nervous system, and modify the functioning of the immune system

These tests showed that MAK did in fact interact with these receptors and one or more of its components blocked the receptors for exogenous opioid compounds. However, it did not block receptors for endogenously produced opioid peptides.

## Reducing Inflammation and Associated Pain

A separate study reported that subjects using MAK-5 for 3 months showed a significant decrease in substance P, another neurotransmitter. Substance P is triggered by pain and is associated with lung and gastrointestinal inflammation. Reduction of substance P thus indicates that MAK may be able to reduce such inflammation and its associated pain. These studies go beyond the free-radical theory and indicate that MAK may have other effects on the physiology.

## Depression

A study carried out at Maharishi University of Management further implicated MAK's mind/body role. Imipramine has been one of the major prescription drugs given for depression. It binds strongly with a receptor in the brain cells that increases the output of serotonin, one of the most thoroughly studied neurotransmitters. Low levels of serotonin correlate with aggression, hostility, and other mental health problems, whereas high levels correlate with a comfortable, even exhilarated, emotional tone. Imipramine, the serotonin trigger, binds not only to brain cells but also to blood platelets, providing another tie between mind and body.

This research showed that MAK interacted with the same receptor on blood platelets as imipramine. This suggests that MAK might bind to the same receptor in brain cells, increasing serotonin levels and thus providing a positive effect on both psychologic mood and immune system functioning.

## Effects and Side Effects

Experience with medicine has taught us always to look for negative results along with the positive. Modern drugs have side effects. Plants also produce not only defenses against pathogens but also toxins to deter predators; they can be toxic to people as well. Ayurveda has long asserted that *rasayanas* have no side effects and that its time-tested herbal pharmacology had already dealt with the issue of toxicity and eliminated it. Beyond that, the mixture of components in *rasayanas* is said to increase potency while also balancing biochemical influences and thus negating destructive side effects. (This balancing effect of multiple ingredients is exactly what is lost with the active ingredient approach; active ingredients act indiscriminately throughout the body.)

To measure toxicity, a blood examination was carried out on 84 subjects who had been using MAK for at least 6 months. Standard tests of biochemical, hematological, and liver enzyme parameters revealed no toxic effects. A separate study performed the same blood tests on nine subjects tested before and after taking MAK-5 for 3 months. Again the blood samples were normal and no toxic effects were found (Sharma et al., 2002).

MAK challenges some preconceptions of modern biomedial science. It is a nonreductive mélange of thousands of different molecules, but it has passed some important scientific tests and produced measurable results. It has been shown that MAK can help control free radicals, thus reducing the constant load of oxidative stress in the body and improving physical health in many measurable ways. The studies indicated that it works more effectively than many of the best known antioxidants and that it may help to combat a wide range of disease. MAK includes natural antioxidants— vitamins, beta-carotene, polyphenols, and bioflavonoids—in high concentration. It also includes a myriad of substances not yet isolated and examined in the laboratory. Although modern medicine leans toward isolated active ingredients, usually produced artificially, Ayurvedic *vaidyas* maintain that complex herbal mixtures of properly chosen prepared ingredients are more effective. They maintain that the natural synergism not only increases the mixtures' potency but also works to mitigate side effects caused by individual components.

In the case of free radicals, and the wide-ranging damage free radicals may cause, the research on MAK apparently upholds the Ayurvedic view. To the extent that these studies are accurate, therefore, they help define a potential new modality for prevention and treatment of disease. Confronted with one common cause of cancer and aging—free radicals—scientists have shown that isolated active ingredients may not work as well as rich natural formulations. An emerging understanding of the complex causes of disease is beginning to lead to demonstration of the benefits produced by natural synergism.

# Other Herbs

## Single Herbs

This chapter has spent a great deal of time on the issue of *rasayanas*, partly because the research is significant and partly because it throws the issue of active ingredients into particularly sharp focus. However, *rasayanas*, like MAK, are not the only use of herbs found in Ayurveda, which has an extensive herbal pharmacopoeia.

MAV uses herbs in a number of formulations based on ancient Ayurveda. Some are taken every day, the herbs being added to the patient's diet. Different taste groups are said to affect the balance of the *doshas* in different ways; herbs and spices are often, by this scheme, used to balance the effects of diet. In addition, many individual herbs are held to have specific medical effects. These are understood in a systematic way; the system involves not only taste groups but also "potency" *(virya)*—that is, whether the herb is heating or cooling—and specific qualities *(gunas)*.

As an example of how this might be used, consider the Ayurvedic herb *ashwagandha* (*Withania somnifera*). A MAV *vaidya* would note that this herb has three tastes: bitter, astringent, and sweet. Its potency (*virya*) is hot and its aftertaste (*vipaka*) is sweet. He or she would also note the specific qualities associated with *ashwagandha*: it is said to alleviate *Vata* and *Kapha*; to be diuretic and sedative; to increase sperm count; and to be useful against edema, cough, skin disease and other diseases. It is also regarded as a general tonic (a *rasayana*).

Such analyses are also applied to more common herbs. Fresh ginger root, for example, has a pungent taste, but a sweet aftertaste; its *virya* is hot; it alleviates *Vata* and *Kapha* but increases *Pitta* mildly. It is widely used in MAV remedies. For instance, it is used to enhance digestive strength (to strengthen the digestive fire or *jatharagni*), which is a central element of health in MAV. It is also said to be helpful in fighting colds, anorexia (because it can be used in specific preparations to stimulate appetite and digestion), chronic arthritis, and constipation (for this, the ginger is dried and powdered). Many other herbs, some of them not well known in the West, whereas others are common and are used in various similar ways in MAV.

## Specific Conditions

Another major use of herbs in MAV is to treat specific imbalances and health problems. There has been a surprisingly large amount of research on this topic, with most of it being in Indian medical journals. To take one study, Khosla, Gupta, and Nagpal (1995) investigated the Ayurvedic claim that fenugreek (*Trigonella foenum-graecum*) is an antidiabetic. In a controlled study, they found that fenugreek produced a significant decline in blood glucose in both normal rats and rats with alloxan-induced diabetes. Another study appeared in the *Lancet* in October 1988 and included among its authors Baruch S. Blumberg, MD, PhD, who won the 1976 Nobel Prize in Medicine for discovering the marker for the hepatitis B virus (Sharma et al., 2002). This study tested the *Phyllanthus amarus*, which "was described in Indian Ayurvedic literature more than 2000 years ago" as being useful for the treatment of jaundice and other diseases. The plant was given for 30 days to patients with hepatitis B; within 15 to 20 days of the end of treatment, 59% of the treated patients had lost hepatitis B surface antigen compared with 4% of controls. The study also demonstrates a lack of toxic side effects from the plant.

Despite such studies, there has been little research and marketing of Ayurvedic herbs in the West. This is partly because of the active ingredient model but also because such herbs are not patentable. Billions of dollars are invested by pharmaceutical companies in research into synthesizing the active ingredient and then testing it in the laboratory and clinic; but there could be no return on investment for similar research on natural substances. You cannot patent a plant. However, emerging research on herbal formulations is changing the orientation.

## How Else Might Herbs Work?

The antioxidant research explains a great deal of the effect of *rasayanas*. It may explain part of the action of individual herbs used for specific illnesses or for general use. But clearly more is involved than free radicals. The study discussed above, for example, makes it clear that at least some of the anticancer effects of MAK are the result of more than free-radical scavenging. For a cancer cell to assume its former, normal state, the DNA within the cell must have been reset. Free radicals damage DNA. Antioxidants by themselves simply stop the damage.

MAV thinks of herbs like tuning forks that vibrate with and harmonize the functioning of different aspects of the physiology. This is based on MAV's understanding of the body as being not so much a piece of matter as a dynamic and orderly pattern of knowledge, which is based ultimately on the underlying vibratory patterns of natural law in the DNA and, before that, in the quantum unified field (Stapp, 1994). The vibratory patterns existing in plants are said to enliven those elements of the human physiology with similar patterns.

In the understanding of MAV, each molecule in an herb is actually an impulse of information, a particular "standing wave" in the underlying field. When carefully chosen, these match the impulses of intelligence in different parts of the human body. When the mind and body go out of balance, there are disruptions in the natural sequence that leads from pure information to DNA, RNA, and proteins and so on to the complete physiology. One such sequence produces liver cells, for example, whereas another produces the heart. Where a sequence is disrupted, disease can occur in that particular part of the body.

The herbal preparations of MAV are said to provide the correct impulse to "reset" a particular sequence, to build a continuous bridge again from the unified field of pure intelligence all the way to the manifest, surface-level expressions of the body. MAK encourages cancer cells to restore themselves to the healthy, functioning cells they once were. Auyrveda indicates that this process of redifferentiation means that the correct sequence is restored, the information flows smoothly, and the *doshas* are rebalanced. The research here suggests that cells too can "regain memory" of their true natures.

This research gives reason to look beyond the "active ingredient" model of modern pharmacology. A *rasayana* (a mélange of dozens of carefully chosen and prepared plants) was found to be 100 times more effective at scavenging free radicals than the isolated active ingredients vitamins C and E and the modern pharmaceutical probucol. The mélange also proved to have a wide range of beneficial effects, many of which result from its antioxidant ability, but some from more profound capacities: Restoring a cancer cell to normal functioning cannot be explained in terms of free-radical scavenging. There is a wide range of other medicinal uses of herbs and plants in Ayurveda, and this chapter discusses only a very small part of the herbal pharmacopoeia.

# Ayurvedic Clinical Approach

The classic practice of Ayurveda can be viewed in light of contemporary scientific evidence and interpretations as above and can also be extracted in a consistent manner from the contemporary translation of interpretation of ancient, classic Ayurvedic texts (Das, 2003; Meulenbeld, 1999–2002; Meulenbeld & Wujastyk, 2001; Pitman, 2004; Sharma, 2002; Srikanta Murthy, 1998–2000; Zysk, 2002).

The first step undertaken in clinical Ayurveda practice is proper diagnosis of the patient and his or her condition. The general diagnostic procedure evaluates the individual's overall health and strength and the specific morbidity from which the person is suffering. The first, *Rogipariksha,* focuses on establishing the patient's *Prakriti* and assessing his or her mental and physical strength. The second, *Rogapariksha,* aims at identifying the illness from which the patient suffers in terms of the *dosha(s)* involved, the *dhatus* involved, and the *srotas* in which it is located.

A specific name for a disease is not necessary if the twofold process of diagnosis is executed properly. The Ayurvedic doctor, *Vaidya,* now knows the patient's strengths and weaknesses and the anatomical and physiologic areas affected. Correct therapeutic treatment follows from this diagnosis.

Ayurvedic therapies are designed to rebalance and reintegrate the individual. They are classified as tonifying and reducing and are intended either to nourish deficiencies and tissue weakness or to detoxify and reduce aggravated doshas. Reduction usually comes first, followed by rejuvenation therapies to rebuild the body's strength.

Reduction is often prescribed for *Kapha* disorders and tonification for *Vata* disorders, whereas *Pitta* disorders normally require a mixture of both therapies. Reduction therapy itself is divided into two parts: palliation and purification. Palliation consists of strengthening the digestive fire, reducing *Ama,* and calming the excess *doshas* so that they can be removed during purification. Purification therapy involves five cleansing therapies (*Panchakarma*): medicated enemas, nasal medications, therapeutic purgation, therapeutic vomiting, and therapeutic release of toxic blood. The specific example of cancer illustrates the traditional Ayurvedic clinical approach although there is no Sanskrit equivalent in classic Ayurveda (see Chapter 3).

## Cancer and Classic Ayurveda

Under the influence of cancer, the three *doshas* destroy rather than preserve and nourish the body. *Vata* causes normal cells to proliferate and become cancerous. *Pitta* steals nutrients from other dhatus to feed cancerous cells, and *Kapha* allows these cells to increase unchecked. Although cancer regulates the activities of all three *doshas,* it usually begins by domination in one. A *doshic* imbalance, accompanied by an overaccumulation of *Ama* and insufficient digestive fire, sets the stage for cancer. In addition, Ayurveda recognizes an intimate link between suppressed emotion and suppressed immunity. Other proposed factors include devitalized foods, a sedentary lifestyle, long-term exposure to radiation or chemical carcinogens, and a lack of spiritual purpose or effort in life.

Because *Ama* is one of the primary causes and enablers of cancer, detoxification is the primary therapy. *Panchakarma* rids the body of both *Ama* and any excessive accumulation of *doshas.* Cancer is classified into *Vata, Pitta,* and *Kapha* varieties, according to the nature of the tumors themselves, the color of the patient's skin, the patient's demeanor, and other symptoms. Patients are put on powerful blood-cleansing herbs, strong circulatory stimulants, immune-strengthening tonics, and special *Kapha*-dispelling herbs. Specific anticancer herbs are administered differently for *Vata, Pitta,* or *Kapha* to obtain maximum assimilation. *Vata* cases are advised to imbibe fresh ginger tea with their herbs; *Pitta* patients should use aloe gel; and *Kapha* cases take honey and black pepper.

# Summary

There are rich traditions and contemporary scientific evidence to support the use of Ayurvedic medicine in the prevention and care of cancer. Transcendental Meditation is a well-organized application of a mind/body therapy approach that has proven benefits. The pharmacopeia of Ayurvedic herbs holds promise for supportive care of cancer patients. Because of the cell differentiation properties (as with certain micronutrients; see Chapters 14–17) of specific traditional herbal combinations, there may also be the promise for the development of effective cancer treatments from this ancient system of knowledge.

## REFERENCES

Alexander, C. N., Langer, E. J., Davies, J. L., Chandler, H. M., & Newman, R. I. (1989). Transcendental Meditation, mindfulness, and longevity: An experimental study with the elderly. *Journal of Personality and Social Psychology, 57*(6), 950–964.

Alexander, C. N., Robinson, P., Orme-Johnson, D. W., Schneider, R. H., & Walton, K. G. (1994a). The effects of Transcendental Meditation compared to other methods of relaxation and meditation in reducing risk factors, morbidity, and mortality. *Homeostasis, 35,* 243–264.

Alexander, C. N., Robinson, P., & Rainforth, M. (1994b). Treating and preventing alcohol, nicotine, and drug abuse through Transcendental Meditation: A review and statistical meta-analysis. *Alcoholism Treatment Quarterly, 11,* 11–84.

Alpha-Tocopherol, Beta Carotene Cancer Prevention Study Group. (1994). The effect of vitamin E and beta carotene on the incidence of lung cancer and other cancers in male smokers. *New England Journal of Medicine, 330*(15), 1029–1035.

Arnold, J. T., Wilkinson, B. P., & Korytynski, E. A. (1991). Chemopreventive activity of Maharishi Amrit Kalash and related agents in rat tracheal epithelial and human tumor cells. *Proceedings of the American Association for Cancer Research, 32,* 128. [abstract]

Bendich, A. (1990). Antioxidant nutrients and immune functions. In A. Bendich, M. Phillips, & R. P. Tengerdy (Eds.), *Antioxidant nutrients and immune functions* (pp. 1–12). New York: Plenum.

Blasdell, K. S., Sharma, H. M., Tomlinson, P. F., & Wallace, R. K. (1991). Subjective survey, blood chemistry and complete blood profile of subjects taking Maharishi Amrit Kalash (MAK). *Journal of the Federation of American Societies for Experimental Biology, 5,* A1317.

Bondy, S. C., Hernandez, T. M., & Mattia, C. (1994). Antioxidant properties of two Ayurvedic herbal preparations. *Biochemical Archives, 10,* 25–31.

Cooper, M. J., & Aygen, M. M. (1978). Effect of Transcendental Meditation on serum cholesterol and blood pressure. *Harefuah, the Journal of the Israel Medical Association, 95*(1), 1–2.

Cooper, M. J., & Aygen, M. M. (1979). A relaxation technique in the management of hypercholesterolemia. *Journal of Human Stress, 5,* 24–27.

Cutler, R. (1985). Dysdifferentiation and aging. In R. S. Sohal (Ed.), *Molecular biology of aging: Gene stability and gene expression* (pp. 307–340). New York: Raven Press.

Das, R. P. (2003). *Indian Medical Tradition Series: Vol 6. The origin of life of a human being.* Delhi: Motilal Banarsidass.

Dillbeck, M. C., & Orme-Johnson, D. W. (1987). Physiological differences between Transcendental Meditation and rest. *American Physiologist, 42,* 879–881.

Dwivedi, C., Sharma, H. M., Dobrowski, S., & Engineer, F. N. (1991). Inhibitory effects of Maharishi Amrit Kalash-4 and Maharishi Amrit Kalash-5 on microsomal lipid peroxidation. *Pharmacology Biochemistry and Behavior, 39,* 649–652.

Engineer, F. N., Sharma, H. M., & Swivedi, C. (1992). Protective effects of M-4 and M-5 on adriamycin-induced microsomal lipid peroxidation and mortality. *Biochemical Arichives, 8,* 267–272.

Gelderloos, P., Ahlstrom, H. H. B., Orme-Johnson, D. W., Robinson, D. K., Wallace, R. K., & Glaser, J. L. (1990). Influence of a Maharishi Ayur-Vedic herbal preparation on age-related visual discrimination. *International Journal of Psychosomatic, 37,* 25–29.

Glaser, J. L., Robinson, D. K., & Wallace, R. K. (1988). Effects of Maharishi Amrit Kalash on allergies, described in Maharishi Ayurveda: An introduction to recent research. *Modern Science and Vedic Science, 2*(1), 89–108.

Glaser, J, Brind, J., Vogelman, J. et al. (1992). Elevated serum dehydroepiandrosterone sulfate levels in practitioners of the Transcendental Meditation (TM) and TM-Sidhi programs, *Journal of Behavioral Medicine 15*, 327–341.

Hennekens, C. H., Buring, J. E., Manson, J. E., et al. (1996). Lack of effect of long-term supplementation with beta-carotene on the incidence of malignant neoplasms and cardiovascular disease. *New England Journal of Medicine, 334*(18), 1145–1149.

Herron, R. E., & Fagan, J. B. (2002). Lipophil-mediated reduction of toxicants in humans: an evaluation of an Ayurvedic detoxification procedure. *Alternative Therapies in Health and Medicine, 8*, 40–51.

Jevning, R., & Wilson, A. F. (1977). Altered red cell metabolism in TM. *Psychophysiology, 14*, 94.

Jevning, R., & Wilson, A. F. (1978). Behavioral increase of cerebral blood flow. *The Physiologist, 21*, 60.

Johnston, B.H., Mirsalis, J., Hamilton, C. (1991). Chemotherapeutic effects of an Ayurvedic herbal supplement on mouse papilloma. *The Pharmacologist 3*, 39 (abstract).

Khosla, P., Gupta, D., Nagpal, R. K. (1995). Effect of *Trigonella foenum-graecum* (fenugreek) on blood glucose in normal and diabetic rats. *Indian Journal of Physiology and Pharmacology, 39*(2), 173–174.

Kushi, L. H., Folsom, A. R., Prineas, R. J., Mink, P. J., Wu, Y., & Bostick, R. M. (1996). Dietary antioxidant vitamins and death from coronary heart disease in postmenopausal women. *New England Journal of Medicine, 334*(18), 1145–1149.

Mazzoleni, G. (2002). Anti-tumor effects of the antioxidant natural products Maharishi Amrit Kalash-4 and -5 (MAK) on cell transformation in vitro and in liver carcinogenesis in mice. *Journal of Applied Nutrition, 52*, 45–63.

Meulenbeld, G. J. (1999–2002). *A history of Indian medical literature* (Vols. *1–3*). Groningen: Egbert Forsten.

Meulenbeld, G. J., & Wujastyk, D. (2001). *Studies on Indian medical history* (Vol. 5). New Dehli: Motilal Banarsidass.

Omenn, G. S., Goodman, G. E., Thornquist, M. A., et al. (1996). Effects of a combination of beta carotene and vitamin A on lung cancer and cardiovascular disease. *New England Journal of Medicine, 334*(18), 1150–1155.

Patel, V. K., Wang, J., Shen, R. N., Sharma, H. M., & Brahmi, Z. (1992). Reduction of metastases of Lewis Lung Carcinoma by an Ayurvedic food supplement in mice. *Nutrition Research, 12*, 51–61.

Pitman, V. (2004). *Indian medical tradition series: Vol. 7. On the nature of the whole.* New Delhi: Motilal Banarsidass.

Prasad, K.N., Edwards-Prasad, J., Kentroti, S., et al. (1992). Ayurvedic agents induce differentiation in murine neuroblastoma cells in culture, *Neuropharmacology 31*, 599–607.

Rodella, L., et al. (2004). MAK-5 enhances the nerve growth factor mediated neurite outgrowth in PC12 cells. *Journal of Ethnopharmacology, 93*, 161–166.

Schneider, R. H., Staggers. F., Alexander, C. N., et al. (1995). A randomized controlled trial of stress reduction for hypertension in older African Americans. *Hypertension, 26*(5), 820–837.

Sharma, H. M. (2002). Free radicals and natural antioxidants in health and disease. *Journal of Applied Nutrition, 52*, 26–44.

Sharma, H. M., Dwivedi, C., Satter, B. C., et al. (1990). Antineoplastic properties of Maharishi-4 against DMBA-induced mammary tumors in rats. *Pharmacology Biochemistry and Behavior, 35*, 767–773.

Sharma, H. M., Guenther, J., Abu-Ghazaleh, A., & Dwivedi, C. (1994). Effects of Ayurvedic food supplement M-4 on cisplatin-induced changes in glutathione and glutahione-S transerase activity. In R. S. Rao, M. G. Deo, & L. D. Sanghvi (Eds.), *Proceedings of the Sixteenth International Cancer Congress 1994* (pp. 589–592). Bologna: Monduzzi.

Sharma, H. M., Hanna, A. N., Kauffman, E. M., & Newman, H. A. I. (1992). Inhibition of human low-density lipoprotein oxidation in vitro by Maharish Ayur-Veda herbal mixtures. *Pharmacology Biochemistry and Behavior, 43*, 1175–1182.

Sharma, H. M., Hanna, A. N., Kauffman, E. M., & Newman, H. A. I. (1995). Effect of herbal mixture Student Rasayana on lipoxygenase activity and lipid peroxidation. *Free Radical Biology and Medicine, 18*, 687–697.

Sharma, H., Mishra, R.K., with Meade, J.G. (2002). *The answer to cancer.* New York: SelectBooks.

Smith, D. E., Glaser, J. L., Schneider, R. H., & Dillbeck, M. C. (1989). Erythrocyte sedimentation rate (ESR) and the Transcendental Meditation program. *Psychosomatic Medicine, 5*, 259.

Srikanta Murthy, K. R. (1998–2000). *Bhavaprakasha of Bhavamishra* (Vols. *1 and 2*). Varanasi: Krishnadas Academy.

Srivastava, A., Samaiya, A., Taraikanti, V., et al. (2000). Maharishi Amrit Kalash (MAK) reduces chemotherapy toxicity in breast cancer patients. *FASEB Journal, 14,* A720.

Stapp, H. P. (1994). *Mind, matter and quantum mechanics.* Berlin: Springer-Verlag.

Wallace, R.K., Dillbeck, M.C., Jacobs, E., Harrington, B. (1982). The effects of the Transcendental Meditation and TM-Sidhi programs on the aging process. *The International Journal of Neuroscience, 16,* 53–58.

Weitzman, S. A., Weitberg, A. B., Clark, E. P., & Stossel, T. P. (1985). Phagocytes as carcinogens: Malignant transformation produced by human neutrophils. *Science, 227,* 1231–1233.

Zysk, K. G. (2002). *Sir Henry Wellcome Asian medical series: Vol 1. Conjugal love in India.* Leiden: Brill.

# 17

Joyce Frye

## Introduction

Treating cancer is the greatest challenge for any form of medical practice. Although homeopathy appears to have much to offer at every stage of disease, there is wide variation in styles of practice and in the rationale used for selection of the homeopathic medicine in any individual case. At present, no single protocol is used by sufficiently large numbers of practitioners to support data collection for outcome comparisons. However, it is useful to review where success has been noted in order to consider how homeopathy may be best incorporated today and what directions in further research might provide added benefit.

To a large extent, the variation in treatment styles arises out of the complexity of homeopathic theory and the need for individualizing treatment to the patient rather than to the tumor type. To better understand this approach, it is helpful to review some basic homeopathic principles and to understand the possible mechanisms of action of homeopathic remedies (Becker-Witt et al., 2003; Belon et al., 2004; Carlston, 2003).

## Background

Samuel Hahnemann, MD, formulated the precepts of homeopathic medicine in Germany beginning in the late 1700s. He laid out his theories in *The Organon of Medicine*, completing the sixth edition shortly before his death in 1843 (Hahnemann, 1843/1996). Following ideas first set forth by Hippocrates; he determined empirically that the medicinal substance most likely to be able to cure a disease in a sick individual is one that could cause symptoms similar to the disease in a healthy individual. Hahnemann called this the *Law of Similars*.

1X = 1 part in 10
3X = 1 part in 1,000
6X = 1 part in 1,000,000
12X (or 6C) = 1 part in 1,000,000,000,000
*Avogadran limit here*
12C = 1 part in 1,000,000,000,000,000,000,000,000,
000
30X = 1,000,000,000,000,000,000,000,000,000,
000
30C = 1,000,000,000,000,000,000,000,000,000,
000,000,000,000,000,000,000,000,000,000,
000

**Commonly sold homeopathic dilutions relative to Avogadro's number.**

Hahnemann vociferously disdained most of the medicine of his day, but noted that where treatments were successful it was because the Law of Similars was at work; for example, mercury was successful for the treatment of syphilis because the symptoms of mercury toxicity are very similar to those of syphilis. However, the mercury was given in such large doses that the patient subsequently became ill from the treatment.

## The Medicines

Following his observation that medicines worked according to the Law of Similars, Hahnemann set about determining what medicines might be good for what. He studied the effect of substances on groups of healthy persons in *provings*, conducting approximately 200 of them in his lifetime. He used the symptoms observed in the proving (often as many as 150 symptoms, including those from the mental and emotional spheres) as the indication for the medicinal use of the substance. To avoid causing further illness, and probably to make them go farther, the medicines (known as *remedies*) were diluted with water. Hahnemann then observed that the more they were diluted, the more effective they seemed to become in their medicinal action.

The dilution process, which became known as *potentization*, is done with a series of dilutions of either 1:10 or 1:100 parts substance to water and alcohol known as X or C potencies respectively (e.g., a 30C potency has been diluted 100-fold, 30 times). Vigorous shaking (*succussion*) between each dilution is integral to the process (see Figure 17.1).

Although the mechanism of action of these highly dilute substances remains undiscovered, it is theorized that in the potentization process, the highly polar water molecules of the diluent become arranged into patterns unique to each medicine (much like a snowflake is a unique form of ice), so that the information of the medicine is retained even though there may be no remaining molecules.

Homeopathic drugs were included in the original Food and Drug Administration (FDA) legislation, so unlike herbal and nutritional supplements, the FDA regulates the manufacture, marketing, and sale of homeopathic drugs. They are delivered in numerous oral and topical dosage forms, including but not limited to liquids, tablets, medicated pellets, ointments, and suppositories. For systemic disease, dosing in the form of medicated sugar pellets that are dissolved in the mouth or by water dilutions is most common.

The Homoeopathic Pharmacopoeia Convention of the United States (HPCUS; www.hpcus.com) determines which medicines have undergone sufficient testing to be considered official homeopathic drugs within the meaning of the Federal Food Drug and Cosmetic Act. Currently, there are approximately 2,000 homeopathic formulations. Medicines are prepared according to Good Manufacturing Practices; and the Latin name of the substance is used for labeling.

Medicinal substances may come from plant, animal, mineral, or chemical sources. Additionally, there are *nosodes*, defined by the HPCUS as "homeopathic attenuations of: pathological organs or tissues; causative agents such as bacteria, fungi, ova, parasites, virus particles, and yeast; disease products; excretions or secretions." Essentially, anything that is toxic enough to cause symptoms in a healthy individual can be potentized to become a homeopathic remedy for treating similar symptoms in a sick individual.

Isopathic (same substance) potentizations are also used—primarily for detoxification. This may be useful when there has been exposure to a known carcinogen. Studies using a rat model have demonstrated decreased tissue levels of arsenic following experimental exposure using homeopathically prepared arsenic dilutions (Cazin et al., 1987). The embryotoxic effects of cadmium have similarly been reduced in the amphibian model (Herkovits & Perez-Coll, 1991).

# Remedy Selection

Hahnemann considered all disease, with the exception of that resulting from direct external forces such as trauma, to arise from disturbances of the *vital force* affecting the entire person, not just the organ or structure where symptoms appeared. Treatment solely of the diseased part still left the organism imbalanced and prone to the next expression of illness. Aphorisms 190–191 of *The Organon* state the following:

> All genuine medical treatment of a malady that has arisen on external parts of the body (and that involves little or no damage from the outside) must therefore be directed towards the whole, towards the annihilation and cure of the general suffering by means of internal remedies.... This is confirmed unambiguously by experience which shows in all cases of a so-called local malady.... that every efficacious internal medicine, immediately after its ingestion, causes significant alterations in the rest of the patient's condition, especially in the external suffering parts (which appear to the ordinary medicinal art to be isolated). To be sure, if one selects an internal medicine, directed at the

whole, which is fittingly homeopathic, it will cause the most salutary alteration, the recovery of the whole human being, along with the disappearance of the external malady,
without the assistance of an external means. (Hahnemann 1843/1996)

The goal in homeopathy is to find a single medicine that matches the *totality* of
symptoms to give the "internal medicine" that will cure the individual rather than simply
removing the obvious disease. Thus, in classical homeopathy, the choice of medicine is
based on an individual's total history and physical symptom complex, including family
history and details of earlier emotional or physical traumas as well as extremely specific
details of local symptoms. Hahnemann developed the concept of *miasmas* (thought at the
time to arise from specific diseases) to explain familial or hereditary predispositions. The
end result is that persons with the same conventional diagnosis are frequently treated
with one of a variety of different medicines because of the unique symptom picture of
each individual.

*Constitutional* homeopathic care often begins with a $1\frac{1}{2}$- to 2-hours interview in
which minute details regarding the individual's symptoms and history are noted. Particular attention is paid to *quality, frequency, sequence,* and *location* of symptoms and to
*modalities*—actions or substances that *aggravate* or *ameliorate* the symptoms (e.g., burning pain ameliorated sore throat that is ameliorated by swallowing cold beverage). All of
the patient's symptoms ideally are found in the proving symptoms of the remedy chosen.

In trauma and in exposure to particularly potent environmental conditions or virulent
organisms, the individual responses become more uniform making it possible to select
one or a very few remedies that will work for most people under those conditions. The
population remedy in such situations is known as the *genus epidemicus*. For example,
during the flu pandemic of 1918, 20% of the entire world population was infected,
and 20–40 million people died. Data from the time compared 24,000 cases of flu treated
allopathically with a mortality rate of 28.2% to 26,000 cases of flu treated homeopathically
with a mortality rate of 1.05%. Almost everyone responded to one of only two or three
remedies, which were the genus epidemicus for that outbreak (American Institute of
Homeopathy, 1921).

# The Cancer Prescription

Most homeopathic physicians advocate primary surgical removal of the tumor followed by
homeopathy, in the belief that homeopathy is less likely to be successful where significant
pathological change has occurred and the tumor burden is too great for the vital force
(Jonas & Jacobs, 1996). Pure homeopathic practitioners insist that homeopathy works
best as a stand-alone treatment along with maintaining a simple diet and avoidance of
toxins.

Historically, this direct regimen was often followed, as, realistically; there were few
alternatives that offered any hope of success. Cowperthwaite of the University of Iowa
in his 1888 text lists homeopathic remedies useful for the treatment of tumors of the
breast, ovary, uterus, and vulva. Arthur Grimmer, MD, practicing in Chicago during
the first half of the 20th century, is said to have treated several thousand cases of cancer
in his 57-year career. Specific data between 1925 and 1929 revealed 150 cured cases of

biopsy diagnosed cancers and prolonged palliation (7–15 years) with excellent quality of life of another 75 cases. The greatest successes occurred where there was little preceding allopathic treatment (Currim, 1996).

Modern homeopathic literature in the United States includes primarily anecdotal case histories—breast cancer (Kreisberg, 1996), carcinoma-in-situ of the cervix, craniopharyngioma (Klein, 1989), and lymphoma (Sommerman, 1992). However, in India where there are over 100 homeopathic medical colleges, larger case series are described (Master 2000, 2001a, 2001b; Ramakrishnan & Coulter, 2001).

Choosing the correct medicine in cancer is the most challenging aspect of using homeopathy. Although treating the whole person with the medicine that matches the *totality* of symptoms as well as the tumor type is ideal, as the stage of disease advances, the symptoms often become more characteristic of the tumor than of the patient, and the homeopath and patient need to extensively explore the patient's memory of the time before cancer to recall the contributing factors and identifying symptoms to choose the constitutional remedy. Additionally, the preceding or concurrent use of radiation and/or chemotherapy alters the symptom picture making the homeopathic prescription even more difficult to discern.

In a young person, where no preceding incidents can be discovered, the homeopath may consider the remedy needed for the parent, which has been passed miasmatically to the child. Ghegas's description of osteosarcoma in a 15-year-old girl is such an example. Seeing no obvious remedy choice, he gave the remedy he knew the father needed. As the tumor regressed, the symptoms more common to the remedy appeared in the child (Ghegas, 1994).

In advanced disease, the remedy of choice for cancer treatment often seems more like genus epidemicus than like constitutional care, but it is difficult to know when that line is crossed. In many cases, only a few remedies are indicated for a particular type of tumor. Often they are *small* (i.e., infrequently used) remedies (Vithoulkas, 1980). The concept of organopathy first described by Paracelsus and adapted for homeopathy by Burnett (2001) may apply when the pathology is extensive and no remedy matches the totality of symptoms. In this case a remedy matching the pathology alone might be initially chosen and the symptoms indicating the constitutional remedy may only appear as the pathology recedes (Sommerman, 1992).

Taking a more formulaic approach, Ramakrishnan, practicing in India, has accumulated several thousand cancer cases. He claims >70% success using methodology that alternates a tumor nosode (carcinocinum or scirrhinum) with another remedy close to the patient's constitution but chosen from a small group that seem to be organ specific. Each remedy is used daily for a week then alternated with the other (Ramakrishnan & Coulter, 2001).

Montfort (2000), in Mexico, theorizes that making remedies from known carcinogens will give more tumor-specific remedies. He has used benzoanthracene for breast tumors, benzopyrene for lung tumors, methylcholantrene for muscle tumors, benzidine for bladder tumors, and fluorenyl acetamide for lung tumors. Results are difficult to evaluate as the remedies have been used alongside conventional radiation and/or chemotherapy. However, bench research involving synthesis of protector proteins at the cellular level found higher levels of tolerance to three different stressors (temperature shock, arsenite, cadmium) following primary low-level exposure (van Wijk & Wiegant, 1998). This kind of research offers a possible explanation for the effect proposed by Montfort (2000).

# Adjunctive Therapy

With the paucity of modern case series, few practitioners or patients choose to forego conventional treatment. Thus, homeopathy currently is most often used in an adjunctive role. Most homeopaths would agree that systemic chemotherapy is more disruptive to the organism's ability to heal, and given the choice, would opt for local radiation alone alongside constitutional homeopathy.

When radiation or chemotherapy is employed, homeopathy may be used for control of side effects. Some amelioration of radiodermatitis during breast irradiation following lumpectomy has been observed in a randomized controlled trial using potencies of belladonna and x-ray (Balzarini, Felisi, Martini, & De Conno, 2000). Others routinely administer a potency of radium or radium bromide isopathically during or after radiation therapy to counteract the presumed deleterious effects of the treatment on the vital force of the organism as a whole (Master, 2000).

The combination remedy Traumeel S has been demonstrated to significantly reduce the severity and duration of chemotherapy-induced stomatitis in children undergoing bone marrow transplantation (Oberbaum et al., 2001). Remedies such as ipecac or tabacum are reasonable considerations for the nausea of chemotherapy, and remedies such as arsenicum or podophyllum may assist with enteritis though many others should be considered.

Supportive care for the emotional aspects of a cancer diagnosis and therapy might be aided by homeopathy (Thompson, 1999). However, it may be difficult to distinguish the effect of the remedy from the effect of the long interviews for remedy selection and subsequent therapeutic relationship with the prescriber that undoubtedly develops. Other sequelae of a cancer diagnosis include limitations in medical therapies for associated conditions. Women undergoing chemotherapy are often thrown into an abrupt menopause. Research is underway to determine whether homeopathy can help with these symptoms (Jacobs, 1999).

# Palliation

Some patients will succumb to their disease. In these cases, the goal is to keep the patient as alert, functional, and comfortable as possible until the very end, when death may come quickly and easily. With homeopathy, this is often possible; however, care of these patients may be very challenging requiring nearly daily attention from the prescriber as the needed remedy may change frequently (Vithoulkas, 1980).

One such case among the author's acquaintances involved a man with disseminated squamous cell carcinoma. The skin had deteriorated to the extent that underlying structures were visible in several areas. Given *pyrogen*, a remedy made from rotten meat, in low (6C) potency, the patient was able to significantly reduce his pain medication, complete a work he was authoring, and enjoy a final picnic on the beach with his friends before his death, which occurred several weeks later than had been predicted (Hescu, personal communication, May 3, 2000). With end-stage cancer, this outcome is often the best for which we can hope.

# Prevention

Grimmer states that in his half-century career, he witnessed no cases of cancer in patients who had undergone homeopathic care for 5 years or more (Currim 1996). Taking one's constitutional remedy generally improves overall energy and emotional and physical health as well as relieving particular local symptoms. When the vital force is strong and the immune system fully functional, the phenomic manifestation of the cancer genotype may be averted. Homeopathy theoretically assists in this capacity; however, large epidemiological studies would be required to demonstrate this claim.

Longitudinal studies of large cohorts of individuals under individualized constitutional homeopathic care should be ideal, but they are potentially confounded by the variable skill of the prescribers in addition to the usual array of factors. Nosode prophylaxis (use of potentized disease material to prevent the disease) is additionally worthy of consideration and may be more easily carried out. It has been successful in infectious disease, for example, protection from smallpox by variolinum—a remedy made from pox fluid (Eaton, 1907). The remedy carcinosinum made from breast cancer tissue might be studied for its prophylactic value in women at risk for this disease. Unfortunately, such studies are unlikely to be undertaken in the current medical politicoeconomic environment.

# Summary

Homeopathy has something to offer at every stage of the cancer disease process. From historical and anecdotal data it appears that the most benefit will be derived when it is instituted as early as possible and continued for health maintenance beyond the apparent cancer "cure" so that the whole person is healed beyond removal of disease. But even in end-stage disease, comfort may be added to the final days.

Much additional research is needed to clarify the process of remedy selection and protocol development. At a minimum, cancer databases should include the homeopathic care rendered so that this can be factored into the assessment of patient outcome.

## REFERENCES

American Institute of Homeopathy. (1921). Vol. 5: 1038.

Balzarini, A., Felisi, E., Martini, A., & De Conno, F. (2000). Efficacy of homeopathic treatment of skin reactions during radiotherapy for breast cancer: A randomised, double-blind clinical trial. *British Homeopathic Journal, 89*(1), 8–12.

Becker-Witt, C., Weißhuhn, T. E. R., Lüdtke, R., & Willich, S. N. (2003). Quality assessment of physical research in homeopathy. *Journal of Alternative and Complementary Medicine, 9*, 113–132.

Belon, P., Cumps, J., Ennis, M., Mannaioni, P. F., Roberfroid, M., Sainte-Laudy, J., et al. (2004). Histamine dilutions modulate basophilic activation. *Inflammation Research, 53*, 181–188.

Burnett, J. C. (2001). Diseases of the spleen. In *Encyclopaedia homeopathica* [Computer software and manual]. Retrieved January 2, 2005, from http://www.archibel.com/homeopathy/encyclopaedia_homeopathica/

Carlston, M. (2003). *Classical homeopathy*. Philadelphia, PA: Elsevier-Churchill Livingstone.

Cazin, J., Cazin, M., Gaborit, J. L., Chaoui, A., Boiron, J., Belon, P., et al. (1987). A study of the effect of decimal and centesimal dilutions of arsenic on the retention and mobilization of arsenic in the rat. *Human Toxicology, 6,* 315–320.

Currim, A. N. (Ed.). (1996). The collected works of Arthur Hill Grimmer, M.D. Norwalk and Greifenberg: Hahnemann International Institute for Homeopathic Documentation, Philadelphia, PA.

Eaton, C. W. (1907). Variolinum. *Journal of the American Institute of Homeopathy, 2.*

Ghegas, V. (1994). *Homeopathic treatment of cancer* [CD]. Amherst, MA: New England School of Homeopathy.

Herkovits, J., & Perez-Coll, C. (1991). Potentised microdoses of cadmium reduce lethal effect of this heavy metal in amphibian embryos. *Berlin Journal of Research in Homeopathy, 1*(2), 93–205.

Hahnemann, S. (1843/1996). *Organon of the medical art* (6th ed.). Redmond, WA: Birdcage Books.

Jacobs, J. J. (1999). Is homeopathy effective for reduction of hot flashes and other estrogen-withdrawal symptoms in breast cancer survivors? *Journal of the American Institute of Homeopathy, 92*(2), 72–77.

Jonas, W. B., & Jacobs, J. J. (1996). *Healing with homeopathy.* New York: Warner Books.

Kreisberg, J. (1996). What is acute? What is chronic? and when?: An ordinary polycrest case with some interesting twists. In S. King, L. Vaughters, & C. Scott (Eds.), *Small remedies and interesting cases: Proceedings of the 1996 Professional Case Conference.* Edmonds, WA: International Foundation for Homeopathy.

Klein, J. (1989). Two cases of cervical dysplasia & a case of cranioopharyngioma. In S. King, L. Vaughters, & C. Scott (Eds.), *Small remedies and interesting cases: Proceedings of the 1996 Professional Case Conference.* Edmonds, WA: International Foundation for Homeopathy.

Master, F. J. (2001a). Homeopathy in cancer. In *Encyclopaedia Homeopathica.* [Computer software and manual]. Retrieved January 2, 2005, from http://www.archibel.com/homeopathy/encyclopaedia_homeopathica/

Master, F. J. (2001b). Tumours and homeopathy. In *Encyclopaedia Homeopathica.* [Computer software and manual]. Retrieved January 2, 2005, from http://www.archibel.com/homeopathy/encyclopaedia_homeopathica/

Montfort, H. (2000). A new homeopathic approach to neoplastic diseases: From cell destruction to carcinogen-induced apoptosis. *British Homeopathic Journal, 89*(2), 78–83.

Oberbaum, M., Yaniv, I., Ben Gal, Y., Stein, J., Ben Zvi, N., Freedman, L. S., et al. (2001). A randomized, controlled clinical trial of the homeopathic medication TRAUMEEL S in the treatment of chemotherapy-induced stomatitis in children undergoing stem cell transplantation. *Cancer, 92*(3), 684–690.

Ramakrishnan, A. U., & Coulter, C. R. (2001). *A homeopathic approach to cancer.* St. Louis, MO: Quality Medical.

Sommerman, E. (1996). Agent orange-induced lymphoma. In S. King, L. Vaughters, & C. Scott (Eds.), *Small remedies and interesting cases: Proceedings of the 1996 Professional Case Conference.* Edmonds, WA: International Foundation for Homeopathy.

Thompson, E. A. (1999). Using homoeopathy to offer supportive cancer care, in a National Health Service outpatient setting. *Complementary Therapies in Nursing and Midwifery, 5*(2), 37–41.

van Wijk, R., & Wiegant, F. A. C. (1998). Homoeopathy and the mammalian cell: Programmed cell recovery and new therapeutic strategies. In E. Ernst & E. G. Hahn (Eds.), *Homoeopathy: A critical appraisal* (pp. 180–187). Woburn, MA: Butterworth Heinemann.

Vithoulkas, G. (1980). *The science of homeopathy.* New York: Grove Weidenfeld.

# 5

**Alternative Therapies
and Practices**

**M**any cancer patients are driven to desperation and the utilization of alternative therapies for which evidence remains elusive (see Chapter 20). There are a variety of alternative therapies for cancer that are relatively well known but have been clouded by controversy. The net result leaves great difficulty in discerning the possible benefits or hazards of these approaches. They are given brief mention in this chapter as illustrations of the challenges inherent in investigating alternative treatments for cancer. Prototypes for controversial therapies are provided by the case of antineoplastons and the case of hydrazine sulfate.

Marc S. Micozzi

## Antineoplastons for Cancer Treatment

The discoverer of antineoplastons, Stanislaw R. Burzynski, earned his MD and PhD degrees together in 1968 from the Medical Academy in Lublin, Poland, at age 24. His research for his doctorate in biochemistry was on peptides, short chains of amino acids that are the building blocks of proteins. Noting that people with chronic kidney failure rarely develop cancer, and that these people have a superabundance of certain peptides in their blood, Burzynski isolated these peptides and they demonstrated antitumor effects; Burzynski named them antineoplastons.

Blood was an inconvenient source of antineoplastons, so Burzynski succeeded in finding them in the urine of healthy humans and gradually identified about a dozen. These simple molecules, many related to phenylacetic acid, were found to activate tumor suppressor genes, that is, those that turn off the activity of oncogenes. Thus the antineoplastons seem to act as a normal control mechanism for cell division, so they are not cytotoxic as are the usual antineoplastic drugs used in cancer chemotherapy (Foye, Lemke, & Williams, 1995). This early work was published in peer-reviewed journals, although many of the early articles were in Polish. Mixtures of these antineoplastons isolated from human urine produced up to 97% inhibition of DNA synthesis and mitosis in neoplastic cells in tissue culture (Burzynski et al., 1976).

Burzynski came to the United States in the early 1970s and worked at Baylor College of Medicine, in Houston, Texas. With others he obtained, in 1974, a 3-year research grant from the National Cancer Institute (NCI). Individual antineoplastons were identified and, by 1980, synthesized. By 1977 he had published a study of the action of antineoplaston A on 21 patients who were considered end stage and untreatable by conventional methods. It was reported that complete remission occurred in 4 cases, more than 50% remission occurred in another 4 cases, and some improvement occurred in another 4 cases. In 2 of the 5 patients who died, there was significant regression of the "neoplastic process," and the deaths were not because of cancer or any toxicity of the treatment (Burzynski et al., 1977). The grant was not renewed.

About this time Burzynski created his own Burzynski Research Institute, in which cancer patients expected to pay for what was correctly labeled as experimental treatment with antineoplastons. Success was claimed to be considerable, especially for brain tumors in children (Burzynski et al., 1999). From the late 1970s to the present, government, state, and medical agencies have questioned the work of Dr. Burzynski's clinic. From the beginning, the prospect was that antineoplaston therapy represented a successful alternative to chemotherapy (Diamond, Cowden, & Goldberg, 1997). Like nutritional supplements, antineoplastons are natural products and should not have been patentable; however, Burzynski obtained the first of several patents in 1984. The NCI had assigned 3 patents on the use of phenylacetic acid for cancer treatment, with Dvorit Samid as the inventor. Burzynski had provided the materials to Samid, with the proviso that phenylacetic acid was among the least effective of the antineoplastons (Haley, 2000).

Attacks on Burzynski, both *ad hominem* and technical, have been directed at him from many sources. Some of the most severe criticisms may be found at www.Quackwatch.com on the page "Stanislaw Burzynski and 'Antineoplastons,'" by Saul Green, PhD, as accessed on October 31, 2001. More serious is the fact that the U.S. Food and Drug Administration (FDA) brought Burzynski to trial several times. Neither patients nor relatives of a deceased patient would testify against Burzynski. The Burzynski Patient Group (www.burzynskipatientgroup.org) appealed to legislators, the NCI, and the FDA and raised money for Burzynski's defense. In addition, the patient group sent antineoplastons across state lines to other needy patients (Elias, 2001).

The NCI had clinical trials of antineoplastons that produced negative results (Diamond et al., 1997; Haley, 2000). After 20 years of struggle, along with publications of many more articles in peer-reviewed journals, Burzynski was asked why he did not leave the United States; he replied that the science would prevail.

According to Green, even Burzynski's claim to a PhD is questionable; Green wrote on his website that

Burzynski attended the Medical Academy in Lubin [sic], Poland, where he received an M.D. degree in 1967 and a D.Msc. degree in 1968... An official from the Ministry of Health in Warsaw informed me that when Burzynski was in school, medical schools did not give a Ph.D.... Faculty members from the Medical Academy at Lubin [sic] informed me that Burzynski received his D.Msc. in 1968 after completing a one-year laboratory project and passing an exam and that he had done no independent research while in medical school... In 1973, when Burzynski applied for a federal grant to study "antineoplaston peptides from urine," he identified himself as "Stanislaw Burzynski, M.D. D.Msc."

In fact, reacting to an article in the *Journal of the American Medical Association* by Green, Burzynski sent the *Journal of the American Medical Association* a sworn statement from the president of the Medical Academy of Lublin confirming Burzynski's PhD in biochemistry and MD with honors (Burzynski, 1993; Haley, 2000). Robert G. Houston, a medical writer, wrote in a letter to the *Journal of the American Medical Association* that, "... Contrary to Green, I found Burzynski's doctoral dissertation in biochemistry listed in the bibliography that Green claims omits it" (Houston, 1993). Contrary to Green's assertions, an online search turned up 11 publications on research by Burzynski from 1964 to 1970, many in Polish.

On the technical side, Green wrote the following: "Tracing the biochemistry [sic] involved in Burzynski's synthesis of antineoplastons shows that the substances are without value for cancer treatment."

By 1985, Burzynski said he was using eight antineoplastons to treat cancer patients. The first five, which were fractions from human urine, he called A-1 through A-5. From A-2 he made A-10, which was an insoluble derivation of phenylacetic acid. He said A-10 was the anticancer peptide common to all his urine fractions. He then treated A-10 with alkali, which yielded a soluble product named AS-2.5. Further treatment of AS-2.5 with alkali yielded a product he called AS-2.1. Burzynski is currently treating patients with what he calls AS-2.1 and A-10.

In reality, AS-2.1 is phenylacetic acid (PA), a potentially toxic substance produced during normal metabolism. PA is detoxified in the liver to phenylacetyl glutamine (PAG), which is excreted in the urine. When urine is heated after adding acid, the PAG loses water and becomes insoluble. Normally, there is none of this insoluble product in human urine.

What Burzynski calls A-10 is really an insoluble product, treated with alkali to make it soluble. However, this does not create a soluble form of A-10. It simply reinserts water into the molecule and regenerates the PAG (Burzynski's AS-2.5). Further treatment of this with alkali breaks it down into a mixture of PA and PAG. Thus Burzynski's AS-2.1 is nothing but a mixture of the naturally occurring substances PA and PAG.

Burzynski claims that A-10 acts by fitting into indentations in DNA. But PAG is too big as a molecule to do this, and Burzynski himself has reported that PAG is ineffective against cancer.

Phenylacetic acid may not be safe. In 1919, it was shown that PA can be toxic when ingested by normal individuals. It can also reach toxic levels in patients with phenylketonuria (PKU); in pregnant women, it can cause the child *in utero* to suffer brain damage.

Clinical effectiveness of substances for cancer is not always related to a complete understanding of their biochemistry. Furthermore, the syntheses were by standard laboratory reactions, not biochemical ones (Burzynski, Mohabbat, & Lee, 1986). From the structures of antineoplaston A-10 and the DNA-intercalating agent Doxorubicin, "the most important anticancer drug available" (Foye et al., 1995), it appears obvious that A-10 (also called PAG) is not too big to fit into (intercalate) with DNA.

According to the *Merck Index*, phenylacetic acid is used as an analgesic, antirheumatic, and urinary antiseptic. Its sodium salt has been approved for human use by the FDA for treatment of hyperammonemia (Burzynski, 1993). Its LD50 lethal dose in mice is 2,710 mg/kg (Burzynski et al., 1986). By comparison from the *Merck Index*, 9th ed., the common antineoplastic drug vincristine has an LD50 lethal dose in mice of 2 mg/kg; this would extrapolate to just 100 mg as the fatal dose for a human.

Green finally states: "Burzynski has never demonstrated that A-2.1 (PA) or 'soluble A-10' (PA and PAG) are effective against cancer or that tumor cells from patients treated with these antineoplastons have been 'normalized.'" Tests of antineoplastons at the National Cancer Institute have never been positive. The drug company Sigma-Tau Pharmaceuticals could not duplicate Burzynski's claims for AS-2.1 and A-10. The Japanese National Cancer Institute has reported that antineoplastons did not work in their studies. No Burzynski coauthors have endorsed his use of antineoplastons in cancer patients. These facts indicate that Burzynski's claims that his antineoplastons are effective against cancer are not credible.

On the contrary, Burzynski has reported promising clinical results with AS2-1 in refractory cancer of the prostate (Burzynski, Kubove, & Burzynski, 1990), and with synthetic A10, and with both in primary brain tumors (Burzynski et al., 1999). According to Robert G. Houston, the NCI saw results of antineoplaston treatments in seven cases and concluded that antitumor responses occurred (Houston, 1993). In a press release, the NCI stated that these were the only patients who had benefited and that Burzynski had sent the NCI incomplete information and when NCI-sponsored trials were done, the patients selected by the NCI were much more advanced and sick than the one Burzynski had agreed to have treated. The NCI used lower doses than Burzynski advised and withdrew two improving patients (Diamond et al., 1997).

The presence of coauthors with Burzynski in at least 11 articles in peer-reviewed journals on the use of antineoplastons in cancer patients seems to contradict Green's assertion. These authors include B. Burzynski, A. B. Conde, J. P. Daugherty, R. Ellithorpe, O. P. Kaltenberg, E. Kubove, M. C. Liau, M. P. Mohabbat, C. H. Nacht, A. Peters, B. Saling, Z. Stolzman, B. Szopa, and M. Szopa.

Antineoplastons do not work all the time—nothing does. But there are enough data and case histories to demonstrate that these medicines may represent a breakthrough (Haley, 2000). A complete summary of results on all of the 650 evaluable patients given antineoplastons is available and shows positive responses in about half the cases (Elias, 2001). For Dr. Burzynski's 3,000 patients, and among alternative physicians, the treatment is gaining respect and credibility (Diamond et al., 1997).

Following raids by the FDA on Burzynski's clinic, confiscation of many of his records, nuisance suits by Aetna Insurance Co., clinical trials by the NCI, an attempt to steal patent rights, and several criminal trials, Burzynski's research continues. Congressional hearings have resulted in fewer restrictions imposed on Burzynski in recent years. However, it is still difficult for patients to obtain treatment with antineoplastons.

# Hydrazine Sulfate

Most conventional therapies are developed systematically with research on animals and small numbers of humans being carried out before they are made available on a widespread basis. Unconventional therapies, in contrast, are often used extensively by the public before research is undertaken to determine the way in which they work (mechanism of action), their safety and their effectiveness (whether they work). Hydrazine sulfate is one of only a few unconventional therapies that was developed in a way that more closely parallels the development of conventional therapies in that a probable mechanism of action was identified and some animal research was carried out before it was made available to patients.

The principal proponent of hydrazine sulfate is Joseph Gold, an American research oncologist, with the Syracuse Cancer Research Institute. Gold was impressed with the research of Otto Warburg, a Nobel prize winner in 1931 who had developed the theory that a major distinction between cancer cells and normal cells is that normal cells obtain their energy through the metabolism of glucose largely aerobically (in the presence of oxygen), whereas cancer cells obtain much of their energy anaerobically (in the absence of oxygen) (Warburg, 1956). When cells function anaerobically, the breakdown of glucose is incomplete and the intermediate products are rebuilt into glucose through a process known as gluconeogenesis—a process that requires a great deal of energy. Dr. Gold's experiments led him to believe that an enzyme, phosphoenol pyruvate carboxykinase (PEP-CK), was critical to gluconeogenesis and that if this enzyme could be blocked the energy-wasting process of gluconeogenesis would be diminished. He considered that this would reduce the severity of cachexia (Henderson & LePage 1958)—the marked lost of body weight and muscle mass often associated with advanced cancer.

Gold then tested a number of chemicals, including the drug L-tryptophan and hydrazine sulfate, in an effort to identify an agent that would inhibit PEP-CK. He found that hydrazine sulfate was the most effective agent for inhibiting PEP-CK, but he noted that it was also an MAO inhibitor (a class of drugs that effect the nervous system and are used to modify mood). As a result of further experiments, Dr. Gold proposed the use of hydrazine sulfate in the treatment of cancer specifically to prevent cachexia. He reported that cancer patients receiving hydrazine sulfate experienced improved appetite, reduced weight loss, and improved survival. It should be noted that other researchers and scientists consider that the mechanisms of cachexia are complex involving more than a disorder of glucose metabolism resulting from cancer cells deriving their energy anaerobically. A prevailing theory is that cachexia results from a combination of metabolic abnormalities, particularly abnormal lipolysis (metabolic breakdown of fat), that are caused by substances called cytokines released by both the body and the tumor as well as from a decrease in food intake. Lipolysis is not affected by hydrazine sulfate.

Gold (1968, 1974) reported antitumor effects, specifically the inhibition of tumor growth, associated with the administration of hydrazine sulfate and recommended it for patients with breast, colorectal, ovary, lung, and thyroid cancers; Hodgkin's and non-Hodgkin's lymphomas; melanoma; and neuroblastoma. Gold recommended that hydrazine sulfate be used in conjunction with any conventional therapeutic agents that were otherwise deemed to be appropriate for the patient. He believed that hydrazine sulfate in combination with these agents would result in an enhanced effect.

Hydrazine sulfate is usually administered by mouth or by injection. Gold's recommended protocol for the administration of hydrazine sulfate is a cycle of 60 mg four times daily for 3 days, 60 mg two times daily for 3 days, followed by 60 mg three times daily for the next 30 to 45 days. The treatment is then discontinued for 2 to 6 weeks before the cycle is repeated. If hydrazine sulfate is taken by mouth it should be taken with a meal. Gold cautions that because hydrazine sulfate has been shown to be an MAO inhibitor, individuals using it should follow the advice usually given to patients using this type of drug, specifically the consumption of hard cheeses should be avoided. In addition, tranquilizers, barbiturates (drugs often used to induce sleep or control epilepsy in cancer patients), or alcohol should not be used in conjunction with hydrazine sulfate.

Hydrazine sulfate can be obtained as 60-mg capsules or in vials for injection containing a solution of 60 mg hydrazine sulfate in each 15 ml. The patient must be under medical supervision.

The costs associated with the administration of hydrazine sulfate are not covered by public or private health insurance. In the United States, hydrazine sulfate has been available to physicians through the Investigational New Drug (IND) program of the U.S. Food and Drug Administration. Hydrazine sulfate is more widely used in Europe, especially in Russia, where it is known as Sehydrin.

Hydrazine sulfate, and its parent chemical, hydrazine, are well-known industrial chemicals used in refining certain metals and as a component of rocket fuel, insecticides, and rust-prevention agents. Industrial quality hydrazine sulfate can be obtained from industrial sources for laboratory research.

The adverse side effects of hydrazine sulfate, when taken as recommended by Gold, have been reported as mild and transient. About 5% to 10% of patients taking hydrazine sulfate complain of nausea, vomiting, anorexia (loss of appetite), pruritis (itching), dizziness, drowsiness, excitation, impaired motor function, or numbness of the extremities. However, convulsions have been noted and one study reported significant neurological toxicity with peripheral neuritis (inflammation and loss of function of nerves in the arms or legs). Liver damage may result from very high doses (i.e., over 80 mg/kg as compared to a therapeutic dose of about 3.5 mg/kg/day).

Some clinical studies have demonstrated that adverse interactions may result if hydrazine sulfate is taken in combination with alcohol, sedatives, or tranquilizes and may lead to increased toxicity and decreased effectiveness of the drug. It is for this reason that proponents advise that these substances should be avoided.

Although there is no evidence that hydrazine sulfate produces any teratogenic effects (abnormalities in the embryo or developing fetus), studies have shown that some other hydrazine derivatives cause teratogenic effects in as many as five animal species. For this reason it would be prudent for pregnant women to avoid the use of this agent.

With respect to cachexia, several laboratory studies have shown that hydrazine sulfate does inhibit the enzyme PEP-CK and thus the process of gluconeogenesis. Some clinical studies have reported a positive effect of hydrazine sulfate in reducing weight loss associated with advanced cancer, especially when used in conjunction with other drugs such as pentoxifylline and megestrol acetate. Other studies report no significant effect.

Animal studies of the possible antitumor effect of hydrazine sulfate were conducted by Gold using rats with transplanted tumors. He described positive effects and also showed, in animal studies, that hydrazine sulfate appeared to enhance the effect of other conventional cancer chemotherapeutic agents.

Since the 1970s, there have been many reports of the effects of hydrazine sulfate in cancer patients. Most of these reports describe the response of individual patients to the administration of hydrazine sulfate. These anecdotal reports have included individuals with advanced cases of cervical, lung, and colorectal cancers, as well as neuroblastomas and lymphomas. Anecdotal reports are useful in generating hypotheses for further research but they are not sufficient for any scientific assessment of the effectiveness of hydrazine sulfate as an antitumor agent.

Subjective and objective evidence of antitumor effects have been observed by Gold (1968, 1974) as well as several Russian researchers observing a series of patients treated with hydrazine sulfate. Some of these studies have reported increased survival rates as well as improvements in appetite and general well-being. One U.S. study reported that hydrazine sulfate increased survival in end-stage lung cancer patients. Other researchers have found no improvement in survival that could be attributed to the use of hydrazine sulfate among patients with cancer. Once again, although these reports are interesting they were not conclusive, although they were not randomized and controlled studies.

However, there have been a number of randomized controlled clinical trials of the use of hydrazine sulfate, mostly conducted in Russia. One of these studies showed significantly improved clinical outcomes—weight gain, increased appetite, pain relief, and tumor regression—among patients treated with hydrazine sulfate when compared with similar patients that received conventional therapy. These improvements were most evident in patients with neuroblastomas.

In the United States, there have been four recent randomized controlled clinical trials of the use of hydrazine sulfate. One study found that hydrazine sulfate was associated with increased survival in patients with lung cancer and three reported no benefit of hydrazine sulfate as a cancer therapy. It was intended that these studies would provide definitive evidence with respect to the effectiveness or lack of effectiveness of hydrazine sulfate. Unfortunately, all three clinical trials had significant methodological flaws and the results were therefore inconclusive.

When hydrazine sulfate is taken as recommended it is usually associated with only mild and transient side effects. However, there have been reports of significant adverse neurological effects and there exists a possibility that it may damage the liver or the developing fetus. Individuals considering the use of hydrazine sulfate should only do so under medical supervision.

There is good evidence that hydrazine sulfate inhibits gluconeogenesis, and thus, it may play a role in reducing the severity of cachexia and in improving the quality of life in cancer patients. However, further research is needed to confirm and quantify these results.

The value of hydrazine sulfate is uncertain as an antitumor agent regarding its capacity to control the rate of growth of tumor cells (tumor stabilization) and to cause a decrease in the size of the tumor (tumor regression) and its effects on overall survival. Many of the observations, particularly in Russia, report beneficial effects of hydrazine sulfate therapy but had methodological flaws. Randomized, double-blind, placebo-controlled studies conducted in the United States showed no benefit from the use of hydrazine sulfate in patients with non-small-cell lung cancer and in advanced colorectal cancer. However, these particular studies also had problems with their methodological design making it difficult to rely on their findings. The use of hydrazine sulfate in cancer has come under serious criticism in the United States and remains controversial (Haley, 2000; Herbert, 1994; Jenks, 1993; Moss, 1999).

# Additional Alternative Treatments

Although not as extensively documented as the foregoing accounts, other selected alternative cancer therapies are discussed herein to illustrate the range of different alternative approaches that have been taken in attempts to address the problem of cancer.

## Cartilage Products

Physician/researcher John Prudden originally set out to determine whether cartilage could assist wound healing. There is now a long list of claimed effects of cartilage preparations that claim to inhibit a wide spectrum of cancers. He has published more than 60 articles on the use of cartilage. Some 50,000 Americans are said to be currently taking shark cartilage at an individual cost of approximately $7,000 or more per year. In 1994, Charles Simone, MD, received IND approval from the FDA for shark cartilage. William Lane, PhD, obtained a use patent on cartilage and published a book entitled *Sharks Don't Get Cancer*. Sharks don't get royalties, either.

## Environmental Medicine

Environmental medicine is an alternative system of medical practice based on the science of assessing the impact of environmental factors on health. It is the result of continuing study of the interfaces among chemicals, foods, and inhalants in the environment and biological function of the individual. Environmental medicine traces its roots to the practice of allergy treatment. In the 1940s, Theron Randolph, the founder of environmental medicine, identified a wide range of medical problems he believed were caused by food allergies.

Cancer is claimed to be caused by a collection of life-style and environmental factors that accumulate over years. Of the 5 million registered chemicals in the world, humans come in contact with over 70,000. Of those, at least 20,000 are known carcinogens. Each year, the United States sprays 1.2 billion pounds of pesticides on food crops, dumps 90 billion pounds of toxic waste in over 55,000 toxic waste sites, feeds 9 million pounds of antibiotics to farm animals to help them gain weight faster, and generally bombards the landscape with electromagnetic radiation. Various environmental toxins potentially lead to the development of cancer, including pollution, pesticides, asbestos, formaldehyde, cigarette smoke, and other common substances found in the immediate environment. Environmental medicine recognizes that illness in the individual can be caused by a broad range of inciting substances, including foods; chemicals found in the home and workplace; chemicals in air, water, and food; and inhalant materials, including pollens, molds, dust, dust mites, and dander. Individual susceptibility to these exposures can vary widely. The response to these exposures over time is specific to each person's own level of susceptibility and can manifest differently from person to person. Therefore, environmental medicine attempts to determine why a particular patient has a particular symptom at a particular time (see Chapter 14 on naturopathy for additional information on environmental medicine).

## Healing Touch

Healing Touch is one of a long line of healing traditions based on the belief in a universal healing energy. Included in these energetic healing techniques are the following: Therapeutic Touch, Polarity, Reiki, Jim Shin Jyutsu, and Reflexology Massage Therapy. The most widely used and accepted are Healing Touch and Therapeutic Touch.

## Immune Augmentation Therapy

According to the Office of Technology Assessment, Immunoaugmentative Therapy (IAT), developed by Lawrence Burton, PhD, is "one of the most widely used unconventional cancer treatments." (see Chapter 20). Burton's theory is that cancer cells multiply when four factors of the immune system fail to recognize and destroy them (see Chapter 20). It has been suggested that tumor antibodies attack the tumor and deblocking proteins remove a "blocking factor" that prevents the patient's immune system from detecting the cancer. Immunoaugmentative Therapy is an experimental form of cancer immunotherapy consisting of daily injections of processed blood products in an attempt to restore normal immune function to the person with cancer. Research has been done to support the efficacy of IAT in mice with leukemia. There has been controversy surrounding possible health risks. In 1985, Burton's clinic in Freeport in the Bahamas was suddenly closed on charges of doses being contaminated with HIV.

## Laetrile

Ernst Krebs, Sr., MD, and Ernst Krebs, Jr., were the developers of laetrile, which is amygdaline, a cyanide-containing compound first isolated from the seeds of pit fruits, such as apricots. The ancient Egyptians, Chinese, Greeks, and Romans all used seed pits, as "sacred seeds" against tumors. Since the 1970s, 70,000 people have used laetrile to treat cancer. Ralph Moss documented the controversy surrounding an alleged cover-up that ended legitimate assessment of laetrile. In 1982 The National Cancer Institute funded a laetrile cancer study that showed that laetrile helped neither cancer nor the symptoms of cancer.

## Neurolinguistic Programming

Neurolinguistic Programming has been shown to provide positive results for patients suffering from a wide variety of serious afflictions, including cancer. The focus of this discipline is to reprogram unconscious thought patterns and behaviors detrimental to the patient's well-being. thus influencing mind-body pathways regulating neurological, hormonal and immune system functioning (see Chapters 4–7)

## Spontaneous Remission

The American Cancer Society's definition of the remission of cancer is as follows:

> . . . a period of time when the cancer is under control. In a complete remission, all the signs and symptoms of the disease disappear. It is also possible for a patient to have partial remission in which the cancer shrinks but does not disappear clinically. Remissions can last anywhere from several weeks to many years. Complete remissions may continue for years and be considered cures. If the disease returns, another remission often can be induced with further treatment. A cancer that has recurred and developed resistance to one anticancer drug or drug combination may respond to different drug regimens.

Norman Cousins reportedly healed himself of leukemia. He spoke of recovery as a two-part system that could be called into active duty by the patient: (1) the healing system and (2) the belief system. His belief was that the healing system is the way the body mobilizes all its resources to combat disease and the belief system is often the activator of "the healing system." In *Spontaneous Remission: An Annotated Bibliography* (coauthored by Caryle Hirshberg), Brandon O'Regan conducted research related to finding evidence of this "healing system" (the spontaneous regression of normally fatal cancers). The bibliography reviews 432 full-text cases of spontaneous remission and 1,574 annotated citations. According to Hirshberg, spontaneous remission is divided into six different categories—no treatment, inadequate treatment, equilibrium, long survival, complementary treatment, and "miracles." Hirshberg identified seven common qualities among patients who experienced a remission.

## Sound Therapy

Pythagoras and Plato both wrote of the healing attributes of sound. Therapeutic sound was first validated in modern times in 1896. Current evidence suggests that the rhythms of the brain, heart, and other organs have a special synchronicity and that disturbances of these rhythms may lead to health disorders (see Chapter 16).

## REFERENCES AND RESOURCES

Burzynski, S. (1993). Letter. *Journal of the American Medical Association, 269*(4), 475.
Burzynski, S. R., Conde, A. B., Peters, A., Saling, B., Ellithorpe, R., Daugherty, J. P., et al. (1999). A retrospective study of antineoplaston A10 and AS2-1 in primary brain tumours. *Clinical Drug Investigations, 18*(1), 1–10.

Burzynski, S. R., Kubove, E., & Burzynski, B. (1990). Treatment of hormonally refractory cancer of the prostate with antineoplaston AS2-1. *Drugs Under Experimental & Clinical Research, 16*(7), 361–369.

Burzynski, S. R., Loo, T. L., Ho, D. H., Rao, P. N., Georgiades, G., & Kratzenstein, H. (1976). Biological active peptides in human urine. III. Inhibitors of the growth of human leukemia, osteosarcoma, and HeLA cells. *Physiological Chemistry and Physics, 8*(1), 13–22.

Burzynski, S. R., Mohabbat, M. O., & Lee, S. S. (1986). Preclinical studies on antineoplaston AS2-1 and antineoplaston AS2-5. *Drugs Under Experimental & Clinical Research, 12*(Suppl. 1), 11–16.

Burzynski, S. R., Stolzman, Z., Szopa, B., Stolzman, E., & Kaltenberg, O. P. (1977). Antineoplaston A in cancer therapy. *Physiological Chemistry and Physics, 9*(6), 485–500.

Diamond, W. J., Cowden, W. L., & Goldberg, B. (1997). *An alternative medicine definitive guide to cancer* (pp. 674–681). Tiburon, CA: Future Medicine.

Elias, T. D. (2001). *The Burzynski breakthrough* (rev. ed.). Nevada City, CA: Lexikos.

Foye, W. O., Lemke, T. L., & Williams, D. A. (Eds.). (1995). *Principals of medicinal chemistry* (4th ed., pp. 822–845). Baltimore, MD: Williams & Wilkins.

Gold, J. (1968). Proposed treatment of cancer by inhibition of gluconeogenesis. *Oncology, 22,* 185–207.

Gold, J. (1974). Cancer cachexia and gluoneogenesis. *Annals of the New York Academy of Sciences, 230,* 103–110.

Haley, D. (2000). Politics in healing: The suppression and manipulation of American medicine (pp. 345–392). Washington, DC: Potomac Valley Press.

Henderson, J. F., & LePage, G. A. (1959). The nutrition of tumors: A review. *Cancer Research, 19*(9), 887–902.

Herbert, V. (1994). Three stakes in hydrazine sulfate's heart, but questionable cancer remedies, like vampires, always rise again. *Journal of Clinical Oncology, 12*(6), 1107–1108.

Houston, R. G. (1993). Letter. *Journal of the American Medical Association, 269*(4), 475–476.

Jenks, S. (1993). Hydrazine sulfate ad is "offensive." *Journal of the National Cancer Institute, 85*(7), 528–529.

Moss, R. W. (1999). *The cancer industry* (pp. 9–19). Brooklyn, NY: Equinox.

Piantadosi, S. (1990). Hazards of small clinical trials. *Journal of Clinical Oncology, 8*(1), 1–3.

Warburg, O. (1956). On the origin of cancer cells. *Science, 123*(3191), 309–314.

Weber, G. (1977a). Enzymology of cancer cells: First of two parts. *New England Journal of Medicine, 296*(9), 486–493.

Weber, G. (1977b). Enzymology of cancer cells: Second of two parts. *New England Journal of Medicine, 296*(10), 541–551.

United States Office of Technology Assessment. (1990). Pharmacologic and biologic treatments. In *Unconventional cancer treatments* (pp. 90–126). Washington, DC: U.S. Government Printing Office.

# Legal and Regulatory Access to Alternative Cancer Treatments

**Alan Dumoff**

## Introduction

Patients facing a cancer diagnosis must confront a wide array of challenges; the spiritual, emotional, and financial struggles and impact on loved ones are never far in the background as patients cope with the ravages of the disease and, for most, aggressive methods of treatment. Patients who do not simply accept their oncologist's recommendations, but seek innovative, complementary, or alternative medical (CAM) treatments, discover a confusing wealth of promise and conflict. Deciding which sources of information are reliable and agonizing over potential therapies and lifestyle changes can be one of the most difficult parts of coping with an uncertain and scary future. As the limitations of conventional oncology are more widely recognized, fewer patients rely solely on their oncologist but rather explore a wide range of CAM approaches or experimental therapies under investigation. Estimates of utilization for patients using physician-based CAM treatments, such as immunoaugmentive therapies, range from 9% to 28%. (Bernstein & Grasso, 2001; Lerner & Kennedy, 1992). When a broad definition of CAM is used that includes self-prescribed herbs, vitamins, or meditation, the number expands to about 80% of cancer patients (Cassileth et al., 1984; Ernst & Cassileth, 1998).

Patients seeking CAM treatments face a sequence of frustrating barriers. Difficulties obtaining reliable, objective information on which to make difficult treatment choices arise not only from the nature of the task and the state of knowledge but also from deeply held professional differences inflamed by vast financial interests. Once a choice to use a CAM therapy is made, many patients discover that these differences of opinion have created a variety of legal barriers that can make accessing these treatments difficult or impossible. Those practitioners seeking to investigate or offer CAM cancer therapies face not only a dearth of resources but also risk professional censure and civil and criminal penalties. Food and Drug Administration (FDA) regulations of drugs and devices can forbid the use of promising therapies or restrict access to clinical trials. The Department of Health and Human Services (DHHS) regulations of Medicare payment can also bar patients directly or through limitations on payment from potentially effective diagnostic methods and treatments. Practitioners must navigate fraud and abuse prohibitions, restrictions on clinical laboratory testing, antikickback measures, and privacy requirements. State restrictions, including those imposed by medical boards, also pose significant risks. And the patients practitioners seek to help, of course, are an ever-present risk in the form of malpractice actions.

Physicians and other practitioners offering CAM treatments face these complex legal challenges, accentuated by closely held differences in theoretical perspectives. These concerns have been addressed in some detail elsewhere (Cohen, 2005; Dumoff, 2004a, 2004b, 2004c). Because regulators focus their efforts where patients are vulnerable, the risks are of particular concern for cancer treatments.

Patients and practitioners have argued in the courts that they should have certain level of freedom to access the therapy of their choice. Seminal cases before federal courts have generally not supported patients' access to treatment based on any hoped for constitutional right of choice. Courts have traditionally deferred to the medical community, not only to their scientific views but also to their views of public policy and the rights of individuals to make choices (Cohen, 1998, 2000, 2003). This deference has created a limited protection, at best, for CAM physicians or the rights of access for their patients.

Given the complexity of evaluating cancer treatments and professional theoretical differences, it is not surprising that the responses of the medical community and regulators have been mixed and, in some cases, seemingly contradictory. Whereas one branch of the FDA was prosecuting Stansilaw Burzynski, MD, for his use of antineoplastins, another branch was assisting him in setting up clinical trials (see Chapter 18). Although the FDA has been largely critical of numerous CAM developments, it has created expedited reviews of investigational new drug (IND) applications and in some cases allowed compassionate INDs (Food and Drug Administration, 1996). When the federal office that oversees laboratory testing (under the Comprehensive Laboratory Improvement Act; CLIA) ruled that live cell blood analysis using dark-field microscopy is an unapproved test that cannot be legally performed, the Office of the Inspector General within the DHHS drafted a public memorandum carefully critical of this decision (Office of the Inspector General, Department of Health and Human Services, 2001).

As Samuel Epstein noted in the late 1970s, "We are not dealing with a scientific problem. We are dealing with a political issue" (Epstein, 1979). As a result, a number of legislative efforts are underway and health policy organizations are trying to tackle these issues. Federal bills that would allow practitioners to use nonapproved treatments with informed consent and limit the FDA's ability to block patients from joining clinical trials have been proposed. State legislation, passed in 15 states so far, offers some protection from medical board discipline for physicians practicing CAM cancer approaches.

Across this health care landscape, this struggle highlights starkly different views about how cancer evolves, how it is diagnosed and treated, methods for studying the value of a therapy, and the relevant endpoints for measuring success. As CAM and conventional efforts have evolved, the differences have perhaps become less dramatic. Investigation of CAM therapies have met with improvements since the advent of the National Center of Complementary and Alternative Medicine (NCCAM) at the National Institutes of Health (NIH). NCCAM provides technical support and funding for clinical studies, explores alternative methodologies appropriate to CAM treatments, and has designated two cancer centers at major medical institutions to act as principle sites for clinical trials: the Johns Hopkins Center for Cancer Complementary Medicine at Johns Hopkins Medical Center and the Specialized Center of Research in Hyperbaric Oxygen Therapy for metastatic cancer treatment at the University of Pennsylvania. Also on the NIH campus, the Office of the Director of the National Cancer Institute (NCI) established the Office of Cancer Complementary and Alternative Medicine in October of 1998. These programs provide technical assistance and research dollars that lend credence as well as support to many of the threads of research and treatment pursued by a variety of CAM practitioners. NCI research has finally suggested possible vindication for some CAM therapies that have been hotly contested. Unfortunately, for those in practice the legal homily remains true that the law is always 10 years behind social changes, with real consequences for those struggling with cancer today.

## Some Historical Notes

Cancer treatments have been controversial since the origins of the organized medical profession, if not since the disease was first recognized. A group of diseases as baffling as they are dangerous, there has been no shortage of creative theories and hopeful efforts reflecting the areas of investigation of the day. Many of these approaches have indeed been outright quackery, as those suffering from cancer are easy targets for scam artists. The proliferation of quack cures in the early 20th century made it even more difficult for legitimate but innovative efforts to gain footing. Differences in views about the etiology of cancer have always reflected deep divisions in the scientific view of biology and health.

The previous century saw a number of hallmark battles that have helped shape the current legal landscape. Some of these battles occurred when federal or state governments restricted practitioners' use of biologic, botanical, or dietary methods of addressing cancer and patients' efforts to access innovative treatments. Other battles have been over research and funding priorities, biases in scientific review and publication, insurance coverage, the right to pain medication, and, perhaps even more disturbing, parental rights to choose therapies for their children.

### Hoxsey and the American Medical Association

In the late 1800s, a farmer noticed that his horse, sick with cancer, sought out unusual herbs and grasses that it didn't ordinarily eat. He experimented with concoctions of these herbs, developing several formulas that his son and then grandson went on to bring to the public in numerous, popular clinics throughout the United States (Chapter 13). In a battle that became intensely personal between Hoxsey and Morris Fishbein, the first editor of the newly formed *Journal of the American Medical Association* (*JAMA*), Hoxsey was painted as the consummate quack, a characterization still made in many circles and in public display at the Smithsonian American History Museum as late as the mid-1990s (Ausebel & Salveson, 1987; Fishbein, 1965).

Hoxsey used a topical treatment for external cancers and an internal elixir for other cancers with some significant successes, acknowledged even by his critics (Ausubel, 1988; *Journal of the American Medical Association*, 1947; Larrick, 1956; Ward, 1990). Like any cancer approach, he had numerous failures as well. Defending his record was a costly process, but he also achieved some successes in his struggle for legitimacy. He sued *JAMA* for defamation and won a jury verdict, in part because of voluminous testimony by patients who believed that his formulas had made a difference. The judge was convinced that the therapy had value but awarded him only token damages. Hoxsey's truer vindication came in the 1990s, when the NCI determined that six of the nine alkaloids in the Hoxsey formula have anticarcinogenic properties. Some critics claimed that Hoxsey resisted clinical trials because he believed the herbs were worthless and painted him as a combative and uncooperative shyster. This claim was belied by Benedict Fitzgerald, a Justice Department attorney who led a government investigation into Hoxsey that began in 1953. Fitzgerald wrote that, to that contrary, it was NCI that "took sides and sought in every way to hinder, suppress, and restrict [The Hoxsey Clinic] in their treatment of cancer" (U.S. Congress Office of Technology Assessment, 1990).

According to medical historian Patricia Spain Ward, who wrote about Hoxsey for the Office of Technology Assessment (OTA), described in some detail below, Dr. Frederick Mohs, a respected surgeon in Madison, Wisconsin, with the help of the Dean of the University of Wisconsin Medical School, developed a topical paste with the same ingredients used by Hoxsey. He used this potion as part of a surgical method that allowed him to isolate and excise suspected tissue in situ. Dr. Mohs published in the *Archives of Surgery* and *JAMA* (Mohs, 1941). During the AMA's assault on Hoxsey's method, the AMA discounted the fact that Mohs's paste and Hoxsey's were identical. As Ms. Ward noted: "Apparently Mohs' use of surgery . . . made his method, in contrast to Hoxsey's, 'scientific' and acceptable. The Council failed to grasp the central fact that both men were using sanguinarine, an alkaloid of bloodroot which has potent anti-tumor properties described in the medical literature as early as 1829." Dr. Ward writes that

> More recent literature leaves no doubt that Hoxsey's formula, however strangely concocted by modern scientific standards, does indeed contain many plant substances of marked therapeutic activity. In fact, orthodox scientific research has by now identified antitumor activity of one sort or another in all but three of Hoxsey's plants and two of these three are purgatives. One of them *(Rhamnus purshiana)* containing the anthraquinone glycoside structure now recognized as predictive of antitumor properties. Between 1964 and 1968 four articles appeared in *Lancet, Pediatrics,* and *Nature,* describing the mitogenic activity of pokeweed, which triggers the immune system by increasing the number of lymphocytes, causing the formation of plasma cells, and elevating levels of immunoglobulin (Ward, 1990).

Hoxsey struggled against the medical establishment his entire career, and then, died of prostate cancer after his own treatment failed him. Hoxsey's battle with the medical establishment is the subject of an award-winning documentary by Kenneth Ausabel, *Hoxsey: When Healing Becomes a Crime* (originally titled *Hoxsey: Quacks Who Cure Cancer?*). To this day, Hoxsey remains a controversial figure, as is the response of the medical community to his treatment.

## Controversy Over Laetrile Research

Another of the early clashes over alternative cancer treatments, one that embroiled major medical institutions, state legislatures, and the Supreme Court in an intense debate, was the use of laetrile, also referred to as amygdalin or vitamin $B_{17}$. In what was hoped to be an effort by established cancer institutes to give a fair evaluation of laetrile, Memorial Sloan-Kettering Cancer Center (MSKCC) in New York and the Mayo Clinic in Rochester, Minnesota, conducted a series of studies over a 5-year period to examine the preventive or tumor-reducing capacity of laetrile. In 1977, MSKCC announced that laetrile had no benefits, a claim that was angrily denied by one of its principle investigators, Kanematsu Sugiura, DSc. Claims were made that data was intentionally manipulated to destroy evidence of laetrile's efficacy. One consequence of these events was the resignation of Ralph Moss, PhD, the public relations director at MSKCC, frustrated over the misrepresentation made about the study data. Dr. Moss wrote a series of books describing the politics underlying disagreements over the management and interpretation of these studies. Data that showed the positive effects in animal studies went unpublished, whereas senior researchers declared to wide publicity that no studies had shown any clinical effect (Moss, 1980, 1989, 1995, 1999).

According to some observers, mice studies at MSKCC demonstrated preventive effects, reduction in organ swelling, and increases in longevity in mice. Human studies demonstrated significant numbers of patients with tumor shrinkages greater that 40%. MSKCC, along with the FDA and the American Cancer Society (ACS), a long-standing critic of CAM cancer therapies, circulated statements flatly claiming that no studies showed any anticancer effects.

Shortly thereafter, the U.S. attorney's office began a grand jury probe against laetrile proponents for smuggling an unapproved drug. The U.S. Supreme Court found in 1979 that terminal patients had no right to access laetrile, and activists in 31 states put legislation on the ballot that would legalize its use. Congressman Dan Burton from Indiana, Chairman of the House Government Reform Committee who held numerous hearings in the 1990s and until 2004 on the barriers faced by CAM treatments, successfully sponsored such legislation when he was freshman in the Indiana General Assembly. Because of these efforts laetrile use for cancer remains legal to this day in Indiana and other states (Indiana Code §§ 16-42-23-1), where interference with use of amygdalin is prohibited by law, MSKCC remains committed to its belief that laetrile has never shown any useful properties in cancer treatment (Cassileth, 2004).

## Dr. Ivy and Krebiozen

Another example of the clash over access to care regards Krebiozen, an alternative cancer formula developed in Argentina by Stevan Durovic, a Yugoslavian physician who brought the formula to the United States in 1949. This caught the attention of Dr. Andrew Ivy, a prominent physician who became convinced that this was an effective treatment. Everything about Krebiozin turned out to controversial; even the nature of the preparation is disputed. Dr. Ivy maintained that it was originally prepared from the blood of horses that had been injected with bacteria. Several federal agencies determined that Krebiozen simply contained mineral oil and creatinine. The FDA determined that there is no scientific evidence that Krebiozen is effective in treating cancer or any other disease, but that it could have dangerous side effects.

Dr. Ivy claimed that Krebiozen stops tumor growth in mice and induces recovery in some people with advanced cancer. Patients on a Krebiozen regime, popular in the 1950s and 1960s, remained on daily injections for the rest of their lives. NCI studied the medical records of 504 cases and found no evidence of anticarcinogenic properties. The FDA determined that the Krebiozen solution contained no creatinine or any substance except mineral oil. Ivy was indicted on a number of criminal charges, including mail fraud, and found guilty but ultimately was acquitted on appeal. As is often the case in such situations, supporters expressed their enthusiasm quite vigorously during this period through protests and sit-ins.

The Krebiozen treatment is the subject of a popular anecdote about the impact of belief on cancer survival that speaks to the interaction of law and treatment. It is said that a man with extensive metastasis went into compete remission under a Krebiozen regime. One day he read that the therapy had been thoroughly discredited. Within months, he was again riddled with cancer. His doctor, who understood the potential impact of the mind over health status, told him that this was mistaken. Within weeks, the man was once again free of cancer. The following year, additional publicity about Krebiozen as a quack cure reached the man, who died within a month.

The mechanism of the placebo effect, and the broader impacts of mental state and belief on health remain mysterious, but there is a great deal of evidence that these impacts are real. The scientific and legal struggle over legitimacy can have unexpected impacts as a result. Policy making should not give false hopes, nor should it unnecessarily dash hopes where the evidence is ambiguous.

## Controversy Over 1990 OTA Report

Responding to demands by patients for a more rational and equitable assessment of CAM cancer treatments, Congress commissioned the U.S. Congressional OTA in 1986 to prepare a report on alternative cancer treatments. The OTA, phased out of existence in 1992, was an independent investigative body that studied the impact of changing technology at the behest of Congress. The OTA had a long-standing reputation for high-quality, independent assessments that was sorely tested when attempting to address the deeply held and emotional differences of opinion about cancer treatment.

Numerous science writers were retained and revised drafts circulated that angered many patients, practitioners, and some of the contract writers of the initial draft. The OTA took the unusual step of allowing public comment in a fiery advisory meeting in March of 1990. Although many in the CAM community felt the OTA had accomplished a significant treatment of the issue that would forward the national conversation, the OTA was broadly criticized for failing to articulate policy approaches that would direct Congress toward increased funding and greater national participation of the CAM voice in developing approaches to cancer. Emotions ran so high during the public meeting that the building had to be evacuated at one point because of a bomb threat (Hildenbrand, 1989–1990). Central concerns were as follows: a perception that OTA supported applying stricter standards of methodology and proof to CAM treatments than to conventional ones, underreported the successes well-known CAM physicians had obtained, overreported the costs of CAM care, and unfairly repeated criticisms without investigation or publication of rebuttals. A frequent professional difference in the field, OTA critics believed the report overly relied on randomized controlled trials (RCTs) as the only reliable method of validation and a failure to support "best case" series as an appropriate means of testing cancer treatments. Critics of the report also argued that the OTA did not appreciate the chilling effect that the legal climate has on legitimate researchers who wish to take innovative approaches to treatment.

One of the contributing science writers of the report, Patricia Spain Ward, PhD, a respected historian of medicine and science at the University of Illinois at Chicago, testified not only before the OTA but also before Congress that the OTA had seriously distorted her writing to downplay the significance of alternative cancer treatments (see box).

These and other criticisms of the OTA report reflect significant concerns that predate the report and continue to this day. The OTA was criticized, for example, for reaching adverse conclusions about therapies without contacting the practitioners researching and delivering that care. The OTA did not contact the Linus Pauling Institute about vitamin C therapy or the Biomedical Hoxsey Center about the Hoxsey remedy (U.S. Congress Office of Technology Assessment, 1990). Testimony at the hearing suggested that when the OTA was unable to find adverse reports on the Hoxsey therapy "the authors resorted . . . to citing toxicity resulting from high doses of individual herbs that are ingredients of the Hoxsey medicines. And arsenic, we are told, can be fatal when ingested, but arsenic is used only topically, and never internally, in the Hoxsey therapy" (Chowka, 1990).

---

*Controversy at the OTA: A Flavor of the Meeting*
The following excerpts from the March 1990 hearing give a flavor of the concerns raised, concerns that remain in the field of CAM cancer therapy.

So I got together five other cases of severe advanced cancer that was medically incurable. Your report breezed over that documentation. I submitted those papers. Those papers were biopsy proven. They were meticulously documented. I submitted them to the *New England Journal*, the *Lancet*, and the *JAMA*, and what did they say? IT IS OF NO INTEREST TO OUR READERSHIP! WHAT KIND OF STATEMENT IS THAT? We looked at eleven cases of prostate cancer. There are 11 cases with the average life of 81 months but that is going. [sic] Most of them are still alive compared to 36 months. And four of those patients, they had complete healing of bone lesions. Do you have ANYBODY? With complete healing of bone lesions? In metastatic prostate cancer, do you have one case? You don't. So why do you ignore what I have? Why do you ignore what macrobiotics or any of these other people can produce. WHAT KIND OF SCIENTISTS ARE YOU? I submit that you are NOT SCIENTISTS. YOU ARE NOT TRUE SCIENTISTS AT ALL.

Vivien Newbold, MD, fellow of the American College of Emergency Physicians (emphasis in original)

I'm somewhat embarrassed as a physician that it took really a response to political pressure instead of scientific zeal to get to this point.

Keith Block, MD

From a report that I had feared being a complete wash out, I think that this report has some balance that I'm pleased with, although a great deal of the writing had some significant negative implications on most of the proponents of unconventional cancer treatments.

Jonathon Collins, an advisor to the OTA and practitioner in Washington State who was an editor of the *Townsend Letter*, a well-established journal of alternative medicine.

Excerpts of transcript, OTA meeting, March 9, 1990

---

*Excerpts of Testimony of Historian and OTA Contributor Patricia Spain Ward, University of Chicago*

My doubts about [the OTA] project grew out of my reading of American medical history. The price we have paid for the professionalization of American medicine is the decline of pluralism in health care. By the time of the Great Depression of the thirties, medical treatments (for cancer or for any other condition) had to secure approval from the American Medical Association or be labeled—and perhaps prosecuted—as quackery.

Over the past half-century the resulting adversarial atmosphere has generated a dreadful chasm between representatives of orthodox medicine and proponents of therapies not yet deemed worthy of acceptance into the conventional fold. I say "not yet accepted," because history offers many examples in which the heresy of yesterday has become the orthodoxy of today: in the words of the great medical historian, Henry Sigerist, "Experience has preceded science in medicine more than once."

By 1987 hostility and distrust so thoroughly pervaded both sides of this chasm, above all in the treatment of cancer, that only an agency of OTA's standing could hope to bridge it.... With the public good as well as OTA's reputation at stake, it saddens me to see that they have failed, apparently because they have not been aware of their own preconceptions.

The authors tell us that "one major reason for wanting to find out whether unconventional cancer treatments work" is the large number of Americans now using them. It was that large number, of course, that initially prompted Congressional demand for this study. The authors do not state—and apparently do not feel—what should, to me, be an equally compelling reason for doing this study: that is, that we need to know whether any of these alternative methods can enhance our none-too-successful track record in the treatment of cancer.

---

These controversies, of course, persist to this day. The government's effort to convict Stansilav Burzynski, MD, medical board sanctions against CAM physicians, denial of claims for coverage of reasonably established CAM approaches, and other difficulties detailed in this chapter are unfortunate highlights in the ongoing struggle for access. By the same token, concerns about potential toxicity, exaggerated claims, and deferred conventional treatments continue to carry real validity. These issues frame the contours of efforts to appropriately integrate CAM therapies into health care delivery.

# Barriers to Access

## Difficulties Accessing Reliable Information

Whether treatment choices made by patients or physicians, or policy choices made by judges or regulators, decisions can only be as good as the information on which they are based. Finding and weighing good information regarding CAM cancer therapies is improving but remains challenging because of the complexity of the science, the politics, and the biases that rule the field.

When a searching inquiry is attempted that goes beyond the views of conventional oncologists, it is quickly discovered that available information is inconclusive at best and contradictory, argumentative, and misleading at worst. Preconceptions about the basis and treatment for cancer predispose interpretation of experimental results, and patients expecting to find helpful information about their choices discover that they are walking into the middle of a vitriolic argument about their disease. The sheer mass of data, the tenor of the argument, and the uncertainty about what all the conflicting data and opinion means, is a very real and frustrating barrier faced by cancer patients. Services that review and condense information about such therapies, such as that operated by Ralph Moss, PhD, are vital links to patients trying to weigh their options.

Should choices be made to use a CAM therapy, patients will likely discover legal, reimbursement, and other barriers that limit their choices. Central to understanding these legal barriers is the recognition that public health officials, legislators, and regulators attempting to make informed judgments in the face of these rancourous disagreements turn to this same body of polarized opinion on which to determine what treatments should be allowed, offered, or reimbursed.

These difficulties arise because of professional disagreement over theories of etiology and methods of patient management. Theories of cancer over the years have spanned a variety of environmental, microbial, immunodysfunctional, and genetic dysregulation and other views of etiology. Whether treatment should directly address these presumed etiologies and target physiological processes such as angiogenesis or immune responses or instead broadly attack cell growth using chemotherapeutic agents or surgical interventions has been a central divide, though a gap that has been shrinking as research advances. Views that were once considered quackery, such as the causative role of immune regulation or the treatment value of autologous vaccines, are now subject to serious research. Current chemotherapeutic and radiation methods of treatment arise from arguably outdated theoretical orientations that remain entrenched, because of institutional reluctance as well as the need for additional development.

The concerns patients have about CAM use can lead to unintended consequences. Patients visiting their oncologists are likely to use various forms of CAM without telling their physician, thus making it more difficult to consider interactive effects and monitor the impacts of treatments for confounding effects. Patients' concern that their efforts will be discouraged or worse by their physicians makes them reluctant to confide in their physicians, a matter of some concern.

*American Cancer Society Operational Statement on Complementary and Alternative Methods of Cancer Management, 2004*

The following is an excert from the American Cancer Society position statement

The American Cancer Society realizes the need to balance access to [CAM] therapies while protecting patients against methods that might be harmful to them. [ACS] supports patient access, but strongly encourages more oversight and accountability by governmental, public, and private entities to protect the public from harm as they seek therapies to complement mainstream cancer care. Harmful drug interactions may occur and must be recognized. Unnecessary delays and interruptions in standard therapies are detrimental to the success of cancer treatment.

*The Pressure Cooker of Oncology Practice: Thoughts on Why Physicians Have Such a Commitment to Conventional Recipes*

When evaluating the mainstream response to CAM therapies, it is helpful to recognize the enormous legal and ethical pressures on physicians to stay within accepted practice. Patients who suffer adverse reactions and poor outcomes have no legal recourse against physicians whose treatment is considered standard of care; malpractice actions can be maintained only where the standards were violated. Physicians thus have a great self-interest in communal agreement and adherence to standards of practice. The commitment to these standards, and to an impassioned defense of the stance that the practices carried on by oncologists are correct, carry enormous emotional weight. Oncologists facing the onslaught of patients, many for whom they have little to offer, must believe that they are providing the best that can be done in the face of their patients' suffering and deaths. For an oncologist to entertain the possibility that they are not providing the best care causes considerable cognitive dissonance. This presents real difficulty for conventional physicians attempting to evaluate therapies arising from unique, nonstandard viewpoints.

## An Alphabet Soup of Opinion: AMA, ACS, NCAHF, and Many More

More than any other area of medicine, the boundaries of accepted practice are patrolled by various medical organizations. The public is informed by the AMA, the ACS, and others whose pronouncements about what therapies are considered safe and effective are generally constrained to conservative, conventional methods of care. The ACS, which pays a lead role in setting standards, has gone through modest evolution. In 1954, it established the Committee on Unproven Methods of Cancer Management, which in 1990 changed its name to the Committee on Questionable Methods of Cancer Management. Although the ACS has aggressively opposed CAM cancer therapies, it has softened some of its language in recent years. The ACS has written that "although many bogus treatments are still being sold to the public, and charlatans continue to promote their 'cures,' there are some nontraditional practices that are well-respected by scientists and the U.S. government believe are worthy of serious study." The ACS notes, however, that the "key word is *study*" (emphasis in original; American Cancer Society, 1971). Alternative methods remain defined as "unproved or disproved methods, rather than evidence-based or proven methods to prevent, diagnose, and treat cancer." This judgment is widely respected and mistranslated as "worthless," creating a vicious circle in which emerging methods cannot obtain funding for research and are crippled in their ability to demonstrate effectiveness or for informed patients to attempt such treatments.

Many historical battles remain entrenched within the ACS review. The ACS lists Hoxsey's treatments as an unproven therapy, though it notes in passing that "a few of the herbs contained in the Hoxsey formula were studied separately and showed some anticancer activity."

Groups such as the National Council Against Health Fraud (NCAHF) take extreme views in opposition to any CAM approach, presuming that treatments that did not originate within NCI and its off-campus research affiliates must be unpromising, if not fraudulent. The NCAHF Web site presents its viewpoint in one of the most thorough compendiums of CAM approaches, written from a position that espouses "zero tolerance" for CAM therapies.

A number of organizations represent specific CAM therapies or the interests of patients seeking CAM therapy. People Against Cancer, The Cancer Control Society, the National Health Federation, the Foundation for Advancement of Cancer Therapies, the Center for Freedom of Choice in Medicine, and many other organizations provide advocacy and support for access to cancer therapies. Patients of many of the more established CAM physicians who have developed their own therapies have organized groups to provide support for patients. These groups, such as the Immuno–Augmentive Therapy Patients' Association, Friends of Dr. Revici, and the Burzynski Patient Group provide information and support for patients. These groups play a vital role in lowering access barriers by educating patients about the nature of therapies, available clinical trials, reimbursement, legal concerns, and other matters patients need to understand. Patients groups have also been quite active in advocating at the federal and state levels for improved freedom of choice and access to CAM therapies. Burzynski patients, for example, have been very effective in assisting the doctor with the FDA by going directly to Congress.

## The War on Cancer and the Battle Over Statistics

It seems no area is without controversy. Even statistics about cancer incidence have sparked debate. One anonymous statistician commented, "I wouldn't be surprised if they are curing a lot of leukemia that never existed" (Greenberg, 1975). NCI reported in June 2001 that there had been an overall decline in U.S. cancer incidence between 1992 and 1998 (National Cancer Institute, 2001). This report was controversial, as critics noted that one of the impacts of such statistics is that it supports the interpretation that medical science is making progress in the "war" on cancer. Yet few cancers, particularly metastatic disease, are amenable to treatment, nor has there been much change in the list of treatable cancers since the "war" was declared in the early 1970s (Moss, 1989).

*Cancer Myths*
Like any struggle in the public mind, the debate over access to CAM therapies involves numerous myths. One such myth is that patients only choose CAM therapies out of desperation and that such choices reflect a depressive and frightened state of mind from which patients need to be protected (American Society of Clinical

Oncology, 1983; Cassileth et al., 1984; Kill, 1988). This is one primary reason given for legal restrictions on access to CAM therapies.

Although it is true that a typical CAM patient has already attempted and failed at least one conventional therapy, patients who choose such therapies are more educated than the general population. The act of making independent decisions to seek CAM approaches is a healthy act that is an active, positive coping mechanism that bodes well for the prognosis and does not suggest poor compliance with conventional treatment (Gordon & Curtin, 2000). Another principle concern of the mainstream cancer community is that patients will defer effective treatment in favor of alternative, unproven approaches. Although there is certainly some reality to this concern, the evidence that patients defer conventional treatment in favor of CAM is weak. Studies provide little support for this view, and most patients instead arrive at CAM physician offices debilitated by both their late-stage cancer and chemotherapy or radiation treatments (Sollner et al., 2000).

Another myth is that all of the therapies used by conventional physicians are in fact proven to be safe and effective. Numerous authors and studies have questioned the value of chemotherapy and radiation treatments for a wide variety of cancers, questioning the efficacy, side effects, methods of research, and interpretation of data (Moss, 1980, 1989, 1995; Bross, 1994; Bross et al., 1996); some criticisms were raised early in the declared war on cancer (Bross et al., 1966). Another way to approach this is to inquire whether oncologists, should they be diagnosed with the cancers that they treat, undergo the therapies they offer (Moore & Tannock, 1988). For example,

> A study was done which shows the majority of oncologists who refer patients for chemotherapy for lung cancer would not themselves take chemotherapy for lung cancer. And in fact if the chemotherapy involved cisplaten. something like 75% of them said they wouldn't take it. But what do these people do all day long? They're sending people for cisplaten. (Moss. 1995)

Another apparent myth is that dietary supplements in some way interfere with chemotherapy. There is evidence for many herbal supplements that they may in fact offer a supportive role, either increasing its cytotoxic ability (Moss, 1989) or protecting the body against the ravages of chemotoxins. A bias against herbal therapies appears to raise a presumption that there is a concern, a presumption that has caused at least one hospital to ban herbal use by its inpatients.

Myths abound among CAM practitioners as well. Some practitioners have such a strong belief in homeopathic remedies, nutritional interventions, various proprietary supplements, or even more arcane remedies, such as colon irrigation, that they believe in such therapies without evidence or even real diagnosis. Much of this belief is predicated on a disdain for reductionist scientific views that discount the more holistic concerns of the role of, for example, immune function, attitude, and lifestyle, on health. Products that agree with these philosophic views can be taken at face value by some without any critical evaluation of their claims. This lack of discernment gives legitimacy to some of the criticisms leveled at CAM approaches, exposes patients to therapies that likely offer insufficient benefit, and furthers the polarization between the two camps.

*Reacting to Medicinal Herbs: The Policy at Children's Hospital of Michigan, Detroit Medical Center*

Although not specifically a matter of oncology, the policy at the Children's Hospital of Michigan to patient use of supplements shows how some health systems are reacting to patient use of herbs. Parents of a child admitted at Children's wanted to continue to provide him melatonin, Valerian root, and algae while hospitalized.

The pharmacy and therapeutics committee reviewed the matter, and although initially favoring patient choice, the health systems' lawyers counseled that the hospital would be liable for reasonably foreseeable problems such as lack of effectiveness, worsening of the underlying medical condition, and potential interactions with conventional therapies and tests. Counsel advised the hospital that informed consent that discloses information about the effectiveness and potential risks associated with alternative therapies would not relieve the health system of liability, given that all potential risks are unknown (Walker, 2000).

This is an extreme position; it is unlikely that the hospital would be held to assume liability for all unknown risks of herbs patients self-prescribe. This presumes courts would adopt an unreasonable burden on the hospital to protect the patients from their own behavior.

# Bias in Research Design, Interpretation, and Funding

The entry requirements for new therapies are very high, and a concern of CAM advocates is that these requirements are higher for CAM approaches than for conventional innovations. This has focused attention on the methods used to evaluate cancer studies, which are evolving but remain controversial.

Research is in some sense at the heart of all obstacles faced in the acceptance of CAM approaches to cancer. Whether a lack of research funding, the rejection of research because of differences of opinion about study design, or wholesale differences in opinion about the nature of cancer, a perceived lack of accepted evidence affects the hospital privileging, insurance reimbursement, medical board and malpractice judgments, and every other part of the legal framework that affects treatment availability. The problem is particularly acute with cancer, as research is presented with unusual differences in about how to document responsiveness to treatment. Choosing the end points for study design alone has been the subject of considerable controversy. The gold standard for study success for some time was the 5-year survival rate, one still used in many studies. For researchers who saw significant reduction in tumor mass over a short span of time, waiting the full 5-year period seemed cruel to patients who could be helped. To more conservative researchers, it was cruel to patients to promise results when it was unclear whether the next years would bring recurrences. For some forms of cancer, tumor shrinkage is an important early sign. Other forms of cancer will respond to various therapies by shrinking, with little effect on long-term survival, so it may be cruel to offer these patients false hopes (Moss, 1995). End points such as tumor shrinkage or other response rates as opposed to long-term survival rates have evolved, in part because of pressures from the

CAM community, but remain controversial. Such complexities make the struggles over deciding which therapies show promise particularly difficult.

The mainstream cancer community continues to set boundaries around what constitutes accepted practice, boundaries that can give rise to personal attacks. More than one well-intended researcher has been labeled a quack, their methods deemed as duping the public. CAM practitioners have fought back with equal vigor, publishing statements about CAM critics that have drawn defamation actions. The temperature of these discussions has cooled in important segments of the community, with centers within NIH/NCI taking a leading role. The ACS and others are more cautious in their statements but remain convinced that most CAM therapies have little to offer but false hopes (Brown, 1986; Murphy et al., 1997).

## Case Study: Barrie Cassileth, PhD, the Livingston-Wheeler Therapy, and Publication Bias

An example of how expectations distort study conclusions involves a journal of no less stature than the *New England Journal of Medicine* (*NEJM*). In an intriguing study comparing the longevity and quality of life of cancer patients treated at the Livingston-Wheeler Clinic, a well-known CAM cancer clinic in San Diego, California, with patients in an oncology clinic at the University of Pennsylvania (Cassileth, 1991), the data showed that the Livingston patients experienced comparable and, in some cases, better longevity than conventional oncology patients (see Chapter 12). The study was conducted by Barrie Cassileth, PhD, currently the director of Integrative Medicine at MSKCC, whose biography notes that she is an "outspoken critic of quack therapies and unproven remedies." In her study, Dr. Cassileth concludes that the Livingston patients' quality of life was worse, a surprising result given the known impacts of surgery, radiation, and chemotherapy. The data in fact showed that each approach had the same effect on quality of life. The misinterpretation arose because the researchers simply compared the posttreatment quality-of-life indexes and found those of the Livingston patients to be lower. Yet, as is often the case given that patients often seek innovative treatments after their quality of life has already suffered, the Livingston group began with a lower quality of life. The data show that the measure declined at the same rate as the conventional comparison group. The proper interpretation of these data is that each intervention had the same impact on quality of life. That the data did not support an adverse conclusion about the Livingston treatment was glaring. A graph published in the article compared the change in quality of life over the course of treatment; the slope of the two lines is identical, graphically demonstrating that they each had the same impact. Yet the conclusion that the Livingston treatment had a more negative impact on quality of life passed peer review muster at *NEJM*. Why? Perhaps it is because the errant conclusion agreed with the expectations of the peer reviewers.

The quality of life was arguably better with the Livingston treatment, as the primary detractor from quality of life in the Livingston study was poor appetite, whereas the Pennsylvania patients had problems with nausea. Although a report of either may yield a similar score on the instrument, nausea is more difficult to endure than loss of appetite. Appetite difficulties may in fact have simply referred to the difficulty sticking to the rather strict Livingston diet.

Other problems existed in analysis; the quality-of-life study, for example, found a highly significant difference at the $p < .001$ level. Such a figure may be misleading because the scale itself is nominal rather than ordinal. Some problems with the study are common to comparisons of CAM and conventional treatment. The design grouped Livingston patients who continued receiving conventional treatments with those receiving only the Livingston treatment in the same cohort. Such cohort confusion is exacerbated because no information is given about overlap between conventional treatments prior to and after enrollment in the program.

Also common to comparative CAM studies, the study used end-stage patients with prognoses of a year or less to live, which acts to select patients who are the least amenable to treatment. This skews the study, especially where the mode being investigated is immunological, whose effects would be predicted to have less power during the end stage of the disease. Despite all these concerns, the Cassileth study has been repeatedly cited as evidence that CAM cancer therapies have a worse impact on quality of life (see, for example, Barrett & Herbert, 2005; Gelb, 2005).

## The Elusive "Level Playing Field": Evaluating Chemotherapy Versus CAM Treatments

When chemotherapy first appeared, it was considered quackery by many physicians (Moss, 1995). This should not be surprising, given the systemic levels of toxicity to which patients are subjected. The evidence that chemotherapy contributes to the control or remission of cancer is itself questionable, and more than one researcher has noted that people with widespread malignancies are being treated with therapies not known to be effective. Some of the major clinical trials testing chemotherapy have been found to be fraudulently biased toward favorable results (Moss, 1989, 1995). This is consistent with the larger problem created by pharmaceutical sponsorship that is much discussed in medical journals (Friedberg et al., 2000; Lenzer, 2004).

Much of the controversy surrounding research revolves around the fit between the methodologies used for a given CAM therapy and the manner in which it is studied. This could be by design, as some have alleged, or because conventional researchers inappropriately apply conventional study designs that do not fit CAM methods, which could generate false negative results. In a study of Linus Pauling's long-term use of high-dose vitamin C therapy, the Mayo Clinic abruptly withdrew patients as soon as there was evidence of tumor progression, when the claim made was of long-term survival. Other criticisms of the study, common to a number of trials of CAM therapies, was an end point requiring an abrupt and rapid response to therapy, an end point that was not claimed for the therapy. When interleukin-2 achieved a minority of responders, it was hailed as a new drug in the fight against cancer, whereas similar numbers for the vitamin C trial resulted in Mayo concluding that there was no effect (Hoffer, 2001). Because CAM studies are so underfunded that they often lack the statistical power to show effects given that a minority response can still be highly significant. This problem is exaggerated when innovative therapies are held to a higher standard of proof.

Another major area of disagreement is the role of RCTs, a design that some CAM researchers believe does not fit the multifactorial nature of cancer and its treatment. Many CAM therapies, for example, are based on the view that a synergistic mix of diet, immune support, and targeted anticarcinogenic actions are needs to gain progress. Some conventional researchers discount such multiple interventions as not subject to proper research, relegating them to the dustbin of "unproven" therapies simply because they do not fit a reductionist model.

In response to criticisms about NCI's overreliance on RCT's, NCI established a Best Case Series Program in 1991 to evaluate data gathered by CAM practitioners who claim success when treating cancer patients outside the context of a formal research trial. The practitioner is asked to submit medical records and primary source materials (such as medical imaging studies and pathology slides) so that NCI can review and assess the overall therapeutic effect of the practitioner's CAM approach. The NCI and the NCCAM then present data from the Best Case Series to the Cancer Advisory Panel for Complementary and Alternative Medicine. The panel reviews the data and suggests whether the approach is worth further exploration and NIH funding.

The best case approach is itself not without controversy. During the OTA review, critics noted that data were frequently rejected by OTA because of negative opinions of orthodox critics. It was argued that reviewers found "flaws" and that favorable results are not even mentioned. The OTA did recommend Best Case Reviews as a way to respond to concerns raised about RCTs, but some in the CAM community noted that many excuses are available to reject documented remissions. NCI has often rejected CAM case reports in the past where the review was not conducted in a blind manner. Blind review or the use of neutral panelists are essential procedures to minimize evaluator bias, especially when an agency has negative positions on a therapy. The climate has improved since the OTA report, and the experience has become more hopeful, but this remains an area of concern.

The Institute of Medicine addressed the issue of research design at length in its 2005 report, *Complementary and Alternative Medicine in the United States*. One of the difficulties with RCTs has been with assigning patients to treatment cohorts randomly because patients often have a strong preference, and researchers have ethical concerns about forcing a patient into a study cohort contrary to their wishes. This is particularly true for cancer patients. IOM stated that observational and cohort studies provide useful data and suggested a number of other study designs, such as outcome tracking (Dumoff, 2005). IOM's report takes a broader view of useful data, reminiscent of the "evidence house" approach of Wayne Jonas, MD, which is composed of six rooms. RCTs are only one way to assess the value of a therapy (Jonas, 2001).

## An Uneasy Truce, Progress Toward an Integrative Conversation

As CAM approaches have gained stature and there is an increasing awareness that some therapies have achieved significant outcomes, a greater level of collegial conversation has begun. One primary meeting ground for physicians and researchers from both the conventional and CAM worlds has been the Center for Mind-Body Medicine's Comprehensive Cancer Care Conference, based on the work of James Gordon, MD., which for 5 years brought the CAM medical world into "productive dialogue with the American cancer establishment." These conferences are cosponsored by the NCI and NIH's NCCAM.

The result of such efforts may continue to be an increasingly improved legal climate for such therapies. Although one may naively wish for a more objective stance, regulators' and prosecutors' attitudes toward practitioners make all the difference in how controversial matters are handled. This is in fact appropriate, as discerning whether a practitioner is taking advantage of patients or truly attempting to help, albeit in an unorthodox fashion, should make a difference in how the legal system responds to a practitioner. The increasing recognition of the value in CAM approaches should create a better climate.

With the establishment of the NCI CAM Office, the NCI is testing the use of some of the most promising CAM therapies against several common cancers, often in collaboration with NCCAM. Trials are underway at Columbia University in New York City to compare the Gonzalez/Kelley regimen of pancreatic proteolytic enzymes plus intense nutritional support with the more conventional chemotherapy for pancreatic cancer (see Chapter 12). Trials have also looked at the safety and efficacy of shark cartilage versus conventional chemotherapy plus radiation therapy for non-small-cell lung cancer and the effect of diet on prostate and breast cancer.

Physicians on both sides of this divide can act from bias rather than from an evaluation of the evidence. Just as conventionally trained physicians may discount a cancer treatment simply because it is based on a nutritional or immunoaugmentive approach, some CAM physicians take to the latest alternative therapy without evaluating its effectiveness or side effects simply because it is consistent with their philosophy. CAM physicians can work through an impressive list of experimental drugs, supplements, and devices as they seek to find the best care for their patients. This can be a legitimate effort to find something where no conventional therapy holds much promise, a rejection of more demanding criteria in the face of such a devastating disease, or, for some, an unwarranted, blind faith in treatments that arise from an alternative viewpoint.

# Judicial Reluctance to Recognize Health Care Freedom

## Consumer Protection Versus Health Freedom

Given the uncertainties about what treatments have value, one might hope that practitioners and patients would have the benefit of the doubt and the ability to make their own choices. Given decisions that reproductive freedom is a fundamental right, one might think that basic decisions about one's own health care would also receive such protection. Although there have been a few remarkable cases supporting such a right, these are exceptions to the legal mainstream. Courts have largely followed the direction of established medicine. The decision to seek an abortion or reject medical treatment, such as heroic efforts at the end of life, is treated with respect for autonomy. Deference to medical judgment continues to overshadow individual choices in between the beginning and ending of life, including dealing with cancer and other vital health issues.

Commentators have argued and hoped that there is indeed a right to choose one's health care treatment, based on a right to privacy. Unfortunately, such a right has not been generally recognized. Instead, struggles over access reflect a number of public policy concerns. Although the evidence for the proposition is weak, critics of CAM therapies are concerned that patients will forego viable conventional treatments while chasing unproven therapies. This is a concern that varies widely by type of cancer. Where particular cancers are amenable to treatment, this is a real concern. Seymour Brenner, MD, while testifying in favor of greater research openness to what he saw as important CAM therapies before the OTA, provided this important counterpoint:

> The only thing I didn't say, and I would like to stress, that we should also tell alternative clinic directors, don't see a patient, for example, I saw patient at one of these clinics that had a stage I breast cancer, a young girl thirty-two years old. A stage I breast cancer treated in a standard fashion today has a 96.5% cure rate. Therefore, they should be told, and somehow we should find a way to implement this, that they should not treat patients who are curable on standard methods. (U.S. Congress Office of Technology Assessment, 1990)

Given the advances that have been made in the conventional treatment of breast cancer since 1990, this statement is even more true today. As the following section makes clear, however, the judicial system treats CAM therapies as if this is always the case.

## Judicial Deference to Conventional Medical Wisdom

Historically, the legal profession has shown great deference to the medical profession in virtually every context. Whether testimony in malpractice actions, ethical dilemmas about the beginning and ending of life, or even social ills, courts rely on their learned, sister profession of medicine and are loath to substitute their judgment for those of medical academia. A classical example of this difference is that of child abuse. Prior to 1962, harsh and abusive discipline was recognized as a social problem, but the courts considered the right of the family to its own beliefs about discipline to be primary. Then an article appeared in the *JAMA* entitled "The Battered Child Syndrome" (Kempe, Silverman, Steele, Groegemuller, & Silver, 1962). This single article converted a community dilemma into a medical condition with a name and is credited with beginning the rapid transition of child abuse from a socially off-limits topic to a recognized medical syndrome openly addressed by society (Pfohl, 1977). This deference to the medical profession reaches legislators as well as judges; within 4 years, all 50 states had laws penalizing child abuse. The deference afforded physicians regarding cancer therapies is no different. As a result, courts have in almost every instance imposed the majority view of physicians, even over the rights of patients to make their own choices about their health.

## The Supreme Court Weighs In: U.S. Versus Rutherford

The issue of whether patients have a right to access the treatment of their choice reached the United States Supreme Court in a class action suit in *United States v. Rutherford* (1979) (Note, 1981). The 10th Circuit Court had ruled that FDA requirements that a drug has to be demonstrated safe and effective has no reasonable application to patients without hope of recovery. The court ordered the FDA to allow laetrile to be available for administration by physicians to terminally ill patients. In an opinion written by Thurgood Marshall, the Supreme Court reversed that decision and held that terminally ill patients had no right to obtain laetrile against FDA requirements that new drugs be approved pursuant to the Food, Drug, and Cosmetic Act (FDCA)(21 U.S.C. § 355), which prohibits the interstate distribution of any "new drug." This decision came in the midst of a public battle resulting in 17 states legalizing laetrile for their citizens, which stood after *Rutherford*. These laws were remarked on by the court, but the will of the citizenry is not an issue before the Supreme Court.

The plaintiffs argued that their rights grew out of their terminal status, removing them from ordinary regulatory considerations about whether products offer safe and effective treatment. Much of the case grappled, therefore, with the meaning of "terminal illness." Because those patients, by definition, would "die of cancer regardless of what may be done," the Court of Appeals concluded that there were no realistic standards against which to measure the safety and effectiveness of a drug for terminal patients. The Court of Appeals on that basis ordered the FDA to allow use of laetrile by cancer patients certified as terminally ill.

In reversing, the Court found that terminal patients also require the protection of the drug approval process. Congress had expressed concern during its passage of the FDCA that individuals with fatal illnesses such as cancer should be shielded from fraudulent cures. The Court said:

> If history is any guide, this new market would not be long overlooked. . . . resourceful entrepreneurs have advertised a wide variety of purportedly simple and painless cures for cancer, including liniments of turpentine, mustard, oil, eggs, and ammonia; peat moss; arrangements of colored floodlamps; pastes made from glycerin and limburger cheese; mineral tablets; and "Fountain of Youth" mixtures of spices, oil, and suet. . . . In citing these examples, we do not, of course, intend to deprecate the sincerity of Laetrille's current proponents, or to imply any opinion on whether that drug may ultimately prove safe and effective for cancer treatment. But this historical experience does suggest why Congress could reasonably have determined to protect the terminally ill, no less than other patients, from the vast range of self-styled panaceas that inventive minds can devise.

With these concerns, it may be less surprising that a privacy right to choose one's treatment from a diverse array of modalities has not been widely adopted by the courts. The Court accepted the widely made argument that if an individual suffering from a potentially fatal disease rejects conventional therapy in favor of a drug with no demonstrable curative properties, the consequences can be irreversible. The counterargument that a terminally ill patient by definition faces no real possibility of reversal was not accepted by the Court, as "[e]ven critically ill individuals may have unexpected remissions and may respond to conventional treatment. . . . " so that we must use only proven remedies with those considered terminal and to do so otherwise "would lead to needless deaths and suffering among . . . patients characterized as 'terminal' who could actually be helped by legitimate therapy." The Court noted that "no one can prospectively define the term 'terminal' with any accuracy." A patient can thus, in the literal eyes of the law, "be said to be terminal only after he dies."

The Court cited congressional concerns about effectiveness as so overriding that "[a]n otherwise harmless drug can be dangerous to any patient if it does not produce its purported therapeutic effect," even in a context where conventional medicine has nothing to offer. It is important to recognize that the deference granted to the medical community is so great that even treatments it believes will not help—these patients were conceded to be beyond the reach of available treatments, after all—are still presumed to have sole legal standing, whereas the CAM treatments, whatever the evidence, cannot be chosen by patients.

Case law grows out of the facts of the cases and the manner in which argument evolves through the courts. In this case, the FDA had found some evidence that laetrile was toxic when consumed orally, making a case for regulatory protection. Critically, the essential right to make medical choices, grounded in a constitutional right of privacy and self-determination, were not raised in *Rutherford*. Although the District Court had held that FDA regulations did indeed impinge on such a freedom, the Court of Appeals' decision focused on whether prior approvals for safety and effectiveness made any sense in the context of terminal patients. The question presented to the Supreme Court was thus narrowed and the larger question never reached.

## Roe Versus Wade

The constitutional right of privacy, established in the 1973 *Roe v. Wade* ruling, written by the late Supreme Court Justic Harry A. Blackmun, *Griswold,* and other cases involving reproductive rights, has never been held to extend to the right to practice unorthodox medicine or for a patient to access the care of their choice. Given that privacy rights are recognized for reproductive freedom, but not for medical choices, a reading of *Roe v. Wade* and other cases that established privacy rights to contraceptive choices offer some surprising guidance. The language in these cases suggest that the Court was not as impressed with the right of a woman to have an abortion as it was distressed at the idea that the State would have the right to impose on the medical judgment of the physician. This reaction by the Court is consistent with the great deference with which courts have treated the judgments of medical physicians in virtually all areas of the law. This deference has been a significant source of the difficulty faced by CAM providers, as the courts turn to the very profession whose professional bodies have opposed CAM approaches for guidance in how these matters should be addressed. This explains why *Rutherford* and *Roe* are actually consistent; neither really address the rights of the patient. What they each do is support and protect the rights of the mainstream physician community.

## Other Cases

Some of the best language supporting a right to access the cancer therapy of one's choice also arose in the laetrile debate and has been quoted by some writers as evidence that the courts recognize such a right. This language is from the Supreme Court of California, which weighed in while *Rutherford* was pending before the United State Supreme Court. Judge Bird, herself a cancer survivor, wrote:

> Cancer is a disease with potentially fatal consequences; this makes the choice of treatment one of the more important decisions a person may ever make, touching intimately on his or her being. For this reason, I believe the right to privacy, recognized under both the state and federal Constitutions, prevents the state from interfering with a person's choice of treatment on the sole grounds that the person has chosen a treatment which the state considers "ineffective." (*The People v. Priviteria, Jr.,* 1979)

Unfortunately, this language was from the dissenting opinion. The majority of the Court held that "the asserted right to obtain drugs of unproven efficacy is *not* encompassed by the right of privacy embodied in either the federal or the state Constitutions." It is significant that *Priviteria* was postured differently than *Rutherford*, as the right to privacy was raised as a defense to a criminal prosecution of the physician rather than a class action on behalf of terminal cancer patients. One consequence of this posture is that in *Priviteria*, unlike *Rutherford*, the assertion that there is a constitutional right of privacy that encompasses a right to choose one's medical treatment. The Supreme Court of California, the highest court to squarely address this question, said no. This is all the more remarkable because California's Constitution has a more clearly delineated right of privacy than in the U.S. Constitution, one that was found to mandate state funding of medically necessary abortions, *Committee to Defend Reproductive Rights v. California* (1981). Yet even in the face of this language, California found no right to laetrile treatment under the state constitution as well.

One remarkable exception to these rulings was *Andrews v. Ballard*, in which the District Court in Texas found a statute restricting acupuncture to only the hands of medical physicians unconstitutional, finding that the right to privacy includes the right to access the health care of one's choice. Much of the court's reasoning was based on those cases in which patients have been found to have a right to accept or decline treatment; the court saw the choice of the type of treatment to be a logical consequence of these holdings. Although there have been some other cases supporting such a right [see, e.g., *Rogers v. State Board of Medical Examiners* (1979)], most courts have declined to follow *Andrews*.

---

Nothing is more disturbing . . . than the spectacle of government power being used to arrest, harass, chasten, and destroy physicians and researchers who, by adopting so-called alternative or unorthodox or unproven approaches, are only trying to help their patients. The vicious system which, on the one hand says "we cannot cure you", and on the other hand says, "but don't try some unproven remedy" and warns you always not to sneak off to Tijuana, must come to an end. It is blatantly immoral. Michael Culbert, Committee for Freedom of Choice in Medicine, at the OTA hearing.

---

*The Ninth Amendment Offers No Protection*
One hope in the fight for medical freedom lay in the Ninth Amendment to the United States Constitution, which provides that:

The enumeration in the Constitution of certain rights shall not be construed to deny or disparage others retained by the people.

The argument that the right to seek the health care of one's choosing was a fundamental constitutional right under the Ninth Amendment was advanced by Conrad LaBeau, who argued that this right is one "retained by the people." Unfortunately, courts have unequivocally ruled that the argument for medical freedom based on the Ninth Amendment has no legal merit. Mr. LeBeau lost the argument when he used it as a defense against food and drug law violations for selling herbal remedies. In *U.S. v. Vital Health Products* (1992, 1993), the court ruled that the Ninth

Amendment does not contain within it a right to choose one's medical treatment. The only rights courts have found within the meaning of the amendment are those that survive scrutiny of the "'traditions and [collective] conscience of our people' to determine whether a principle is 'so rooted [there] . . . as to be ranked as fundamental'" [*Griswold v. Connecticut* (1965) (J. Goldberg, concurring)].

The Ninth Amendment is unfortunately interpreted in a very narrow sense; those few accepted rights must be demonstrated to be at the core of common conceptions of freedom. Although those seeking alternatives to Western care would certainly rank such freedom as fundamental, the courts limit "retained" freedoms to such clearly, fundamentally, and universally held beliefs as the right to have a family, or, as in *Griswold* and its protection of birth control dissemination, to decide when to have a family. Although even this language would seem to sweep in such a basic right as health care choices, the fundamental nature of this right has essentially been trumped by medical opinion. Implicit in these judicial views is a sense that professional views of health choice are so encompassing that they override autonomous choices about one's own health.

The judicial opinions rejecting the Ninth Amendment as a constitutional right to medical freedom are consistent with a vast and definitive array of case law that allows states the greatest possible latitude when protecting public health. Potential rights under the Ninth Amendment must be balanced against the Tenth Amendment, which reserves all nonenumerated powers to the states; this includes the so-called police power, which allows the states virtually exclusive power to regulate matters of public health and safety. The state's police power will almost always outweigh a call to what practitioners and clients alike might hope to see in the shadows of the Ninth Amendment.

*A Bright Spot: Choosing Therapy Where Informed*
The doctrine of informed consent is one that arises from a recognition that one has a right to control what happens to one's own body. It was noted by Judge Benjamin Cardozo, who later ascended to the Supreme Court, as long ago as 1914 in *Schloendorff v. The Society of the New York Hospital*. Underlying principles of informed consent is the view that a doctor performs an assault if a treatment is performed without the consent of a patient fully appraised of the risks. It does not directly allow access to alternative treatments, but a patient's signature on an informed consent form that explains the procedure, its status as a nonconventional treatment, its risks and benefits, and the nature of other treatments that could be attempted does provide some protection not only for informed consent but also against actions in malpractice and can help against regulatory disagreements.

The informed consent doctrine offers malpractice protection because the patient is presumed to assume the risk of those harms for which they have been warned. One well-known CAM cancer treatment was tested when Immanuel Revici, MD, offered his nonconventional treatment for breast cancer to a patient who had been advised by numerous doctors to undergo a biopsy. She refused, sought Dr. Revici's treatment, and after the tumor increased in size and metastized the plaintiff underwent a bilateral mastectomy at Memorial Sloan-Kettering. She sued him for fraud, premised on Dr. Revici's alleged promise to cure Mrs. Schneider of breast cancer, as well as malpractice and a claim for lack of informed consent. An appeals court found that the jury should have been instructed that the consent form constituted an express assumption of risk. [*Schneider v. Revici, M.D., and Institute of Applied Biology, Inc.* (1987)]. The jury found that Mrs. Schneider was equally responsible for the damages she suffered.

It is important to note that good basic medical practice is always an important part of such defenses. In addition to the informed consent form, Dr. Revici documented that he recommended to the patient that she have the tumor surgically removed.

Some medical boards see fully developed informed consent forms as an important way of protecting patients; if patients are fully aware of the innovative or experimental nature of a treatment and its risks, and if applicable, the risks of deferring conventional treatments, these boards are more tolerant of CAM activities by physicians. Such a policy does not surmount federal issues regarding unapproved drugs or devices.

An issue of informed consent of great concern that has not received the attention it deserves is the poor quality of informed consent forms for conventional cancer treatments. The significant risks and limited benefits that many chemotherapeutic, radiation, and surgical interventions offer are often poorly documented and explained to the patient. Oncology treatments are offered as if no choices really exist, and many patients undergo these serious treatments unaware of the extent and nature of the risks they face. Many patients do not realize the debilitating nausea and weakness, loss of appetite and sex drive, hair loss, and other problems that conventional therapies quite often deliver, nor do they realize the poor statistical odds many therapies deliver. Yet many medical boards single out alternative cancer therapies as requiring unique levels of consent stating that they lack of evidence and detailing possible risks. This lack of a level playing field stilts patients toward conventional therapies, when the direct risks of side effects is arguably much higher with these aggressive approaches.

## Free Speech: Protected Where Just Speech

Free speech protections under the First Amendment allow a significant amount of educational materials about cancer therapies to be widely disseminated. The Internet, magazines, books, and other publishing sources make available enormous amounts of data, some useful and some seriously misleading. Such informational discussion is protected speech. Once speech is tied to a product or a healing relationship, however, the extent that such protections are available is drastically reduced.

Some practitioners who are not licensed to treat cancer patients frame their discussions as educational. When one tells a client "If I had these symptoms, I would suspect a liver deficiency, and would try to assist the liver using milk thistle" or "This herbal mixture is known to alleviate the ravages caused by radiation therapy," this is the provision of information and is arguably protected by the First Amendment. Although the protections of free speech are some of the most honored and respected by our courts, these statements will likely be seen by a disciplinary body and the courts as an artifice meant to allow the practice of medicine.

The protections of free speech are limited because speech can be interpreted as an act rather than as speech that is protected under the First Amendment. Speech about a product can be an expression of intent; an unapproved product sold with the intent that it be used to treat cancer cannot legally be sold, and the speech about the claim is evidence of intent and as such is not protected. This argument has, for the moment, trumped what had been a successful challenge to FDA restrictions on health claims made on dietary supplements. In *Pearson v. Halala* (1999), the U.S. Court of Appeals for the District of Columbia Circuit ruled that the FDA must permit health claims, even if they do not meet FDA's ambiguous "significant scientific agreement" standard, as long as the claim can be rendered nonmisleading by a disclaimer. The court examined possible disclaimers in some detail and suggested that FDA concerns regarding misleading information could under many circumstances be addressed by a disclaimer as simple as "the evidence in support of this claim is inconclusive."

After *Pearson*, the FDA proposed a final rule that limited *Pearson's* reach. Commentators to the proposed rule argued in light of *Pearson* that the FDA may not prohibit disease claims but must choose the less restrictive alternative of permitting such claims provided that they are accompanied by disclaimers. The FDA concluded that even if the rule were viewed as a direct restriction on speech, it would not violate the First Amendment as interstate marketing of a drug without preapproval is illegal. The FDA argued that its final rule does not prohibit speech but rather clarifies when labeling claims are evidence of intended use. As such, the First Amendment is not implicated because the FDA is merely enforcing laws regarding the intent of sales, and it is the intent and not the speech that places the regulatory burden on the speaker.

This argument was in the context of FDA regulations implementing the Dietary Supplement Health and Education Act of 1994 (DSHEA), which was enacted as a compromise about what health statements may be made for dietary supplements. The law has always disallowed claims that a product be used to "diagnose, cure, mitigate, treat, or prevent disease," (21 U.S.C. §§ 343(r)(6)) but the DSHEA allows an explanation of the impact a product has on the structure/function of the body. An example of this distinction is that antioxidants can be sold as helping to remove oxidized material in the body, but could not, without prior approval as a health claim, state that antioxidants have a beneficial effect in preventing cancer. Disease and structure/function claims clearly overlap; where a statement includes a disease claim, it cannot be made under the DSHEA. Nonphysician health care practitioners are well advised to stay within this rubric when discussing herbs and other supplements. Although physicians have much broader rights when dealing with patients, they should also follow these guidelines when discussing or advertising supplements to the public (see box).

---

*How to Speak: Implications for Practitioners*
Nutritional advice has been problematic throughout the alternative health care community. Although physicians face some risk, the problem is much greater for nonphysician practitioners. The FDA does not regulate the practice of medicine, so what a physician tells his or her patient about an herb or other supplement in the treatment room is unregulated by the FDA and physicians should not have qualms about making specific recommendations for medicinal herbs and compounds to their patients. Where a physician should take care is in statements to the general public,

which are not protected. Advertisements, interviews, and so forth discussing the medicinal value of herbs can be problematic. General statements that are merely educational, such as "there is some evidence that mushroom-derived polysaccharides have demonstrated capacity to suppress tumor growth" (Spencer & Jacobs, 1999) are educational and acceptable. Urging patients to come to you for such treatment can be seen as a drug claim made for an unapproved drug.

Nonphysician practitioners, such as acupuncturists in a state whose scope of practice does not include herbal practice, walk an ambiguous line when discussing herbs and other supplements with their patients. Although the DSHEA does not regulate practitioners, staying within this rubric is more defensible.

Nonmedical practitioners have been successfully prosecuted for giving nutritional recommendations. Many of these cases contain facts that may have added to a court's willingness to find the providers culpable of practicing medicine without a license. A chiropractor, for example, found guilty of medical practice act violations for giving nutritional advice was selling a line of nutritional products. Although the language of the court suggests it may have upheld his conviction in any event, these sales undercut the argument that the statements were informational rather than prescriptive. This has happened even in states in which chiropractors are entitled to give "dietary advice," particularly where remedies are suggested for particular ailments. These disciplinary actions occur because of a belief that the chiropractor's conduct is counter to the established history of chiropractic as a "drugless art." Courts are particularly concerned where blood work is used as a basis for nutritional guidance or where the provider has otherwise exceeded their scope of practice. The DSHEA may have a positive effect here, as it is now more clear that supplements are not treated as drugs. The benefit of this legal protection, however, is available only if the same type of language counseled by the DSHEA is used, couching recommendations in terms of structure and function rather than for a disease (Dumoff, 2000).

Discussing structure rather than disease where the substance is a food or dietary supplement serves to make the conversation more clearly educational and lessens, if not removes, the intent to prescribe for a particular illness.

# Direct Barriers to Practice

## Federal Regulation of Drugs, Devices, and Dietary Products

### The Approval Process and Its Political Aspects

Under the FDCA, drugs and devices that diagnose or treat cancer or other diseases must be approved by the FDA. The approval requirement is driven in most instances by the intended use of products rather than the nature of the product itself. If one offers Chlorella as a food source, it is unregulated, but when it is offered for its antitumor activity, it becomes a drug. The FDA regulates pharmaceuticals and biological substances, such as antineoplastons, Ukraine, or hydrazine sulfate; biologics, such as immunoaugmentive therapy or autologous vaccines; or devices such as hyperbaric chambers.

To market a drug, biologic, or medical device in interstate commerce, it must be approved by the FDA. Violation of the FDCA can result in significant civil or criminal penalties. This process involves stepping a drug through phases of clinical trials from animal safety through human safety and efficacy, a process that generally costs well in excess of $500 million. Given these financial requirements, research is generally limited to the major pharmaceutical houses. The financial and political impact of these entry barriers makes it very difficult for therapies not arising from mainstream currents of thought to achieve sufficient testing and proof to gain FDA approval (Goldberg, 1997).

**Case Study: Burzynski Prosecution.** A major battle over patient access to innovative and highly promising cancer treatments erupted in the struggle among the FDA, the Texas Medical Board, and Stansilav R. Burzynski, MD, developer of a cancer therapy he terms *antineoplastins*. Burzynski, who developed his approach while a researcher at Baylor College of Medicine in the late 1970s, isolated certain peptides in human urine that appear to act as biochemical switches that "turn off" cancer genes by interrupting signals for cells to multiply. He set up a clinic in Houston, Texas, and began treating patients and distributing the drug without FDA approval (Kolata, 1996). In 1983, the FDA sought to close his clinic, but because their jurisdiction is limited to items shipped in interstate commerce, they were successful only in enjoining Burzynski from introducing antineoplastins into interstate commerce as an unapproved drug. Burzynski maintained that he could treat patients in Texas, a position that brought numerous grand jury investigations and repeated FDA raids seeking evidence of interstate commerce. Texas bought suit against Burzynski in 1992, charging that he was treating cancer patients with an unapproved drug and advertising that the drug is effective against cancer. The matter eventually reached the Supreme Court of Texas, which expressly rejected Burzynski's argument that he could legally treat Texas residents.

In 1998, the Texas Attorney General obtained a court agreement that required Dr. Burzynski to stop soliciting cancer patients for his treatments. Under the agreement, Burzynski agreed to abide by conditions that limited his ability to distribute his drugs, including an agreement that he distribute antineoplastins only to patients enrolled in FDA-approved clinical trials, unless or until FDA approves his drugs for sale, and not advertise antineoplastins for the treatment of cancer.

In addition to this state action, FDA pressed charges against Dr. Burzynski for 75 criminal counts, including mail and insurance fraud and violating prohibitions of using unapproved drugs in interstate commerce. The fight between Dr. Burzynski and various government agencies has been long, loud, and often acrimonious. His attorney, Richard Jaffe, raised numerous concerns about the tactics employed by both the federal government and the state. Harris County Attorney Mike Driscoll, for example, was on Dr. Burzynski's Board of Directors and a vocal supporter. In response to his supportive testimony at trial, Mr. Jaffe believes FDA issued a subpoena for his already public campaign contribution records to raise the specter of an investigation. (Jaffe, 1995). Other questionable subpoenas included one to Dr. Ralph Moss, a noted proponent of fair evaluations of CAM cancer therapies, and for all of Dr. Burzynski's patient records.

The federal prosecutors had to convene four grand juries before they were finally able, in 1995, to get one to approve charges (Burzynski Patient Group, 1996). Dr. Burzynski received a considerable outflow of public support during this trial, including rallies outside the courthouse, in large part because of the tireless efforts of many of his patients who effectively organized public and political opposition to the government's prosecution (Starr & Siegel, 1996). After a 2-month trial, the jury was equally divided between finding Dr. Burzynski guilty and innocent on all counts, resulting in a mistrial. The judge acquitted Dr. Burzynski of 34 counts, and the government retried Dr. Burzynski in 1997 on the remaining charges. He was cleared of all charges except for one count of contempt of court.

One of the government briefs argued against admitting patient testimony so damaging to them in the first trial by arguing that these witnesses were nothing more than a thinly veiled attempt to win the sympathy of the jury by demonstrating that the drug is effective against cancer. Although this argument makes sense from a technical standpoint—the FDA is the arbiter of what is effective, not the jury—it does provide a sense of the Kafkaesque quality of the government's action.

The Kafkaesque nature of the action goes deeper: as FDA's enforcement branch conducted this effort to curtail Dr. Burzynski's activities and put him in jail, other branches in FDA were working with him to develop IND clinical trials. The first ones were approved as early as 1994 to test the safety and efficacy of antineoplastins (National Cancer Institute, 2002). These approvals developed through an increasing consensus in the medical community that the results Dr. Burzynski was obtaining indicated anticancer activity, including a site visit by NCI scientists in 1991. As early as 1991, years before the criminal charges were brought, an internal FDA memo noted that the "human brain tumor responses are real" (Friedman, 1991). FDA's view of this dual approach is that it is not opposed to serious study of antineoplastins but that physicians must go through this process before offering treatments to the public (Gordon & Curtin, 2000).

The first early study done on Dr. Burzynski's work was done by NCI in 1983 using the P338 mouse leukemia tumor model, which showed no activity. Dr. Burzynski's attorney, Rick Jaffe, points out that because antineoplastins have never been offered to treat leukemia, which is quite a different disease than the tumors targeted by antineoplastins, such tests are designed to fail rather to provide a true test of this work.

Some in the news media cast Dr. Burzynski, and the 72 clinical trials approved after the trial for various forms of cancer, as something "he did . . . very reluctantly and only after many years. . . . " Burzynski first applied for permission to conduct clinical trials while an associate professor at Baylor University College of Medicine in 1976 and again in 1983. His first permits were not approved by the FDA until 1995, after the government had begun prosecuting him on the charges from which he was eventually exonerated. There are currently 35 protocols for cancer Phase II clinical trials for antineoplastons at the Burzynski clinic.

The scientific controversy over antineoplastins has found strong voices on both sides of the debate. Robert E. Burdick, MD, a respected oncologist, did an independent evaluation of the record and testified that antineoplastins as a treatment for brain cancer are "astounding" and need to be intensively investigated. Dr. Burdick, a Seattle oncologist with 27 years of experience, and a faculty member of the University of Washington, reviewed the case records of all the brain cancer patients included in Burzynski's FDA approved CAN-1 trial initiated in February 1996. Dr. Burdick told the court that he was "very impressed with the number of complete and partial responses that I have seen here . . . [t]he responses here are also far in excess of any prior series of patients published in the medical literature." Unfortunately, Dr. Burdick's testimony was not considered germane, as Judge Sim Lake precluded any discussion of the efficacy of the treatment in Burzynski's trial.

One concern about the clinical trials is that patients cannot participate unless they have first undergone conventional treatments. Some of these conventional treatments can cause a range of adverse side effects that can make recovery more difficult, undermining trials of any follow-up therapy. This requirement is predicated on a belief that conventional treatments have something to offer, a proposition in dispute. This leads directly to ironic and frustrating allegations researchers of CAM therapies frequently encounter: that Dr. Burzynski's responses resulted from the residual effects of conventional therapy. The consensus in the medical community is that any benefit from chemotherapy or radiation occurs within 2 months of the cessation of these modalities. Antineoplastins are introduced after this period to ensure that later responses can be properly attributed to the antineoplastin therapy. Researchers are often placed in this dilemma, as patients who have not exhausted conventional treatment are considered off-limits ethically, but then any improvements in patients who have received conventional treatment are claimed to have obtained their results from the conventional care.

Dr. Burzynski's clinical trials represent a wide range of cancer types in children and adults treated by both intravenous injection and oral routes. All patients treated at the clinic must be enrolled in a clinical trial, or, if they do not qualify for admission to a clinical trial, they may be treated in many cases pursuant to a "special exception."

---

*An Inside View of the Burzynski Trial: A Letter from a Juror to Janet Reno, United States Attorney General*
The following are excerpts from a letter written by one of the jurors in the first Burzynski criminal trial to Janet Reno, United States Attorney General

Dear Attorney General Reno,

I was recently a juror on a Federal trial in Houston, Texas. . . . This letter is to inform you of how upset I am at how my time and tax dollars were wasted on this trial.

This case, which began on January 6, 1997, involved the FDA and their apparent anger at Dr. Burzynski for continuing to make available his unapproved new drug, Antineoplaston, to persons living out of the state of Texas. . . .

A second reason I feel this case should not have gone to trial is because while the trial was going on the FDA had already approved 71 clinical trials, thereby allowing Dr. Burzynski full release to ship Antineoplaston to persons living out of the State of Texas. This was not known to the jurors at the time. After the trial ended, I gleaned this information and felt I had been involved in something that was a ridiculous waste of two months of my life. After all, wasn't this a moot point at this time? Surely our government has real 'criminals' to prosecute. . . .

In addition, the prosecution failed to introduce even one witness who could say anything defamatory about Dr. Burzynski's character. One would think after four years of preparing for this trial they would have found at least one disgruntled patient, former employee, business associate, or colleague who had something negative to say about him.

Also, since the prosecution had been working on the case for four years, I expected the exhibits, witnesses and evidence to be compelling. It was not, and they didn't come close to proving their case.

Since the trial I have learned much about the history of this man and the attempts by the FDA to shut him down. It is my heartfelt belief that a person confronting a life-and-death situation, either for himself or for a dependent child, should be allowed to make these tough decisions himself. Once the FDA has said that a drug is non toxic and that it will not harm a person (which they had), it should be left up to the patient to choose what he or she feels is the best treatment available. The FDA should be supporting Dr. Burzynski in his valiant effort to cure and ease the suffering of cancer patients. Incredibly promising results have taken place already with the remission of brain tumors, non-Hodgkins lymphoma, and breast and prostate cancers. The lives and quality of life of cancer patients should be uppermost in the minds of the FDA—not what rules were allegedly broken in the past.

Since the end of the trial, I have done independent research and have learned many disturbing facts about the FDA's antics (sic) in this case. Some notable incidents are:

- The FDA convened four or five different grand juries before the last one agreed to indict Dr. Burzynski.
- On two separate occasions the FDA confiscated a total of 300,000 documents (i.e., patient records, MRI scans, progress charts, etc.) and for Dr. Burzynski to be able to continue to treat his patients, he had to purchase a Xerox machine, install it at the FDA office, hire someone to make copies, and to make it even more difficult, he was required to call a day in advance to make an appointment for copies to be made. To this day these documents have not been returned.
- Amy Lecocq, the lead prosecutor in this case, violated at least six federal laws governing subpoenas of journalists when she subpoenaed a Dr. Richard Moss. When he pointed this out to her, she withdrew the subpoena.
- Patients and their families met with the House Commerce Subcommittee on Oversight and Investigations, headed by Representative Joe Barton of Texas. After hearing the collective plight of these brave people and also hearing from Dr. Burzynski's lawyer, Rick Jaffe, Rep. Barton used the word "vendetta" in describing the actions of the FDA over the past 12 years in regards to Dr. Burzynski. I would agree with this assessment.

I do feel so very fortunate to have been allowed the opportunity to serve on a federal jury and would do it all over again. I saw first hand that our system of trial by jury, which says that a person is innocent until proven guilty, does work, and for this I will always be grateful.

Sincerely,

L. Darlene Phillips

*FDA and Congress at Cross-Purposes: The FDA Reconsiders Its Mission*

When the wife of Congressman Dan Burton (R–Indiana) was diagnosed with breast cancer, her physician told her that she had a 50% chance to live 5 years. Congressman Burton found this statement to be callous. He read an article about Dr. Springer, a physician from Germany now living in Illinois, who was conducting an experimental program with 71 women, stimulating their immune system to fight off cancer recurrence. Congressman Burton's wife enrolled in the study. Congressman Burton started speaking with a significant number of Dr. Springer's patients. Many told him that his program had enabled them to far outlive their prognoses. As chair of the Government Oversight Committee, Congressman Burton informed the FDA about the importance of Dr. Springer's program. He asked that Dr. Springer's treatment be allowed to be administered by the women's hometown physicians to spare them the regular travel to Chicago.

After looking into Dr. Springer's program, the FDA decided to close it down. It reported that Dr. Springer had not complied with a number of FDA requirements. The FDA's decision "went through all the 71 women like a knife," recalled Congressman Burton. In response to this decision, Congressman Burton told the head of the FDA that if the agency closed Dr. Springer's program, he would hold a congressional hearing every week in which the FDA would be asked to explain to the American people why it had taken away a promising cancer treatment. The FDA reconsidered its position and agreed to assist Dr. Springer in meeting its requirements. Dr. Springer died in 1998, but his program is still in operation, thanks to the efforts of Dr. Springer's patients and Wayne Jonas, MD, at the Finch University/Chicago Medical School, and most of the women enrolled in it are doing very well (Burton, 1999).

## FDA Efforts to Create More Open Policies

The FDA has come under a great deal of criticism for the lengthy delays in the drug approval process; even experimental drugs that are within the accepted rubric of conventional approaches take considerable time for approval. Activists from the AIDS and cancer communities have raised concerns about these delays, particularly where drugs show some promise for treating a terminal condition where there is no approved alternative. As a result of numerous meetings with FDA and congressional inquiries, the FDA and Congress have both taken steps to alleviate these barriers. FDA policies are principally aimed at experimental drugs under approved INDs within conventional views of oncology, but some of these policies allow for some improved access to CAM treatments as well.

## Expedited Reviews, Compassionate and Sole Investigator INDs

These demands led to expedited review and approval of promising new cancer drugs, reforms that included the FDA Modernization Act of 1997 whose purpose is to generate the "prompt approval of safe and effective new drugs and other therapies is critical to the improvement of the public health so that patients may enjoy the benefits provided by these therapies to treat and prevent illness and disease."

The FDA had, even before this act, taken steps to improve patient access to promising new cancer therapies. The FDA worked to

- shorten approval times for cancer treatments by recognizing that tumor shrinkage is often an early indicator of a treatment's effectiveness
- make promising cancer therapies approved by foreign countries available to cancer patients even before the product is approved in the United States
- ensure that all FDA cancer therapy advisory committee meetings include an ad hoc member who has personal experience with the illness for which a new product is being considered
- make it easier for investigators to test new uses for cancer therapies already on the market

The FDA had usually required that a cancer therapy's sponsor demonstrate improvements in survival time or quality of life before a therapy could be approved. Based on accumulating evidence, the FDA determined that it is appropriate to approve products that show evidence of tumor shrinkage as long as there is no satisfactory alternative therapy. Because sponsors can more quickly demonstrate tumor regression than improvements in survival time or quality of life, and do so in studies that are relatively easy to carry out, this can substantially shorten the time needed to obtain marketing approval. Reliance on shrinkage as an end point only where there is no alternative therapy provides a balance to the concerns, discussed earlier, about bringing therapies to market earlier without overvaluing the impact of tumor shrinkage on longevity (Food and Drug Administration, 1996).

An exception to cost-intensive IND requirements is sole investigator INDs, in which the FDA may assist a physician in the filing requirements for creating a small, single investigator IND for a few subjects. This is ordinarily done with the support of the drug manufacturer or sponsor. Where there is an IND in place, but the eligibility criteria in the protocol are not suitable for a particular patient for whom other options don't exist, a special exception may be granted to allow that patient access to the treatment under study, an allowance known as a *compassionate exemption*. Treating a patient as an exception is at the discretion of the investigator and sponsor and usually requires filing extra paperwork, including sending a request to the FDA, modifying the consent form, and obtaining permission from the local Institutional Review Board. Sponsors may generally not charge for unapproved drugs, although charges for costs associated with the administration of the drug and patient care may be passed on to the patient.

# Personal Import

One policy adopted by the FDA to ease restrictions on cancer patients seeking drugs unapproved in the United States, but that are approved in other countries, is to allow patients to import such drugs for personal use. Such importations must be no more than a

3-month personal supply and be shipped directly to the patient's home and a supervising physician must be available. The FDA designed this policy primarily for patients who have been treated overseas and wish to continue that treatment back home, though this is not a requirement. Autologous vaccines and other cancer therapies are imported in this fashion.

This is not an absolute right but a discretionary policy on the part of the FDA. Some items that the FDA believes are dangerous and should not be admitted into the country are banned for import and listed on import alerts. Items on this list, maintained at the FDA's Web site, will be interdicted by customs officials.

Patients can bring unapproved drugs obtained by import for personal use into their physician's office to be administered and monitored. For a physician to recommend to patients as a matter of course that they should import an unapproved drug to bring into the office for administration, however, can be problematic. The FDA can take the position that the physician is required to have IND approval before participating in treatment with such drugs.

## Laboratory Regulations: Restrictions on Diagnosis

Given that the differences between conventional and CAM approaches to cancer originate in theoretical differences in the nature of cancer, it is not surprising that these differences arise in diagnosis as well as treatment. One of the most direct arenas in which this appears are federal and state regulations of laboratory testing. CLIA sets forth a detailed federal regulatory scheme. CLIA operates as an office within The Center for Medicare and Medicaid Services (CMS, formerly the Health Care Financing Administration). The goal of CLIA is to ensure laboratory proficiency and accuracy. CLIA requirements are based on the level of complexity of a test, with simple tests being performed under a simple application that exempts the physician office or lab from full CLIA requirements. Tests of high complexity can be performed only in laboratory settings that demonstrate proficiency, have procedures to maintain and validate their testing equipment, have personnel training in place, and so forth. Many physicians with a CAM practice are not aware that tests they use, based on controversial views of cancer physiology and biochemistry, may be tests not approved by CLIA and subject to sanctions.

## Case Study: CLIA and OGC Examination of Live Cell Dark-Field Microscopy

One test that provides an example of this situation is live blood cell analysis (LBA), a test that uses dark-field microscopy to examine blood for a wide array of pathologies, including the presence of parasites, lipid and other metabolic deficiencies, and other factors that include diagnoses of various cancers.

LBA is performed by placing a drop of blood from the patient's fingertip onto a microscope slide under a glass coverslip to keep it from drying. The slide is then viewed at high magnification with a dark-field microscope, which illuminates the slide in a manner that preserves the blood as a living fluid without fixing and staining it so that the rich cellular activity can be viewed. Some limited uses of dark-field are approved, but LBA proponents' claims to be able to deduce the quality of metabolic and immune function and see parasites and a range of other physiological functions are considered unfounded by conventional hematologists.

In January 1996, CLIA determined, with the advice of the Centers for Disease Control (CDC), NIH, and several major medical centers, that the LBA test procedure did not make scientific sense. No manufacturer of dark-field, practitioner, or researcher who uses LBA was consulted as part of the decision making in an effort to understand the rationale for this approach, because, in the words of CLIA director Judy Yost, MD, "they did not choose to make themselves known to us."

CLIA regulation is based on the level of complexity and proficiency that a test requires. CLIA determined that LBA automatically defaulted to high complexity because it had not been categorized by CDC. CLIA also determined that, because the test does not make sense according to conventional views of biochemistry, proficiency could never be demonstrated. LBA was thus effectively made illegal.

It is estimated that there are approximately 10,000 to 15,000 sites using LBA, of which 80% are unregistered with CLIA. Many of these sites are within the offices of chiropractors, naturopaths, herbalists, and other nonphysicians that are less aware of CLIA requirements. These sites are subject to civil and criminal prosecution for performing LBA, whereas those physician's offices that are registered are primarily subject to a cease and desist order. A few states also have laws that effectively prohibit LBA as it is currently performed.

Because of concerns arising within CMS as well as by those who find the test highly useful, a regional Office of General Counsel (OGC) office studied the manner in which CLIA has regulated CAM testing and issued a report, which was made public in August 2001. This report addressed LBA as a case study of the larger issue of what it termed "unestablished" lab tests, a term that encompasses the range of CAM testing that includes Biological Terrain Analysis and other metabolic tests not recognized as acceptable tests by CLIA. The OGC surveyed all of the state CLIA offices and consulted with the conventional scientific community and with numerous providers and trainers of LBA. Although many CLIA staff did not believe that the claims made for LBA make biological sense, the range of opinion about how to regulate such tests fell across a broad range. Some felt that public safety required more aggressive enforcement, whereas others felt that as long as Medicare or Medicaid were not billed the test should be afforded legal status. Many felt that unestablished tests should be regulated, but half of the states felt it should be under a targeted program that could better and more fairly assess such testing than CLIA was able to do. The OGC recommendations, which have been accepted by CLIA, include both the need to better evaluate the diagnostic validity of LBA as well as to improve laboratory disclosure and enforcement.

## Malpractice Risk

Physicians deviating from standards of care are justifiably concerned about their exposure to malpractice liability. Such liability is by definition a risk in offering CAM cancer therapies, because CAM is by definition nonstandard care. The reality in practice, generally, for physicians offering CAM therapies is that they are rarely sued and the real legal risks of such practice lie elsewhere. Because patients seeking CAM care are generally educated, have explored a variety of choices, and made a careful decision to seek such care, they are more likely to take responsibility for their choices (Freimuth, 1988). Malpractice actions generally require not only a bad result caused by a violation of a standard of care but also an angry patient who feels that the doctor was callous in his or her treatment (Adamson et al., 2000; Dumoff, 1995; Pfifferling, 1994). CAM physicians, particularly those who offer compassionate support to their patients, are seen as doing their best in a difficult situation and thus are rarely held responsible by their patients.

Cancer treatment, however, is a significant risk for malpractice, and oncologists are generally quite conservative as a group and hew tightly to defined standards of care given the high risks of morbidity and mortality associated with cancer. When classified by diagnosis, cancer accounts for the second, third, and fourth most likely malpractice claims (cancer of bronchus and lung, breast, and colon and rectal cancer) (Weiss, 2002). The most significant risks occur when offering a CAM treatment for those types of cancer that have high longevity rates with conventional treatment.

Negligence can arise from commission, such as a therapy outside the standard of care that interferes with other treatment or is itself toxic, or omission, such as failing to diagnose a tumor or metastacy or providing necessary treatment. It is important that patients provided CAM therapies sign a carefully prepared consent form, acknowledging an understanding that the therapy is in fact nonconventional and not supported by the medical community. Many physicians offering such therapies do so in a complementary rather than alternative fashion; the patient has a conventional oncologist as well, and the CAM therapy is offered in a supportive role. This is a legally safer method, but many physicians who offer immunosupportive and other therapies believe that chemotherapy and radiation cause wasting and contribute to the inability of the body to heal itself because of its damaging impacts on the immune system and require patients to discontinue conventional care. Even for these physicians, malpractice actions have not been common. The legal preparation for physicians offering CAM care should primarily focus not on patients suits but on a wide variety of regulatory restrictions (Dumoff, 2004a, 2004b, 2004c).

Physicians need to keep their conventional diagnostic skills sharp and follow patients with a conventional eye, even when pursuing a strictly alternative course of treatment. Good documentation of diagnostic impressions and the use of conventional testing in addition to any CAM methods of diagnosis are essential. Good medical documentation is always important, and this is certainly true when using any form or complementary or alternative cancer care. Even where the focus is on an alternative method of care, a review of the chart by a conventional physician should show that sound evaluation and reasoning lay underneath any CAM method that may also be used.

Physicians can be subject to liability for negligent referral, which arises where either the approach referred to is inappropriate or the physician knew or should have known of competency problems with the practitioner (Cohen, 1998, 2000; Dumoff, 1995). Physicians should have confidence in and know the credentials of any health care practitioner to which they refer. These suits are not common and physicians should simply approach collaborative opportunities by becoming educated and comfortable with the strengths and weaknesses of chiropractors to whom they wish to refer or work.

An easily overlooked risk management requirement is the notification of one's malpractice carrier of any unusual additions to one's practice. Where nonstandard therapies are adopted without notice, and a claim is filed, the carrier may refuse coverage because of a material misrepresentation of the nature of the practice. If the carrier balks at covering the practice, and the physician is willing to go bare with regard to practices that are reasonably safe but merely unknown to the carrier, it may be possible to negotiate an exclusion that would allow the core coverage to continue.

# Federal, State, and Private Regulation of Payment

Even where regulatory barriers don't prevent care, financial barriers can as effectively bar treatment. Insurance benefit coverage limitations or exclusions often bar innovative, experimental, or alternative methods of care. Treatments that are not considered medically necessary are not covered. Challenging denials can be quite foreboding, particularly where one is ill. Although there have been some real inroads in the coverage of various CAM therapies, generally, these inroads have had little impact on payment for CAM cancer therapies. In a survey of 114 HMOs, 67% report offering at least one type of alternative health care (Landmark Healthcare, 1999). Most of these coverages are for chiropractic and, to a lesser extent, acupuncture, massage therapy, and, for some HMOs, vitamin therapy and relaxation therapy. Very few offer coverage of experiemental, herbal, or other therapeutic approaches that could be applied to cancer treatment.

Many patients seeking CAM therapies are willing to pay out of pocket without expecting reimbursement. Unfortunately, this does not entirely alleviate the physician from a considerable body of regulation about what services can be billed. Where payment could occur in some circumstances, billing must conform to the law. Patients may submit in the hopes of coverage, or in the case of Medicare, where it is known that CMS will not pay, claims may still be submitted to get a denial that can be presented to a secondary insurer. Billing must conform to legal requirements in these cases as well. Although CAM therapies can be done and billed for with legal safety, it does require knowledge of a complex array of federal laws and requirements.

Medicare requirements include the use of Current Procedural Terminology codes that accurately reflect this services being performed. This includes making it clear that a therapy is experimental if that is the case. Because these codes were developed to reflect conventional choices, it is easy to unintentionally misrepresent a service by improperly using a code. An example occurs in the delivery of insulin potentiated chemotherapy (IPT), an experimental therapy that, if billed as mainstream therapy, would likely be considered fraudulent. IPT uses a 10% fractional dose of a standard chemotherapeutic agent along with insulin, which is thought to help target cancer cells that have many more insulin receptors than healthy cells. Not billing for insulin to make the therapy appear standard of care would misrepresent the therapy. Similarly, the J-codes, used to represent the agent itself, must show the fractional amount. By reporting the insulin, particularly when tied to a cancer diagnostic code, and the amount of the agent used, the insurer is on notice that the treatment is nonstandard.

Medicare recognizes that there are many experimental regimens being tried with patients and expects these various cocktails to be reported fully, with support in journals if available to support the practice. There are a variety of low-dose chemotherapeutic approaches, most if not all of which are considered experimental.

Some physicians whose practices are principally based on the delivery of CAM services that are not reimbursed in any event chose to opt out of Medicare. This allows physicians to enter into private contracts with patients, in which they agree that no claims will be submitted to Medicare. Physicians can then charge for services without regard to Medicare judgments about validity or to the level of the fee. Since January 1998, physicians have been able to opt out of the Medicare program for a 2-year interval. The patient agrees not to submit claims to Medicare but instead to pay the physician's fees directly. If a physician has responsibilities other than working in a CAM setting, this should be done with great care as this is not a case-by-case election but applies to all patients seen in any setting except for those seen in an emergency. To opt out, the physician must submit an affidavit to Medicare and have each Medicare-eligible patient sign a contract explaining the situation, including agreeing not to submit claims and acknowledging that they are responsible for payment.

## Case Study: Livingston and Medicare Prosecution

The response of federal authorities to the efforts of Virginia Livingston, MD, to develop and provide treatment for cancer is an unfortunately clear example of the legal issues involved in accessing such therapies. Dr. Livingston, who died in 1992 but is survived by the Livingston-Wheeler Clinic in San Diego, believed that a ubiquitous, cell wall-deficient bacteria she named *Progenitor cryptocides* triggered cancer when the immune system was no longer able to contain the growth factors produced by the bacterium. She produced an autologous vaccine, which she used in conjunction with vitamin I.V.s and a strict dietary regimen. When studied for outcomes, this approach was favorably compared to conventional oncological treatment (Cassileth, 1991).

Despite clear instructions to patients that these services were not covered by Medicare, a number of patients submitted claims in hopes of getting reimbursement. Though less than a $100 was paid in error, the government moved to sanction Dr. Livingston, excluding her from Medicare for the maximum period of 10 years. At the administrative hearing, the issue that emerged was whether the delivery of *nonstandard* care necessarily meets the Medicare concern for *substandard* care. Operating from a conventional perspective, the prosecutors in the case presumed that these were legally equivalent. This arises because of the presumption that if a procedure were valuable it would be accepted by conventional medicine, a presumption that fails to recognize either the time line of innovation or the bias against approaches that arise from unique views of etiology.

The administrative law judge (ALJ) ruled in this case that Dr. Livingston's care was innovative and appropriate; even though it was nonstandard, it was not substandard. What happened next highlights the extent to which these views are entrenched. Although the ALJ ordered that CMS reinstate Dr. Livingston as an approved Medicare provider, CMS refused to follow the order. A writ of mandamus was filed in federal court to force CMS to reinstate Dr. Livingston, but, unfortunately, she died during the pendency of this action.

## Noncoverage and Medical Necessity

CAM or other experimental cancer treatments may be denied either because of express policy exclusions or because nonstandard therapies cannot be demonstrated to be medically necessary, virtually by definition. Claims personnel and utilization review staff are generally not aware of those CAM approaches that have acquired more accepted status, such as nutritional support as a complementary treatment, so that claims are generally denied.

One of the pacesetters for insurance reimbursement is the Blue Cross and Blue Shield Committee for Technology Evaluation and Coverage (TEC). The TEC Committee reviews treatments to see if and under what circumstances they are medically necessary and may be covered. One of the criteria for TEC approval is that any FDA approvals be obtained and that well-designed studies be published in peer-reviewed journals (Blue Cross and Blue Shield Association, 1987). These criteria provide an intentionally high threshold for treatments for which payment will be made.

## Litigation With Private Insurers

Whether private insurers have to pay for experimental treatments has been hotly contested and subject to extensive litigation. Litigation seeking coverages of experimental therapies generally revolve around policy language; the matter is primarily a contractual issue. Some cases hinge on medical opinion as to the validity of a given therapy, raising the specter of dueling experts. But most cases instead revolve around drier issues of contract language. Unless a policy includes a rider at a higher premium allowing for coverage of some experimental therapies, policy language almost universally excludes "unproven" and "experimental" treatments. These treatments are seen, by definition, as unable to rise to the level of medically necessary as they have not yet been proven safe and effective.

Experimental treatments can have two meanings in the insurance context; some courts hold the term refers to treatments subject to a formal study [see, for example, *Lewis v. Trustmark Insurance Company* (1999)], whereas others see the term as referring to treatments not accepted by the medical community [see, for example, *Healthcare America Plans v. Bossemeyer* (1998)]. Most litigation has been around cutting-edge conventional efforts such as high-dose chemotherapy with autologous immune support. But CAM therapies will often be considered unproven and by default "experimental" from a conventional perspective even if it not subject to a study. There have been exceptions, however, in which payment for immunoaugmentive therapies and others have been supported by the courts despite exceptions for experimental therapies [see, for example, *McLaughlin v. Connecticut General Life Insurance Company* (1983)].

Controversies arise in a number of contexts. Any therapy that is yet subject to continuing clinical trials will likely be argued by an insurer to remain experimental virtually by definition, even if it may be generally accepted for a particular indication. Such a case could turn on the sense of the medical community about a given treatment. Where a CAM therapy has not undergone formal clinical trials, it might be argued that best case series and other clinical support should cause them to be accepted as sufficiently demonstrated to avoid "experimental" exclusion language. Where the issue is the accepted role or available support for such therapies, one key legal issue is the extent to which the insurance contract gives discretion to the insurer. Some contracts explicitly assign discretion as to which therapies are experimental to the administrator of the policy, discretion the courts honor and which will likely end the matter in the insurer's favor (see, for example, *Healthcare America Plans v. Bossemeyer* (1998)]. An argument that has been successful for patients, on the other hand, is that where contracts are ambiguous about the standards by which exclusions for experimental treatments should be judged, they should be interpreted in the insureds' favor, which places a high burden on the insurer who is denying claims [see, for example, *Pirozzi v. BCBS of Virginia* (1990)]. In an insurance matter prior to *Rutherford,* for example, an insurer was required to pay for laetrile treatment (Note, 1983).

Given that patients face an evolving picture, both in their health status and with regard to what the medical community accepts, insurers cannot reject a preauthorization request and hold to that decision as the situation evolves. It must give a full and fair consideration as new information warrants [see, for example, *Killian v. Healthsource* (1998)].

One source courts defer to is the CMS to see if it considers a treatment covered. This creates rather severe restrictions because CMS is notoriously conservative, to be expected given its role in allocating government health dollars. Therapies require widespread acceptance before being approved by CMS.

A common source of litigation is whether an exclusion for tissue transplant bars payment for various experimental or CAM therapies. Many policies do exclude tissue transplants, an exclusion used by insurers to deny claims for autologous vaccines, stem cell research, and other work involving blood products. Rather than engage this as a battle between experts as to medical necessity, courts generally consider this a contractual issue, in which case the question is whether the average person would understand the term "tissue transplant" to encompass blood products [see, for example, *Simkins, M&K Enterprises, Nevadacare, Inc.* (2000)].

## Medicare Payment for Clinical Trials

Medicare payments are limited to a narrow interpretation of what is medically necessary, so not surprisingly, payments have generally not been available for experimental trials and not at all for CAM therapies. In June 2000, President Clinton directed Medicare to revise its payment policy and reimburse the routine patient care costs of approved clinical trials. The change provides greater access for seniors to cancer clinical trials. In addition to supporting Medicare beneficiaries, this move was also intended to help speed new treatments into regular use. Many clinical trials have not had enough patients enroll, in large part because of costs. One study that swayed Clinton was a report that seniors are underrepresented in cancer clinical trials. Sixty-three percent of all cancer patients are older than 65, yet this group comprises just 33% of enrollees in cancer clinical trials.

Although not covering the costs of the experimental drugs themselves, Medicare will now cover anything normally covered even if it is a service or item associated with the experimental treatment. For example, Medicare will pay for the intravenous administration of a new chemotherapy drug being tested in a trial, including any therapy to prevent side effects from the new drug. Cancer treatment and diagnosis trials are covered if they are funded by the NCI, NCI-Designated Cancer Centers and sponsored clinical trials, and all other federal agencies that fund cancer research. Some states have also passed legislation providing insurance coverage for clinical trials of cancer treatments. Virginia passed such legislation in 1999, attached to a patient bill of rights.

# State Regulation of Medical Practitioners

## State Boards of Medicine and the Federation of State Medical Boards

State medical boards enforce peer review-determined standards of care, particularly where there is the potential that patients may be harmed, a term that can encompass diversion from conventional treatment. With the urging of the Federation of State Medical Boards, many state medical boards have taken positions critical of CAM practice and in some case launched investigations resulting in discipline against physicians. Some of these cases have involved physicians who have developed their own approaches to cancer, such as the case mentioned earlier of Immanuel Revici, MD, in New York. Because CAM therapies are by definition nonstandard care, physicians are at risk for practicing such care. Even in states that have legislation protecting CAM practice, medical boards have still disciplined some physicians for issues of record keeping, informed consent, billing, or other matters without, ostensibly, sanctioning their CAM practice [see, for example, *Clark, M.D., v. Department of Professional Regulation, Board of Medical Examiners* (1985)].

The Federation hosted a number of meetings in which the NCAHF presented their viewpoint, essentially a "zero tolerance" policy toward CAM methods. As a result, the Federation adopted policies that reflect a rejection of CAM, beginning with the very definition:

> . . . for the purposes of this report, the terms "alternative medicine/therapy" and/or "complementary medicine" have not been utilized by the committee due to a lack of consensus among both practitioners and the public as to their meaning. The committee has chosen to use the term "questionable health care practices" to include those treatments, procedures and/or promotions, conventional or unconventional, which may be unsafe and thereby considered a risk to the public's health, safety and welfare and/or which may be worthless and thereby likely to deceive or defraud the public.

Although not exactly sponsoring "questionable health care practices" as a synonym for CAM, the point has not been lost on state medical boards.

In a positive turn of events, FSMB reevaluated its position in 2002. Although some of these new policies will likely continue to plague CAM physicians, the guidelines represent a sea change in how the medical establishment is responding to the emergence of innovative, nonstandard therapies. FSMB acknowledges that ". . .standards [of medicine] allow a wide degree of latitude in physicians' exercise of their professional judgment and do not preclude the use of any methods that are reasonably likely to benefit patients without undue risk." The guidelines also recognize that "patients have a right to seek any kind of care for their health problems."

These guidelines are voluntary and their impact on state board decisions has not yet been felt to any great extent. Physicians have been disciplined by their state boards for providing various alternative cancer therapies, including laetrile, Krebiozen, the Revici approach, and others (Evers, 1988). The guidelines do, however, represent part of a positive trend toward an improved climate for CAM practices.

*State Legislation Protecting CAM Physician Practice*
Fifteen states have adopted legislation that expressly forbids their medical boards from disciplining physicians for their use of CAM practices. First enacted in the State of New York, these laws bring a variety of approaches to bear in an effort to give patients access to CAM therapies. These laws offer limited protection, as boards may still investigate and bring charges against physicians without making the CAM practice the *per se* basis for the charges.

Examples of language include the following excerpts.

*Alaska*
Professional incompetence, gross negligence, or repeated negligent conduct; the board may not base a finding of professional incompetence solely on the basis that a licensee's practice is unconventional or experimental in the absence of demonstrable physical harm to a patient [Alaska Statute, Section 08.64.326(a)(8)(A); enacted June 14, 1990].

*New York*
(4) This article [Article 131.] shall not be construed to affect or prevent the following:
(e) The physician's use of whatever medical care, conventional or non-conventional, which effectively treats human disease, pain, injury, deformity, or physical condition [Education Law, Section 6527(4)].

*North Carolina*
Unprofessional conduct . . . The Board shall not revoke the license of or deny a license to a person solely because of that person's practice of a therapy that is experimental, nontraditional, or that departs from acceptable a prevailing medical practices unless, by competent evidence, the Board can establish that the treatment has a safety risk greater than the prevailing treatment or that the treatment is generally not effective [North Carolina General Statute, Section 90-14(a)(6); enacted June 29, 1993].

*Texas*

*Standards for Physicians Practicing Integrative and Complementary Medicine*
. . . § 200.3. Practice Guidelines for the Provision of Integrative and Complementary Medicine. A licensed physician shall not be found guilty of unprofessional conduct or be found to have committed professional failure to practice medicine in an acceptable manner solely on the basis of employing a health care method of integrative or complementary medicine, unless it can be demonstrated that such method has a safety risk for the patient that is unreasonably greater than the conventional treatment for the patient's medical condition . . . (Texas Administrative Code: 22 TAC §§ 200.1–200.3).

## Pain Medication and State Board Discipline

An area in which physicians have clearly felt chilled in their treatment choices is pain management. Intractable cancer pain is very difficult to manage, and terminal patients have little to lose from doses of pain medication that might provide relief. The Maryland Board of Physician Quality Assurance has noted that they are "concerned that fear of disciplinary action may lead to inappropriately restrictive prescribing of controlled drugs" and have offered guidelines for physicians. The Board states that "whereas it is inappropriate to prescribe analgesics to maintain addiction, it is good medical care to provide relief from chronic pain even in the face of habituation and tolerance."

Physicians have, however, been disciplined by a number of states, including Maryland, for prescribing what the state considers "excessive" amounts of painkillers. This issue has been highly controversial, with a number of national associations representing patients in pain who believe that the medical profession is unnecessarily ignoring patients' pain.

## State Regulation of Cancer Therapies

As noted, some states have entered the debate over controversial cancer treatments by legalizing the use of laetrile. Other states have directly addressed concerns about fraudulent cancer therapies by criminalizing those therapies that are not FDA approved. The State of California, for example, enacted the following law in 1967:

> Section 1707.1 provides: "The sale, offering for sale, holding for sale, delivering, giving away, prescribing or administering of any drug, medicine, compound or device to be used in the diagnosis, treatment, alleviation or cure of cancer is unlawful and prohibited unless (1) an application with respect thereto has been approved under Section 505 of the Federal Food, Drug and Cosmetic Act, or (2) [Full reports of investigations for safety and effectiveness, ingredients, and other aspects of therapeutic evaluation.]

## Legislative Efforts

### Access to Medical Treatment Act

The Access to Medical Treatment Act has been before Congress since 1996. The act would establish a basic right for patients to receive treatments, even if not approved by the FDA, if offered by a licensed health care practitioner. The bill would require informed consent that would offer certain protections to practitioners using CAM approaches. The bill would create an adverse reporting databank, to which practitioners would be required to report difficulties so that dangerous therapies could be tracked. This is conceived of as acting as an informal clinical trial that would involve practitioner's offices across the nation. Versions of this bill would change the import restrictions on approved drugs or devices from other countries and change the interstate shipment restrictions on experimental drugs or devices.

## Infrastructure: Evolving Needs

One of the core barriers to the more complete integration of CAM cancer therapies into health care delivery systems is a lack of completed infrastructure. Infrastructure, such as credentialing mechanisms designed to offer some assurances of credibility and safety, provides legal defenses against litigation as well as from professional censure. Although many organizations address CAM cancer methods, clinical development has not reached a point where respected training, fellowship, and certification programs in alternative cancer approaches could be expected to have developed. Once these developments progress, it will become clearer where the boundaries of substandard care lie, and such care will be more defensible and more accessible. In the meantime, it will remain difficult for medical centers to credential practitioners or privilege particular methods of care with any certainty given their controversy and lack of academic credentials.

The broader field of CAM has developed a broader professional support network than commonly recognized, including national credentialing bodies and certification programs, a variety of state licenses, accredited core and continuing education training programs, and recognized bodies of research and considerable legislative activity preserving, even if in a limited fashion, patients rights of access. The CAM cancer field has developed much more limited support because of the professional and clinical difficulties presented by the nature of cancer itself, a constellation of diseases whose serious consequences have led to social investment in mainstream medicine as the arbiter of treatments. Given these, it is not surprising that a primary source of support for CAM therapies are the patients themselves, whose activism is surpassed only by AIDS activists.

# Summary

Although the scientific and political landscape of CAM treatments for cancer has rapidly evolved, the schism between mainstream views that dominate practice, research, and regulation remain. The conversation between conventional and CAM approaches has become more open, and there is greater recognition that some CAM approaches are making important contributions.

Skepticism about alternative treatments, based in part on legitimate concerns and in part on institutional biases against botanical, immunoaugmentive, and other methods of grappling with cancer. Such biases are quite likely limiting viable and important options. Both sides of the debate at times polarize the issue, making it more difficult to separate legitimate areas of investigation and treatment from those that have no promise.

The legal establishment of orthodox medical views affects treatment across the board—restrictions on accepted standards of medical practice, drug and device approvals, laboratory procedures, reimbursement for services, publication and investments in research—making it difficult for patients to exercise choice over their own destiny. That the courts have not yet recognized a fundamental right for patients to receive controversial treatments places a great deal of power in the hands of the conventional community of physicians. Given the lack of resounding success that has been achieved against many cancers, and the finality of the decision, it is critical that physicians and regulators educate themselves about CAM findings and respect the wishes of patients to explore approaches that offer promise.

The efforts of NCCAM, NCI, the Center for Mind–Body Medicine, and many other institutions making efforts to further the conversation between conventional and CAM practitioners at the Comprehensive Cancer Conference are all important steps. As these institutional efforts evolve, access to therapies that have increasing chances to prove their value will also increase.

## REFERENCES

Adamson, T. E., Bunch, W. H., Baldwin, D. C., Jr., et al. (2000). The virtuous orthopaedist has fewer malpractice suits. *Clinical Orthopaedics, 378*, 104–109.

American Cancer Society. (1971). *Unproven methods of cancer management.* New York: Author.

American Cancer Society. (2004). *American Cancer Society operational statement on complementary and alternative methods of cancer management.* Retrieved May 13, 2005, from http://www.cancer.org/docroot/ETO/content/ETO_5_3x_American_Cancer_Society_Operational

American Society of Clinical Oncology. (1983). Ineffective cancer therapy: A guide for the layperson. *Journal of Clinical Oncology, 1*, 154–163.

Ausubel, K. (1988). The troubling case of Harry Hoxsey. *New Age Journal, July–August*: 43–47, 49, 78–79, 86.

Ausubel, K., & Salveson, C. (Producers). (1987). *When healing becomes a crime (originally titled Hoxsey: Quacks who cure cancer?)* [Motion picture]. United States: Realidad Productions.

Barret, S., & Herbert, V. (2005). *Questionable cancer therapies.* Retrieved May 12, 2005, from http://www.quackwatch.com/01QuackeryRelatedTopics/cancer.html

Bernstein, B. J., & Grasso, T. (2001). Prevalence of complementary and alternative medicine use in cancer patients. *Oncology, 10*, 1267–1272.

Blue Cross and Blue Shield Association. (1987). *Technology evaluation criteria.* Chicago, IL: Author.

Bross, I. D. (1994). *Fifty years of folly and fraud in the name of science.* Buffalo, NY: Biomedical Metatechnology Press.

Bross, I. D., et al. (1996). Is toxicity really necessary? II. Sources and analysis of data. *Cancer, 19*, 1785–1795.

Bross, I. D., et al. (1966). Is toxicity really necessary? III. Theoretical aspects. *Cancer, 19*, 1976–1804.

Brown, H. G. (1986). Worthless methods of cancer management. In *Cancer manual* (7th ed.). Boston: American Cancer Society.

Burton, D. (1999). *Complementary and alternative medicine (CAM) in cancer care: A progress report.* Retrieved May 12, 2005, http://www.cmbm.org/conferences/ccc99/transcripts99/burton.html

Burzynski Patient Group. (1996). Correspondence to members of the United States Senate and House of Representatives.

Cassileth, B. R. (1991). Survival and quality of life among patients receiving unproven as compared with conventional cancer therapy. *New England Journal of Medicine, 324*, 17.

Cassileth, B. R., & Deng, G. (2004). Unorthodox treatments for cancer. *Oncologist, 9*(1), 80–89.

Cassileth, B. R., et al. (1984). Contemporary unorthodox treatments in cancer medicine: A study of patients, treatments, and practitioners. *Annals of Internal Medicine, 101*(1), 105–112.

Cassileth, B. R., et al. (1987). *Report of a survey of patients recieving immunoaugmentative therapy.* Unpublished manuscript.

Chowka, P. B. (1990). Presentation to the panel on Unconventional Cancer Treatments. *Office of Technology Assessment of the United States Congress.* Washington, DC: U.S. Government Printing Office.

*Clark, M.D. v. Department of Professional Regulation, Board of Medical Examiners,* 463 So. 2d 328 (Fla. Ct. App. 1985).

Cohen, M. (1998). *Complementary and alternative medicine: Legal boundaries and regulatory perspectives.* Baltimore, MD: Johns Hopkins University Press.

Cohen, M. (2000). *Beyond complementary medicine: Legal perspectives on health care and human evolution.* Ann Arbor: University of Michigan Press.

Cohen, M. (2003). *Future medicine: Ethical dilemmas, regulatory challenges, and therapeutic pathways to health care and healing in human transformation.* Ann Arbor: University of Michigan Press.

Cohen, M. (2005). *Legal issues in integrative medicine: A guide for clinicians, hospitals, and patients* (NAF Publication). Washington, DC: U.S. Government Printing Office.

*Committee to Defend Reproductive Rights v. California*, 29 Cal. 3d 252; 625 P.2d 779 (1981).

Dumoff, A. (1995). Malpractice liability of alternative/complementary health care providers: A view from the trenches. *Alternative and Complementary Therapies 2*, 151–156 and 239–243.

Dumoff, A. (2000). Defining"disease": The latest struggle for turf in dietary supplement regulation. *Alternative and Complementary Therapies, 6*(2), 95–104.

Dumoff, A. (2004a). Legal and ethical issues in integrative practice. In B. Kligler, & R. Lee, (Eds.), *Integrative medicine*. New York: McGraw-Hill.

Dumoff, A. (2004b). Legal issues presented by integrative practice. In *Seminars in integrative medicine*. New York: Elsevier.

Dumoff, A. (2004c). Recognizing and working with legal issues: A legal audit for integrative practices and CAM practitioners: Parts I & II. *Alternative and Complementary Therapies, 10*(2/3), 109–115, 175–179.

Epstein, S. (1979). *The politics of cancer*. New York: Anchor Press/Doubleday.

Ernst, E., & Cassileth, B. R. (1998). The prevalence of complementary/alternative medicine in cancer: A systematic review. *Cancer, 83*(4), 777–782.

Evers, M. (1988). *Legal constraints on the availability of unorthodox cancer treatments: Freedom of choice viewpoint*. U.S. Congress Office of Technology Assessment. Washington, DC: U.S. Government Printing Office.

Fishbein, M. (1965). History of cancer quackery. *Perspectives in Biology and Medicine, 8*, 139–166.

Food and Drug Administration. (1996). FDA, cancer therapies: Accelerating approval and expanding access. Retrieved May 14, 2005, from http://www.fda.gov/opacom/backgrounders/cancerbg.html

Freimuth, V. (1988). *The public's search for information on unorthodox cancer treatments: The CIS experience*. U.S. Congress Office of Technology Assessment. Washington, DC: U.S. Government Printing Office.

Friedberg, M., et al. (1999–2000). Evaluation of conflict of interest in economic analyses of new drugs used in oncology. [comment in *Journal of the American Medical Association*, 1999, *282*(15), 1474–1475] [comment in *Journal of the American Medical Association*, 2000, *283*(11), 1423–1424] [comment in *Journal of the American Medical Association*, 2000, *283*(11), 1423; author reply 1424].

Friedman, M. (1991). Internal FDA memo from later acting FDA commissioner, October 31.

Gelb, L. (2005). *Unproven cancer treatments: Hope or hoax? FDA consumer*. Retrieved May 12, 2005, from http://www.fda.gov/bbs/topics/CONSUMER/CON00128.html

Goldberg, B. (Ed.). (1997). *An alternative medicine definitive guide to cancer*. Tiburon, CA: Future Medicine.

Gordon, J. S., & Curtin, S. (2000). *Comprehensive cancer care: Integrating alternative, complementary, and conventional therapies*. Cambridge, MA: Perseus.

Greenberg, D. (1975). Critical look at cancer coverage. *Columbia Journalism Review, 74*: 40–44.

*Griswold v. Connecticut*, 381 U.S. 479, 493 (1965).

*Healthcare America Plans v. Bossemeyer*, 1998 U.S. App. Lexis 31323 (10th Cir. 1998).

Hildenbrand, G. (1989–1990). Bomb threat quells cancer demonstration and OTA. *The Gerson Institute Healing Newsletter, 5*, 4.

Hoffer, L. J. (2001). Proof versus plausibility: Rules of engagement for the struggle to evaluate alternative cancer therapies. *Canadian Medical Association Journal, 164*(3), 351–353.

Illich, I. (1976/1999). *Limits to medicine: Medical nemesis, the expropriation of health*. New York: Marion Boyars.

Institute of Medicine. (2004). *Complementary and alternative medicine in the United States*. Washington, DC: U.S. Government Printing Office.

Jaffe, R. (1995). FDA abuse and retaliation: Dr. Stanislaw Burzynski. *Townsend Letter for Doctors, August/September*.

Jonas, W. B. (2001). The evidence house: Something we all can live in. *Western Journal of Medicine, 175*, 79–80.

Fishbein, M. (1947). Editorial: Hoxsey cancer charlatan. *Journal of the American Medical Association, 133*, 774–775.

Kempe, C. H., Silverman, F., Steele, B., Groegemuller, W., & Silver, H. (1962). The battered child syndrome. *Journal of the American Medical Association, 181*, 107–112.

Kill, K. A. (1988). Unproven cancer therapies. *American Pharmacology, NS28*, 18–22.

*Killian v. Healthsource*, 152 F.3d 514 (6th Cir. 1998).

Kolata, GB. (1996, July 24). Doctor's cancer "cure" attacked by F.D.A.. *The New York Times*.

Larrick, G. P. (1956). Public warning against Hoxsey cancer treatment. *Consumer Reports, 21*, 303.

Landmark Healthcare. (1999). *Landmark report II of HMOs and alternative care*. New York: Landmark Healthcare, Inc.

Lenzer, J. (2004). Scandals have eroded US public's confidence in drug industry. *British Medical Journal, 329*, 247.

Lerner, I. J., & Kennedy, B. J. (1992). The prevalence of questionable methods of cancer treatment in the United States. *CA: A Cancer Journal for Clinicians, 42*, 181–191.

Lerner, M. (1994). *Choices in healing: Integrating the best of conventional and complementary approaches to cancer*. Cambridge, MA: MIT Press.

*Lewis v. Trustmark Insurance Company*, 1999 U.S. App. Lexis 15746 (4th Cir. 1999).

*McLaughlin v. Connecticut General Life Insurance Company*, 565 F. Supp. 434 (N.D. Cal. 1983).

Memorial Sloan-Kettering Cancer Center. (n.d.). *Expert biography, Barrie R. Cassileth, Ph.D.* Retrieved May 13, 2005, from http://www.mskcc.org/prg/mrg/bios/525.cfm

Mohs, F. E. (1941). Chemosurgery: A microscopically controlled method of cancer excision. *Archives of Surgery, 42*, 279–295.

Moore, M. J., & Tannock, I. J. (1988). How expert physicians would wish to be treated if they developed genito–urinary cancer. *Proceedings of the American Society of Clinical Oncology, 7*, 118. [Abstract No. 455]

Moss, R. W. (1980). *The cancer syndrome New York*. New York: Grove Press.

Moss, R. W. (1989). *The cancer industry: Unraveling the politics*. New York: Paragon House.

Moss, R. W. (1995). *Questioning chemotherapy*. Brooklyn, NY: Equinox.

Moss, R. W. (1999). *The cancer industry*. Brooklyn, NY: Equinox.

Murphy, G. P., Morris, L. B., & Lang, D. (1997). *American Cancer Society: Informed decisions—The complete book of cancer diagnosis, treatment, and recovery*. New York: Viking.

National Cancer Institute. (2001). *Annual report to the nation finds cancer incidence and death rates on the decline: Survival rates show significant improvement*. Bethesda, MD: National Institutes of Health.

National Cancer Institute. (2002). *Cancer facts, antineoplastons*. Retrieved May 20, 2002, from http://www.cancer.gov/cancertopics/factsheet/Therapy/antineoplastons

National Institutes of Health. (1994). *Alternative medicine: Expanding medical horizons*. A Report to the National Institutes of Health on Alternative Medical Systems and Practices in the United States (NIH Publication No. 94-066). Washington, DC: U.S. Government Printing Office.

Note: (1981). "The uncertain application of the right of privacy in personal medical decisions: The laetrile cases." *Ohio State Law Journal, 42*(2), 523–550.

Note: (1983). "Selected recent court decisions: Third-party reirnbursement—Laetrile treatment—Free v. Travelers Insurance Co." *American Journal of Law and Medicine, 9*(1), 103–116.

Office of the Inspector General, Department of Health and Human Services. (2001). Clinical Laboratory Inspection Act (CLIA) Regulation of Unestablished Laboratory Tests, OEI-05-00-00250.

*Pearson v. Halala*, 164 F.3d 650 (D.C. Cir. 1999).

Pfifferling, J. H. (1994). Ounces of malpractice prevention. *Physician Executive, 20*(2), 36–38.

Pfohl, S. J. (1977). The "discovery" of child abuse. *Social Problems, 24*(3), 310–323.

*Pirozzi v. BCBS of Virginia*, 741 F. Supp. 586 (E.D. Va. 1990).

*Rogers v. State Board of Medical Examiners*, 371 So.2d 1037 (Fla. Dist. Ct. App. 1979).

*Schloendorff v. The Society of the New York Hospital*, 211 N.Y. 125; 105 N.E. 92 (N.Y.S. 1914).

*Schneider v. Revici, M.D., and Institute of Applied Biology, Inc.*, 817 F.2d 987 (2d Cir. 1987).

*Simkins, M&K Enterprises, Nevadacare, Inc.*, 229 F.3d 729 (9th Cir. 2000).

Sollner, W., Maislinger, S., DeVries, A., Steixner, E., Rumpold, G., & Lukas, P. (2000). Use of complementary and alternative medicine by cancer patients is not associated with perceived distress or poor compliance with standard treatment but with active coping behavior: A survey. *Cancer, 89*(4), 873–880.

Spencer, J. W., & Jacobs, J. J. (1999). *Complementary/alternative medicine: An evidence-based approach*. St. Louis, MO: Mosby.

Starr, R., & Siegel, S. (1996). An open letter to the *New York Times*, Burzynski Patient Group. *The New York Times*, New York, NY.

Studdert, D. M., Eisenberg, D. M., Miller, F. H., Curto, D. A., Kaptchuk, T. J., & Brennan, T. A. (1998). Medical malpractice implications of alternative medicine. *Journal of the American Medical Association, 280*, 1610–1615.

*The People v. Priviteria, Jr.*, 23 Cal. 3d 697; 591 P.2d 919 (Ca. 1979).

*United States v. Rutherford,* 442 U.S. 544, 99 S. Ct. 2470, 61 L. Ed. 2d 68 (1979).

U.S. Congress Office of Technology Assessment. (1990). *Unconventional cancer treatments* (Publication OTA-H-405). Washington, DC: U.S. Government Printing Office.

U.S. Department of Health and Human Services, Public Health Service, Food and Drug Administration. (1986). Immuno-augmentative therapy (IAT). Import Alert 57-04. In *Regulatory procedure manual. Part 9. Imports* (chapters 7–79). Washington, DC: Author.

*U.S. v. Vital Health Products,* 786 F. Supp. 761, 777-78 (E.D. Wisc. 1992), *aff'd* 985 F.2d 563 (1993).

Walker, P. C. (2000). Evolution of a policy disallowing the use of alternative therapies in a health system. *American Journal of Health-System Pharmacy, 57*(21), 1984–1990.

Ward, P. S. (1984). Andrew C. Ivy and Krebiozen: "Who will bell the cat? *The Bulletin of the History of Medicine, 58*(1), 28–52.

Ward, P. S. (1990). History of Hoxsey treatment. *Cancer Journal for Clinicians, 40*(1), 51–55.

Weiss, G. G. (2002). Malpractice: Don't wait for a lawsuit to strike. *Medical Economist, 6,* 82.

# A Patient's Experience and Perspective

20

Anonymous

**Y**ears ago, I was watching a television special on a teenage boy named Billy who was talking about his experience with cancer. He was diagnosed with lymphoma and subsequently shunned chemotherapy to pursue unproven alternative cancer treatments. He explained in the interview that he was convinced it was the use of these treatments that put him into remission. Then there was an interview with his incarcerated physician. The physician was prosecuted for treating Billy with 714-X (see Chapter 13), an alternative cancer treatment that at that time was illegal for a physician to administer to a patient. The physician claimed to have saved Billy's life with this treatment yet he found himself behind bars.

That was the last that I heard of these alternative cancer treatments until I myself was diagnosed with non-Hodgkin's lymphoma. I was preparing to begin medical school when I discovered a swollen cervical lymph node. Having a complete medical workup, I was fortunate to catch this cancer at Stage I. Histologically, it was a large diffuse high-grade lymphoma. Translated into layperson's terms, this means a fairly aggressive cancer, but one that is highly responsive to surgery, chemotherapy, and radiation.

My medical education was temporarily put on hold. Being at Stage I, the very first step was to remove the tumor. I found a very good surgeon at New York Hospital of Special Surgery, who did an excellent job in removing quite a large tumor, which was roughly the size of an egg.

While waiting for my scheduled surgery, which was in 2 weeks, I happened to come across the world of alternative cancer treatments. It seems almost every cancer patient has some kind of exposure to these treatments. The public is getting constant exposure through books, magazines, the Internet, and friends. I was checking my e-mail one day and received a message claiming apricot seeds can cure cancer. A young man with kidney cancer claimed it was the apricot seeds that were responsible for his miraculous cure. This person was also the feature on a television special edition of *Extra* years back when he discussed his use of the apricot kernel after failing standard treatment. I didn't really know what to think of this. The advertisement came across as a typical scam. Was this person trying to make money selling apricot seeds or do these seeds really have anticancer activity? When I began to read about the different alternative cancer treatments, I learned that it was the contents within the apricot seeds that can be given in the drug form known as laetrile. This highly controversial cancer treatment back in the 1970s was proven to have no clinical value in extending survival in patients with advanced metastatic disease that had not been cured by standard treatments.

I had a recent conversation with a fellow doing research at Sloan-Kettering Memorial Hospital. Ironically, it was at this hospital where the laetrile controversy first made headlines throughout the country. This fellow was one of a number of researchers conducting clinical trials evaluating alternative cancer treatments at Sloan-Kettering. One of their studies was the evaluation of the apricot kernel, which is known to be partially composed of arsenic and cyanide. Researchers in this study found that in patients with nonmetastatic disease who were previously treated with standard treatments, the apricot kernel had a significant benefit in these patients. However, there was a failure to show any activity against metastatic disease. With the new war on terror, government funding for this project was subsequently terminated and the study was put on hold. So in the end, the laetrile controversy may not be dead after all.

There is no short list of the alternative cancer treatments available today. I realized this when I visited the health food store. While waiting to undergo surgery, I figured the one useful thing I could do was begin to eat healthy food and start taking some vitamins. Little did I know what I was about to discover. One couldn't possibly miss an entire wall filled with over 100 books on this topic. Everything was there: books on healthy eating, juicing, herbal therapy, treatment for all kinds of chronic illnesses from arthritis and headaches to cancer and heart disease. I don't disregard something until I've researched it. Noticing that there were countless books claiming success with cancer treatment, I decided to begin reading. Perhaps there was something here that I might find useful. So I picked up some vitamins, purchased a couple of books, and went home.

After a few days of reading extensively on this topic, I found that in these books, doctors make the argument that many forms of cancers can be treated by strengthening the body's biochemical terrain and supporting the body's natural processes, fortifying it so that it can fight cancer on its own. It is a theory based on developing optimal functioning of all body systems and maintaining this optimal health for the rest of a patient's life through the means of a sound nutritional diet, vitamins and antioxidants, herbal and enzyme therapy, systemic detoxification, and enhancement of the immune system.

The doctors in these books questioned the use of chemotherapy and radiation and blasted drug companies and government agencies, accusing them of constructing a multibillion-dollar business that not only put profits first but also suppressed development of and access to effective alternative treatments. The viewpoints given in some of these books were extreme and biased to say the least. Chemotherapy and radiation have successfully saved many lives and this cannot be denied. However, you have the mainstream medical field claiming that alternative medicine is quackery and that these physicians are profiting from desperate cancer patients who believe anything and are willing to try any treatment to survive. Both sides accuse each other of having profit as a motive. One can argue that mainstream medicine, with decades of medical research, is certainly more dependable than many forms of these "unproven" alternative forms of treatment. But in reality almost all these treatments have never been evaluated with adequate studies.

I couldn't help but feel anger and disappointment at the medical establishment for their inability to work together and come to an agreement. And I'm certain that many cancer patients feel the same. And the blame doesn't rest on just the shoulders of government agencies. Many practitioner of complementary and alternative medicine share this blame as well for their stubbornness and inability to work with the National Cancer Institute (NCI). It's bad enough that cancer patients are dealing with a potentially lethal illness. But to have doctors on one side saying one thing and doctors on the other side saying something else is, in my opinion, ludicrous. Some of these treatments have been around for decades. Why haven't they been properly evaluated? I didn't blame the oncologists. I found them to be very caring physicians and, unfortunately, there are no studies for them to help guide cancer patients. As a result, the oncologist and their cancer patients are left out in the cold not knowing what's effective. Fortunately, attitudes are changing and the future seems brighter. The National Institutes of Health (NIH), the NCI, and physicians of complementary and alternative medicine are finally working together to scientifically investigate many of these treatments.

## Choosing Between Conventional and Alternative Cancer Treatments

I decided that I would take my time and carefully analyze all my options. My parents were very supportive while I decided whether to pursue the alternative treatments or the conventional ones. Having many family friends who are physicians, I found myself in daily telephone conversations with doctors who were concerned that I may reject chemotherapy and radiation and pursue only alternative treatments. They were all convinced that I was in great danger if I passed up conventional therapy.

I found myself in a precarious situation. I decided to make appointments with physicians on both sides of the spectrum. I first visited two oncologists, one at Columbia Presbyterian and the other at Memorial Sloan-Kettering. They did a very nice job in explaining to me the prognosis of my cancer and the treatments, which were needed. While I was listening to these doctors, I was waiting for my chance to pop the big question and ask them about these alternative cancer treatments and their opinion. To my surprise, they did not discourage the use of these treatments. The doctor referred to these treatments as *complementary medicine* rather than *alternative medicine*. He explained how many of these treatments are unproven but unlikely to do any harm and that they could possibly help. Moreover, if I wanted to use these treatments along with chemotherapy and radiation, there shouldn't be any problem.

Following my meeting with the oncologists, I visited a number of physicians practicing alternative medicine. They discussed my different options and informed me of their treatment protocol. One of the physicians suggested that if the need arises such that my cancer does not respond to treatment, he could refer me to an oncologist who combines both chemotherapy and well as complementary treatments.

I came eventually to the point where I had to make a decision whether to combine both conventional chemotherapy and radiation with complementary treatments or whether to pursue only the alternative treatments as a sole modality. It was an extremely difficult decision to make. I decided to go with the alternative treatments and if my cancer continued to progress, I could always come in with the conventional treatments. Was I taking a risk? Absolutely! With surgery, chemotherapy, and radiation, I was told that the 5-year survival rate with my cancer was 80%. With surgery alone, which I had opted for, that figure drops dramatically. Lymphoma is by definition a systemic disease and surgery alone is not curative, especially with an aggressive high-grade lymphoma. I was heavily criticized by many for the decision that I made. My parents were very supportive of my decision, which was very helpful. Everyone else thought I was crazy and that making the decision that I did was just a stupid move. But they didn't know what it's like to be told that you must visit a sperm bank before treatment because of the risk of infertility as a side effect of the chemotherapy or to be told that there is a risk of cardiomyopathy and heart failure. I figured I'd go for the gold. If I could cure this cancer with surgery and alternative medicine alone, I wouldn't have the risk of developing a secondary cancer as a long-term side effect of the chemotherapy.

## Getting Started

I now needed a physician who would be able to provide me with a comprehensive alternative treatment plan. I ended up receiving in the mail a brochure from an organization called People Against Cancer. They provide cancer patients with useful information with regard to effective alternative cancer treatments. They not only give patients useful information but also connect patients to practicing physicians. In the world of alternative cancer therapies choosing the best therapy and approach to offer the best chance of a cure is extremely difficult in. One has no idea where to start and how to know which is the most effective. This is where People Against Cancer were very helpful. They informed me that the best approach to treating cancer is one that takes into consideration many different means of achieving optimal health. This includes a sound nutritional diet, along with nutratherapy that includes vitamins, minerals, herbs, enzymes, glandular extracts, detoxification, immunotherapy, exercise and stress reduction, as well as the avoidance of toxins in our food, air, water, and workplace as best as possible.

I got in touch with a physician who worked with me and guided me through this treatment protocol. I also worked with a nutritionist who stressed the importance of diet. I completed a questionnaire that gave my physician the proper information he needed to recommend a diet and supplement regimen. I was told that fruits and vegetables should make up approximately 60% of my food intake and to eat as many raw vegetables as possible. Green vegetables such as lettuce, green beans, broccoli, spinach, and asparagus were of particular importance though I was told that no vegetable should be avoided. Blueberries, strawberries, pineapples, grapes, apples, and papaya were additionally stressed as well. Grains were to make approximately 20% of my food intake. Intake of high-quality grains was stressed in the form of wheat, rice oats, barley, millet, rye, and corn in the form of breads, cereals, pastas, and so on. High-protein foods such as meats or other complete proteins were to make up 10% of my diet. Vegetarianism was not recommended and

I was told that I would feel better if I included some seafood (all types), chicken, and turkey along with some nuts and seeds. Red meats were to be used only once or twice per week, if at all. Dairy products were to make up the last 10% of my food intake in the forms of yogurt, cottage cheese, and other cheeses. I was to avoid processed cheese and so-called cheese foods. I was to use honey, molasses, and pure maple syrup when a sweetener was needed. I was also told to drink eight glasses of water per day. Spring, mineral, distilled, or other bottled waters were preferred to tap water. Foods that I choose were to be organically grown and pesticide free, with whole and natural ingredients whenever possible. Finally, I was to avoid as best as possible a long list of items that included white sugar and flour, heavily processed and deep fried foods, artificial flavorings and colorings, presalted and prepared foods, soft drinks, caffeine, and so on.

I followed this diet without any problem. I've never been a fan of fast foods and my diet had always been well rounded so the adjustment was easy for me to make. On top of this, I added three glasses of fresh juice consisting of apples, carrots, beets, and green vegetables daily. Green tea, well known as a powerful antioxidant with proven anticancer activity, became a regular drink. I was a very compliant patient and was enjoying my new healthy way of life. There was no doubt that my energy level had dramatically increased. To me, that was an indication that my body's level of functioning had improved.

Along with this diet, I was placed on a nutritional supplement program. This included high-dose vitamins and antioxidants, anticancer herbs, essential minerals, as well as enzymes and glandular extracts from New Zealand consisting of pancreas, bone marrow, lymph, liver, and thymus extracts. Finally, I was put on a 48-day detoxification program for improved metabolism and nutrient assimilation. I found this concept of detoxification to make a lot of sense. We are all exposed to a great deal of toxins daily. Ridding the body of these harmful toxins predisposing to physical disease and metabolic imbalances was essential.

It should be noted that this regimen, a dietary approach that matches a patient to their metabolic type, was proposed by two physicians, William Donald Kelly, DDS, and Bill Wolcott, MD. This treatment of diet, supplements, enzymes, and detoxification has also been used by Nicholas Gonzalez, MD, whose patient records were reviewed by the National Cancer Institute, resulting in a government-subsidized grant for further research on pancreatic cancer. A study is currently underway at Columbia University on the Gonzalez therapy in pancreatic cancer (see Chapter 12).

# Leaving the United States for Treatment

The last thing needed to complete my anticancer treatment protocol was an effective means of immunotherapy. Although an adequate diet as well as the nutritional supplements I was following at that time certainly played a role in immune enhancement, I decided that perhaps it may be wise to take another step in that direction. When I first began reading about the different alternative cancer treatments available, I came across a form of therapy that played a large role in my decision to put chemotherapy and radiation on hold and pursue an alternative treatment. I soon found myself leaving the United States for a treatment that U.S. physicians are not permitted by law to give to their patients.

## Immuno-Placental Therapy

The treatment is called Immuno-Placental Therapy (IPT), a form of embryonal stem cell therapy. Russian immunologist Valentine I. Govallo, MD, PhD, had been conducting research and clinical studies on the anticancer effects of placental tissue for over 20 years. He is the author of over 250 scientific articles and 20 books, including *The Immunology of Pregnancy and Cancer*.

Understanding the way a fetus relates to its mother on an immunological level, Dr. Govallo used pregnancy as a model to study cancer. In his book, Dr. Govallo explains this relationship in detail. According to him, a fetus contains both maternal as well as paternal antigens. During a miscarriage, a mother's immune system recognizes the paternal antigens as foreign to her and the fetus is rejected. Therefore, during pregnancy, there is a physiologic immunosuppression protecting the fetus. It is the placenta, which synthesizes "blocking factors," that blocks the mother's immune system at the level of the fetal/placental immune system. In other words, placental immunity helps protect a fetus against rejection by the mother's immune system. In women with repeated miscarriages, Dr Govallo was able to stimulate the development of the placenta and protect the fetus. In working with these women, he was able to prevent miscarriages with a 91% success rate. Through his research with spontaneous abortions, Dr. Govallo reasoned that just as a fetus is protected by "blocking factors" synthesized by the mother's immune system, tumors also shield themselves from a cancer patient's immune system, allowing unrecognized proliferation. He theorized that the placenta contains factors suppressing the defense mechanism of malignant cells, removing the tumor's immunological shield and permitting a patient's immune system to neutralize the tumor. Dr. Govallo states the following in his book:

> Antigens from fetal tissue and from malignant tumors have many common antigenic determinants as well as stage-specific expression of the same oncogenes. Embryonic products and embryo antigens associated with tumor cells leads to immunosuppression and malignization. With immunization of placental cells, the B cells of oncological patients produce antisuppressory (anti-blocking) antibodies which neutralize numerous embryo-like products formed by malignisized cells: isoferritin, HCG-like products, CEA, alpha-fetoprotein, TSF, and others. In other words, the antibodies form complexes with blocking factors and with immunosuppressory agents on circulating lymphocytes and tumor cells resulting in the removal of suppressory embryo-like products. Therefore, placental extracts of the chorionic villi, which contain a broad spectrum of trophoblast antigens can stimulate, through cross-reactive antigens, a tumor specific effector cell immunity (CTL, LAK, NK cells, and macrophages).

At the end of Dr. Govallo's book is a six-page summary. The following are excerpts taken from this summary, which are explained in much greater detail throughout his book:

> If one keeps in mind that malignancy, a synthesis of different embryonic substances (numerous enzymes, alpha-feto protein, chorionic gonadotropin, carcinoembryo antigens, etc.) takes place, it is possible that the indicated facts only complement the existing concepts about embryolization of cancer. Diverse data of dedifferentiation of cancer cells,

embryonic-type organization of cytoplasmic structures in cancer cells, expression of identical oncogenes on malignant and embryonic cells, participation of the same types of growth factors in oncogenesis and embryogenesis, and the similar morphofunctional characteristics (invasive growth, metastasizing, etc.) of cancer and trophoblast cells can be referred to as the embryolization of cancer.

The absence of efficient effector immunity in malignization can be explained from the standpoint of the embryonic theory of cancer. Hormones and lymphokines produced by placental or cancer cells selectively activate suppressory CD8 lymphocytes and inhibit CTL and LAK generation. Cancer and embryonic tissues stimulate migration of bone marrow suppressory cells whose residents are local suppressors. Suppressory lymphocytes from the spleen and regional lymph nodes also migrate to these tissues, and reinforce local protection. Spleen suppressory cells and intratumor lymphocytes produce suppressory factors, which have remote effects. This results in a situation in which even the existing cytotoxic lymphocytes are unable to overcome the anti-tumor barrier of the tumor. B cells synthesize humoral blocking antibodies, which independantly, or together with an antigen, mask the determinants of embyonic and cancerous cells. The products of extraembryonic tissues and those of malignant cells block the afferent link of immunity. The molecules or hormones, sialo acids, transferrin, and metabolites participate in the process of antigenic mimicry, also providing afferent blockage of immunity.

The idea of an immunosuppressory "shield," generated by cancer, forces us to modify approaches to the immunotherapy of cancer. It is known from experimental data that the immunization of pregnant females with embryonic cells or their extracts, when the trophoblast is intact and the placenta is not injured, is not al all dangerous to the embryo. In cases of incomplete development of the trophoblast and the placenta (primary and secondary spontaneous abortions), the immunization of pregnant women with alloantigents increases immunosuppresion and may prevent rejection of the fetus.

While in the case of spontaneous abortions, cellular LAI response to embryo antigens, blocking serum activity, nonspecific suppressory lymphocytes and the deficit of small lymphocytes in the lymphocytogram are absent. All of these indicators change after immunotherapy, and the normal reproductive function of women is restored (that is, the development of the placenta is stimulated). On the contrary, in cancer patients, the LAI response to embryo antigens, serum blocking factors, suppressory lymphocytes, and a deficit of small lymphocytes are all present. Therefore, the task of cancer immunotherapy is to create a reactivity level that is characteristic of a spontaneous abortion.

It became evident that in fighting cancer, deblocking therapy, aimed at the suppression of endogenic immunosuppression, must become a leading component of the immunological strategy. For this therapy, we used an extract of the fetal portion of the placenta-the chorionic villi-containing a concentrate of immunosuppressory and deblocking products. Even a single immunization with a large dose of placental extract achieved a reverse development of lung cancer metastases. Later on, a program of repeated placental extract injection was developed. This treatment was conducted with the immunological reaction controlled and simultaneous enhancement of functional T cells by using the products of embryonic thymuses. A comparative study of the blocking characteristics of different samples of placental extracts allowed selection of the extract most suitable for a particular patient. This study was conducted using LAI tests with the blood cells of the patient and embryo antigens.

The consequences of the above-mentioned effects were termed by us as *immu-noembryotherapy*. In patients immunized with placental extracts, the intensity of the LAI response to embryo antigens decreased, humoral and cellular suppressory factors were eliminated from the blood, and small/large lymphocyte ratio in the lymphocy-togram gradually became normal. Clinically, in a number of cases, this process was accompanied by a reverse development of metastases and the absence of further pro-gression of the disease. In 60–80% of patients with breast, lung, uterine, kidney, and other cancers, a stable remission (observed over more than 10 years of medical care) was achieved. The longest period of observation for patients with lung cancers as of 1992 has been 17 years.

Many aspects concerning the application of placental extracts in the treatment of on-cological patients require further study in order to achieve greater accuracy. The source of the effect of chorionic tissue extract, its influence on the effector immunocompetent cells (CTL, NK, LAK cells, and macrophages) and on the system of natural and induced suppressory lymphocytes, the participation of MHC antigens in this process (the role of HLA compatibility between the cancer patient and female donors of the chorion), the participation of fetal and trophoblast antigens, and the relationship of this phenomenon to other embryonic cells and tissues are not entirely clear.

Representatives from People Against Cancer made a trip to Russia to review the work of Dr. Govallo. He began a study in 1974 on 45 patients with a variety of advanced cancers ranging from malignant melanoma, lung, breast, kidney, and colorectal cancers. As of 1997, 29 of the original 45 patients remained alive, a 64.4% survival rate after 20 years. After verifying Dr. Govallo's work by reviewing his patient records as well as meeting some of his long-term survivors, People Against Cancer brought the treatment to the Immuno-Augmentative Therapy (IAT) clinic in Freeport, the Bahamas. It was at this clinic where I received IPT. IPT is also available in Germany, Switzerland, and other countries in Europe. Unfortunately, no studies are underway at present to verify Dr. Govallo's therapy. His immunological theories in his book are well referenced and documented, but there are few clinical trials evaluating this therapy.

# Off to the Bahamas

IAT is a treatment developed by Lawrence Burton, PhD, a biologist and cancer researcher from St. Vincent Hospital in New York City. According to him, he found measurable deficiencies of certain immune proteins in the blood of people with cancer. Isolating and extracting the substances, he injected them into patients, bringing about remissions in many forms of cancer. He focused his work on certain factors that he and his col-leagues identified as blocking proteins, deblocking protein tumor antibody, and tumor complement that were isolated from the human blood.

Dr. Burton claimed impressive recovery statistics, especially in patients with ad-vanced colon cancer and mesothelioma of the lungs, as well as cancers of the bladder, prostate, pancreas, and lymphomas. Because lung mesothelioma, an asbestos–related can-cer is known to be incurable with rapid disease progression, Dr. Burton's claims were immediately dismissed by many of his peers. Surrounded by controversy, he set up a research center in Freeport, the Bahamas, and began to treat cancer patients. The clinic has treated over 5,000 patients with cancer, with the claim that a large group of patients has survived over 20 years. At present, John Clement, MD., is the director of the IAT clinic.

As I was flying to the Bahamas, I recalled a telephone conversation I had with a family friend, who happened to be an oncologist. He told me that in all his years of practice, he has never known one patient who was cured by their treatment. When I arrived at the clinic, I understood why this was so. Almost all the patients had cancer that was so advanced that I don't believe anything was going to cure their disease. Perhaps treatment may help extend survival, but a cure was a long shot for many of these unfortunate people.

In my first meeting with Dr. Clement, we discussed the treatment of Immuno-Placental Therapy his clinic was offering. Because I was only the 50th patient to receive this therapy in his clinic, his experience with treatment and outcome of this therapy was minimal and he therefore did not make any guarantees. I decided to go ahead with the therapy, which cost $7,500. The therapy was quite easy. It consisted of two intramuscular injections, spaced 1 week apart. It was that simple and there were no side effects whatsoever. In the meantime, I had a week to hang around the clinic and talk to some of their patients.

The majority of patients coming in to the clinic for daily treatment were those who had been diagnosed within the past few years and their disease had progressed with standard conventional therapy. Aside from these patients, there were a few patients I met during that week who had been returning to the clinic for several years for follow-up therapy after successful treatment of their cancer by IAT. The first of such patients I met was a young lady who must have been in her twenties. She was diagnosed with lymphoma several years ago and was being treated in the United States by standard therapy. Unfortunately, her cancer was progressing and she was near death. The treatment she received at the clinic worked, and since then she has been in stable remission. The second lady I saw was in her sixties. I saw her standing outside the clinic one afternoon and began talking to her. Twenty years ago, she was diagnosed with Stage III colon cancer. Like me, she opted for the alternative approach first. She was cured of her disease and, like the other survivors, she returns often for evaluation and maintenance therapy. The last patient I saw was by far the most fascinating of all. He was an elderly gentlemen who had been receiving IAT treatment for 9 years for mesothelioma of the lung.

As I was leaving this clinic, I realized everything I read about this place was true. It was no gimmick and the treatment that was being offered for so many years had helped many. Dr. Clement was a kind and, above all, an honest physician, who I had a great deal of respect for. He truly believes IAT is an effective cancer therapy. As we spoke over dinner one night, he told me how many of his colleagues in the United Kingdom severed their relationship when he decided to treat cancer using IAT. In his mind, he believed he was doing the right thing. A year later, a physician I knew had a patient with ovarian cancer. She wanted to send her patient to the Bahamas for treatment. When she spoke to Dr. Clement, he told her that they don't accept patients with ovarian cancer because this cancer does not respond to IAT. This physician said to me, "I thought those people in the Bahamas were all about money, but I guess I was wrong." As a former patient, I couldn't agree with her more.

The NCI and the National Center for Complementary and Alternative Medicine (NCCAM) at the NIH have recently contracted the Rand Corporation to evaluate IAT.

# Complete Remission and Cure

I recently had the opportunity to attend a 2-day seminar at the Center for Integrative Medicine at Thomas Jefferson University Hospital (TJUH). Jefferson integrative physicians incorporate nutritional, herbal, homeopathic, and traditional Chinese medicine therapies into a comprehensive patient care approach. At this seminar, a review of the "evidence" was presented by medical doctors practicing integrative medicine as well as oncologists. Topics covered included the use of high-dose micronutrient supplementation, botanical medicine, immune stimulants, including mistletoe (Iscador) and mushrooms, enzymes, and the controversy of combining high-dose antioxidants with conventional chemotherapy and radiation.

What is unique to TJUH is the way in which the Center for Integrative Medicine works in conjunction with Jefferson's Kimmel Cancer Center counseling patients and developing treatment plans. They discuss each individual recommendation with an oncologist to determine the best course of treatment. In this way, patients are guided by experienced physicians from both sides of the spectrum. Successfully, they are overcoming many of the barriers between conventional oncology and alternative medicine.

As an example, a case was presented at the seminar of a 54-year-old female with colorectal cancer. She presented with a 4-cm mass with muscularis involvement with no nodal involvement or distant metastasis. The patient first received recommendations from an outside nutritionist who placed her on a high-fiber diet, raw vegetables, a high-dose antioxidant regimen, seeds, nuts, and numerous herbal supplements. When this patient came to the Integrative Center at TJUH, the physicians consulted with the oncologists and informed the patient of a 97% cure rate with the use of pre-op radiation and chemotherapy, surgery, and post-op chemotherapy. The patient underwent the conventional treatments and new dietary recommendations were made to alleviate side effects. Because of this favorable prognosis, antioxidants were withheld during radiation and chemotherapy to prevent possible unwanted interaction. After treatment, this patient was given advice on how to safely use complementary and alternative therapies to help maintain a long-term remission. From my own experience as a patient, taking one's health into one's own hands by utilizing these treatments can psychologically transform and heal not only physically but also emotionally and mentally.

Since being treated in 1998, I have been free of cancer for nearly 8 years. I will never really know what cured my cancer, whether it was the surgery, IPT, juicing, the antioxidants, or the herbs. But the need for objective testing, case review, and clinical investigation of such therapies is obviously clear. Alternative cancer therapies with therapeutic potential must be differentiated from worthless remedies. And through medical research, oncologists can be given additional modalities in cancer therapy, shifting the survival curve further to the right. If this issue is not confronted, potential lives will certainly be lost. Patients will continue to run away from standard treatments and at times begin self-prescribing ineffective remedies they find in health food stores.

With the establishment of the Office of Alternative Medicine in 1991, now known as NCCAM, a new direction was potentially taken in the fight against cancer. Until recently, the output of this agency has been relatively poor. But the future looks more promising. NCCAM is presently funding John's Hopkins Medical Center with a 5-year $7.8 million grant to evaluate alternative cancer therapies, including the herbal formula

PC-SPES for prostate cancer (see Chapter 13). Along with the studies underway at Columbia University and many other research projects, the medical community will soon be given scientific evidence on the validity of these treatments. Physicians will then be able to better utilize safe and effective complementary treatments in combination with conventional treatments. In the future, a diagnosis of cancer may mean seeing an oncologist, a nutritionist, an herbalist, and an acupuncturist, consulting each other to determine the best course of treatment for the patient.

# Index

Abrahamsen, A. F., 103
Academy for Guided Imagery, 69, 75, 76
ACAOM. *See* Accreditation Commission for Acupuncture and Oriental Medicine
Access to Medical Treatment Act, 439
Accreditation Commission for Acupuncture and Oriental Medicine (ACAOM), 339
Ackerknecth, E. H., 26
Acklin, M. W., 103
active-cognitive coping strategy, 104
activity (physical), and colon cancer, 127, 128
acupuncture, 228, 298, 316–317
    American Cancer Society's support of, 316
    as analgesia, 317–318
    *Andrews v. Ballard* and, 419
    Berlioz's book (1816) on, 306
    integration promoted by, 337
    medicine v., 317
    myelosuppression/hormonal markers and, 318–319
    for nausea/vomiting, 316, 318
    NIH's support of, 307, 316, 318
    physician's recommendations for, 308
acute promyelocytic leukemia (APL), 176
Adachi, S., 108
adaptation
    cancer as, 15–17
    cellular, 13
    human beings dietary, 126, 128
Adriamycin, MAK and, 366
Adult Growth Examination, 346
aging, MAK and, 367–368
agriculture
    influence of irrigation on, 143
    nutrition and, 143
alcoholism, TM and, 347–348
*Alcoholism Treatment Quarterly,* 347–348
Alcott, William, 287
Alexander, C. N., 347, 348
Alpha Tocopherol Beta Carotene (ATBC) study, 177
Alternative Medicine Office (U.S. Congress), 81
American Cancer Society (ACA), 316, 408
American Chemical Society, 252

American College of Physicians-American Society of Internal Medicine Consensus Panel Statement on End-of-Life issues, 114
American Dance Therapy Association, 90
American Medical Association (AMA), 41, 408
    CAM Operational Statement by, 408
    Hoxsey and, 401–402
American Psychological Association, 40
American School of Chiropractic, 283
American School of Naturopathy, 283
amines, as causative in cancer, 133–134, 136
analgesia, hypnosis-induced, 44
anatomic pathology, 23
ancient cancers, 23
Ancient Egypt/Nubia
    cancer evidence from, 27–28
    medical papyruses of, 22, 29
Ancient Middle East, cancer evidence from, 28
*Andrews v. Ballard* acupuncture case, 419
anthroposophy (of Steiner), 244
antibiotics
    era of, 18
    as "magic bullet," 18
antineoplastons. *See also* Burzynski, Stanislaw R.
    for cancer treatment, 387–391
    as possible cancer breakthrough, 390
antioxidant(s). *See* green tea; red tea; Vitamin C; Vitamin E
    enzymes and, 355
    rasayanas and, 371
    synergism of, 359–360
anxiety
    about future, 102
    biofeedback for, 52, 54
    cognitive therapy and, 54
    expressive therapy and, 86
    hypnosis management of, 43
    imagery's influence on, 67
    religion and, 103
    TM and, 345
APL. *See* acute promyelocytic leukemia
apocrine gland function, and breast biology, 156–157

*arbuda* (glands and tumors), 46. *See also Atharvaveda;* Sushruta
Aristotle, on function of art, 84
Armstrong, B., 151
aromatherapy. *See* essential oils therapy
*Artemesia anuua* herb, and breast cancer, 333
Art Recovery program (California Pacific Medical Center), 92
art therapies
  for children, 92
  humanizing influence of, 86–87
  symbolic language of, 82
ascorbic acid. *See* Vitamin C
*ashwagandha* herb, 371
Assagioli, R., 73
assay, for carcinogenicity, 15
*Astragulus* study, 332
*Atharvaveda,* 30
atmospheric cure (Rickli), 286
Australia, breast cancer/lactation study, 153
Authentic Movement (Adler), 87
autohypnosis, 43
autonomic nervous system, stressor's influence on, 106
autotoxicity, 288–289
autumn crocus, used as drug, 30
Ayurvedic medicine. *See also Charaka Samhita; dravyaguna;* herbs, of Ayurvedic medicine; Maharishi Amrit Kalash; *ojas; rasayanas;* Transcendental Meditation
  behavioral rasayanas of, 351–352
  clinical approach of, 372–373
  diet/digestion in, 349–351
  *dosha* concept of, 370
  *dravyaguna* (Ayurvedic pharmacology), 352
  herbal medicines of, 352–355
  herbal rasayanas of, 357–359
  physician's beside manner in, 352

Baider, L., 104
Balraj Maharishi, 358
Bartenieff, Irmgard, 90
basal cell carcinoma, and Pacific Yew, 251
Bateson, Mary Catherine, 88
Baylor College of Medicine (Houston, TX), 388
Beach, Wooster, 290
behavioral rasayanas, 351–352
Benson, Herbert, 48–49
Berg, J. W., 151
Berkel, J., 98
Berlioz, Louis, 306
beta-carotene, 177, 215. *See also* Alpha Tocopherol Beta Carotene (ATBC) study; Beta Carotene and Retinol Efficacy (CARET) study
  breast cancer and, 191
  cancer influenced by, 123, 167

  endometrial cancer and, 201
  free radicals and, 355
  lung cancer and, 191
  toxicity of, 215
  Vitamin A v., 215
Beta Carotene and Retinol Efficacy (CARET) study, 178
BHT (butylated hydroxytoluene), and carcinogenesis, 171, 203
bias, in research design/interpretation/funding, 411–415
Bilz, F. E., 286
biochemical individuality, 293
biofeedback, 51–55
  blood pressure and, 52
  cancer applications of, 53–55
  early history of, 51–52
  methodology of, 52–53
  nausea/vomiting control through, 53
  neuroendocrine/immune effects of, 54–55
  pain reduction via, 52
  physical/psychological benefits of, 38
  postsurgical incontinence and, 54
  prostate cancer and, 54
  videoendoscopic, 53
bioflavonoids
  free radicals and, 355
  synergism of, 359–360
biologic adaptation, and cancer, 125–127
biological dualism, 241
biology
  breastfeeding and reproductive, 152–154
  as mediating factor, 106–111
  nutrition and evolutionary, 143
Biomedical Hoxsey Center, 405
black tea, 248
blood pressure
  biofeedback's usefulness for, 52
  expressive therapy's influence on, 84
  meditation's influence on, 50
Blumberg, Baruch S., 371
BMA. *See* bone marrow aspirations
BMT. *See* bone marrow transplant
body image, and expressive therapy', 84
body scan/progressive muscle relaxation, 70
Boik, John, 320
bone marrow aspirations (BMA), 44–45
bone marrow transplant (BMT), 44
*Book of Changes* (*Yi Jing*), 305
books/tapes, self-help, 69
botanical medicines, 298
*botanics* doctors, 290
Braid, James, 39
Branch Davidians, 112

Bras, G., 150, 151
breast biology
    apocrine gland function and, 156–157
    dietary protein and, 156
breast cancer
    age variations in, 144
    apocrine gland function and, 156–157
    *Artemesia anuua* herb and, 333
    beta-carotene and, 191
    birth mother's age and, 148
    breastfeeding and, 141–142, 143, 152
    CAM study (San Francisco) and, 304
    causative factor variability in, 131
    coping mechanisms for, 108
    dietary fat intake and, 149–150
    dietary restriction's influence on, 135
    drugs v. nutrition for, 142
    early life dietary patterns and, 147
    estrogen's influence on, 135
    fatigue/depression/lack of social support and, 108
    fertility association with, 124
    fiber's protective effect in, 135, 201
    genetic factors in, 110–111
    height/frame size and, 149
    high-progesterone-type oral contraceptives and, 155
    hormonal influences on, 154–155
    inbreeding and, 110
    increasing incidences of, 142
    Japanese-American women *vs.* native Japanese women and, 144
    Japan's increase in, 133, 149
    Jews and, 97, 110
    Latter-Day Saints and, 99
    macronutrients and, 149
    MAK and, 363–364
    menarche onset/menopause and, 152, 153
    migrant's and, 132, 146
    milk consumption and, 151
    mortality/morbidity, international differences, of, 144
    obesity and, 147
    olive oil and, 133
    overnutrition and, 141, 147, 152
    pregnancy and, 124, 153
    premenopause v. postmenopause and, 154
    protein/tumors and, 141, 147
    as prototypical malignant condition, 17
    reproductive variables/reproductive history and, 152
    retinoids and, 216
    risk factors for, 146–149
    social support study, 105
    spiritual expression's influence on, 108
    as third leading cause of death, 96

    total food consumption as variable, 150
    total protein v. animal protein, 150
    Vitamin E and, 191
    western-style diet's influence on, 145
Breast Cancer Fund, 91, 334
breastfeeding
    and cancer, 141–142, 143, 152
    overnutrition and, 148
    reproductive biology and, 152–154
    single breast, 153–154
breasts
    fluid composition of, 157–158
    secretory activity of, 156, 157
    tissue microenvironment of, 158–159
Brenner, Seymour, 416
Bross, I. J., 98, 205
Brothwell, D., 26, 28, 29
Brown, D., 102
Brown, E. C., 103
browning (of meat/fish). *See* amines
Brunet, J. S., 110
Brusch, Charles, 259
Buber, Martin, 95
Buchbauer, G., 274
burdock root (*Arctium lappa*), 258–259, 260
Burkitt, Denis Parsons, 129
Burkitt's lymphoma, 7, 9, 26
Burnett, J. C., 381
Burton, Dan, 428
Burton, Lawrence, 395, 452–453
Burzynski, Stanislaw R., 387
    *ad hominem*/technical attacks on, 388
    FDA challenges of, 388, 390, 400, 424–427
Burzynski Patient Group, 409
Burzynski Research Institute, 388
Bushwick, B., 113
B vitamins, and carcinogenesis, 193

cachexia, hydrazine sulfate's and, 391, 393
Cacioppo, John, 106
Caisse, Rene, 259
calcium
    cancer cell cycling influenced by, 135, 187
    tumors and, 188
    Vitamin D regulation of, 187
caloric restriction, 151
CAM. *See* complementary alternative medicine
Camerino, M., 107
camphor, 255. *See also* 714-X
    immune system and, 256
    Naessens selection of, 256
cancer. *See also* breast cancer; colon cancer; colorectal cancer; esophageal cancer; Japan-Hawaii Cancer Study; lung cancer; oral cancer; ovarian cancer; penile cancer; stomach cancer

cancer (*cont.*)
   as adaptation, 15–17
   ancient, 23
   Ancient Egypt/Nubia evidence of, 27–28
   Ancient Middle East evidence of, 28
   antineoplastons for treatment of, 387–391
   beta-carotene's influence on, 123, 167
   biologic adaptation and, 125–127
   Blacks to White ratios for, 96
   causative factor variability in, 131
   causes of, 7, 15
   Cenozoic Era evidence of, 25–26
   complementary/integrative modalities and, 8
   in contemporary society, 31
   definition/description, 3, 125
   dietary aberrations influence on, 125
   dietary etiology of, 129
   dietary restrictions on, 135
   as disease of older age, 127
   as disease of organs (cell populations), 13
   as disease of postreproductive years, 126
   etiology/epidemiology of, 4
   expressive therapies and symbolism of, 88
   factors specific to, 132–133
   fiber and, 200–202
   food additives influence on, 203
   historical perspective on, 21–31, 143
   and human body, 13–14
   Hutterites and, 99–100
   hypnosis applications for, 43–47
   Israeli Jews lower rates of, 6
   Jews and, 97–98
   Latter-Day Saints and, 99
   macronutrients promotion of, 147
   male to female ratios for, 96
   as metaphor, 88–89
   micronutrients protective influence from, 147
   migrants and, 132, 145, 146
   as multistep disease, 136
   myths about, 409–410
   naturopathy and, 292–294
   New World evidence of, 28–29
   occupational hazards association with, 6
   Paleozoic/Mesozoic Eras evidence of, 25
   patterns of occurrence, 21
   as preventable disease, 168
   prevention levels in, 168–169
   prolonged remissions of, 9
   and religious commitment, 100–102
   retinoids/Vitamin A and, 173–175
   retinoid therapy for, 176
   as second leading cause of death, 96
   Seventh Day Adventists and, 98–99
   socioeconomic status and, 151
   soft-tissue, 22

   *speed* image of, 88–89
   TM, free radicals, and, 345–347
   U.S. statistics, 96, 167
   vegetable intake links with, 129–130
   virus association with, 18
cancer, antiquity of
   clay tablets/papyruses references, 22, 23
   documentary evidence, 29–30
   Islamic civilizations early references, 23
   study of, 23–24
Cancer Advisory Panel for Complementary and
       Alternative Medicine (CAPCAM), 414
*Cancer and Natural Medicine* (Boik), 320
Cancer and Steroid Hormone Study (U.S.), 152
cancer care
   Chinese medicine and, 303–338
   Interactive Guided Imagery uses in, 70–74
   mind/body modalities relationship to, 37
cancer cells
   cytoplasmic to nuclear ratio, 6
   MAK's reversal of, 365, 368
   phases of growth, 10
   pleomorphism of, 5
   resistance developed by, 9
   response to drug therapy variations, 9
Cancer Control Society, 409
cancer patient (Hodgkin's Lymphoma) case study, 455
   conventional v. complementary treatment choice,
       447–448
   dietary choices, 448–449
   Immuno-Placental Therapy choice, 450–452
   supplement choices/detoxification program, 449
cancer patients
   biofeedback's application for, 53–55
   challenges faced by, 399
   concerns of, 38
   desperation of, 387
   hypnosis application for, 43, 44, 45
   meditation's application for, 50–51
   Vitamin C for, 217–218
   withholding CAM information by, 407
cancer prevention, diet/lifestyle possibilities, 21
Cannon, Walter, 37
CAPCAM. *See* Cancer Advisory Panel for
       Complementary and Alternative Medicine
carcinogenesis, 6. *See also* chemical carcinogenesis;
       gene expression model; somatic mutation
       hypothesis; viral carcinogenesis
   BHT 's reduction of, 171
   B vitamins and, 193
   estrogens and, 134
   fatty/bile acids as promoters of, 135
   host factors, 17–18
   models of, 14–15
   nutrition's influence on, 168, 169, 170

phases of, 170–171
plant food's influence on, 171
two-stage model of, 131–132
Vitamin A and, 171–175
Vitamin C and, 171
yogurt's influence on, 151
carcinogens
defined, 168
difficulties in studying, 174–175
environmental, 17
industrial, 169
metabolic variability reactiveness to, 17
vegetables/plant foods as source of, 130
cardiovascular disease (CVD), and dietary fat, 124
carotinoids, 174, 177. *See also* Alpha Tocopherol Beta
Carotene (ATBC) study
cancers influenced positively by, 183
stomach cancer and, 191
Vitamin E association with, 175
Carroll, B. E., 101
cartilage preparations, 394
Carver, C. S., 102
Cassidy, C. M., 29
Cassileth, Barrie, 412–413
CCAOM. *See* Council of Colleges of Acupuncture and
Oriental Medicine
cell-mediated immunity, 107
cells
adaptation by, 13
"bomb squads" (antioxidant enzymes) of, 355
calcium/wheat bran's influence on cycling of, 135
colon's high replication rates of, 128
nutrition's influence on, 126
sensitivity/resistance of, 14
cellular affinity, 5
cellular dedifferentiation, 5, 14, 15
cellular differentiation, 5–6, 14
cellular growth, factors stimulating, 16–17
Cenozoic Era, cancer evidence from, 25–26
Center for Freedom of Choice in Medicine, 409
Center for Integrative Medicine at Thomas Jefferson
University Hospital, 454
cervical cancer
Kanglaite injection and, 333
Latter-Day Saints and, 99
micronutrient deficiency links with, 129
Vitamin C and, 183
chaplains, clinicians/physicians referrals to, 114
*Charaka Samhita,* 349
chemical carcinogenesis, 15, 17
chemosensitivity
chemotherapy and, 18–19
in vitro testing for, 18
chemotherapy, 9–10
agent choice for, 18

CAM v., 413–414
and chemosensitivity, 18–19
Chinese medicine and, 304
current principles of, 18
imagery's influence on adverse effects of, 67
immune system and, 432
MAK and, 365–367
side effects of, 38
*Yin-Yang* perspective on, 315–316
young people's greater success, 18–19
Chen, Sophie, 268
Cheung, C. S., 312
children
art therapy for, 92
hypnosis susceptibility of, 43, 44
overnutrition's influence on, 147
Children's Hospital of Michigan, 411
China, breast cancer and, 153
Chinese herbal mixtures. *See also* PC-SPES Chinese
herbal mixture
FDA/FTC monitoring of, 266
integration promoted by, 337
safeness of, 266, 334–336
U.S. FDA approval of, 333
*Chinese Materia Medica,* 305
Chinese medicine, 303–338
anecdotal (present day) reports, 336–338
body's composition according to, 308
cancer types/diagnostic patterns, 314–315
chemotherapy/radiation and, 304
conventional protocol enhancement, 330–334
current utilization of, 307–308
herbs, formulas, 321–328
herbs, individual, 320
historical origins of, 305–306
individuals as resilient, dynamic ecosystems,
303
research, modern, on, 319–320, 329–330
theories of, 308–311
treatment strategies, 320
Western references to, 306–307
*Yin-Yang* perspective on chemotherapy/radiation,
315–316
chiropractic, 291
choline deficiency, 193–194
Christian Science, 291
Ciampa, R. C., 113
Circle the Earth healing dance (Tamalpa Institute), 91
cisplatin, MAK and, 367
citrus fruit
colorectal cancer and, 182
pancreatic cancer and, 183
Clement, John, 453
CLIA. *See* Clinical Laboratory Improvement
Amendments

Clinical Laboratory Improvement Amendments (CLIA)
  laboratory testing regulations of, 430
  Live Blood Analysis/Dark-field microscopy case study, 430–431
clinicians
  chaplain referrals by, 114
  efficacy of, 114–115
*Closing in on Cancer: Solving a 5000-Year Old Mystery* (National Cancer Institute), 21–22
Coenzyme Q10, 241
coffee enemas
  in Gerson diet, 230
  in Kelley-Gonzales diet, 239
  in Livingston-Wheeler diet, 236
cognitive/attentional distraction procedures, 55
cognitive therapy, and anxiety reduction, 54
Cohen, Sheldon, 74
Cole, B., 104
Collector, M. I., 107
colon
  energy increases relation to, 128
  high cell replication rates of, 128
  internal ecology of, 129
  low dietary intake influence on, 128
colon cancer, 96
  African's lower rates of, 129
  exercise and, 136
  fiber/cereals and, 129, 133, 200–201
  Finland's rates of, 133, 135
  high fat intake promotion of, 134
  Japan's rates of, 133
  migrant's and, 132
  physical activity's relation to, 127, 128
  types of, 131
colorectal cancer. *See also* Melbourne Colorectal Cancer (CRC) Study
  citrus fruit and, 182
  Jews and, 97
  Seventh-Day Adventists low incidence of, 98
  Vitamin E and, 182
  Vitamins A/C and, 182–183
Committee on Unproven Methods of Cancer Management (ACA), 408
community healing projects, 90, 91
complementary alternative medicine (CAM)
  AMA Operational Statement about, 408
  antineoplastons for, 387–391
  controversial therapies, 387–396, 445
  conventional v., 447–448
  environmental medicine, 394–395
  FDA possible restriction of, 400
  financial barriers to, 433–434
  FSMB critical stance against, 437

growing collegiality towards, 414–415
insurance coverage denied for, 433–434, 435
Krebiozen cancer formula, 403–404
Laetrile treatment, 395
legal challenges to, 400
organizations representing, 409
patient's seeking of, 399
physician based, 399
side effects of, 21
state regulations protective of, 438
complementary alternative therapies, 8, 21, 81, 241, 304
  art therapies, 82
  barriers to integration of, 440
  cartilage preparations, 394
  dance therapy, 84, 85, 87, 90
  healing touch therapies, 395
  Immuno-Augmentative Therapy, 395
  Neurolinguistic Programming (NLP), 396
  self-care component of, 88
  sound therapy, 396
  talking/narrative therapies, 84
  usage statistics, 82
*Complementary and Alternative Medicine in the United States* (IOM), 414
conflict resolution, 91
connection, disconnection v., 89
*The Conquest of Cancer* (Livingstone), 237
control/secondary control
  patient issues of, 104
  redirection of, 104
controversial therapies, 387–396, 445
  antineoplaston therapy, 387–391
  hydrazine sulphate, 391–394
coping
  active-cognitive strategies for, 104
  for breast cancer, 108
  death as result of negative religious, 112
  negative religious strategies for, 111–112
  prayer and, 105
  religion and, 102–103
  religious patterns of, 103–106
  social support for, 105
copper, tumors influenced by, 194
coronary artery disease, and body fat distribution, 127
cortisol
  prayer/faith's influence on, 108
  spiritual expression's influence on, 108
  stress influenced activation of, 106
Council of Colleges of Acupuncture and Oriental Medicine (CCAOM), 339
Cousins, Norman, 396
CPT. *See* Current Procedural Terminology
creation stories, 83
creative energy, releasing of, 87–88

Cunningham, A. J., 66, 72
curing, healing v., 81
Current Procedural Terminology (CPT), 433
Cutler, Richard, 368
CVD. *See* cardiovascular disease

D'Angelo, T., 108
D'Aquili, E., 109
Davis, H. J., 100
Dawson, W. R., 27
Day, N. E., 154
dehumanization
    art's counteracting influence on, 86–87
    negative impact of, 86
dehydroepiandrosterone sulfate (DHEA-S), and TM,
    347
Dein, S., 112
depression
    breast cancer influenced by, 108
    DNA influenced by, 108
    expressive therapy"s influence on, 84
    imagery's influence on, 67
    MAK and, 369
    as stressor, 108
    tumor growth influenced by, 108
Deri, Susan, 88
detoxification, 299
deWaard, F., 98
De Wolff, Herman J., 292
Dharmananda, Subhuti, 320
DHEA-S. *See* dehydroepiandrosterone sulfate
diabetes
    body fat distribution linked to, 127
    garlic and, 254
diagnosis, restrictions on, 430–431
diet. *See also* fat (body); nutrition; protein
    aberration possibilities in, 125
    as adaptation to environment, 124
    Ayur Vedic medicine and, 349–351
    and cancer (modern perspective), 130–131
    carcinogenesis influenced by, 168, 169
    as cause of cancer, 22
    deficiency disorders, 126
    energy imbalances in, 127–129
    evolution theories and, 124
    geographic/temporal variability in contemporary,
        125–126
    high-fat v. low-fat, 134
    human being's adaptations in, 126, 128
    tumors and, 170
diethylstilbestrol, 7
dilutions ( *potentization*), of homeopathic medicine, 378
disconnection
    connection v., 89
    from self/others, 89

disease
    free radicals/ROS and, 353–354
    sedentism and, 143
    unified understanding of, 353
distress, psychological, and immune system, 57
*Divine Husbandman's Classic of the Materia Medica*
        (attributed to Shen Nong), 305
DNA
    cancer's alteration of, 14
    depression's influence on, 108
    environmental influences of, 15
    nuclear, 15
Doll, R., 151, 167
*doshas* (of Ayurvedic medicine). *See kapha* dosha; *pitta*
        dosha; *vata* dosha
*dravyaguna* (Ayurvedic pharmacology), 352, 358
Drew University (Los Angeles) mushroom study, 331
drug(s)
    antineoplastic agents, 9
    autumn crocus used as, 30
    as carcinogen (*See* diethylstilbestrol), 10
    FDA approval of, 423–424
    genetic differences in metabolizing, 17
    for malignant diseases, 7–9
    methotrexate, 10
    reason for effectiveness of, 9
    side effects of, 18
Dundee, J. W., 318
Dunkel-Schetter, C., 105
Dunn, J. K., 110
Durovic, Stevan, 403
Dwivedi, Chandradhar, 361
dysdifferentiatlon theory, 368

Earth
    as living organism, 90
    reconnecting with, 90
East Finland Heart Survey, 192
*East-West Journal*, 226
eclectic medicine, 290
ecologic body, 89–90
Eddy, Mary Baker, 291
Egan, K. M., 98
Ehman, J. W., 113
Eleusian Mysteries celebrations, 83
Elias, S., 110
Elision, C. G., 101
Elkins, T., 102
Elliot-Smith, G., 27
embryonic products/embryo antigens, and tumors, 450
emotions
    expressive therapy processing of, 85–86
    healing influenced by, 85
    "metabolizing" of, 350
    *ojas* and, 350

emotions (*cont.*)
    perceived control of, 56–57
    physical health influenced by, 37
endogenous hormones, 154–155
endometrial cancer, and beta-carotene, 201
enemas. *See* coffee enemas
energy
    cancer and imbalances in, 127–129
    colon surface area increases and, 128
Enstrom, J. E., 99
environmental influences
    asbestos fibers, 15
    on cancer, 168
    as cause of cellular adaptation, 13
    of DNA, 15
    on human behavior, 143
    individual hypersusceptibility to, 17
    statistics regarding, 22
environmental medicine, 394–395
enzymatic diets, 241
enzymes
    digestive, for treating cancer, 238
    pancreatic (Kelley-Gonzales diet), 240
epidemiological studies
    of Chinese populations, 205
    in Israel, 206
    of Japan/Japanese populations, 206
    of older Americans, 207
    in United States, 207
epidemiology, of cancer, 4, 6
epigallocatechin gallate (EGCG), 249
Epstein, Samuel, 400
Epstein-Barr virus, 7
Erewhon natural foods, 226
Erickson, Milton, 39
erythrocyte sedimentation rate (ESR), and TM, 347
Esdaile, James, 39, 44
esophageal cancer, 134, 181
Esper, E. J. C., 25
ESR. *See* erythrocyte sedimentation rate
essential oils therapy, 270–275
    analgesic properties of, 274
    antimicrobial effects of, 273–274
    central nervous system influenced by, 272
    clinical applications of, 272
    digestion influenced by, 274
    essential oils, composition, 270–271
    intensive/palliative care and, 274–275
    sedative effects of, 274
    touch/massage component of, 272
    treatment/administration, 271–272
Essiac, 258. *See also* burdock root; Indian rhubarb;
      sheep sorrel; slippery elm
    as complementary treatment, 259
    herbal components of, 258–259

Memorial Sloan-Kettering lab studies of, 261
estrogens
    Asian/American women, variability of, 17
    breast cancer influenced by, 135, 154
    carcinogenesis and, 134
etiology, of cancer, 4, 6
Eveleth, P. B., 148
evocative imagery, 73–74
exercise, and colon cancer, 136
existential angst, of patients, 112
exogenous hormones, 154–155
expressive therapies. *See also* art therapies; Authentic
      Movement; dance therapy; storytelling
    applications of, 84–85
    benefits of, 84, 85–86
    blood pressure and, 84
    description of, 82–83
    family involvement in, 89
    improvisatory nature of, 83
    origins of, 83–84
    primary goal of, 83
    psychologic functions influenced by, 85
    resources, 94
    symbolic processes of, 83
    usefulness of, 82
expressive therapists, 82
    physicians association with, 82, 86
extended survival characteristics, 66
extrinsic religiousness, 102

Fair, William, 268
faith
    problematic role of, 111
Falke, R. L., 105
families
    healing of, 89
fat, dietary. *See also* fish oil; olive oil
    breast cancer and, 149–150
    cancer cell growth influenced by, 131–132
    colon cancer and, 134
    CVD association with, 124
    human ancestors lower intake of, 128
fat (body)
    diabetes/coronary artery disease linked to, 127
    hormones and, 155–156
fatigue
    breast cancer influenced by, 108
Fawzey, F. I., 66, 106
Fawzey, N. W., 66
FDA. *See* Food and Drug Administration
fear
    about future, 102
Federation of American Societies for Experimental
      Biology (FASEB)
    Report on Dietary Fiber and Health, 198

Federation of State Medical Boards (FSMB), 437
Felter, Harvey Wickes, 290
Fernsler, J. I., 105
Fernstein, L. G., 105
fertility
    historical shifts in, 124
fiber, dietary, 198–203
    breast cancer protective effect of, 135, 201
    cancer cell growth influenced by, 129, 131–132, 133
    colon cancer an, 200–201
    colon cancer and, 129
    definitions of, 198
    dietary consumption of, 200
    discovery of/observation of effects, 198
    dosage/requirements, 203
    endometrial cancer and, 201
    foods and, 199
    as macronutrient, 129
    measurement of, 199–200
    mechanisms of action, 202–203
    ovarian cancer and, 201
    pancreatic cancer and, 202
    prostate cancer and, 201–202
    types of, 198–199
Fields, Jeremy, 360, 367
"fight-or-flight" response, 106
fight-or-flight response, 37–38
Finland
    colon cancer rates of, 133, 135
First Amendment (free speech), 421–422
Fishbein, Morrils, 401
fish oil
    protective influence of, 133
Fitzgerald, Benedict, 402
flowering periwinkle
    as source of chemotherapeutic agents, 8
food additives
    and cancer, 203
Food and Drug Administration (FDA)
    Burzynski challenged by, 388, 390, 400, 424–427
    Chinese herbal mixtures monitoring by, 266
    Congress v., 428
    drugs/devices and approval by, 423–424
    homeopathic drugs monitoring by, 379
    increasing openness of, 428–430
    IND program, 392
    therapies forbidden by, 400
Foulkes, W. D., 110
Foundation for Advancement of Cancer Therapies, 409
free radicals. *See also* oxygen
    body's balance of, 356–357
    cancer-causing, 353
    defenses against, 355–356
    diseases linked to, 353–354
    factors generating, 345

    importance of knowledge of, 353
    MAK and, 360–361
    positive influence of, 354
    SOD and, 355, 357, 360
    TM and, 345–347
Freud, Sigmund, 272
Friends of Dr. Revici, 409
FSMB. *See* Federation of State Medical Boards
*Fundamentals of Complementary and Integrative Medicine* (Micozzi), 21
future
    stress/fear/anxiety concerning, 102

Gaia hypothesis (Earth as living organism), 90
Gallagher, T. F., 108
Ganzheitstherapie. *See* whole body therapy
garlic, 252–255
    adverse effects of, 254
    and diabetes, 254
    LDL/triglycerides and, 253
    long-term use of, 254–255
Gaskill, S. P., 151
gastric cancer
    macrobiotics and, 229
gene expression model, 14, 15
Gerson, Max B., 230, 231
Gerson Clinic (Mexico), 230
Gerson diet, 213, 230–235
    as adjunctive treatment, 234
    American Medical Association's opposition to, 232
    cancer case successes, 231–232
    contemporary concerns regarding, 235
    elements of, 233
    high potassium component, 234
    low sodium component, 233–234
    as "quack " cancer therapy, 233
    rigors of, 230
Gerson Institute (California), 230, 233
Ghalioungui, P., 29
Gisler, R. H., 107
Glaser, J. L., 346–347
God
    American's belief in, 97
    coping strategies and, 111
    IR as search for, 102
    patient's feeling abandoned by, 113
    seen as having control over disease, 103
    Western religion on, 95
Gold, Joseph, 391
Goldstein, M. S., 26
Gonzales, Nicholas, 238, 239
Govallo, Valentine I., 450–452
Graham, S., 177, 207, 287
Graham-Poole, John, 92
Granville, A. B., 27

Green, Saul, 388
green tea, 249, 449. *See also* epigallocatechin gallate
    antioxidant value of
    composition of, 248
    epidemiological studies of, 249
Gregg, J. B., 29
Grief Experience inventory, 103
Grimmer, Arthur, 380
growth rate
    protein intake's influence on, 148
    relation of maturation to body size/shape, 148
*Guernica* (Picasso), 82
Gupta, D. D., 371

Hahn, J., 112
Hahnemann, Samuel, 290, 377
Haight, B., 85–86
Hall, H., 65, 110
Halprin, Anna, 91
Halprin, Daria, 91
Halstead, M. T., 105
Hanks, Amy, 320
Hannisdal, E., 103
Hansen-Flaschen, J., 113
Harbeck, R., 107
Hazelnut, 250–252
head/neck cancers
    retinoids and, 177–178
healing
    community rituals, 90
    curing v., 81
    emotions influence on, 85
    of families, 89
*Healing and the Mind* (Moyers), 81
healing imagery, 71–72
healing touch therapies, 395
health, mental
    *ojas* and, 350
health, physical
    mind/body modalities influence on, 37
    *ojas* and, 350
health care freedom
    consumer protection v., 415–416
    First Amendment and, 421–422
    informed consent doctrine and, 420–421
    judicial reluctance in recognizing, 415–422
    Ninth Amendment and, 419–420
    *People v. Priviteria, Jr.*, 418
    *United States v. Rutherford*, 416–418
"Health Food Store"
    Lust's origination of, 283
health outcomes, negative
    religion and, 111–112
Hellman, L., 108
Hendrix, S., 85–86

herbal rasayanas, 357–359
    synergism of, 359–360
Herberman, R. B., 108
herbs
    FDA/FTC monitoring of, 266
    formulas, Chinese, 321–328
    impulses of intelligence in, 372
    individual, Chinese, 320
    reacting to medicinal, 411
    safety of/herb–drug interactions, 265–268, 334–336
    vibratory patterns of, 372
herbs, of Ayurvedic medicine, 352–355
    *ashwagandha* herb, 371
    *Phyllanthus amarus* herb, 371
    resequencing of intelligence impulses by, 372
heritability
    of cancer, 15
Heuch, I., 153
Higher Power
    IR as search for, 102
Hike Against the Odds, 91
Hildebrand, Gar, 235
Hippocrates, 285
Hirayama, Takeshi, 229
Hirshberg, Caryle, 396
*The History of Cold Bathing* (Floyer, John), 285
*A History of Pathology* (Long), 29
Ho, J. H. C., 153–154
Hodgkin's lymphoma, 103
Hoffman, A., 107, 252
Hoffman, F. L., 97
Holbrook, Martin Luthier, 287
holotropic principle, 75
Homeopathic/Eclectic College (Illinois), 286
Homeopathic Medical College (New York), 283
homeopathic medicine, 290, 298, 377–383
    as adjunctive therapy, 382
    background of, 377–378
    cancer recommendations of, 380–381
    dilutions (*potentization*) of, 378
    goal in, 380
    medicinal sources, 379
    *miasmas* of, 380
    *nosodes* of, 379
    as palliative measure, 382
    preventive aspects of, 383
    *provings* of, 378
    remedy selection, 379–380
Homeopathic Pharmacopoeia Convention of United States (HCPUS), 379
Hooton, E. A., 28
hopelessness
    imagery's influence on, 67
hormonal markers
    acupuncture effects on, 318–319

TM and aging, 346–347
hormones
  body fat and, 155–156
  endogenous/exogenous, 154–155
host factors, in carcinogenesis, 17–18
Houston, Robert G., 389
Howe, P. R., 172
Hoxsey, Harry, 262, 405. *See also* Biomedical Hoxsey
    Center
  and AMA, 401–402
  vindication of, 402
Hoxsey dietary regime, 259, 262
*Huang-di Nei-jing. See Inner Classic of the Yellow
    Emperor*
Hull, Clark, 39
human behavior, as environmental adaptation, 143
human beings
  cancer and body of, 13–14
  dietary adaptations of, 126, 128
  lengthy infant/juvenile dependence of, 126
human genetic sequence, 16
*Human Intestinal Flora* (Drasar and HIll), 288
Hummer, R. A., 101
humoral immunity, 107
Hutterites
  and cancer, 99–100
  and childhood leukemia, 110
hydrazine sulphate, 391–394
  administration of, 392
  adverse effects of, 392
  cachexia and, 391, 393
  Russian studies of, 393
  tumors and, 392, 393
  U.S. studies on, 393
*Hydropathic Encyclopedia* (Trall), 287
hydrotherapy, 281, 285, 298–299
Hygienic System, 286, 287–288
hyperplasia, 16–17
hypertropy, 16–17
hypervitaminosis A (overdose), 173
hypnosis, 38. *See also* Braid, James; Mesmer, Franz
    Anton
  as altered state of consciousness, 40
  American Medical Association's recognition of, 41
  American Psychological Association's definition of,
    40
  auto-, 43
  BMA utilization of, 44–45
  cancer applications of, 43–47
  children and, 43
  historical perspective of, 39–40
  immune-enhancing effects of, 46–47
  LP utilization of, 44–45
  myths/misconceptions regarding, 42–43
  nausea/vomiting control via, 45–46

  pain management via, 44–45, 105
  pediatric cancer patients and, 43, 44, 45
  physical/psychological benefits of, 38
  physiologic changes during, 41
  potential mechanisms of, 47–48
  procedures for inducing, 41–42
  Spiegels pain control studies involving, 66
  stress/anxiety management via, 43
  study of BMT and, 44
  surgery and, 39, 44
  theoretical perspectives on, 40–41
hypnosis-induced analgesia, 44
hypnotic induction profile, 42
hypnotizability factor, and patient outcomes, 45, 47
hypothalamus, as "pharmacological laboratory," 351

IARC. *See* International Agency for Research on
    Cancer
IAT. *See* Immuno-Augmentative Therapy
Ideal Model imagery, 72
Ideda, M., 102
Ikeda, J., 28
IL-6 (Interleukin-6)
  religious belief/behavior influence on, 109
  stressor's influence on, 107
imagery, 43, 47. *See also* Interactive Guided Imagery
  books about, 78
  categories of use, 68–69
  choosing approach to, 69
  conventional medicine's relationship with, 76
  description/importance of, 67–68
  evocative, 73–74
  Fawzey's malignant melanoma studies involving, 66
  grounding procedure, 74
  groups, 77
  guided, 69
  healing, 71–72
  Ideal Model, 72
  immune system influenced by, 65
  medical counterweight, 72
  medical/surgical interventions v., 74
  multi-sensory involvement in, 71
  patients unsuitable for, 74–75
  precautions/contraindications, 74–75
  professional training resources, 77
  quality of life improvements via, 67
  self-help books/tapes, 69
  Shrock's breast/prostate cancer study involving, 66
  Simonton's studies involving, 66
  support v., 67
  treatment/self-care options with, 68–69
imagery relaxation, 70–71
immune system
  *Astragalus* herb and, 332
  biofeedback's influence on, 54

immune system (*cont.*)
    cancer growth mediation by, 46
    chemotherapy/radiation's influence on, 432
    chronic stress impairment of, 106
    Essiac and, 259
    guided imagery's influence on, 65
    hypnosis influence on, 46–47
    "innate," 107
    Iscador and, 246
    laughter's influence on, 351
    MAK and, 362–363, 369
    mushrooms/polysaccharides and, 269
    psychological distress's influence on, 57
    religion, stress, and, 108–109
    spirituality's influence on, 109
    Vitamin A's influence on, 216
immunity, humoral/cell-mediated, 107
Immuno-Augmentative Therapy (IAT), 395,
    452–453
Immuno-Augmentative Therapy Patient's Association,
    409
immunoembryotherapy, 452
*The Immunology of Pregnancy and Cancer* (Govallo),
    450
Immuno-Placental Therapy (IPT), 450–452
inbreeding,
    breast cancer and, 110
    cancer development and, 99
    childhood leukemia (Hutterites) and, 110
incontinence (postsurgical), and biofeedback, 54
India. *See also* Ayurvedic medicine
    ancient medical texts of, 30
Indiana University, 364
Indian rhubarb (*Rheum palmatum*), 258–259, 260–261
inflammation, MAK and, 368–369
information
    care in disseminating, 422–423
    difficulties accessing reliable, 407
informed consent doctrine, 420–421
Ing, R., 153–154
"innate" immune system, 107
*Inner Classic of the Yellow Emperor* (*Huang-di Nei-jing*),
    305
Institute for Traditional Medicine (Portland, Oregon),
    320
Institute of Health and Healing (California Pacific
    Medical Center), 88–89
Institute of Medicine (IOM), 414
Insulin Potentiated Chemotherapy (IPT), 433
insurance
    and experimental treatments, 435
    and lack of CAM coverage, 433–434, 435
    litigation and private, 435–436
Interactive Guided Imagery,
    books about, 78

cancer care and, 70–74
    described, 69–70
    dialogue in, 73
    dialogue of, 72–73
    insurance company's reimbursement for, 76
    nonjudgmental/content-free language of, 70
    professional training resources, 77
    qualities of, 70
    training/certification/quality assurance issues,
    75–76
International Agency for Research on Cancer (ARC),
    249
*International Journal of Human Development*, 85–86
intrinsic religiousness, 102
    church attendance and, 103
Investigational New Drug (IND) program, 392
IPT. *See* Immuno-Placental Therapy
IPT. *See* Insulin Potentiated Chemotherapy
Iron/Bronze Ages, cancer evidence from, 26–27
Iscador (mistletoe), 243–247
    administration/dosage of, 245–246
    clinical studies on, 247–248
    evidence of effectiveness, 246–247
    immune system and, 246
    as part of "holistic" therapies, 245
    preparation of, 245
    Steiner's studies of, 244
    viscumin/viscotoxin, as key components of, 247
    in vitro experiments on, 247
Ishisuka, Sagen, 225
Israeli Jews, and cancer, 6
Issels, Josef, 235
    whole body therapy of, 238
Ivy, Andrew, 403–404

Jansen, A. M., 273
Japan
    diet/cancer relationships of, 132, 133, 144–146,
    149
    lactose intolerance in, 151
Japan-Hawaii Cancer Study, 145
Jehovah's Witnesses, blood transfusions refused by, 111
Jenklns, R. A., 103, 104
Jews, and cancer, 6,
    97–98
Jia Kun (Chinese traditional medicine oncologist), 312,
    328
Johns Hopkins Center for Cancer Complementary
    Medicine, 401
Johnson, S. C., 102, 105
*Journal of Alternative and Complementary Medicine*, 339
*Journal of Behavioral Medicine*, 346–347
*Journal of the American Medical Association* (JAMA),
    233, 389, 401
*Journal of Theoretical Biology*, 233

Kaczorowski, J. M., 103
Kaiser Health Maintenance Organization study, 308
Kanglaite injection, 333
*kapha* dosha, 371, 373
Kaplan, G. A., 101
Kato, I., 98
Katz, J. L., 108
Kawamura, K., 108
Kaye, J. M., 43
Keller, S. E., 107
Kelley-Gonzales diet, 239–240. *See also* Gonzales, Nicholas
    case studies
    clinical trials, 240
    components of, 239
Kellog, J. H. (American hydropath), 285, 287–288
Khosla, P., 371
Kiecolt-Glaser, J. K., 106–107
King, H., 101–102, 113, 158
*King's American Dispensary* (Felter and Lloyd), 290
Kneipp, Sebastian, 281, 285
Kneipp Water-cure, 283
Kneipp Water-Cure Institute (New York City), 283
*The Kneipp Water-Cure Monthly* (Lust), 283
Koenig, Harold, 95, 103, 111, 112
Koopman, C., 108, 109
Koresh, David, 112
Krebiozen cancer formula, 403–404
Krebs, Ernst, Jr., 395
Krebs, Ernst, Sr., 395
Krogman, W. M., 28
Kuhne, Louis, 286
Kuratsune, M., 102
Kushi, Aveline, 226
Kushi, Lawrence, 226, 230
Kushi, Michio, 225
Kushi Institute, 226
Kvale, G., 150

Laakso, K., 157
Laben, Rudolph von, 90
lactose intolerance, 151
Laetrile treatment, 395
    controversies of, 403
    MSKCC/Mayo Clinic evaluation of, 403, 446
    *United States v. Rutherford* decision on, 416–418
Laht, H., 157
Lane, William, 394
Langer, E. J., 347, 348
Larson, D. B., 102, 103
larynx cancer
    Vitamins A/C and, 181
Latter-Day Saints, and cancer, 99
laughter, and stress/immune system, 351
Law of Similars, 378

*Law of Similars* (Hahnemann), 377
LDL. *See* low-density lipoprotein
*Lectures on the Science of Human Life* (Graham), 287
Lee, J., 108
legal challenges, to CAM, 400
Lemon, F. R., 98
lesions, and choline deficiency, 193–194
leukemia (acute)
    retinoid therapy and, 176
    Vitamin D and, 187
Levy, S. M., 108
Lilienfield, A., 100
Lindlahr, Henry, 286
Lindlahr College of Natural Therapeutic, 286
Linus Pauling Institute, 405
Lippman, M., 108
Littlewood, R., 112
Livingston, Virginia C., 235
    Medicare prosecution of, 434
Livingston-Wheeler Therapy, 213, 235–238
    components of, 236
    conventional treatment v., 238
    history of, 235–236
    publication bias and, 412–413
    quality of life and, 238
    three diets aspect of, 237
    treatment recommendations/research, 237
Lloyd, J. W., 101
Lloyd, John Uri, 290
Locke, F. B., 101–102
Long, Esmond R., 29–30
low-density lipoprotein (LDL), 361
Loyola University Medical School, 360, 367
LP. *See* lumbar punctures
Lull, R. S., 25
lumbar punctures (LP), and hypnosis, 44–45
Lundin, F. E., Jr., 100
lung cancer
    beta-carotene and, 191
    fruit consumption/Vitamin C and, 180–181
    Hutterite's low incidence of, 99
    Jews and, 97
    Kanglaite injection and, 333
    MAK and, 363–364
    micronutrients deficiency links with, 129
    mortality rates for, 96
    Seventh Day Adventists low incidence of, 98
    Vitamin A and, 174–175
    Yunan Tin Mines (China) and, 206
    Zen-Buddhist priests and, 102
Lust, Benedict, 281
    "Health Food Store" originated by, 283
    schools founded by, 283
Lyon, J. L., 99

MacCurdy, G. G., 28
MacMahon, B., 177
macrobiotic diet, 213, 225. *See also East-West Journal;*
 Erewhon natural foods; Ishisuka, Sagen;
 Kushi, Michio; Ohsawa, George
 as cancer diet, 226, 227
 case histories, 228
 clinical studies, 228
 dietary recommendations, 226–227
 and gastric cancer, 229
 history of, 225–226
 lack of medical foundation, 227
 and pancreatic cancer, 228–229
 and prostate cancer, 229
 seaweeds in, 229
 as spiritual philosophy, 225
 unexpected recoveries and, 230
macronutrient(s)
 and breast cancer, 149
 as cancer promoting, 147
 cancer risk and, 123
 dietary fiber as, 129
 micronutrient's modulation of, 137
"magic bullet"
 antibiotics as, 18
 search for cancer's, 18
Maharishi Amrit Kalash (MAK)
 Adriamycin and, 366
 aging and, 367–368
 breast cancer and, 363–364
 cancer cell reversal and, 365, 368
 chemotherapy and, 365–367
 cisplatin and, 367
 depression and, 369
 free radicals and, 360–361
 immune system and, 362–363, 369
 LDL and, 361
 lung cancer and, 363–364
 side effects and, 369–370
 skin tumors and, 364
 toluene and, 367
maitake mushrooms, 269
MAK. *See* Maharishi Amrit Kalash
Malcolm's law, 148
malignant diseases, drugs for, 7–9
malpractice risks, for physicians, 431–433
manipulative therapies, 291
Marcow-Speiser, V., 91
marital discord, and cortisol fluctuations, 106–107
Marshall, J., 181
Martin, A. O., 110
Martinson, I. M., 105
massage, and essential oils therapy, 272
Matsunaga, E., 156
Matthews, D., 103

Mauger, P. A., 103
May, Rollo, 82
May apple, developed as podophyllin, 8
Mayo Clinic, 403
MBSR program. *See* mindfulness-based stress
 reduction (MBSR) program
McFadden, Bernarr, 291
McGuire, W. L., 151
MD Anderson Hospital and Tumor Institute, 332
Meares, Ainslie, 50
medical counterweight imagery, 72
medical practitioners
 state legislation protective of, 438
 state regulation of, 437–438
medical texts, of ancient India, 30
medical treatment
 refusal of, 111
 unhealthy practices v., 111
Medicare
 clinical trial payments and, 436–437
 CPT required by, 433
 Livingston, Virginia C., prosecution by, 434
 reporting expectations of, 433–434
medicine (conventional)
 acupuncture v., 317
 art v., 86–87
 CAM v., 447–448
 evolving views of, 81
 high-technology scientific, 82
 imagery/visualization's relationship with, 76
 judicial deference to, 416
 state board discipline and pain, 439
medicine (unconventional). *See* complementary
 alternative medicine; complementary
 alternative therapies
meditation, 51. *See also* mindfulness meditation;
 Transcendental Meditation
 blood pressure reduction via, 50
 cancer application of, 50–51
 physical/psychological benefits of, 38
 physiological changes during, 48–49
 potential mechanisms of, 51
 self-directed, 49
 types of, 49
megavitamin therapy, 297
Melbourne Colorectal Cancer (CRC) Study, 190
Memorial Sloan-Kettering Cancer Center (MSKCC),
 268, 403
 Essiac studies, 261
 Laetrile evaluation, 403, 446
menarche, onset of
 animal protein and, 148
 breast cancer and, 152, 153
Mendeloff, A., 100
menopause

breast cancer and, 152
   red clover studies, 262–263
Mesmer, Franz Anton, 39
mesmerism, 39
metabolism
   of chemical carcinogens, 17
   fast acetylators/slow acetylators, 17
   of therapeutic drugs, 17
Metchnikoff, Elie, 288
Mettlin, C., 177
*miasmas*, of homeopathic medicine, 380
Michel, Y., 85–86
micronutrients, 129
   cancer cell growth influenced by, 131–132
   as cancer protective, 147, 167, 168
   macronutrients modulated by, 137
   role of, 169
   selenium's interactions with, 196
   Vitamin A interactions with, 175–176
   Vitamin C interactions with, 184
migraine headaches
   biofeedback's usefulness for, 52
   expressive therapy's influence on, 84
migrants, cancer rates of, 132, 145, 146
migrant studies, 22
milk (of mother), cow's v. human, 148
Miller, Neil, 51–52
mind/body modalities. *See also* biofeedback; hypnosis;
      meditation
   cognitive/attentional distraction, 55
   mechanisms underlying, 55–57
   physical health influenced by, 37
   relaxation techniques, 55
mindfulness-based stress reduction (MBSR)
      program, 50
mindfulness meditation, 49, 51
Minnes, L., 65
mistletoe. *See* Iscador
Moadel, A., 113
Mohs, Frederick, 402
Monjan, A. A., 107
Monk, M., 100
monoterpenes, 241
Montfort, H., 381
Moodie, R. L., 25
moods. *See* Profile of Mood States
Moolgavkar, S. H., 154
Moore, R., 56
Mormons. *See* Latter-Day Saints
mortality rates
   for Blacks/Whites, 96
   for lung cancer, 96
   for males/females, 96
Moss, Ralph, 403
movement choirs, 90–91

Moyers, Bill, 81
MSKCC. *See* Memorial Sloan-Kettering Cancer
      Center
mummies, examination of, 27
mushrooms/mushroom extracts, 269–270
   Drew University study, 331
   natural killer (NK) cells activated by, 269, 331
   shiitake/maitake mushrooms, 269, 331
   Sun soup mushroom mixture, 269
Musick, M. A., 103, 105
myelosuppression, and acupuncture, 318–319
myths
   about cancer, 409–410
   of male independence, 89
   regarding hypnosis, 42–43

Naessens, Gaston, 255. *See also* 714-X; somatids;
      somatoscope
Nagpal, R. K., 371
Naguib, S. M., 100
Nam, C. B., 101
Narod, S. A., 110
National Cancer Institute (NCI), 177, 240, 250, 388,
      402
National Cancer Research Institute (Japan), 229, 269
National Center for Complementary and Alternative
      Medicine, 81
National Certification Commission for Acupuncture
      and Oriental Medicine (NCCAOM), 339
National Council Against Health Fraud (NCAHF),
      409
National Health and Nutrition Examination Survey
      (U.S.), 158
National Health Federation, 409
National Health Interview Survey, 101
National Institute on Aging, 368
National Institutes of Health (NIH), 81, 307, 316,
      318
*Natural Compounds in Cancer Therapy* (Boik), 320
natural killer (NK) cells, 46
   mushroom activation of, 269
*The Natural Method of Healing* (Bilz), 286
natural selection, and reproductive success, 126
Nature Cure, 285–287
*Nature Cure Magazine* (Lindlahr), 286
*Nature's Path* (De Wolff), 292
*The Naturopathic and Herald of Health* (Lust), 282
naturopathic medicine/naturopathy. *See also*
      autotoxicity; eclectic medicine; Holbrook,
      Martin Luthier; homeopathic medicine;
      hydrotherapy; Hygienic System; Kellog, J. H.;
      Kneipp, Sebastian; manipulative therapies;
      Metchnikoff, Elie; Nature Cure; Suggestive
      Therapeutics; Thompsonianism; Tilden, John
      H.; Trall, Russell

naturopathic medicine (*cont.*)
   and cancer, 292–294
   clinical approach of, 300
   Hippocrate's influence on, 285
   history of, 281–284
   hydrotherapy as basis of, 285
   preneoplastic conditions, management of, 300–301
   as preventive medicine, 296
   principles of, 294–296
   therapeutic modalities of, 297–299
   varied therapies of, 284–292
Naturopathic Society of America, 284
nausea/vomiting
   acupuncture for, 316, 318
   biofeedback's control of, 53
   hypnosis control of, 45–46
NCCAOM. *See* National Certification Commission for
   Acupuncture and Oriental Medicine
Neolithic Period, cancer evidence from, 26–27
neoplasia, and Vitamin A, 172
neoplasm
   definition of, 3
   functional v. benign, 3
   Mesozoic era evidence of, 25
   Neolithic era evidence of, 26
   tumors synonymous with, 4
neuroendocrine system, stressor's influence on, 106
Neurolinguistic Programming (NLP), 396
neurologic changes, during spiritual activity, 109
Newberg, A., 109
Newbold, Vivien, 228
*New England Journal of Medicine,* 81, 412
*New Guide to Health* (Thompson), 289
*New Science of Healing* (Kuhne), 286
New World, evidence of cancer, 28–29
New York School of Massage, 283
*New York Times,* 307
Nielson, J., 111
NIH. *See* National Institutes of Health
Ninth Amendment, and health care freedom, 419–420
nitrosamines, as causative in pancreatic cancer, 133
Niwa, Yukie, 354, 360
Niwa Institute (Japan), 360
Nixon, Richard, 307
NK cells. *See* natural killer (NK) cells
NLP. *See* Neurolinguistic Programming
*nosodes,* of homeopathic medicine, 379
nuclear DNA, as target of carcinogens, 15
Nurses Health Study, on lactation/breast cancer, 153
nutrition. *See also* beta-carotene; macronutrients
   agriculture/animal domestication's influence on,
     143
   for breast cancer, 142
   cell's dependence on, 126
   disease prevention/management via, 123

   evolutionary biology on, 143
   medical profession's rejection of, 231
   sedentism's influence on, 143
   therapeutic, 293
   western-style diet, 145

obesity
   and breast cancer, 147
   cancer risk increased by, 127
   human ancestor's lower rates of, 128
   prenatal influences on, 147
occupational hazards, cancer's association with, 6
Oda, Tatsuya, 357
Office of Cancer Complementary and Alternative
   Medicine (OCCAM), 401
Office of Technology Assessment (OTA), 395, 404
Ogata, A., 102
Ohio State University College of Medicine, 361
Ohsawa, George, 226
*ojas*
   consciousness-matter connected by, 349
   emotions and, 350
   as end-product of perfect digestion/metabolism,
     349
   factors for decreasing, 350
   rasayanas and, 357
olive oil, breast cancer rates and, 133
Olness, K., 65
omega-3 fatty acids, 208
Omenn, G. S., 178
oncogenes
   definition of, 16
   retinoid's influence on, 216
oncology, definition of, 4
*One Man Alone: An Investigation of Nutrition, Cancer,*
   *and William Donald Kelley* (Gonzales), 239
oral cancer, 134
   Vitamins A/C and, 181
oral contraceptives, 155
O'Regan, Brandon, 396
"organic repression" idea (Freud), 272
*The Organon of Medicine* (Hahnemann), 377,
   379
organopathy, 381
Ornish, Dean, 84
orthomolecular medicine (Pauling), 293
Osborne, C. K., 151
Osler, William, 307
osteopathic medicine, 291
OTA. *See* Office of Technology Assessment
Ott, B. B., 113
ovarian cancer, 98
   fiber's influence on, 201
   Jews and, 97, 110
   Latter-Day Saints and, 99

overnutrition
    and breast cancer, 141
    breastfeeding and, 148
    childhood and, 147
    overview of, 152
oxygen
    dark side of, 345
    ROS of, 353

Pacific Yew (*Taxus brevifolia*), 251. *See also* Taxol®
    and basal cell carcinoma, 251
    Native American uses of, 251
    taxanes (anti-cancer chemicals) from, 251
    tea/capsules/salves, 251
pain
    acupuncture and, 317–318
    biofeedback's reduction of, 52
    expressive therapy's influence on, 84
    hypnosis management of, 44–45, 105
    imagery's influence on, 67
    MAK and, 368–369
    Spiegel's hypnosis studies for control of, 66
paleopathology, 22, 25–29
Paleozoic/Mesozoic Eras, cancer evidence from, 25
Palmer, Daniel David, 291
pancreatic cancer
    citrus fruit/Vitamin C protective effect on, 183
    fiber and, 202
    macrobiotic diet and, 228–229
    nitrosamine and, 133
papyruses
    medical evidence on, 23, 29
    tumor evidence on, 22
Paracelsus, 381
Pargament, K. I., 103, 104, 111
Pasteur Institute, 288
Patel, Vimal, 364
patient outcomes
    believability's influence on, 51
    hypnotizability factor and, 45, 47
patients
    cancer's challenges to, 103
    control/secondary control issues of, 104
    existential angst of, 112
    guided imagery's influence on, 67
    imagery's unsuitability for some, 74–75
    metaphysical viewpoint needs of, 104
    philosophical/theological/worldviews of, 104
    quality of life issues, 104
    spiritual distress of, 112
    straight talk preferred by, 113
    as treatment partners, 86–87
Pauling, Linus, 293
PC-SPES Chinese herbal mixture, 264–265
    development of, 268

UCSF/Sloan-Kettering prostate cancer study, 264–265
Peabody Museum at Harvard University, 28
pediatric cancer patients, and hypnosis, 43, 44, 45
penile cancer, 97
Pennebaker, J., 85
People Against Cancer, 409, 448, 452
PEP-CK. *See* phosphoenol pyruvate carboxykinase
Perlis, Cindy, 92
Pert, **Cancace**, 85
Peto, R., 167
Petrakis, N. L., 153–154, 156, 157, 158
Phillips, R. L., 98
philosophy
    patient's reorientation of, 104
*Philosophy of Natural Therapeutics* (Lindlahr), 286
phosphoenol pyruvate carboxykinase (PEP-CK), 391
*Phyllanthus amarus* herb, 371
physcultopathy. *See* Physical Culture school of health/healing
Physical Culture school of health/healing, 291
physical medicine, 299
physicians (conventional). *See also* medical practitioners
    chaplain referrals by, 114
    conventional treatment commitments of, 408–409
    expressive therapists association with, 82, 86
    malpractice risks of, 431–433
    patients desires from, 113
    patients withholding CAM information from, 407
    state legislation protective of, 438
*pitta* dosha, 371, 373
pituitary, as "pharmacological laboratory," 351
plants. *See also* Essiac; green tea; Iscador; red clover
    for cancer care, 243
    carcinogenesis and, 171
    vibratory patterns of, 372
Plato, 396
pleomorphism, of cancer cells, 5
polyphenols
    chemopreventive effect of, 249
    as component of Essiac, 260
    as component of green tea, 248
    as component of red tea, 250
polysaccharides, of mushrooms, 269
polyunsaturated fatty acids (PUFAs), 193
Pomeranz, Bruce, 317
POMS. *See* Profile of Mood States
prayer
    as coping strategy, 105
    cortisol levels influenced by, 108
pregnancy, breast cancer influenced by, 124, 153
preneoplastic conditions, management of, 300–301
Profile of Mood States (POMS), 108
progressive muscle relaxation, 70

prostate cancer
　and biofeedback, 54
　fiber and, 201–202
　migrant's and, 132
　PC-SPES Chinese herbal mixture study, 264–265
protein
　breast biology and dietary, 156
　breast cancer/tumors and, 141, 147, 150
　human growth and need for, 148
　menarche onset and animal, 148
　total v. animal, 150
*provings*, of homeopathic medicine, 378
Prudden, John, 394
Puchalski, C. M., 113
PUFA. *See* polyunsaturated fatty acids
Pythagoras, 396

Quackwatch.com, 388
quality of life issues, 104

Rabin, B. S., 107
Race for the Cure, 90
radiation treatment
　Chinese medicine and, 304
　effectiveness of, 6
　immune system and, 432
　*Yin-Yang* perspective on, 315–316
radiotherapy, hypnosis v. general anesthesia for, 45
Raleigh, E. D., 103
Ramakrishnan, A. U., 381
*Ramayana*, 30
rasayanas (Ayurvedic medicine). *See also ashwagandha*
　　herb
　antioxidants and, 371
　behavioral, 351–352
　herbal, 357–359
Rassnicke, S., 107
*Rational Hydrotherapy* (Kellog), 285, 288
Rause, V., 109
Raynaud's disease, and biofeedback, 52
reactive oxygen species (ROS), 353
　diffusion of, 355
　diseases linked to, 353–354
*Recalled by Life* (Sattilaro), 228
red clover (*Trifolium pratense*), 262–263
　composition of, 262
　menopausal studies, 262–263
red tea (*rooibos*), 250
Reite, M., 107
relaxation response, 48–49
relaxation techniques, 55
　body scan/progressive muscle relaxation, 70
　imagery relaxation, 70–71
religion
　anxiety's relation to, 103
　and coping, 102–103
　immune system, stress and, 108–109
　and negative coping strategies, 111–112
　negative health outcomes and, 111–112
　spirituality's interchangeability with, 95
　in United States, 97
religious commitment
　and cancer, 100–102
　health benefits of, 111
　IL-6 influenced by, 109
religiousness
　intrinsic/extrinsic, 102
　worship attendance as measure of, 100–102
remains, human/animal
　paleopathological evidence from, 25–29
　postmortem preservation/transformation of, 31
　studies of, 24–25
reproductive biology, and breastfeeding, 152–154
research
　bias in design/interpretation/funding of, 411–415
　on cancer causing compounds, 7
Reston, James, 228, 307
retinoids (synthetic Vitamin A), 173, 215
　and breast cancer, 216
　and cancer, 173–175
　cell differentiation influenced by, 215
　head/neck cancers and, 177–178
　oncogenes influenced by, 216
　and tumors, 176, 215
retinol. *See* Vitamin A
Revici, Immanuel, 241, 437
Revici therapy, 241
Reynolds, P., 101
Rickli, Arnold, 285
*Rigveda*, 30
Riley, Joe Shelby, 291
Ring Dance (of Mediterranean), 83
risk factors
　for breast cancer, 146–149
　for obesity, 127
　for physician malpractice, 431–433
　for prostate cancer, 201–202
Robbins, A., 83
Roberts, J. A., 102,
　　113
*Roe v. Wade*, and right to privacy, 418
Rogers, R. G., 101
*rooibos*. *See* red tea
ROS. *See* reactive oxygen species
Ross, M. H., 150, 151
Roszak, T., 90
Rous sarcoma virus, 7
Rowling, J. T., 27
Rozen, F., 110
Ruffer, M. A., 27

Sakurazawa, Yukikazu. *See* Ohswawa, George

Samid, Dvorit, 388

Sandison, A. T., 26

Santo, G. E., 110

Sattilaro, Anthony, 228

Schaal, M. D., 108, 109

Scheel, John, 281

Schindler, B. A., 43

Schleifer, S. J., 107

Schneider, Robert, 346

Schweitzer, Albert, 235

*Science and Health with Key to the Scriptures* (Eddy), 291

*The Scream* painting (Munch), 82

seaweeds, 229

sedentism, and disease/nutrition, 143

Sehydrin. *See* hydrazine sulfate

selenium (sodium selenite), 194–197
    discovery of/observation of effects, 195
    and human cancer, 195–196
    mechanisms of action, 194
    micronutrients and, 196
    People's Republic of China experiments with, 197
    tumors influenced by, 194, 196

self-help books/tapes, 69

Sephton, S. E., 108, 109

714-X
    administration of, 257
    availability of, 256–257
    clinical studies of, 258
    diseases treated with, 257
    Naessen's development of, 256
    side effects/successes with, 257

Seventh Day Adventists
    and cancer, 98–99
    diet/breast cancer study, 149
    prostate cancer risk study, 201–202

sexual energy, releasing of, 87–88

Shands Hospital (Florida), 92

*Sharks Don't Get Cancer* (Lane), 394

Sharma, H. S., 346, 361

shee sorrel (*Rumex acetosella*), 258–259, 261

*Shen Nong Ben Cao Jing. See Divine Husbandman's Classic of the Materia Medica*

Shen Nong (originator of herbal medicine), 305

shiitake mushrooms, 269

Short, T. H., 113

Shrock, Dean, 66

side effects
    of chemotherapy, 38
    of drugs, 18, 21
    MAK and, 369–370
    nonpharmacologic methods for treating, 38
    of Vitamin C, 217

Simone, Charles, 394

Simonton, O. Carl, 66, 72

Simonton, Stephanie, 66, 72

Simpson, J. L., 110

Singer, C., 29

skeletal remains, preservation/study of, 24, 28, 29

skin cancer
    MAK and, 364
    retinoid therapy and, 176

slippery elm (*Ulmus fulva/Ulmus rubra*), 258–259, 261

Smithsonian Institution, 29

smoking, and cancer, 169

social support
    breast cancer and, 108
    for coping, 105
    interventional studies, 105

Society for the Arts in Healthcare, 87

socioeconomic status
    and breast secretory activity, 156
    cancer and, 151

SOD. *See* superoxide dismutase

Sodestrom, K. E., 105

soft-tissue
    cancers of, 22
    post-mortem preservation of, 24–25

somatic mutation hypothesis, 14–15

somatids (blood entities), 255–256

somatoscope (Naessen's invention), 255, 258

Soulie, R., 26

sound therapy, 396

South Dakota State University, 361

soy products, 207–208, 229

Specialized Center for Research in Hyberbaric Oxygen Therapy, 401

Speiser, P., 91

Spiegel, D., 56, 66, 105, 108

Spilka, B., 102, 105

spiritual dialogue, role of, 113–114

spiritual distress, potential for, 112

spirituality
    immune system influenced by, 109
    religion's interchangeability with, 95
    in United States, 97
    women's cortisol levels influenced by, 108

*Spontaneous Remission: An Annotated Bibliography* (Hirshberg & O'Regan), 396

spontaneous remissions, 396

state regulation(s)
    Access to Medical Treatment Act, 439
    of cancer therapies, 439
    of medical practitioners, 437–438
    pain medication and, 439
    protecting CAM physician practice, 438

Stathopoulos, E., 26

Stein, M.,

Steinberg, K. K., 98
Steinbock, R. T., 28, 29
Steiner, Rudolph, 225, 244
Stern, M. P., 151
Stevens, R. G., 154
Stifoss-Jassen, H., 103
Still, Andrew Taylor, 291
stomach cancer, 134
    Chinese herbs and, 332
    Kanglaite injection and, 333
    starchy foods association with, 202
    Vitamins A/C and, 182, 191
storytelling, as healing art, 84
straight talk, patient preference for, 113
stress
    about future, 102
    cancer diagnosis and cause of, 38
    cell-mediated immunity and, 107
    definition of, 37
    humoral immune system influenced by, 107
    hypnosis management of, 43
    immune system influenced by, 108–109
    laughter's influence on, 351
    TM's influence on, 346, 347
stressor(s)
    bereavement as, 107
    cortisol production stimulated by psychological,
        106
    depression as, 108
    elicitation of autonomic/neuroendocrine responses,
        106
    IL-6 influenced by, 107
    T-lymphocyte production influenced by, 107
    tumor growth influenced by psychological, 108
substance abuse, and TM, 348
Suggestive Therapeutics (Weltmer), 291
Sugiura, Kanematsu, 403
superoxide dismutase (SOD), 355, 357, 360
support, relaxation/stress reduction/imagery v., 67
support groups
    for coping support, 105
    UCSF based, 91–92
    usefulness of, 87, 88
Supreme Court
    and health care freedom, 416–418
    People v. Priviteria, Jr. (health care freedom), 418
    Roe v. Wade (right to privacy), 418
    United States v. Rutherford (health care freedom),
        416–418
surgery
    hypnosis used during, 39, 44
    imagery's influence on adverse effects of, 67
survival. See extended survival characteristics
Susan G. Komen Foundation, 90
Sushruta (Indian physician), surgical treatise of, 30

Suzuki, T., 28
Sved, A. F., 107
Swieten, Gerhard van, 306
symbolism
    expressive therapies use of, 83
    as language of art therapies, 82
Syracuse Cancer Research Institute, 391

Takemoto, K., 108
Tamalpa Institute, 91
Tanner, J. M., 148
taphonomy, 22, 23
Tarakeshwar, N., 112
taxanes (from Pacific Yew), 251
Taxol® (Briston-Meyers Squibb)
Taylor, Kim, 306
Taylor, S. E., 101, 105
tea (Camellia sinensis). See black tea; green tea; red tea
Thomas, D. B., 154
Thompson, Samuel, 289
Thompsonianism, 289–290
Thoreson, C., 108
Thornton, C., 107
thoughts, physical health influenced by, 37
Tilden, John H., 288
T-lymphocytes, stressor's influence on, 107
TM. See Transcendental Meditation
toluene, MAK and, 367
Toniolo, P. G., 98
Torbjornsen, T., 103
Toxic Substances Control Act (1976), 7
Trall, Russell, 287
Transcendental Meditation (TM), 49. See also
        Ayurvedic medicine
    alcoholism and, 347–348
    clinical results, 347–348
    DHEA-S and, 347
    ESR and, 347
    "fourth state" of consciousness of, 348
    free radicals, cancer, and, 345–347
    metabolizing "peace and contentment" through,
        351
    stress reduction and, 346, 347
    substance abuse and, 348
Tripathy, Debu, 304
tumors
    calcium and, 188
    caloric restriction and, 151
    camphor's influence on, 256
    copper's influence on, 194
    depression's influence on, 108
    diet modification and, 170
    Egyptian medical papyruses reference to, 22, 23
    11th century B.C.E. description of, 311
    embryonic products/embryo antigens and, 450

homeopathic recommendations for, 380
hydrazine sulphate and, 392, 393
Lower/Middle Pleistocene evidence of, 26
Paleo-Eskimo skull evidence of, 29
protein and, 141, 147, 150
psychological stressor's influence on, 108
retinoids and, 176, 215
selenium's influence on, 194, 196
as *swelling* (Latin derivation), 22, 29
as synonymous with neoplasm, 4
Vitamin A/retinoids and, 176
Vitamin C and, 171
Vitamin D and colon, 187
zinc's influence on, 194

UCSF/Sloan-Kettering prostate cancer study,
    264–265
*Unconventional Cancer Treatments* (Congressional
    Office of Technology Assessment), 229
uniformitarianism, geologic law of, 24
United States (U.S.)
    Alternative Medicine Office of Congress, 81
    Cancer and Steroid Hormone Study, 152
    cancer statistics of, 17, 96, 167
    hydrazine sulphate studies of, 152
    National Health and Nutrition Examination
        Survey, 158
    spirituality/religion in, 97
*United States v. Rutherford* Laetrile decision, 416–418
Universal Osteopathic College (New York), 283
University of California, San Francisco, 91–92, 320,
    334
University of Texas Center for Alternative Medicine
    Research in Cancer, 329
Unschuld, Paul, 305

*vata* dosha, 371, 373
Vedanta, 226
vegetables/plant foods
    anticancer properties of, 129–130, 181
    Chinese populations and, 205
    green/yellow vegetables, 205
    as major fiber source, 200
    raw v. cooked, 208
    as source of carcinogens, 130
videoendoscopic biofeedback, 53
viral carcinogenesis, 16
Virchow, Rudolph, 22
viruses
    cancer's association with, 18
    as causative factors, 7
    Epstein-Barr virus, 7
    Rous sarcoma virus, 7
    treatment of, 18
viscotoxin, 247

viscumin (mistletoe lectin), 247
*vis medicatrix naturae* (healing power of nature), 285
Vitamin A (retinol), 171, 214. *See also* Alpha
        Tocopherol Beta Carotene (ATBC) study;
        beta-carotene; retinoids
    and cancer, 173–175
    colorectal cancer and, 182–183
    discovery of/observation of effects, 172
    dosage/requirements, 176
    epidemiological studies involving, 177
    hypervitaminosis A (overdose), 173
    immune system and, 216
    interactions with micronutrients, 175–176
    larynx cancer and, 181
    lung cancer and, 174–175
    mechanisms of action, 172
    natural preformed, 177
    oral cancer and, 181
    sources of, 172
    stomach cancer and, 182, 191
    toxicity symptoms of, 173, 214
    and tumors, 176
    zinc interactions with, 175
Vitamin C (ascorbic acid), 178–186, 219
    antioxidant properties of, 217
    cervical cancer and, 183
    colorectal cancer and, 182–183
    deficiency of, 217
    discovery of/observation of effects, 179–180
    dosage/requirements, 184–185
    esophageal cancer and, 181
    free radicals and, 355
    high dose, 185, 218–219
    kidney stones from high dosage of, 186
    larynx cancer and, 181
    LDL and, 361
    Linus Pauling Institute and, 405
    lung cancer/fruit consumption and, 180–181
    mechanisms of action against cancer, 178–179
    micronutrients interactions with, 184
    non-carcinogenic influence of, 171
    oral cancer and, 181
    pancreatic cancer and, 183
    physiologic levels and effects of, 185–186
    side effects of, 217
    stomach cancer and, 182, 191
    Vitamin A interactions with, 175
Vitamin D
    anticancer properties of, 187
    calcium regulation by, 187
    leukemia and, 187
Vitamin E (alpha-tocopherol), 219–220
    anticancer properties of, 189–190, 219–220
    antioxidant action of, 188
    breast cancer and, 191

Vitamin E (*cont.*)
    colorectal cancer, 182
    deficiency of, 189
    dietary sources of, 193
    discovery of/observation of effects, 189
    epidemiological studies of, 190
    formulation variety, 192–193
    free radicals and, 355
    LDL and, 361
    low toxicity levels, 189, 219
    PUFAs impact on, 193
    Vitamin A interactions with, 175
vitamins. *See also* megavitamin therapy
    free radical defense by, 355
    importance of, 130, 213
    natural v. synthetic, 214
    synergism of, 359–360

Wada, Y., 28
Wallace, Robert Keith, 346, 347
Wang, Xu-Hui, 268
Warburg, Otto, 391
Ward, Patricia Spain, 402, 405
Watkins, J. G., 73
Weiner, H., 108
Weiss, J. M.
Wells, C., 26
Weltmer, Sidney, 291
Wendel, Hugo R., 283
*Western Journal of Medicine*, 308
wheat bran, cancer cell cycling influenced by, 135

whole body therapy (Issels), 238
whole foods, 204
    cancer protective, 204
    epidemiological studies, 205
    green/yellow vegetables, 205
    omega-3 fatty acids, 208
    soy products, 207–208
Willet, W. C., 177
Williams, Roger, 293
Willmore, J. G., 27
Winder, E. L., 98
Wolbach, S. B., 172
Wolbarst, A. L., 97
Wolff, G., 97
women, as gatherers (early humans), 143
Wong, N., 110
worldviews, patient's reorientation of, 104
Wynder, E. L., 98, 157, 205

*Yearbook of Drugless of Health* (Lust), 284
*Yin-Yang* perspective, 315–316
Yogi, Maharishi Mahesh, 49
yogurt, and carcinogenesis, 151

Zammit, T., 29
zinc
    tumors influenced by, 194
    Vitamin A interactions with, 175
Zisook, S., 107
Zone Therapy (Riley), 291

SPRINGER PUBLISHING COMPANY

# Complementary/Alternative Therapies in Nursing, 5th Edition

## Mariah Snyder, PhD, RN, FAAN
## Ruth Lindquist, PhD, RN, FAAN, APRN, BC, Editors

*"…guides nurses in the art and science of holistic nursing and healing. It builds upon and extends previous editions with the essential philosophical knowledge, self as healer, and current evidence-based practices…It is crucial that nurses continue to become more informed about complementary and alternative therapies so they may safely and appropriately become integrated into current nursing practice, education, and research."*

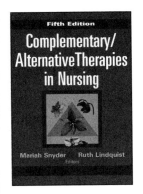

—**Barbara Dossey,** PhD, RN, AHN-BC, FAAN, Director, Holistic Nursing Consultants, Santa Fe, New Mexico

**A uniform format used throughout the book gives easy access to information about each therapy. Each chapter contains:**

- A description of the therapy
- Scientific basis for use of the therapy
- Inclusion of one or two techniques that can be used to implement the therapy
- Conditions and patient populations in which the therapy has been used
- Suggestions for research
- Precautions to be aware of when using a therapy are noted in the intervention section.

### Partial Contents:

Self As Healer • Presence • Therapeutic Listening • Imagery • Music Intervention • Humor • Yoga • Biofeedback • Meditation • Prayer • Storytelling as a Healing Tool • Journaling • Reminiscence • Animal-Assisted Therapy • Healing Touch • Therapeutic Touch • Reiki • Acupressure • Massage • Tai-Chi • Aromatherapy • Herbal Medicines • Functional Foods/Nutraceuticals • Exercise • Groups • Progressive Muscle Relaxation

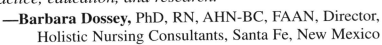

*2006 · 464pp · 0-8261-1447-4 · softcover*

**11 West 42nd Street, New York, NY 10036-8002** • **Fax: 212-941-7842**
**Order Toll-Free: 877-687-7476** • **Order On-line: www.springerpub.com**

CL